Basics of Modern Statistical Genetics

Basics of Modern Statistical Genetics

Editor:

Linda Lait

Delve Publishing

www.delvepublishing.com

Basics of Modern Statistical Genetics

Editor: Linda Lait

708 3rd Avenue, 6th Floor
New York, NY 10017
United States of America
www.delvepublishing.com

ISBN: 978-1-68095-742-6

Library of Congress Control Number: 2016951496

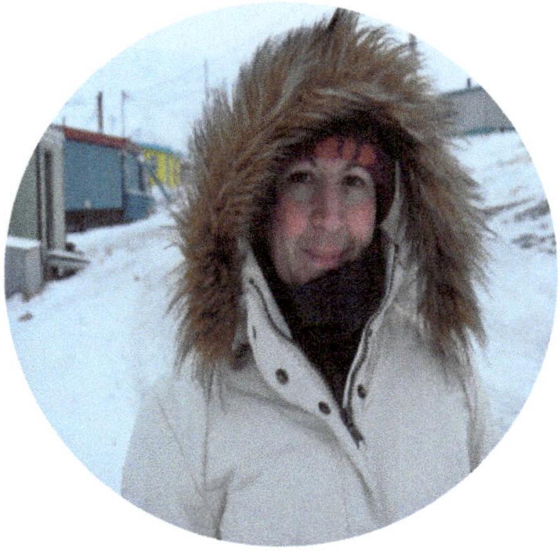

About the Editor

Linda Lait

Linda obtained her MSc from the University of Lethbridge in 2011 and will be completing her PhD at Memorial University of Newfoundland in 2016. Her interests include the evolutionary history of species, particularly those of conservation concern, which she studies with molecular markers. Increasingly complex questions can be answered with the improved technologies that are emerging. She is currently finishing up her PhD in molecular genetics, and will be starting as a Postdoctoral Fellow studying phylogeography and molecular evolution in insects.

Contents

List of Contributors

Zheyang Wu
Department of Epidemiology and Public Health, Yale University School of Medicine, New Haven, Connecticut, United States of America,

Hongyu ZhaO
Department of Epidemiology and Public Health, Yale University School of Medicine, New Haven, Connecticut, United States of America,
Department of Genetics, Yale University School of Medicine, New Haven, Connecticut, United States of America

Nick Patterson
Broad Institute of Harvard and MIT, Cambridge, Massachusetts, United States of America,

Alkes L. Price
Broad Institute of Harvard and MIT, Cambridge, Massachusetts, United States of America,
Department of Genetics, Harvard Medical School, Boston, Massachusetts, United States of America

David Reich
Broad Institute of Harvard and MIT, Cambridge, Massachusetts, United States of America,
Department of Genetics, Harvard Medical School, Boston, Massachusetts, United States of America

Daniel C Eastwoo
Warwick HRI, University of Warwick, Wellesbourne, Warwickshire, CV35 9EF, UK

Andrew Mead
Warwick HRI, University of Warwick, Wellesbourne, Warwickshire, CV35 9EF, UK

Martin J Sergeant
Warwick HRI, University of Warwick, Wellesbourne, Warwickshire, CV35 9EF, UK

Kerry S Burton
Warwick HRI, University of Warwick, Wellesbourne, Warwickshire, CV35 9EF, UK

Sara J. Larsson
Department of Plant Breeding and Genetics, Cornell University, Ithaca, New York, United States of America,
USDA–Agricultural Research Service, Robert W. Holley Center for Agriculture and Health, Ithaca, New York, United States of America

Alexander E. Lipka
USDA–Agricultural Research Service, Robert W. Holley Center for Agriculture and Health, Ithaca, New York, United States of America

Edward S. Buckler
Department of Plant Breeding and Genetics, Cornell University, Ithaca, New York, United States of America,
USDA–Agricultural Research Service, Robert W. Holley Center for Agriculture and Health, Ithaca, New York, United States of America

Minghui Wang[1]
School of Agriculture and Biology, Shanghai Jiao Tong University, Shanghai, People's Republic of China,
Shanghai Key Lab of Animal Biotechnology, Shanghai, People's Republic of China

Qishan Wang
School of Agriculture and Biology, Shanghai Jiao Tong University, Shanghai, People's Republic of China,
Shanghai Key Lab of Animal Biotechnology, Shanghai, People's Republic of China

Yuchun Pan
School of Agriculture and Biology, Shanghai Jiao Tong University, Shanghai, People's Republic of China,
Shanghai Key Lab of Animal Biotechnology, Shanghai, People's Republic of China

Joseph K. Pickrell
[1] Department of Human Genetics, University of Chicago, Chicago, Illinois, United States of America,

Jonathan K. Pritchard
Department of Human Genetics, University of Chicago, Chicago, Illinois, United States of America,
Howard Hughes Medical Institute, University of Chicago, Chicago, Illinois, United States of America

Cameron Palmer
Department of Systems Biology, Columbia University Medical Center, New York, New York, United States of America

Itsik Pe'er
Department of Systems Biology, Columbia University Medical Center, New York, New York, United States of America
Department of Computer Science, Columbia University, New York, New York, United States of America

Jiandong Ding
Shanghai Key Lab of Intelligent Information Processing, Fudan University, Shanghai, China.
School of Computer Science, Fudan University, Shanghai, China.

Danqing Li
Shanghai Key Lab of Intelligent Information Processing, Fudan University, Shanghai, China.
School of Computer Science, Fudan University, Shanghai, China.

Uwe Ohler
Institute for Genome Sciences & Policy, Duke University, Durham, North Carolina, USA.
Department of Biostatistics & Bioinformatics, Duke University, Durham, North Carolina, USA.

Jihong Guan
Department of Computer Science & Technology, Tongji University, Shanghai, China

Shuigeng Zhou
Shanghai Key Lab of Intelligent Information Processing, Fudan University, Shanghai, China.
School of Computer Science, Fudan University, Shanghai, China.

Jianjun Hu and Jia Xu
Department of Computer Science and Engineering, University of South Carolina

Catherine M. Stein
Department of Epidemiology and Biostatistics, Case Western Reserve University, Cleveland, OH, USA
Uganda – Case Western Reserve University Research Collaboration, Kampala, Uganda

Noémi B. Hall
Department of Epidemiology and Biostatistics, Case Western Reserve University, Cleveland, OH, USA

LaShaunda L. Malone
Uganda – Case Western Reserve University Research Collaboration, Kampala, Uganda

Ezekiel Mupere
Department of Epidemiology and Biostatistics, Case Western Reserve University, Cleveland, OH, USA
Uganda – Case Western Reserve University Research Collaboration, Kampala, Uganda
Mulago Hospital, Makerere University School of Medicine, Kampala, Uganda

Yushi Liu
Lovelace Respiratory Research Institute

Toru Nyunoya
Lovelace Respiratory Research Institute
VA Medical Center

Shuguang Leng
Lovelace Respiratory Research Institute

Steven A Belinsky
Lovelace Respiratory Research Institute

Yohannes Tesfaigzi
Lovelace Respiratory Research Institute

Shannon Bruse
Lovelace Respiratory Research Institute

Peter M Visscher
Genetic Epidemiology Group, Queensland Institute of Medical Research, Brisbane, Australia

Sarah E Medland
Genetic Epidemiology Group, Queensland Institute of Medical Research, Brisbane, Australia

Manuel A. R Ferreira
Genetic Epidemiology Group, Queensland Institute of Medical Research, Brisbane, Australia

Katherine I Morley
Genetic Epidemiology Group, Queensland Institute of Medical Research, Brisbane, Australia

Gu Zhu, Belinda K Cornes
Genetic Epidemiology Group, Queensland Institute of Medical Research, Brisbane, Australia

Grant W Montgomery
Genetic Epidemiology Group, Queensland Institute of Medical Research, Brisbane, Australia

Nicholas G Martin
Genetic Epidemiology Group, Queensland Institute of Medical Research, Brisbane, Australia

Cheongeun Oh
Department of Epidemiology and Public Health, Yale University School of Medicine, New Haven, CT, USA,

Kenny Q Ye
Department of Applied Mathematics and Statistics, State University of New York at Stony Brook, Stony Brook, New York, USA and

Qimei He
Department of Preventive Medicine, State University of New York at Stony Brook, Stony Brook, New York, USA

Nancy R Mendell
Department of Applied Mathematics and Statistics, State University of New York at Stony Brook, Stony Brook, New York, USA and

Jinmyung Choi
Department of Neurology, Yale School of Medicine, New Haven Connecticut, United States of America,

Parisa Shooshtari
Department of Neurology, Yale School of Medicine, New Haven Connecticut, United States of America,

Kaitlin E. Samocha
Analytic and Translational Genetics Unit, Department of Medicine, Massachusetts General Hospital and Harvard Medical School, Boston, Massachusetts, United States of America,
Program in Medical and Population Genetics, Broad Institute of Harvard and MIT, Cambridge, Massachusetts, United States of America,
Stanley Center for Psychiatric Research, Broad Institute of Harvard and MIT, Cambridge, Massachusetts, United States of America,
Program in Genetics and Genomics, Biological and Biomedical Sciences, Harvard Medical School, Boston, Massachusetts, United States of America,

Mark J. Daly
Analytic and Translational Genetics Unit, Department of Medicine, Massachusetts General Hospital and Harvard Medical School, Boston, Massachusetts, United States of America,
Program in Medical and Population Genetics, Broad Institute of Harvard and MIT, Cambridge, Massachusetts, United States of America,
Stanley Center for Psychiatric Research, Broad Institute of Harvard and MIT, Cambridge, Massachusetts, United States of America,

Chris Cotsapas
Department of Neurology, Yale School of Medicine, New Haven Connecticut, United States of America,
Analytic and Translational Genetics Unit, Department of Medicine, Massachusetts General Hospital and Harvard Medical School, Boston, Massachusetts, United States of America,
Program in Medical and Population Genetics, Broad Institute of Harvard and MIT, Cambridge, Massachusetts, United States of America,
Stanley Center for Psychiatric Research, Broad Institute of Harvard and MIT, Cambridge, Massachusetts, United States of America,
Department of Genetics, Yale School of Medicine, New Haven CT, United States of America

Fredrik Boulund
Department of Mathematical Sciences, Chalmers University of Technology and University of Gothenburg

Anna Johnning
Institute of Neuroscience and Physiology, the Sahlgrenska Academy at the University of Gothenburg

Mariana Buongermino Pereira
Department of Mathematical Sciences, Chalmers University of Technology and University of Gothenburg

DG Joakim Larsson
Department of Infectious Diseases, Institute of Biomedicine, the Sahlgrenska Academy at the University of Gothenburg

Erik Kristiansson
Department of Mathematical Sciences, Chalmers University of Technology and University of Gothenburg

Marinela Capanu
Memorial Sloan-Kettering Cancer Center, New York, NY, USA

Iuliana Ionita-Laza
Department of Biostatistics, Columbia University, New York, NY, USA

Megan H. Brewer
Northcott Neuroscience Laboratory, ANZAC Research Institute, Concord, New South Wales, Australia,
Sydney Medical School, University of Sydney, Camperdown, New South Wales, Australia,

Rabia Chaudhry
Northcott Neuroscience Laboratory, ANZAC Research Institute, Concord, New South Wales, Australia,
Sydney Medical School, University of Sydney, Camperdown, New South Wales, Australia,

Jessica Qi
Northcott Neuroscience Laboratory, ANZAC Research Institute, Concord, New South Wales, Australia,
Discipline of Pathology, University of Sydney, Camperdown, New South Wales, Australia,

Aditi Kidambi
Northcott Neuroscience Laboratory, ANZAC Research Institute, Concord, New South Wales, Australia,

Alexander P. Drew
Northcott Neuroscience Laboratory, ANZAC Research Institute, Concord, New South Wales, Australia,

Manoj P. Menezes
The Institute for Neuroscience and Muscle Research, The Children's Hospital at Westmead, Westmead, New South Wales, Australia,
T.Y. Nelson Department of Neurology and Neurosurgery, The Children's Hospital at Westmead, Westmead, New South Wales, Australia,
Paediatrics and Child Health, University of Sydney, Camperdown, New South Wales, Australia,

Monique M. Ryan
Department of Neurology, Royal Children's Hospital, Parkville, Victoria, Australia,
Murdoch Childrens Research Institute, Parkville, Victoria, Australia,
Department of Paediatrics, University of Melbourne, Parkville, Victoria, Australia,

Michelle A. Farrar
Department of Neurology, Sydney Children's Hospital, Randwick, New South Wales, Australia,
School of Women's and Children's Health, UNSW Medicine, University of New South Wales, Kensington, New South Wales, Australia,

David Mowat
School of Women's and Children's Health, UNSW Medicine, University of New South Wales, Kensington, New South Wales, Australia,
Department of Medical Genetics, Sydney Children's Hospital, Randwick, New South Wales, Australia,

Gopinath M. Subramanian
Department of Paediatrics, John Hunter Children's Hospital, Newcastle, New South Wales, Australia,

Helen K. Young
Department of Paediatrics, Royal North Shore Hospital, St Leonards, New South Wales, Australia,
Northern Clinical School, Sydney Medical School, University of Sydney, St Leonards, New South Wales, Australia,
Department of Neurogenetics, The Children's Hospital at Westmead, Westmead, New South Wales, Australia,

Stephan Zuchner
John P. Hussman Institute for Human Genomics, University of Miami Miller School of Medicine, Miami, Florida, United States of America,
Dr. John T. Macdonald Department of Human Genetics, University of Miami Miller School of Medicine, Miami, Florida, United States of America,

Stephen W. Reddel
Department of Neurology, Concord Repatriation General Hospital, Concord, New South Wales, Australia,

Garth A. Nicholson
Northcott Neuroscience Laboratory, ANZAC Research Institute, Concord, New South Wales, Australia,
Sydney Medical School, University of Sydney, Camperdown, New South Wales, Australia,
Molecular Medicine, Concord Repatriation General Hospital, Concord, New South Wales, Australia

Marina L. Kennerson
Northcott Neuroscience Laboratory, ANZAC Research Institute, Concord, New South Wales, Australia,
Sydney Medical School, University of Sydney, Camperdown, New South Wales, Australia,
Molecular Medicine, Concord Repatriation General Hospital, Concord, New South Wales, Australia

Richarda M. de Voer
Department of Human Genetics, Radboud University Medical Center, Nijmegen, The Netherlands,

Marc-Manuel Hahn
Department of Human Genetics, Radboud University Medical Center, Nijmegen, The Netherlands,

Robbert D. A. Weren
Department of Human Genetics, Radboud University Medical Center, Nijmegen, The Netherlands,

Arjen R. Mensenkamp
Department of Human Genetics, Radboud University Medical Center, Nijmegen, The Netherlands,

Christian Gilissen
Department of Human Genetics, Radboud University Medical Center, Nijmegen, The Netherlands,

Wendy A. van Zelst-Stams
Department of Human Genetics, Radboud University Medical Center, Nijmegen, The Netherlands,

Liesbeth Spruijt
Department of Human Genetics, Radboud University Medical Center, Nijmegen, The Netherlands,

C. Marleen Kets
Department of Human Genetics, Radboud University Medical Center, Nijmegen, The Netherlands,

Junxiao Zhang
Department of Human Genetics, Radboud University Medical Center, Nijmegen, The Netherlands,

Hanka Venselaar
Center for Molecular and Biomolecular Informatics, Radboud Institute for Molecular Life Sciences, Radboud University Medical Center, Nijmegen, The Netherlands,

Lilian Vreede
Department of Human Genetics, Radboud University Medical Center, Nijmegen, The Netherlands,

Nil Schubert
Department of Human Genetics, Radboud University Medical Center, Nijmegen, The Netherlands,

Marloes Tychon
Department of Human Genetics, Radboud University Medical Center, Nijmegen, The Netherlands,

Ronny Derks
Department of Human Genetics, Radboud University Medical Center, Nijmegen, The Netherlands,

Hans K. Schackert
Abteilung Chirurgische Forschung, Technische Universität Dresden, Dresden, Germany,

Ad Geurts van Kessel
Department of Human Genetics, Radboud University Medical Center, Nijmegen, The Netherlands,

Ad Geurts van Kessel
Department of Human Genetics, Radboud University Medical Center, Nijmegen, The Netherlands,

Marjolijn J. L. Ligtenberg
Department of Human Genetics, Radboud University Medical Center, Nijmegen, The Netherlands,
Department of Pathology, Radboud University Medical Center, Nijmegen, The Netherlands

Roland P. Kuiper
Department of Human Genetics, Radboud University Medical Center, Nijmegen, The Netherlands,

Brett Deml
Department of Pediatrics and Children's Research Institute at the Medical College of Wisconsin and Children's Hospital of Wisconsin, Milwaukee, Wisconsin, United States of America,
Department of Cell Biology, Neurobiology and Anatomy, Medical College of Wisconsin, Milwaukee, Wisconsin, United States of America,

Ariana Kariminejad
Kariminejad-Najmabadi Pathology and Genetics Center, Tehran, Iran,

Razieh H. R. Borujerdi
Qom Welfare Organization, Qom, Iran

Sanaa Muheisen
Department of Pediatrics and Children's Research Institute at the Medical College of Wisconsin and Children's Hospital of Wisconsin, Milwaukee, Wisconsin, United States of America,

Linda M. Reis
Department of Pediatrics and Children's Research Institute at the Medical College of Wisconsin and Children's Hospital of Wisconsin, Milwaukee, Wisconsin, United States of America,

Elena V. Semina
Department of Pediatrics and Children's Research Institute at the Medical College of Wisconsin and Children's Hospital of Wisconsin, Milwaukee, Wisconsin, United States of America,

Preface

Over the past 40 years we have seen significant advances in the use of genetics to study subjects from evolution and ecology to medicine and human health. Early protein and restriction analysis studies have given way to high-throughput sequencing and genome-wide studies. With these advances has come the need for increasingly complex statistical analyses. This has come in the form of multifaceted algorithms such as eigenanalysis and Bayesian analysis. Bayesian analysis has become one of the most widely used techniques in modern statistical genetics as the use of Markov chain Monte Carlo (MCMC) methods have made it relatively quick and simple to incorporate prior information into the model. Gene mapping studies have also become increasingly widespread as candidate genes are being found for a number of phenotypes, conditions, and diseases. In this book we look at a number of novel techniques used to study populations, phenotypes, and gene expression in organisms as diverse as humans and plants. We end with three case studies applying statistical genetics to identify genes associated with human diseases.

Editor
Linda Lait

INTRODUCTION

Probability and statistics play an important role in genetics. The mechanism of "meiosis", the forming of sperm or egg cells, is thought to be probabilistic in nature, as is the process of mating in large populations. The relationship between "genotypes" (DNA-sequence) and "phenotypes" (observable traits or diseases) can be modelled by probability distributions. The analysis of genetic determinants is based on random samples from a population, often biased, and various statistical methods are necessary to analyses such data. This course provides an introduction to stochastic models and methods used in genetics, directed at students in mathematics. We do assume a good working knowledge of probability and statistics (e.g. likelihood and Bayes inference, asymptotic, testing), but do not assume prior knowledge of genetics. In particular, the jargon in this description will be explained.

Statistical genetics is a classical branch of applied probability and statistics, which has recently gained much new interest, due to the significant breakthroughs in genetics, both experimentally and theoretically. With modern techniques and significantly increased data it is hoped to link diseases and other traits to genes (pieces of DNA) that can be precisely located on the genome in an unprecedented manner. One could safely say that this area is among the hottest in applied stochastic, and in science in general. There are plenty of opportunities for mathematicians interested in life sciences. This course incorporates parts of many different areas of statistics.

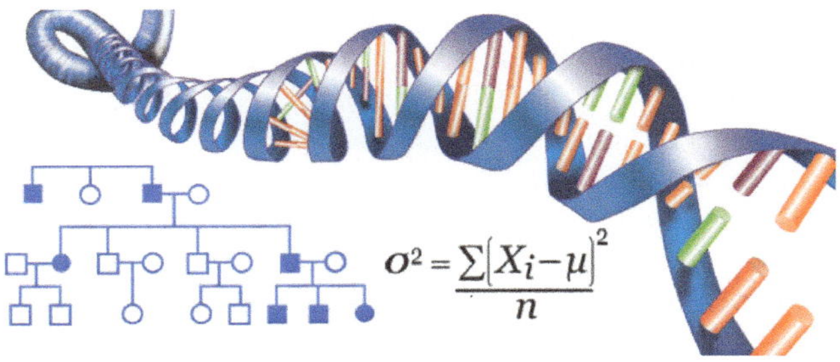

Of course we start with Mendel's laws of "segregation", which stipulate that each parent passes a randomly chosen gene on to his/her offspring from each pair of genes, independently across genes. The latter independence was later found out to be untrue, and replaced by "linkage models", which stipulate positive dependence between genes sitting close together on the genome. The most popular model is based on a Poisson process model for "crossovers" during meiosis. The resulting models combined with "penetrance models" (conditional distributions for phenotypes given genotypes) allow to write likelihoods for the observed phenotypes in families (or "pedigrees"), and thus to estimate the dependence of phenotypic traits on genetic factors. Because a full likelihood analysis requires the specification of many probability densities and is computationally intensive, other methods with the same aim are based on reduced data, in particular "IBD" (identity by descent) status, and/or on clever sampling plans. "Association" studies are based on the idea that, under a random mating assumption, a population should tend to equilibrium, with deviations in pairs of genes (possibly) in a random sample of individuals indicating that these genes are close together on the genome. Finally, "biometric analysis" is directed at decomposing phenotypic variation into genetic and environmental parts.

Statistical genetics is a scientific field concerned with the development and application of statistical methods for drawing inferences from genetic data. The term is most commonly used in the context of human genetics. Research in statistical genetics generally falls into one of three areas:

- population genetics - Study of evolutionary processes affecting genetic variation between organisms
- genetic epidemiology - Studying effects of genes on diseases
- quantitative genetics - Studying the effects of genes on 'normal' phenotypes

An understanding of the basic ideas of inheritance has been evident throughout the history of mankind, ever since the domestication of animals or the practice of farming began. The Babylonians and ancient Egyptians utilized cross pollination of crops and selection of domesticated animals for breeding, but did not develop a formal theory for the principles underlying the inheritance of traits. Later, ancient Greek philosophers developed elementary theories to explain how inheritance worked in humans, grappling unsuccessfully with the apparent paradox that inherited characteristics can sometimes differ between offspring and parents. Some diseases in humans, such as sickle cell anemia and hemophilia, have been recognized as inherited disorders for centuries and, as the science of medicine developed, so too did the recognition that many diseases are heritable. Yet, bipolar disorder, one of the oldest known disorders in humans, was not widely regarded as heritable until the 1950s. Although we can document an awareness of the basic concept of inheritance for millennia, most of our current knowledge about inherited human diseases has been acquired only in the last century. As the concept of inherited disease gradually developed, Genetics, the science of inherited variation and heritable biological material in living organisms, became an integral part of the search for the origin of disease. Today stories of gene discovery for many diseases dominate the news landscape. Despite centuries of formal and informal observation of patterns of inheritance in humans, the discipline of human genetics is relatively young. Humans are difficult to study because, in contrast to plant and animal genetics, experimental crossings are not possible, environmental factors are hard to control, and humans have small families with many years required for a new generation to develop. Environmental and genetic factors broadly overlap during childhood, making it difficult to separate the relative contributions of the environment and genetics to the development of disease. As a result, much of our understanding of basic genetic principles and how genes affect variation in organisms comes from experimental studies in plants (Mendel's experiments with garden peas in the 1860s) and animals (Morgan's experiments in the 1920s with flies). Mendel's laws were initially largely ignored, but 'rediscovered' by scientists in the 1900s and hotly debated by geneticists, biologists, statisticians and biometricians. Part of this debate centered on the apparent conflict between Mendel's work Experiments in Plant Hybridization (1865) and Darwin's theories set forth in the Origin of the Species (1859), which was published just prior to Mendel's paper. Darwin used the notion of inherited traits as the basis for natural selection, but he believed that traits in parents were 'blended' in the offspring. Mendel's work verified the inheritance of traits, but he deliberately used discrete traits that were not blended in offspring. Developing models and theories for how Mendel's discrete inherited units could explain variation in continuous human characteristics was a subject of much debate during these early years of statistical genetics. In this text we use the term trait broadly to encompass both measured and discrete characteristics, as well as disease outcomes.

Basic Concepts in Genetic Disease

Statistical Genetics is a branch of statistics that deals with the analysis of inherited traits and genetic data. We use genetic data loosely here to refer to the biological material that is inherited during reproduction via egg and sperm cells. In early days, statistical genetics was largely dominated by statistics for experimental studies in plants and animals. Galton's statistical work in the 1880s on the inheritance of height in humans is an important exception to this rule. Over the years, the methodological focus of statistical genetics has changed to keep pace with the different kinds of genetic data that technology has made available. Most recently, new technologies arising from the Human Genome Project and HapMap Project have generated a surge of methodological development to address unsolved problems in human genetics. The development of statistical models and methods to explain how genes influence traits continues to be a common goal in plant, animal and human genetics. When the discipline of statistical genetics was just beginning, we had little understanding of the basic biological underpinning of genetics and inheritance apart from the fact that humans had 'units'–later termed 'genes'–that were inherited from their parents and that 'units' could differ from person to person. Most important from the statistical point of view, there was no standardized way to assay or characterize the genetic information at the molecular level in an individual. The available data for most statistical investigations consisted only of traits, also known as phenotypes. We use the terms traits and phenotypes here to mean individual characteristics, not observed at the molecular level, which are thought to have a heritable basis. For example, a person's blood type at the ABO locus is a phenotype which depends upon their variants at the ABO gene. A person's phenotype (here blood group) can be obtained without knowledge of their gene variant. However, knowing a person's blood type will imply something about the information encoded in their ABO gene. In these early years, statistical genetics was focused on methods for determining if traits or diseases were inherited and measuring the degree of inheritance (studies of familial aggregation), and to determine the underlying genetic model that explains the relationship between the phenotype and the underlying disease (segregation analysis). For these analyses, individuals with the disease, called probands, were identified; information on relatives of the probands was used to form family or pedigree structures. The term ascertain is used when referring to probands to indicate that the selection of individuals for study may depend on their phenotypes; depending upon study objectives, all available relatives of probands may be included in the study regardless of phenotype. The phenotypes or traits of the relatives and their familial relationships were exploited in a segregation analysis to infer the underlying genetic model. Advances in our understanding of the biology of genetics and in laboratory technology have enabled us to now readily obtain data directly on gene variants, called genetic markers, at specific locations in the genome. Having marker data for samples of families has enabled gene mapping, which encompasses a variety of methods used to find the chromosomal location of a disease-causing gene. An early statistical approach to gene mapping was to use linkage analysis of pedigrees. Linkage analysis uses marker data and the traits of a pedigree; by studying the patterns of co-inheritance of the marker and the disease throughout the pedigree, we can infer how far the disease gene is from the marker.

Linkage analysis relies on both Mendel's laws discovered in his pea experiments and the concept of genetic distance elucidated in Morgan's fly experiments. Many variants underlying genetic disorders have been discovered using the basic idea of linkage analysis, e.g., cystic fibrosis, Huntington's disease and rare variants underlying early onset Alzheimer's disease. The genetic architecture of diseases in humans ranges from diseases that are caused by just a single disease variant in a single gene to settings where multiple variants in multiple genetic loci can contribute to the disease risk, often interacting with environmental factors. Diseases or disorders which are initiated by variants in a single gene are typically rare and severe conditions, e.g., Cystic Fibrosis, Duchenes' Muscular Dystrophy and Sickle Cell Anemia. Such diseases are often referred to as Mendelian disorders or diseases. Mendelian disorders and diseases follow simple Mendelian patterns of inheritance in families and generally do not have any other causes other than the genetic disease variant. Linkage analysis has been very successful in finding genes for Mendelian disorders. Most common diseases, e.g., asthma, obesity, Alzheimer's disease, bipolar disorder, etc., fall into the category of multi-factorial diseases or complex genetic diseases. Here, disease risk is thought to be influenced by a set of genes and environmental factors which may interact with each other. Although this book is focused on the concepts of gene mapping for complex diseases, the basic genetic principles of inheritance of genetic material are the same for both Mendelian and complex diseases. Linkage analysis has been less successful with finding genes for complex disorders. Today gene mapping involves scanning the entire human genome at hundreds or thousands or even millions of genetic markers in the genomes of large samples in order to look for genetic variation associated with disease traits (Genome Wide Association Studies (GWAS)). Such studies have led to new findings for many complex diseases: cancer, diabetes, eye disease, obesity and others. These Genetic Association studies are also a component of gene mapping; their current popularity stems from the advances in genotyping and from information about the structure of genetic variation captured in the HapMap Project. Genetic association analysis is distinct from virtually all other types of statistical genetics analyses in that it can be carried out using samples of unrelated individuals rather than families or pedigrees. Genetic association analysis using both unrelated samples, and using samples of families, is the main focus of this book. Population Genetics is concerned with the genetic variation within and between populations, over time and space. This includes modeling variation in genes due to many factors: selection of certain variants due to response to environmental conditions, in- and out-migration, drift occurring in small populations, and mutations, as well as understanding genetic differences in populations. Genetic Epidemiology is a branch of epidemiology that deals with both genetic and environmental contributions to disease. Genetic epidemiology uses methods from statistical genetics and epidemiology to understand the interplay between genes, environment and disease. Sometimes data on geographic, spatial, temporal and/or racial, as well as familial, variation in disease rates can provide insight into the genetic nature of disease. We close this section with two examples of genetic diseases which illustrate some of the ideas discussed in this section. Sickle Cell Anemia. Sickle cell anemia is a Mendelian disorder that affects red blood cells and is associated with severe morbidity, including pain, hemolytic anemia and infections; without proper medical management, the death rate is high. This disorder is a common textbook example of a genetic disease because it was the first to be labeled a molecular disorder resulting from a genetic mutation. The disorder was widely recognized as an inherited disorder for centuries by indigenous people in sub-Saharan Africa because of the way it occurred in families, but reports did not appear in the Western medical literature until the early twentieth century. By this time, the shape of red blood cells could be seen under a microscope, and scientists discovered that the red blood cells of those suffering from sickle cell disorder had a sickle shape, rather than the normal round shape. This phenomenon was calling 'sickling' and individuals with red blood cells which could be made to sickle were labeled 'sicklemics'. Segregation analyses of African and African-American pedigrees (see Section 4.4) played an important early role in demonstrating that the disorder was genetic and in understanding its inheritance mechanism. Segregation analyses of African and African-American pedigrees done in the 1920s used the sickling trait, ignoring the fact that not all sicklemics had sickle cell disorder. Some 25 years later, segregation analyses using sickle cell disease as the trait correctly identified the genetic nature of sickle cell disorder. About this time, laboratory studies showed that sickling was due to a genetic variant which changed the molecular structure of hemoglobin, enabling scientists to limit their search to the hemoglobin gene without any linkage studies. A decade later, the specific variant in the hemoglobin gene on chromosome 11 was located.

Review of Molecular Genetics

This section and the next serve as the basic background material in biology needed for the remainder of the book. Individuals with no prior exposure to the concepts may find these sections difficult to absorb on first reading. It may be necessary to reread these sections while covering later material. The human genome refers to all of the basic biological material that is transmitted from parents to offspring, determining their inherited characteristics. The heritable material is stored on chromosomes in the nucleus of every cell. There are 23 pairs of chromosomes in the human genome; 22 of the pairs are autosomal, consisting of non-identical copies (i.e., the two copies may have different variants) of the same chromosome while the 23rd pair contains the sex chromosomes (Fig 1). The two non-identical chromosomes in an autosomal pair are referred to as homologous chromosomes. For the sex chromosomes, females have two non-identical copies of the X chromosome, while males have one X and one Y. The centromere of a chromosome is a region found near the middle of the chromosome; it plays an important role in cell division and reproduction. It also is used to specify genetic locations as it divides each chromosome into a short arm (p for petit) and a long arm (q, next after p in the alphabet). The banded regions shown in Fig 1 can be seen under a microscope after staining; they are also used in specifying genetic locations. Each chromosome is composed of long strands of DeoxyriboNucleic Acid (DNA). DNA is the basic biological material of inheritance; it determines how proteins are manufactured in the body. DNA is composed of complementary base pairs (Fig 2). There are four distinct bases (A, C, T, G) which compose DNA in pairs. The pairing is obligatory: G and C are always paired, and A and T are always paired.

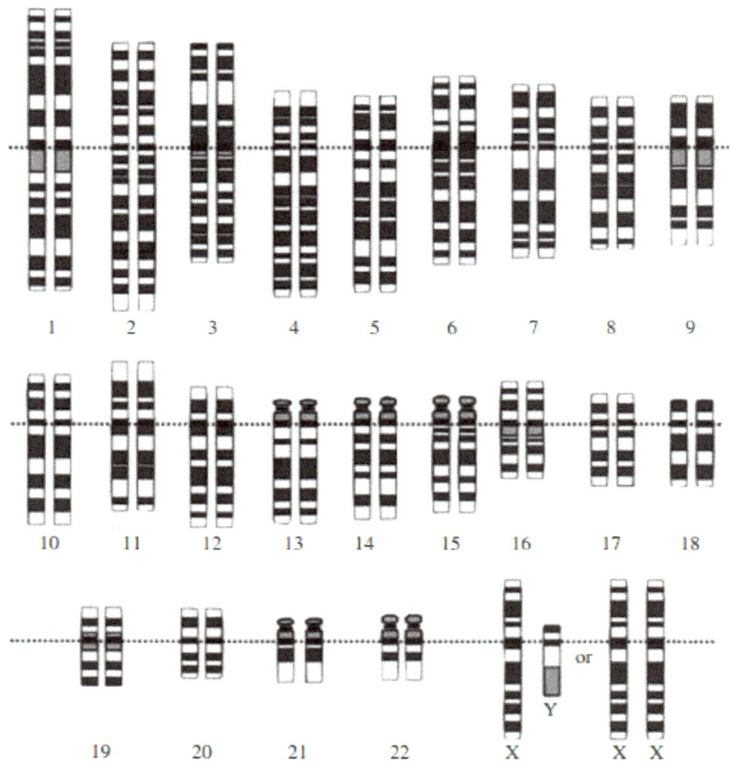

Figure 1. A Graphical representation of the human genome. Source: National center for biotechnology information.

Genes are largely contiguous stretches of DNA that are responsible for making proteins; the beginning and end of a gene are signaled by specific, short DNA sequences. Current estimates suggest that there are about 20,000–30,000 genes distributed throughout the genome. This estimate has varied wildly over the years, mostly getting much smaller; older books quote 80,000 or even 100,000 genes. The DNA sequence in a gene consists of coding and non-coding regions, or exons and introns. DNA sequences that make up the exons code for specific proteins determined by the DNA sequence; DNA sequences lying in introns, or sequences lying outside of genes, do not code for proteins, but are thought to play other important roles in regulating the manufacture of proteins. Most of the three billion base pairs in humans are in non-coding regions. Genes vary widely in size, some being as small as a few thousand base pairs, and some containing millions of base pairs. The number and size of both exons and introns also varies between genes. For instance, the APOE gene has four exons and three introns in 3611 base pairs and the gene coding for the human ABO blood type has seven exons and six introns in 5171 base pairs.

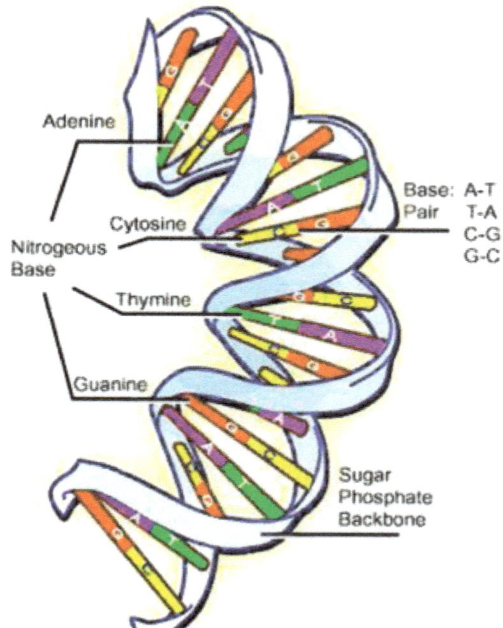

Figure. 2 A strand of DNA showing complementary base pairing. Source: Courtesy of Jane Wang.

The focus of gene mapping has historically been to find the location of one or more of the protein coding regions which have variants affecting disease. However, increased appreciation of the role that non-coding DNA plays in gene regulation and expression, and the many recent association studies that implicate non-coding regions as associated with disease suggest that complex disorders may be influenced by genetic variants in non-coding regions as well. A genetic locus refers to a particular location in a chromosome that is polymorphic. Polymorphic means that the data at that locus can have more than one possible variant; a polymorphism refers to a polymorphic genetic locus. The different variants at a locus are called alleles. Historically the minor allele frequency at a locus was required to have population frequency of at least 1% in order for a locus to be considered polymorphic, but more recently the term is used loosely to indicate any locus where two or more variants are found, regardless of frequency. When there are only two possible variants, it is conventional to refer to them as 'A' and 'a'. When dealing with the autosomes, an individual with two copies of A, one on each of the two chromosomes, is called homozygous A, or AA; an individual with one A and one a is called heterozygous, or Aa, and aa is homozygous a. The terms homozygote and heterozygote are also used to denote individuals who are homozygous A or a, or who are heterozygous. The genotype of an individual refers to the pair of alleles at a location, i.e., AA, Aa, or aa.

A Comment on Notation: Since Mendel's paper, it has been conventional to use the capital and lower case forms of a letter to describe the 2 versions of an allele but this has limitations for more than two alleles. Other conventions which are used include capital letters, A, B, C, etc., or numbers, 1, 2, 3, etc., for different alleles at a single locus. Generally, with a number or letter designation, the choice of label is arbitrary. In some cases a specific designation is given to a disease allele, e.g. S in the Hemoglobin gene which causes sickle cell anemia. With SNPs (see below) we sometimes use base pairs, e.g., G or A to describe alleles. We do not adopt a single labeling convention in this book, but will use the most convenient notation in a given discussion. In most cases, a particular convention will be obvious.

Types of Genetic Variants

A key feature in the success of gene mapping is having information on genetic variation in humans. Genetic variation means that different copies of homologous chromosomes can have different DNA sequences in specific regions; this definition covers a multitude of possibilities for how DNA sequences differ. In the living cell, DNA undergoes frequent chemical change, especially when it is being replicated. Most of these changes are quickly repaired; those that are not repaired result in mutations. All new genetic variation in humans arises as a result of these mutations. Variation in DNA sequence from person to person also arises as a result of the process of reproduction; this will be discussed in Section 2.3. Mutations can arise de novo during the process of meiosis, meaning they are present in the offspring but not in either parent, or they can be inherited from parents. Generally we reserve the term mutation for the de novo occurrence; subsequently we refer to it as a variant, or a disease variant if it causes increased disease risk. Gene mapping is concerned with finding inherited disease variants. We use the term genetic marker, or just marker, to describe genetic data, observed at the molecular level, at a particular locus that allows us to distinguish genetic differences in individuals. Variants that arise in the coding region of a gene can cause the protein encoded by that gene to malfunction and cells that rely on this protein cannot function properly. This can cause problems for the tissues or organs. Such conditions related to gene mutations, or variants, are called genetic disorders or diseases. Genetic variants which cause a genetic disorder are often referred to as disease mutations. A disease susceptibility locus (DSL) indicates a gene, or specific genetic locus, which has a variant associated with a disease.

This nomenclature has arisen as a convenient way to distinguish the underlying disease gene (usually unknown) which one is searching for, from the marker data used in the search. The term mutation is often used to refer to the event which creates a new variant at the genetic locus and not to the variant itself; we will subsequently adopt that convention here. Single Nucleotide Polymorphisms (SNP). The simplest type of genetic marker is a single nucleotide polymorphism (SNP). The double helix structure of DNA requires that each chromosome has complementary base pairs at each location, as illustrated for each of the two chromosomes in Fig 3, which shows a SNP at a pair of nonidentical but homologous chromosomes. For simplicity, one chromosomal variant is labeled 'A', and one is labeled 'a'. The A allele should not be confused with the A base in the DNA sequence; rather it is standard notation for an allele and denotes nothing about the underlying biology. In distinguishing the A allele from the a allele, there is a lot of redundant information; a single chromosome is made up of one strand of base pairs. However, for each base in a pair, the other base in the pair is determined by complementarity; thus it is necessary to 'read' only one base. In order to unambiguously read a sequence of base pairs, we define a 5' and a 3' end according to the asymmetrical bonding of sugar and phosphate residues that form the backbone structure of DNA. By convention, a chromosomal sequence is read, left to right, from the 5' strand, which is depicted as the top strand in both chromosomes in Fig .3. Thus the sequence for allele A at this location is CCGATCTAGCGAT and the corresponding sequence for a is CCAATCTAGCGAT; they differ only at the third base pair.

The two alleles depicted in the figure differ at the third base pair, where an A base is substituted for a G. As we discuss in the next section, whether or not this difference is biologically meaningful depends on where they occur in the DNA sequence and the nature of the letter change. SNPs play a very important role in modern gene mapping; they occur commonly throughout the genome and the financial cost of genotyping multiple SNPs at different locations is relatively modest, making them very attractive markers for large scale genetic studies. SNPs occur once in every 300 base pairs on average, for approximately 10 million SNPs in the human genome. Most commonly, SNPs are found in intronic or non-coding DNA sequences. SNPs which occur in these non-coding regions have not thus far been shown to have direct genetic effects on disease or traits, but within a coding region, they can be disastrous, as we discuss in the next section.

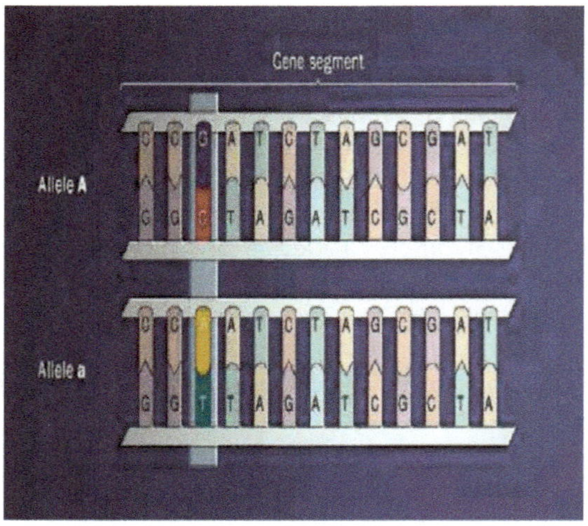

Figure. 3 Illustration of a single nucleotide polymorphism (SNP) on a pair autosomal chromosomes. The third base pair of each chromosome shows variation; it can either be G-C or A-T. The labels A and a are used to denote the two variants, or alleles. Source: Courtesy of Professor Lyle Palmer

Indels. Extra base pairs (between 1 and 1000 in number) can be inserted or removed (deleted) in between two specific base pairs in a DNA sequence. Collectively, such variants are called indels. They differ from SNPs in that a SNP is merely a substitution and does not change the number of base pairs in the DNA sequence. Variable Number of Tandem Repeats (VNTRs). A common type of variation in DNA consists of specific DNA sequences that are repeated immediately adjacent to each other a variable number of times. See Fig 4. Microsattelites are an important class of VNTRs which have a small (1–6) number of base pairs which are repeated. When exactly two nucleotides are repeated, it is called a 'dinucleotide repeat'; when three are repeated, it is called a 'trinucleotide repeat'. Because the number of repeat base pair sequences can vary widely from one person to the next, microsattelites are excellent markers for distinguishing one person from the next. As such, they are widely used in forensic DNA and paternity testing. They also have been used as the basis of most linkage mapping.

Structural Variants. Structural variants include many types of chromosomal changes, including rearrangements, duplications, translocations, inversions, deletion or insertions of genetic material. Many structural variations in chromosomes involving very large segments can be seen under the microscope. These typically arise de novo during the formation of egg and sperm cells and often give rise to substantial disease burden. As these are largely not inherited, they will not be covered in this book. Duplications and deletions involving large segments of DNA that can contain many different genes are usually defined as Copy Number Variants (CNVs) because in such cases, individuals appear to have too many (more than 2) or too few (0 or 1) copies of the gene or chromosomal segment. The origin of most CNVs present in individuals (de novo versus inherited) is generally unknown. Methods for discovering and detecting CNVs in individuals are now being developed.

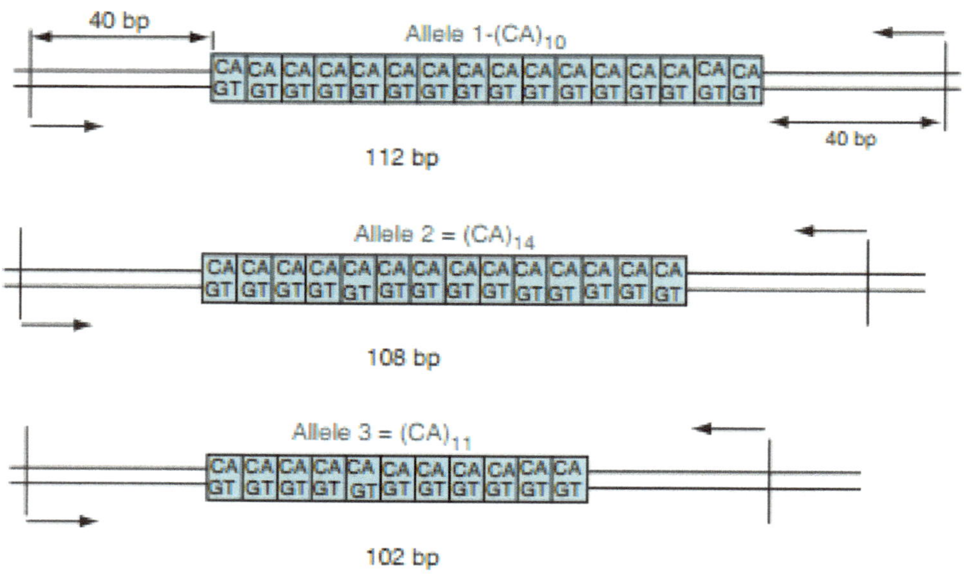

Figure 4. Example of three different alleles at a short tandem repeat of CA.

Effects of Genetic Variants on Disease

Many genetic variants have no known effects on disease or disorders in humans, but all types of variants can interfere with normal biological functioning and cause diseases of varying levels of severity. SNPs occurring outside a coding region are thought not to play a role in disease, and even SNPs occurring in a coding region may not have any biological effects because of some flexibility built into coding sequences. As depicted in Fig 5, amino acids are encoded by codons, which are three base pair sequences. Most codons have a many-to-one relationship with an amino acid, that is, several three base pair sequences can code for the same amino acid. For example, if the third base in the TCT codon for serine is changed to any one of the other three bases, e.g., TCA, serine will still be encoded. Such variants are said to be silent or synonymous because they cause no change in their product, but they can still be useful as genetic markers. Sickle cell anemia is caused by a single base pair change in the hemoglobin gene on chromosome 11. Figure 5 shows the coding sequence of the normal hemoglobin gene (A) and the sickle hemoglobin gene (S). The two sequences differ by a change of an A base in the normal Hemoglobin sequence which codes for glutamine, to a T base. The sickle allele (called S for Sickle) changes the sequence coding so that it codes for valine instead of glutamine. This is an example of a missense mutation as it changes the DNA sequence to code for a different amino acid. Individuals with SS genotype develop sickle cell anemia; AS and AA individuals are not affected by the disease. AS (and SS) individuals have a better resistance to malaria because some of their hemoglobin is type S. SNPs can also cause nonsense mutations, for example, by changing a coding sequence for an amino acid into a stop sequence which can result in too little protein being produced. Tandem repeats can also cause diseases and disorders.

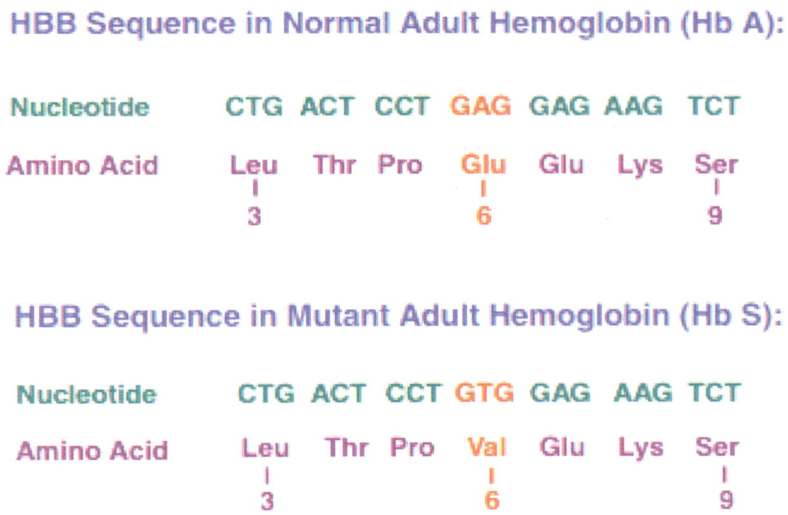

Figure 5. A variant in the hemoglobin gene causing sickle cell anemia.

The non-coding region on the human X chromosome contains a locus where the triplet CGG is repeated (CGGCGGCGGCGG, etc.) in individuals from 5 to 100 times without causing a harmful phenotype. These longer repeats tend to grow longer still from one generation to the next (to as many as 4000 repeats). This causes a constriction in the X chromosome, which makes it quite fragile, and leads to Fragile X Syndrome. Males who inherit such a chromosome show a number of harmful effects including mental retardation. Females who inherit a single fragile X chromosome are only mildly affected. Huntington's is another disease characterized by excessive short sequence repeats in the coding region of the Huntingtin gene. The Huntington gene (HTT) is located on the short arm of chromosome 4. It contains a sequence of three DNA bases, CAG, repeated multiple times (i.e., ...CAGCAGCAG...) on its 5' end. If the number of repeats of CAG is less than 27, normal protein is produced, but with more than 36 repeats, a form of protein is produced that increases the rate of neuron decay in the brain and elsewhere, causing the onset of Huntington's disease symptoms. Deletion of a sequence of DNA which interrupts a coding sequence can also have effects on disorders. For example a deletion of 32 base pairs in the cytokine receptor-5 (CCR5) gene disables receptors on the surface of cells and disrupts the ability of the HIV-1 virus to infect the cell. In this case, the deletion is beneficial to humans exposed to the HIV-1 virus. Structural variants involving large segments of DNA can cause substantial disease burden. For example, Down's syndrome arises as a result of errors in meiosis, causing an extra copy of chromosome 21. Although characterized as a genetic disorder, it is not heritable. However, many structural variants can be inherited, and can cause increased disease burden. At the present time, some associations have been found between various complex disorders and CNVs, although none can be considered definitive as yet. Many CNVs appear to be benign, and it is not clear to what extent CNVs are heritable, or largely de novo.

CHAPTER 1

STATISTICAL POWER OF MODEL SELECTION STRATEGIES FOR GENOME-WIDE ASSOCIATION STUDIES

Zheyang Wu, Hongyu Zhao

AUTHOR SUMMARY

Almost all published genome-wide association studies are based on single-marker analysis. Intuitively, joint consideration of multiple markers should be more informative when multiple genes and their interactions are involved in disease etiology. For example, an exhaustive search among models involving multiple markers and their interactions can identify certain gene–gene interactions that will be missed by single-marker analysis. However, an exhaustive search is difficult, or even impossible, to perform because of the computational requirements. Moreover, searching more models does not necessarily increase statistical power, because there may be an increased chance of finding false positive results when more models are explored. For power comparisons of different model selection methods, the published studies have relied on limited simulations due to the highly computationally intensive nature of such simulation studies. To enable researchers to compare different model search strategies without resorting to extensive simulations, we develop a novel analytical approach to evaluating the statistical power of these methods. Our results offer insights into how different parameters in a genetic model affect the statistical power of a given model selection strategy. We developed an R package to implement our results. This package can be used by researchers to compare and select an effective approach to detecting SNPs.

Citation: Wu Z, Zhao H (2009) Statistical Power of Model Selection Strategies for Genome-Wide Association Studies. PLoS Genet 5(7): e1000582. doi:10.1371/journal.pgen.1000582

INTRODUCTION

In genome-wide association studies (GWAS), hundreds of thousands of markers are genotyped to identify genetic variations associated with complex phenotypes of interest. The detection of truly associated markers can be framed as a model selection problem: a group of statistical models are considered to assess how well each model predicts the phenotype, and the selected models are expected to include all or some of the truly associated genetic markers and few, if any, markers not associated with the phenotype. In the literature, three model-selecting procedures have been advocated: marginal search, exhaustive search, and forward search.

Marginal search analyzes markers individually and is the simplest and computationally least expensive among these three search methods. Under certain assumptions, such as no interactions among covariates (or markers in the GWAS context), Fan and Lv [1] proved that the truly associated covariates will be among those having the highest marginal correlations. However, Fan and Lv acknowledged that marginal search may suffer when an important covariate is jointly associated as a group but marginally unassociated as individuals with the response (phenotype). In GWAS, the phenotypes are likely associated with multiple genes, their gene-gene interactions (i.e. epistases), and gene-environment interactions. Therefore, marginal search may not be optimal for the analysis of GWAS data.

In contrast to marginal search, exhaustive search and forward search simultaneously consider multiple markers in the model. Exhaustive search examines all possible models within a given model dimension, and forward search identifies markers in a stepwise fashion. As they consider interactions, they may gain statistical power compared to marginal search [2]–[5]. In practice, exhaustive search bears a much larger computational burden because the number of models that need to be explored is an exponential function of the number of markers jointly considered. For example, if 500,000 markers are genotyped, an exhaustive search of all marker pairs would study around 10^{11} candidate models. This requires significant computational resources, especially when permutations are needed to establish overall significance levels, e.g. for the purpose of appropriately accounting for dependencies among markers. Because of this computational burden, it is difficult or even impossible to assess the power of exhaustive search through simulation studies.

Based on limited simulations and real data analysis, conflicting results exist in the literature on the relative merit of exhaustive search and forward search. Because exhaustive search considers many more models, it may increase the probability that the truly associated markers do not rise to the top as more models involving unrelated markers may outperform the true models simply due to chance. Forward search explores a smaller model space, allowing a less stringent threshold for significance. However, forward search may miss the markers that have a strong interaction effect but weak marginal effect. Through limited simulation studies, Marchini and colleagues [4],[5] concluded that exhaustive search is more powerful in finding truly associated markers in the presence of epistasis. On the contrary, based on the analysis of a real data set for yeast, Storey and colleagues [2],[3] recommended sequential forward search. They reported that exhaustive search suffers from lower power because a substantial increase in the number of models. By analytically demonstrating the conditions under which exhaustive search is better than forward search, and the reverse, our research systematically explains these contradictory results.

It is clear that the optimal model selection strategy depends on the underlying genetic model, which is unknown to researchers. In the most extreme case, if the underlying genetic model has no marginal association, an exhaustive search is the only way to find influential genes. On the other hand, for a model with purely additive genetic effects, marginal or forward search will be the most effective. For the cases between these two extremes, the optimal model selection strategy should achieve a delicate balance between computational efficiency, statistical power, and a low false positive rate. Without the knowledge of underlying models, it is necessary to evaluate the different methods by thoroughly comparing them across a large genetic model space, in which both computationally intensive simulations and limited real data analysis are difficult to fully explore.

In this article, we derive the analytical results for statistical power of marginal search, exhaustive search, and forward search. These formulas can significantly reduce the computational burden in power estimation. To implement the formulas, we developed an R package *markerSearchPower*. We demonstrate through simulations that our results are accurate. Through our results, we can systematically assess different SNP search methods across a large model space and efficiently identify the optimal one. Our derivation approaches are general and can be applied to the model selection procedures in other random predictor settings.

The rest of this article is organized as follows: in the Results section, we present the model set-up, the validation of our analytical results through simulations, and the comparisons among three model selection strategies; in the Discussion section, we summarize the power comparison results and discuss our methodological contributions; and in the Methods section, we outline the derivations of asymptotic distributions and power calculations.

RESULTS

Model Setup

A genetic model relates phenotype to genotypes, and this relationship can be rather complex. In general, statistical power depends on the effects of risk alleles, allele frequencies in the population, epistasis, as well as environmental risk factors and their interactions with genetic factors. We focus on a model commonly used in the literature, which offers valuable insights into the relative performance of model selection methods.

Assume that genotype data are available from p independent single nucleotide polymorphisms (SNPs). Our results can be generalized to other types of markers. We use $X_{i1}, \ldots, X_{ip}$, $i=1, \ldots, n$, to denote the genotypes for the ith sampled individual, for SNPs $1, \ldots, p$, respectively. Let the alleles at the jth SNP be M_j and m_j with frequencies p_j and $q_j=1-p_j$, respectively. Under the assumption of Hardy-Weinberg equilibrium and additive allelic effects, we use the following coding for this SNP:

$$X_{ij}=\begin{cases} 1 & Genotype=M_jM_j, \text{ with probability } p_j^2 \\ 0 & Genotype=M_jm_j, \text{ with probability } 2p_jq_j \\ 1 & Genotype=m_jm_j, \text{ with probability } q_j^2 \end{cases}. \tag{1}$$

We focus on the scenario that two of these SNPs, indexed by 1 and 2, are truly associated with a quantitative outcome Y through the following genetic model

$$Y_i=b_0+b_1X_{i1}+b_2X_{i2}+b_3X_{i1}X_{i2}+\varepsilon_i, \tag{2}$$

where $\varepsilon_i \sim N(0, \sigma^2)$ is independent of the genotypes. The interaction term represents the epistatic effect, and its coefficient b_3 measures the direction and magnitude of this effect.

Based on the observed data, we fit the following models using Ordinary Least Squares (OLS) involving one or two SNPs:

$$\hat{Y}_{i(j)}=\hat{\beta}_{0(j)}+\hat{\beta}_{1(j)}X_{ij}, \tag{3}$$

$$\hat{Y}_{i(jk)}=\hat{\beta}_{0(jk)}+\hat{\beta}_{1(jk)}X_{ij}+\hat{\beta}_{2(jk)}X_{ik}+\hat{\beta}_{3(jk)}X_{ij}X_{ik}. \tag{4}$$

The subscripts in the above models index the SNP(s) included in these models. Based on models (3) and (4), three model selection methods seek candidate markers according to the corresponding test statistics. In marginal search, we fit simple linear model (3) and compare the T-statistics [6] T_j for $j=1, \ldots, p$. A model, and thus its involved SNP, is selected if the corresponding T-statistic is among the largest from all tests. In two-dimensional exhaustive search, we fit regression model (4) for all SNP pairs and compare the F-statistics [6] F_{jk} for all $j<k$ where $j, k \in \{1, \ldots, p\}$. The models with the highest values of the F-statistics are selected. In forward search, we first conduct a marginal model selection through model (3) and select the jth SNP if $|T_j|$ is the largest. With X_j, we then add

another SNP X_k ($k \neq j$) for different SNPs, and choose models in format (4) which generate the highest F-statistics.

Two criteria are adopted to decide if the chosen models are correct. On one hand, we could be rather stringent and call a model correct only if it matches the true underlying genetic model. This is consistent with the concept of "joint significance" in Storey et al. [2]. On the other hand, we could be more generous and call a model correct if it contains at least one of the truly associated markers. This is consistent with the null hypothesis used in some published simulation studies [4],[5]. Accordingly, we consider two definitions of power for a model selection procedure:

- the probability of identifying exactly the true model (in marginal search, it is the probability of detecting both true SNPs);
- the probability of detecting at least one of the true SNPs.

Under power definition (A), the null model is any model other than the true genetic model; under power definition (B), the null model is any model containing neither true SNP.

Comparison Between Analytical and Simulation Results

We evaluated the accuracy of the asymptotic results derived in the Methods section by comparing the analytical results with those from simulations. To estimate power through simulation studies, we generated 1,000 data sets with n subjects and p candidate SNPs assuming Hardy-Weinberg equilibrium, as indicated in (1). The quantitative trait values were generated through true model (2) involving two true SNPs. We then used marginal search, exhaustive search, and forward search to identify SNPs associated with the trait. Under power definition (A), the target model(s) were the true model (or models with one true SNP in marginal search), and the other models were considered null models. Under power definition (B), the target models were those containing at least one true SNP, and the rest were considered null models. The empirical power estimated from these simulations was the proportion of that datasets that we were able to successfully find the target model(s) through model selection procedures, under the control of a pre-specified number (R) of falsely discovered null models. Such control offers a fair comparison of power among the three model selection methods and is numerically equal to the detection probability (DP) control [7], which is the probability of including a "correct model" when selecting R (or R+1 in marginal search under power definition (A)) of the most significant models.

In the first set-up for model (2), we considered n=100 subjects, p=300 SNPs, genetic effects $b_1=b_2=0.1$, $b_3=2.4$, allele frequency of each SNP $q_j=0.3$, $j=1, \ldots, p$, and variance $\sigma^2=3$. Table 1 summarizes the calculated power and the simulated power under definitions (A) and (B). The second set-up is the same as the first except $b_3=1.4$. For this set-up, Table 2 shows the results under definitions (A) and (B). The two values of b_3 represent large and small interaction terms with which the simulation generated a broad spectrum of power values. In both set-ups, the analytical power is very close to the empirical power based on simulations.

Table 1: The probability of detecting the exact true model (or both true SNPs in marginal search) under power definition A, and the probability of detecting at least one of the true SNPs under power definition B, with the false discovery number R varying. $b_1=b_2=0.1$, $b_3=2.4$

Category	Strategy	Source	$R=1$	$R=5$	$R=10$	$R=15$	$R=20$	$R=30$
Definition A	Marginal search	simulation	0.268	0.556	0.683	0.754	0.790	0.851
		calculation	0.279	0.552	0.673	0.738	0.781	0.836
	Exhaustive search	simulation	0.987	0.998	1.000	1.000	1.000	1.000
		calculation	0.978	0.995	0.998	0.998	0.998	1.000
	Forward search	simulation	0.780	0.788	0.789	0.789	0.789	0.789
		calculation	0.795	0.800	0.800	0.800	0.801	0.801
Definition B	Marginal search	simulation	0.790	0.950	0.980	0.985	0.993	0.995
		calculation	0.806	0.958	0.982	0.990	0.993	0.997
	Exhaustive search	simulation	0.993	0.999	1.000	1.000	1.000	1.000
		calculation	0.985	0.999	0.999	1.000	1.000	1.000
	Forward search	simulation	0.843	0.910	0.944	0.961	0.974	0.986
		calculation	0.828	0.906	0.938	0.952	0.966	0.983

doi:10.1371/journal.pgen.1000582.t001

Table 2: The probability of detecting the exact true model (or both true SNPs in marginal search) under power definition A, and the probability of detecting at least one of the true SNPs under power definition B, with the false discovery number R varying. $b_1=b_2=0.1$, $b_3=1.4$

Category	Strategy	Source	$R=1$	$R=5$	$R=10$	$R=15$	$R=20$	$R=30$
Definition A	Marginal search	simulation	0.055	0.180	0.291	0.359	0.425	0.512
		calculation	0.053	0.179	0.289	0.355	0.424	0.515
	Exhaustive search	simulation	0.394	0.586	0.667	0.706	0.715	0.753
		calculation	0.399	0.567	0.638	0.681	0.707	0.728
	Forward search	simulation	0.242	0.308	0.331	0.340	0.343	0.348
		calculation	0.238	0.308	0.331	0.342	0.349	0.354
Definition B	Marginal search	simulation	0.394	0.695	0.802	0.869	0.899	0.935
		calculation	0.406	0.698	0.807	0.862	0.894	0.932
	Exhaustive search	simulation	0.533	0.757	0.823	0.850	0.880	0.910
		calculation	0.569	0.738	0.809	0.848	0.874	0.906
	Forward search	simulation	0.422	0.561	0.654	0.731	0.769	0.841
		calculation	0.433	0.554	0.647	0.711	0.758	0.821

doi:10.1371/journal.pgen.1000582.t002

We chose these two set-ups in which the power was reasonably large to approximate most practical settings. The chosen value of p is much smaller than that in GWAS (in the 100,000's) for the feasibility of simulation. As discussed in the Methods section, the asymptotic results are derived by assuming a large p. Therefore, we expect better approximations if p has a value similar to those in a real GWAS.

Power Comparisons of Model Selection Methods

The simulation results shown in Table 1 and Table 2 demonstrate that our analytical results provide good approximations to the true power, which is the basis for comparing the performance of these model search methods in a practical GWAS. We now consider a more realistic setting with a sample size of 1000 individuals (n) and a total of 300,000 SNPs (p). We assumed a genetic model of form (2) with $\sigma^2=3$ and varied the values of $b_1=b_2$ as well as that of b_3 from −1 to 1 by a step size of 0.1. To simplify the discussion, we assumed all SNPs had the same allele frequency of $q_j=0.3$, $j=1, \ldots, p$. Note that this setting can be changed without affecting the qualitative nature of the comparison results.

Figure 1 gives the 3D plots of statistical power over the genetic model space for different model selection methods (in columns) under two power definitions (A) and (B) (in rows), when controlling the number of false discoveries to be $R=10$. These figures illustrate that marginal search and forward search cannot detect the marginal association of the influential SNP 1 or 2 in a certain region of the model space, while exhaustive search can. This portion of the model space is represented by the region where the power of marginal search and that of forward search are very close to 0, no matter how large the genetic effect is. According to formulas (8) and (16) in the Methods section, the marginally non-detectable region for SNP 1, where $b_1+b_3(p_2-q_2)=0$, depends on the additive genetic effect b_1, epistatic effect b_3, and the allele frequency p_2 of SNP 2. The non-detectable region for SNP 2 is analogous by symmetry. In exhaustive search, such region does not exist, as indicated by formula (12). So, exhaustive search can better identify the signals when they are counterbalanced.

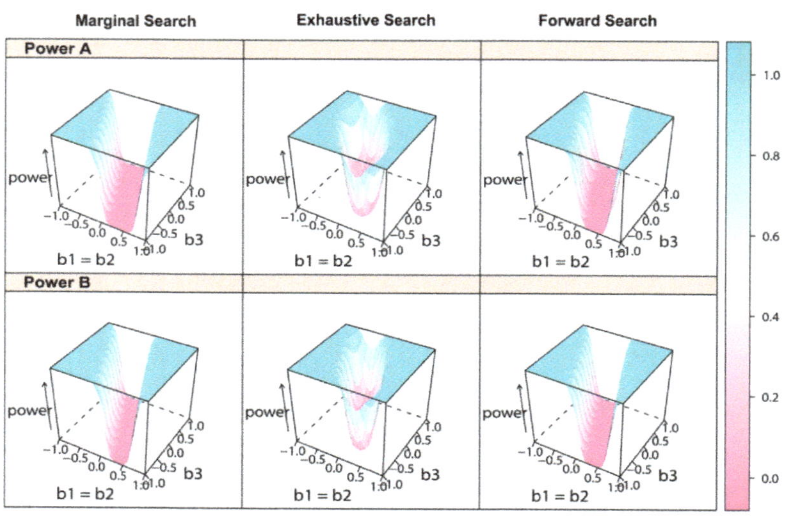

Figure 1: 3D plots of statistical power over genetic model space. The results of power for the three model selection methods: marginal search in the left column, exhaustive search in the middle column and forward search in the right column. Two definitions of power (A) for detecting

the true model or both true SNPs in marginal search in row 1, and (B) for detecting either true SNP in row 2 are considered. We consider genetic models with the main effects $b_1=b_2$ varying from −1 to 1 and the epistatic effect b_3 varying from −1 to 1. The allele frequency $q_j=0.3, j=1, \ldots, p$, and the false discovery number R is set to be 10.

In order to better visualize the difference of model selection methods, we show the power differences between different methods. The left, middle, and right columns of Figure 2 and Figure 3 present the power difference between marginal search and exhaustive search, between marginal search and forward search, and between forward search and exhaustive search, respectively. For a specific comparison, the red areas represent negative values, indicating the former method has lower power, and the green areas represent positive values, indicating the former method has higher power. The dashed contours in these plots represent the heritability of the genetic model, i.e., the proportion of the total variation due to genetic effects, which is defined as

$$H^2 = \frac{\text{genetic variance}}{\text{total variance}}.$$

Under our model set-up,

$$\begin{aligned}\text{genetic variance} = {} & 2b_1^2p_1q_1 + 2b_2^2p_2q_2 + 4b_1b_3(p_2-q_2)p_1q_1 \\ & + 4b_2b_3(p_1-q_1)p_2q_2 \\ & + \left[(p_1^2+q_1^2)(p_2^2+q_2^2) - (p_1-q_1)^2(p_2-q_2)^2\right]b_3^2,\end{aligned}$$

$$\text{total variance} = \text{genetic variance} + \sigma^2.$$

In each plot, there are two areas in which the difference of power is close to 0. First, in the central area where the signal is weak (small H^2), all model selection procedures have low power and tend to fail to pick up the true SNPs. Second, in the edge areas where the signals are strong, all model selection procedures have similarly good power. The light colored areas represent these two special situations in which there is little difference in power among model selection methods.

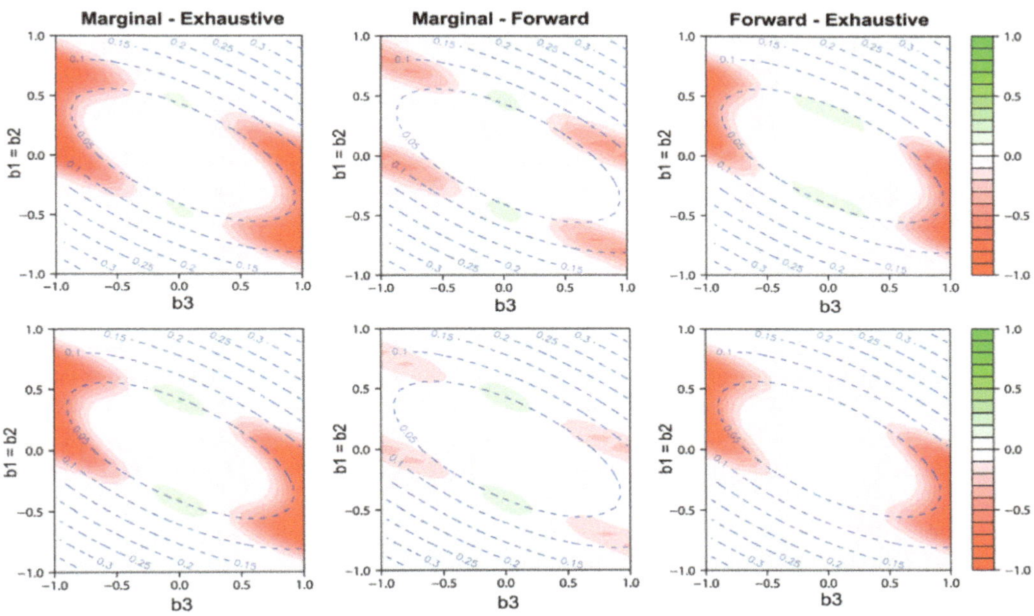

Figure 2: Comparisons among model selection power for detecting the true model or both true SNPs in marginal search over genetic model space.

The power differences between marginal search and exhaustive search in the left column, between marginal search and forward search in the middle column, and between forward search and exhaustive search in the right column. Green areas indicate positive values of difference, and red areas indicate negative values of difference. We consider genetic models with the main effects $b_1=b_2$ varying from −1 to 1 and the epistatic effect b_3 varying from −1 to 1. The allele frequency $q_j=0.3, j=1, \ldots, p$, and the false discovery number R is set to be 1 in row 1 and 10 in row 2.

http://dx.doi.org/10.1371/journal.pgen.1000582.g002

To compare marginal search and exhaustive search, the left columns of Figure 2 and Figure 3exhibit the power difference under power definitions (A) and (B), respectively. Exhaustive search has significant advantage in the red areas where the interaction effect b_3 is large or $b_1+b_3(p_2-q_2)$ is small. Such advantage is more pronounced under power definition (A) than under power definition (B). Marginal search performs better in the green areas where b_3 is small and b_1 and b_2 are both moderate. There are two reasons for the better performance of marginal search. First, with a small interaction term b_3 in these green areas, marginal search well detects the signals when the two-marker genetic effects are projected onto a marginal space through the simple regression of form (3). At the same time, with moderate b_1 and b_2, the power for these two methods is not close to 0 or 1, so that they are distinguishable. Second, marginal search considers fewer models so that the desired models are more likely to be found from the models with the best fit.

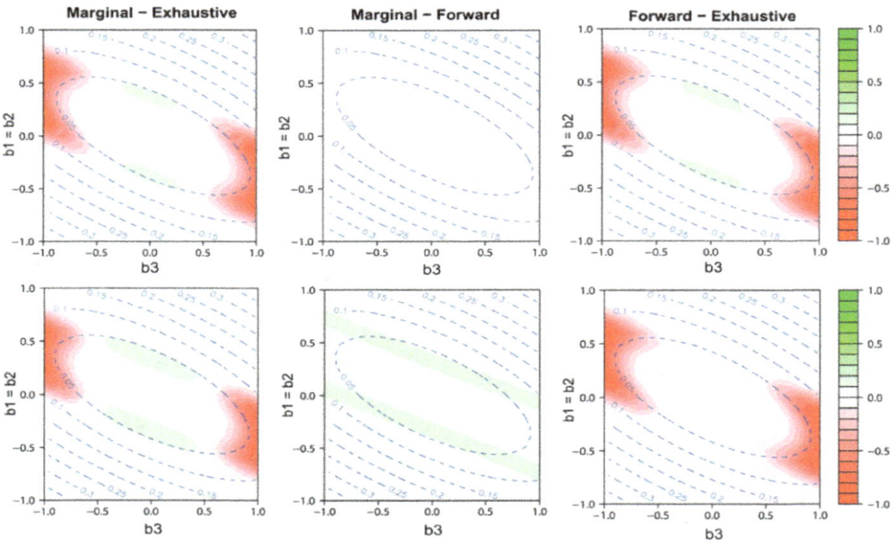

Figure 3: Comparisons among model selection power for detecting either true SNP over genetic model space. The power differences between marginal search and exhaustive search in the left column, between marginal search and forward search in the middle column, and between forward search and exhaustive search in the right column. Green areas indicate positive values of difference, and red areas indicate negative values of difference. We consider genetic models with the main effects $b_1=b_2$ varying from −1 to 1 and the epistatic effect b_3 varying from −1 to 1. The allele frequency $q_j=0.3, j=1, \ldots, p$, and the false discovery number R is set to be 1 in row 1 and 10 in row 2.

Under different power definitions, the performance of forward search relative to that of marginal search can change. Capable of including interaction terms, forward search has an advantage over marginal search in finding the full correct model under power definition (A), as shown by the red areas in the middle column of Figure 2. Based on the analytical formulas in the Methods section, there is a positive correlation between the test statistics in the first and second steps of forward search. Therefore, if one of the associated SNPs can be picked up in the first step, the contribution of the epistatic term makes forward search more powerful to identify the second correct SNP. Under power definition (B), the middle column of Figure 3shows that marginal search always has similar or slightly better power than forward search, because forward search is less likely than marginal search to pick up a true SNP if an incorrect SNP is chosen first. The power of forward search will not improve greatly even if the number of false discoveries R increases.

As shown in the right column of Figure 2, exhaustive search under power definition (A) always has a similar or higher power to detect the true model when compared to forward search. Although forward search can also detect the interaction terms through joint analysis, its ability to capture the interaction terms is restricted, especially when marginal effect is small in the deep red areas of $b_1+b_3(p_2-q_2)\approx 0$. Under power definition (B), forward search is more powerful than exhaustive search when R, the number of controlled false discoveries, is small, but is less powerful when R is large. With small R (e.g. $R=1$), forward search benefits from considering fewer models and is better than exhaustive search in the green areas of Figure 3. This benefit is reduced for larger R and will eventually be dominated by the advantage of exhaustive search. Since the first step of forward search is essentially a marginal search, the advantage of exhaustive search over marginal search also applies to forward search. This is reflected in the right columns of Figure 2 and Figure 3, where the red areas are similar to those in the left columns. As reflected by the change of red/green areas between the first and the second rows in both Figure 2 and Figure 3, if we raise the number of allowed false discoveries R, the power of marginal search will increase the most, followed by the power of exhaustive search, and then the power of forward search. With the same increase in R, marginal search includes a much higher proportion of the models with true SNPs than exhaustive search. For forward search, the increase of power is smaller because it is more difficult to identify a correct SNP in the second step when an incorrect SNP is more likely to be selected in the first step.

We also explored additional model set-ups with $n=100, p=1000, R=1, 5$, and $10, q_j=0.3$ and $0.5, j=1, \ldots, p$, and $\sigma^2=3$. The values of the genetic effects $b_1=b_2$ and $b_3$varied from −2 to 2 by a step size of 0.2. When $q_j=0.5$, the graphs are symmetric about $b_1=b_2=0$ and $b_3=0$. In general, the patterns are similar to those shown in Figure 2 and Figure 3.

An Example of Power Comparisons Motivated from Real GWAS

In the following we provide an example to show how to apply our approach to calculating and comparing the power of model selection methods in empirical analysis. Because there are no consistently replicated interaction effects from real studies, we constructed hypothetical interaction models based on real data so that the marginal associations between traits and markers were matched, while allowing the interaction term to vary. Specifically, we calculated power based on a set of genetic models derived from a genome-wide association study of adult height by Weedon et al. [8]. Based on the reported 20 loci that putatively influence adult height, we set up a two-marker genetic model composed of SNPs rs11107116 and rs10906982, each of which showed moderate marginal effect. According to the Supplementary Table 4 in the original publication, the estimated marginal effects of rs11107116 and rs10906982 are respectively 0.045s.d. and 0.046s.d. with a sample standard deviation (s.d.) of height of 6.82 cm. Assuming different levels of interaction between the two SNPs (quantified by b_3), we estimated the parameters b_1, b_2, and σ^2 using model (2) so that the marginal effects matched the observed values. The Methods section gives the details of how these parameters were estimated. We used the set-up of Weedon's study: sample size n=16,482, number of candidate SNPs p=402,951, and the frequencies of the height-increasing allele for rs11107116 and rs10906982 p_1=0.77 and p_2=0.48, respectively.

Figure 4 shows the comparisons among the power of the three model selection methods over different values of b_3. For the detection of both SNPs, graphs A (R=1) and C (R=20) indicate that if the magnitude of epistasis b_3 is large, exhaustive search (red dashed curve) has significant advantage over forward search (green dotted curve), which is better than marginal search (black solid curve). If b_3 is small, marginal search has higher power than the other two. For the detection of at least one of the two SNPs, graphs B (R=1) and D (R=20) indicate that marginal search is similar or better than forward search; both methods are not affected by the variation of b_3. The relative performance of exhaustive search strongly depends on the magnitude of epistasis. Comparing graphs B (R=1) and D (R=20), it is clear that marginal search is superior over a larger region when a larger false discovery number R is tolerated.

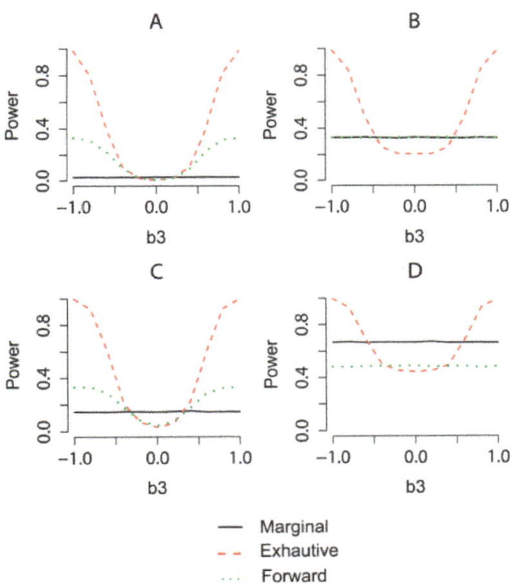

Figure 4: Plots of model selection power with given observed marginal effects.

Power comparisons of three model selection procedures over a sequence of epistatic effect b_3: marginal search by black solid curve, exhaustive search by red dashed curve, and forward search by green dotted curve. We assume the true SNPs to be rs11107116 and rs10906982, which influence adult height with their marginal effects set to be the same as those observed in Weedon et al. 2008. Graphs A with R=1 and C with R=20 indicate the power of finding both SNPs; graphs B with R=1 and D with R=20 indicate the power of finding at least one of the two SNPs.

With R=20, graphs C and D indicate that exhaustive search is better than marginal search to find both or at least one of the SNPs when the magnitude of b_3>0.3 or 0.6, respectively. We studied the statistical significance of the interaction terms with the simulated data (1,000 runs) when b_3 equals these two cutoffs. When b_3=0.3, 11.4% of the simulations had the Bonferroni p-values (adjusted by the number of all possible pairs of the 20 found loci) that exceeded the significant threshold at 0.05. Therefore, a small epistatic effect, rarely showing significance from the observed data, can still make an exhaustive search more powerful than a marginal search under power definition (A). Under power definition (B), when b_3=0.6, 87.3% of the Bonferroni adjusted p-values were significant. That is, to make exhaustive search more powerful than marginal search for finding either SNP, a true epistatic effect needs to be large enough to often identify a statistically significant interaction.

This example demonstrates that the value of the interaction term and the number of false discoveries affect the relative performance of model selection methods, which can be one of the reasons for the conflicting results about the power of model selection methods in the existing literature [2],[4]. Therefore, the suspected values of parameters such as epistatic effects can affect the researchers' choice of model selection methods.

DISCUSSION

In this article, we have derived rigorous analytical results for the statistical power of three common model selection methods, and applied these results to compare the methods' performance for GWAS data. These results not only make the computationally expensive simulations unnecessary, but also systematically reveal how different genetic model parameters affect the power.

The comparison results among the three model selection methods illustrate the trade-off between searching the full model space and a reduced space. In one extreme, exhaustive search explores the full 2-dimensional space covering all possible epistatic effects, but it may reduce the probability that the true model(s) ranks among the top models because many more models are considered. In the other extreme, marginal search casts the true 2-dimensional model onto a 1-dimensional space without considering epistasis at all. However, we have a better chance to find more true positives when the marginal association is retained in the 1-dimenisonal space, because fewer models are examined and the false positive control appears comparatively liberal. Between these two extremes, forward search first considers marginal projection, and then partially searches the 2-dimensional space via residual projection given the chosen predictor in the first step. Thus, forward search has the partial benefit of joint analysis which considers epistatic effects conditionally. The stringency of its false positive control exists between those of exhaustive search and of marginal search.

The relative performance of these model selection methods also depends on the definition of power. Based on definition (A), exhaustive search performs the best in finding the true underlying genetic model in most of the model space considered. Under power definition (B), marginal search is a good choice: it is not much worse than exhaustive search for a large proportion of the model space, and it is always better than the classic forward search through which only one SNP is picked up in the first step. For most geneticists, finding at least one of the truly associated SNPs under power definition (B) is a primary concern, especially in the first stage of GWAS.

Because we do not have prior information about the true genetic model in the beginning, marginal search, which is easy to compute, is a good start in the first stage of GWAS to find one or some of the main genetic effects. In the later stage(s), if the promising SNP candidates are limited, exhaustive search can be applied with less demanding computation, especially when epistasis among loci is of interest. Our conclusions based on the analytical studies justify this multi-stage strategy in GWAS.

Difference between Our Methods and Traditional Power Calculation and Simulations

Our power calculation for model selection strategies is different from a traditional power calculation for multiple regression models [9]. The traditional approach is to calculate the probability of accepting a specific multiple-regression model and rejecting the null hypothesis that the response and the covariates have no association, when controlling the type I error rate. This power calculation focuses on models instead of model selection methods, as it does not address any procedure of model selection. In contrast, our analytical approach is to calculate the probability that a model selection method can pick up the models that contain the true covariates (true SNPs in GWAS).

Our analytical approach leads to new insights into model selection methods than simulations and limited real data analysis. Furthermore, our approach addresses a critical limitation of prior studies [4],[5] that do not distinguish the models with all correct predictors from those with only a subset of the correct predictors. In those studies, the null distribution assumes the test statistic is from a model without any of the true predictors, and the alternative distribution assumes the statistic is from any model containing at least one true predictor (or, when considering the power for finding both true loci, the models with either true locus are ignored from the null distribution). This is a common problem of traditional multiple testing for model selection method, as pointed out by Storey et al. [2], who stated that "there is no statistically rigorous method to test for joint linkage, which exists only if both loci have nonzero terms in the full model." To address this issue, all involved models (including true, partially true, and wrong models) are considered and ranked by how well they fit the observed data. Our power calculation distinguishes the case that model selection procedures find the true model based on power definition (A) from the case that the procedures find a partially true model based on definition (B). We have derived the null and alternative distributions for each case, and thus provide the basis for model performance comparisons.

To compare the power of model selection methods, our approach explicitly considers the correlation structures among the test statistics for the null and alternative hypotheses, which achieves more accurate assessment of model selection methods than Bonferroni-corrected type I error control that is commonly used in the literature [4],[5]. Bonferroni-based control is usually a conservative control when the test statistics are dependent on each other. As illustrated by both simulations (results not shown) and the theoretical derivations in the Methods section, the considered models and their test statistics usually exhibit complex correlation structures. Therefore Bonferroni-based control is not optimal as it only considers the number of models evaluated (that is, the number of hypothesis tests) and ignores correlation structures generated by different search strategies. The adequacy of our approach has been demonstrated through a good agreement between the analytical and the simulation results shown in Table 1 and Table 2. Furthermore, our study of correlation structures improves the understanding of the mechanism of different search strategies discovering genetic signals. For example, in forward search, the failure of the first stage is likely to cause the failure of the second stage even if there is a large epistatic effect, because the test statistics for the true predictors are positively correlated between the two stages.

Control Related to Type I Error Rate and False Discovery Proportion

To obtain the significance threshold, we control the number of false discoveries at R depending on how the power is defined. This control is practically meaningful and equals to the detection probability (DP) control [7] as discussed in the Results section. Furthermore, controlling the number of false discoveries is related to controlling the type I error rate. Since the type I error rate is defined as the probability of rejecting a hypothesis given it is a true null, with the definition of null models corresponding to the power definition (A) or (B), the estimation of component-wise type I error rate could be considered as

$$\hat{\alpha} = \frac{R}{\text{total \# of null models}}.$$

The model selection problem is also a large-scale simultaneous hypothesis testing problem. A widely applied significance control criterion in this scenario is the false discovery rate (FDR) [10]. The false discovery number control in our study is also related to the control of the false discovery proportion (FDP), which is an estimate of FDR. Under power definition (A)

$$FDP = \frac{R}{R + i \times power(R)},$$

where $power(R)$ denotes the power calculated based on the number of selected null models R, and i indicates the number of correct models: i=2 for marginal search, and i=1 for exhaustive search and forward search.

On the Derivation of Asymptotic Distributions

Through the simulations in the Results section, our derivation of asymptotic distributions is shown to be accurate for moderately small genetic effects when the sample size n=100. Since the asymptotic derivation assumes large sample size, the power calculation results should provide accurate approximations for reasonably smaller genetic effects in GWAS which have a much larger number of observations in general. The asymptotic derivation has several benefits. First, we can derive the results for the models with random predictors. Because genotypes are randomly observed in genetic studies, it is necessary to consider such models. Traditional methods for deriving the non-central F distributions for the test statistics are based on fixed predictors [7],[11],[12]. As functions of predictor variables, these non-central parameters are not statistically consistent when genotypes are random. Although one may integrate the power over all possible configurations of markers [13], it is very cumbersome unless n is small. Our method, based on asymptotic theorems, provides a satisfactory solution for models with random predictors. Our novel approach presented here can be applied to derive the distributions of such models' test statistics. Second, the derived asymptotic multivariate normal distributions for theoretical null and alternative hypotheses allow us to incorporate complex correlations among the test statistics into power calculation based on population parameters. For a given GWAS data set, the correlations presented in the data may also be addressed by empirical estimation of the null hypothesis [14],[15]. Third, the ideas behind the asymptotic derivation can be applied to study the distributions for hypothesis testing and power calculation in general as long as the statistics have certain functions of random variables.

On Simplifying Assumptions

We have assumed that the markers are independent in this paper. There may be linkage disequilibrium (LD) among SNPs. However, LD in general is weak among tagging SNPs [16]–[18]. Furthermore, simulations based on real GWAS data (results not shown) indicate that even in the presence of LD, our analytical results are quite accurate when more false positives are acceptable, i.e. a large R value. In addition, the analytical power approximations are more accurate for power definition (B) than for definition (A). In general, when the dependency among true SNPs and the ensemble of unrelated SNPs is weak or moderate, our power calculation provides acceptable approximations.

In reality, the underlying true model could be more complicated than model (2) with more related SNPs and interactions. Our analytical results of power calculation can be extended through the approaches similar to the one we developed here. Although the genetic models studied are simple, our results provide insights into the relative performance of different model selection procedures.

METHODS

Asymptotic Distribution Results

To calculate the power of model selection procedures shown in the Results section, we first derive general results on the asymptotic distributions. Let $\mathbf{Z}_i=(Z_{i1}, \ldots, Z_{is})$, $i=1, \ldots, n$, be n independent and identically distributed (iid) random vectors of dimension s. Assume the mean vector is $\boldsymbol{\theta}=E(\mathbf{Z}_i)=(\theta_1, \ldots, \theta_s)$ with $\theta_j=E(Z_{ij})$ and the variance-covariance matrix is $\Sigma=Cov(\mathbf{Z}_i)$ with $(\Sigma)_{jk}=Cov(Z_{ij}, Z_{ik})$, j, $k=1, \ldots, s$. Let $\bar{\mathbf{Z}}=(\bar{Z}_1,\ldots,\bar{Z}_s)$, where $\bar{Z}_j=\frac{1}{n}\sum_{i=1}^{n} Z_{ij}$. Considering a real valued function $h(\bar{\mathbf{Z}})$ of $\bar{\mathbf{Z}}$

if $\nabla h(\boldsymbol{\theta})=\left(\frac{\partial h(\boldsymbol{\theta})}{\partial\theta_1},\ldots,\frac{\partial h(\boldsymbol{\theta})}{\partial\theta_s}\right)\neq 0$, we have

$$\sqrt{n}[h(\bar{\mathbf{Z}})-h(\boldsymbol{\theta})] \xrightarrow{L} N(0,\tau^2), \tag{5}$$

where $\tau^2=[\nabla h(\boldsymbol{\theta})]'\Sigma[\nabla h(\boldsymbol{\theta})]$ and $\xrightarrow{L}$ denotes the convergence in law [19].

We extend the above result in two ways to suit our needs of deriving the distribution of test statistics that are examined in model selection procedures . First, we consider two real valued functions $h_1(\bar{\mathbf{Z}})$ and $h_2(\bar{\mathbf{Z}})$ of the same sample mean $\bar{\mathbf{Z}}$. If $\nabla h_1(\boldsymbol{\theta})\neq 0$ and $\nabla h_2(\boldsymbol{\theta})\neq 0$, we have the convergence in probability that:

$$Cov\left(\sqrt{nh_1}(\bar{\mathbf{Z}}),\sqrt{nh_2}(\bar{\mathbf{Z}})\right) \xrightarrow{P} [\nabla h_1(\boldsymbol{\theta})]'\Sigma[\nabla h_2(\boldsymbol{\theta})]. \tag{6}$$

Secondly, if $\nabla h(\theta)=0$, the asymptotic distribution of $nh(\bar{\mathbf{Z}})$ is:

$$n[h(\bar{\mathbf{Z}})-h(\boldsymbol{\theta}) \xrightarrow{L} c\chi_d^2, \tag{7}$$

where if $A\equiv D^2h(\boldsymbol{\theta})\Sigma$, with $D^2h(\boldsymbol{\theta})=\frac{\partial^2}{\partial\theta^2}h(\boldsymbol{\theta})$ being the Hessian matrix of $h(\boldsymbol{\theta})$, we have

- $c=1/2$, $d=rank[A]$, if A is idempotent;
- $c\approx trace(A^2)/2trace(A)$, $d\approx trace(A)^2/trace(A^2)$, if A is not idempotent.

Power Calculations

With the results above, we derive the relevant distributions of T- and F-statistics associated with three types of regression models, which will be used for calculating the power of model selection methods. Specifically, F_{12} is the F statistics for the correct model in which both SNPs are true. T_i and F_{ij}, $i=1$, 2, $j=3$, …, p, are test statistics for "half" correct models in which only one SNP is truly associated. T_j and F_{lk}, $3\leq l<k\leq p$, are the statistics for incorrect models in which neither SNP in the models is associated with the phenotype. Complex correlations exist among the models even with the assumption of independence among SNPs. The correlations come from two sources. First, since the quantitative trait is associated with both SNPs 1 and 2, the fitted regression models containing either of these SNPs have correlated test statistics. Second, models sharing a common SNP (no matter it is true or wrong) also have correlated test statistics. To allow correlations, we therefore explore the marginal and the joint distributions of various test statistics for different models, and then derive how likely a "half" correct model would stand out from incorrect models, as well as how likely a correct model would outperform "half" correct models or incorrect models.

Marginal Search

Statistics and Asymptotic Distributions

To calculate the power of marginal search, we need to obtain the distributions of the involved test statistics. We first derive the T-statistic for the two true SNPs in the marginal model. In the simple regression model involving the first true SNP (SNP 1), i.e. $\hat{Y}_{i(1)}=\hat{\beta}_{0(1)}+\hat{\beta}_{1(1)}X_{i1}$, the corresponding T-statistic has the following asymptotic distribution $T_1-\sqrt{nh_1}(\boldsymbol{\theta}) \xrightarrow{L} N(0,\tau_1^2)$,

where

$$h_1(\boldsymbol{\theta})=\frac{\sqrt{2p_1q_1}(b_1+b_3(p_2-q_2))}{\sqrt{2p_2q_2(b_2^2+2b_2b_3(p_1-q_1)+b_3^2(p_1^2+q_1^2))+\sigma^2}}, \tag{8}$$

and the formula of τ_1^2 (a constant of n). For the marginal model of the second SNP (SNP 2), the asymptotic distribution of T_2 is gotten by symmetry between indices 1 and 2. Based on the asymptotic mean of T_1 derived above, we can quantify the influence of genetic parameters of SNP 2 and epistasis on the power of marginal search to pick up SNP 1. As for some genetically interesting observations, when there is no epistatic effect (i.e. $b_3=0$), we have $h_1(\boldsymbol{\theta})=\frac{b_1\sqrt{2p_1q_1}}{\sqrt{2p_2q_2b_2^2+\sigma^2}}$, which means the magnitude of marginal association of X_1 and thus the power of marginal search to find X_1 are decreasing functions of the main effect of X_2, the minor allele frequency (MAF) of X_2, and the random error variance σ^2, with the decreasing rate specifically given by $\sqrt{2p_2q_2b_2^2+\sigma^2}$. When epistasis exists (i.e. $b_3\neq 0$) but $b_1=0$, $h_1(\boldsymbol{\theta})$ reflects the marginally projected signal of epistasis, which is still a decreasing function of the MAF of X_2. The influence of b_2 depends on the allele frequencies p_1 and q_1. On the other hand, if $b_1\neq 0$, it is possible that $b_1+b_3(p_2-q_2)=0$ when the main effect b_1 and interaction effects b_3 have opposite directions (assuming q_2 is the MAF). With such epistatic pattern, marginal detection surely fails to detect the true genetic variants no matter how strong the true genetic effects are.

Now we derive the joint distribution of T_1 and T_2. Since Y is a function of both X_1 and X_2 in the underlying true model (2), T_1 and T_2 are correlated even when X_1 and X_2 are independent and do not interact, i.e. $b_3=0$. The correlation between T_1 and T_2 can be substantial in certain genetic models. The asymptotic joint distribution of $(T_1, T_2)'$ is

$$(T_1,T_2)'-\boldsymbol{\mu}_{T_1,T_2}\xrightarrow{L} MVN(\mathbf{0},\boldsymbol{\tau}_{T_1,T_2}), \quad (9)$$

where $\boldsymbol{\mu}_{T_1,T_2}=\sqrt{n}(h_1(\boldsymbol{\theta}),h_2(\boldsymbol{\theta}))'$, $\boldsymbol{\tau}_{T_1,T_2}=\begin{pmatrix}\tau_1^2 & \tau_{1,2}\\ \tau_{1,2} & \tau_2^2\end{pmatrix}$, $\tau_i^2=Var(T_i)$,

The covariance $\tau_{1,2}$ is gotten based on the result in (6), and its formula (as a constant of n).

Let T_j, $j=3, \ldots, p$, be the T-statistic from model (3) for a wrong SNP j, according to the asymptotic result in (5),

$$T_j \xrightarrow{L} N(0,1), \quad (10)$$

which holds regardless of the allele frequencies and the underlying true genetic model. It can be shown that T_j is also independent of T_1 and T_2 according to the result in (6). Under the assumption of fixed design matrix, T_j has a T distribution with $n-2$ degrees of freedom based on a traditional linear model analysis [6],[12]. This null distribution is still asymptotically valid for random predictors since the T distribution converges to the standard normal as $n\to\infty$.

Power of Marginal Search Procedure

Based on the above results for the distributions of T-statistics, we first calculate the power of marginal search under power definition (A). If the marginal search is allowed to contain R wrong SNPs, i.e. the number of false discoveries is controlled by R, the power of identifying both true SNPs is just the probability that both $|T_1|$ and $|T_2|$ are greater than the Rth largest value in the set $\{T_j, j\geq 3\}$:

$$P(|T_1|\wedge|T_2|\geq|T|_{(r)})=\iint P(|T|_{(r)}\leq|t_1|\wedge|t_2|)g(t_1,t_2)dt_1dt_2$$

where $|T_1|\wedge|T2|=\min\{|T_1|,|T_2|\}$, $r=p-2-R+1$, $|T|_{(r)}$ is the rth smallest (or the Rth largest) order statistics of $|T_j|$, $j=3, \ldots, p$, and $g(t_1, t_2)$ is the joint probability density function (PDF) of $(T_1, T_2)'$ given in (9). Let $\Phi(\cdot)$ be the cumulative distribution function (CDF) of $N(0, 1)$, then

$$P\left(|T|_{(r)}\leq|t_1|\wedge|t_2|\right)=(1-2\Phi(-|t_1|\wedge|t_2|))^r \sum_{l=0}^{p-2-r}\binom{r+l-1}{l}(2\Phi(-|t_1|\wedge|t_2|))^l.$$

To get the power of marginal search under definition (B) that either SNP 1 or SNP 2 is selected, we calculate the probability that either $|T_1|$ or $|T_2|$ is larger than the random cutoff point: $P(|T_1|\vee|T_2|\geq|T|_{(r)})$, where $|T_1|\vee|T_2|=\max\{|T_1|, |T_2|\}$.

Exhaustive Search

Statistics and Asymptotic Distributions

The distributions of the relevant test statistics are derived first for calculating the power of exhaustive search. We first get the joint distribution of the test statistics involving true SNPs 1 and 2: T_1, T_2, and F_{12}. Define $T_{12}\equiv\sqrt{F_{12}}$. Based on the asymptotic distribution result in (5), we have

$$(T_{12},T_1,T_2)'-\boldsymbol{\mu}_{T_{12},T_1,T_2}\xrightarrow{L} MNV(\mathbf{0},\boldsymbol{\tau}_{T_{12},T_1,T_2}), \quad (11)$$

where $\boldsymbol{\mu}_{T_{12},T_1,T_2}=\sqrt{n}(h_{12}(\boldsymbol{\theta}),h_1(\boldsymbol{\theta}),h_2(\boldsymbol{\theta}))'$ and $\boldsymbol{\tau}_{T_{12},T_1,T_2}=\begin{pmatrix}\tau_{12}^2 & \tau_{12,1} & \tau_{12,2}\\ \tau_{12,1} & \tau_1^2 & \tau_{1,2}\\ \tau_{12,2} & \tau_{1,2} & \tau_2^2\end{pmatrix}$.

The formula of $h_1(\boldsymbol{\theta})$ is given in (8), and

$$h_{12}(\boldsymbol{\theta})=\left(\frac{2}{3\sigma^2}(b_1^2p_1q_1+b_3^2p_1q_1(p_2^2+q_2^2)+2b_1b_3p_1q_1(p_2-q_2)+p_2q_2(b_2+b_3(p_1-q_1))^2\right)^{1/2}. \quad (12)$$

The formulas of $\tau_{12}^2=Var(T_{12})$ and $\tau_{12,i}=Cov(T_{12}, T_i)$, $i=1, 2$, are independent of n.

We then derive the F-statistics for the incorrect models in form (4) to fit Y with X_j and X_k, $3\leq j<k\leq p$. Following the result in (7), F_{jk} has a common marginal asymptotic distribution:

$$F_{jk}\xrightarrow{L}\frac{1}{3}\chi_3^2. \quad (13)$$

With F_{34} as an example

Based on the traditional power calculation for regression models, the null model is the incorrect model with neither SNP associated with the phenotype. When the design matrix is fixed, the null distribution of F_{jk} is an F distribution with degrees of freedom $(3, n-4)$ [12]. Result (13) indicates the F distribution for null is also valid when the genotypes are treated as random variables, because $F(3, n-4)$ converges to $\frac{1}{3}\chi_3^2$ when n is large.

In order to calculate the power of model selection methods, we need to address the correlation structures among involved statistics. The statistics are correlated when two epistatic models in form (4) share a common SNP. Also, F-statistics involving X_1 and those involving X_2 are correlated because the true underlying model includes both SNPs. Consequently, the elements in the set $\{F_{12}, F_{ij}, i=1, 2, j=3,\ldots,p\}$ are all correlated with each other. To capture the important dependency, we decompose F-statistics as follows:

$$F_{ij} \to \frac{1}{3}F_i + \frac{2}{3}\left(h_i^2(\boldsymbol{\theta})+1\right)F_{j|i}, \tag{14}$$

when i=1, $h_1(\boldsymbol{\theta})$ is given by equation (8). The detailed proof for decomposing F_{13} . Through this decomposition, the correlation between F_{ij} and F_{ik}, can be explained by F_i while we treat $F_{j|i}$ and $F_{k|i}$ to be independent. Furthermore, with the result (14) we can use the joint distribution (11) to capture the correlation between $F_{12}$and F_{ij}.

Based on the asymptotic distribution in (7), we have $F_{j|i} \overset{(d)}{\cong} c\chi_d^2$.**(15)**where i=1, 2, j=3, …, p, c=v/2e, and d=2e^2/v, with $E(F_{j|i})$→e and $Var(F_{j|i})$→v.. Based on our numerical studies (results not shown), c is close to 1/2 and d is close to 2 in a large proportion of the parameter space of $\{q_i, q_j, \mathbf{b}, \sigma^2\}$ (e.g. when allele frequencies q_i and $q_j$do not converge to 0 or 1, genetic effect $\mathbf{b}=(b_1, b_2, b_3)'$ and random error variance σ^2 are not too large). When c=1/2 and d=2, $c\chi_d^2$ is asymptotically equivalent to an F distribution with degrees of freedom 2 and n–4. $F(2, n–4)$ is the distribution of $F_{j|i}$ when X is fixed [6],[12]. Our results demonstrate that for the random design matrix, the weighted chi-square distribution (15) is more appropriate.

Power of Exhaustive Search Procedure

With the distribution of test statistics derived above, we first calculate the probability of exhaustive search to identify the exact true model. Under power definition (A), the test statistic F_{12} for the exact true model corresponds to the "alternative" distribution, whereas the F-statistics for all other models such as totally incorrect models and "half" correct models are combined together to generate a mixed "null" distribution. Let $S_1 \equiv \{F_{ij}, i=1, 2, j=3,\ldots,p\}$, $S_2 \equiv \{F_{jk}, 3 \leq j<k \leq p\}$, and $F_{S,[R]}$ denote the Rth largest variable in a set S. When controlling the false discovery number by R, the probability of detecting the exact true model (2) is

$$P(F_{12} \geq F_{S_1 \cup S_2,[R]}) = \iiint P\left(t_{12}^2 \geq F_{S_1' \cup S_2,[R]}\right) g(t_{12},t_1,t_1)d(t_{12},t_1,t_1),$$

where $g(t_{12},t_1,t_2)$ is the PDF of (11), $S_1' = \left\{ \frac{t_i^2}{3} + \frac{2(1+h_i^2(\boldsymbol{\theta}))F_{j|i}}{3}, i=1,2; j=3,\ldots,p \right\}$ from the decomposition (14), and

$$P\left(t_{12}^2 \geq F_{S'_1 \cup S_2,[R]}\right) = \sum_{r=0}^{R-1} \sum_{\{r_1,r_2,r\} \in S_r} P_1 P_2 P_3,$$

in which

$$S_r = \left\{ \{r_1,r_2,r_3\} : \sum r_i = r,\ 0 \leq r_1,\ r_2 \leq p-2,\ 0 \leq r_3 \leq N \right\},$$

$$P_1 \binom{p-2}{r_1} \left[1 - G_{11}\left(\frac{3t_{12}^2 - t_1^2}{2(1+h_1^2(\boldsymbol{\theta}))}\right)\right]^{r_1} G_{11}\left(\frac{3t_{12}^2 - t_1^2}{2(1+h_1^2(\boldsymbol{\theta}))}\right)^{p-2-r_1},$$

$$P_2 \binom{p-2}{r_2} \left[1 - G_{12}\left(\frac{3t_{12}^2 - t_2^2}{2(1+h_2^2(\boldsymbol{\theta}))}\right)\right]^{r_2} G_{12}\left(\frac{3t_{12}^2 - t_2^2}{2(1+h_2^2(\boldsymbol{\theta}))}\right)^{p-2-r_2},$$

$$P_3 \binom{N}{r_3} \left[1 - G_2\left(t_{12}^2\right)\right]^{r_3} G_2\left(t_{12}^2\right)^{N-r_3},$$

$N = \binom{p-2}{2}$ is the number of variables in S_2, $G_{1i}(\bullet)$ is the CDF of distribution (15) for i=1, 2, and $G_2(\bullet)$ is the CDF of distribution (13). The test statistics within the sets $S^* \equiv \{F_{j|1}, F_{j|2}, j=3,\ldots,p\}$ and $S_2 \equiv \{F_{jk}, 3 \leq j<k \leq p\}$ are treated as asymptotically independent as $p \to \infty$.

According to the power definition (B), the probability of exhaustive search to detect at least one of the associated SNPs is $P(\max(\{F_{12}\} \cup S_1) \geq F_{S_2,[R]}) = 1 - \iiint P_{t_{12},t_1,t_2} g(t_{12},t_1,t_2) d(t_{12},t_1,t_2)$,

Where

$$\begin{aligned} P_{t_{12},t_1,t_2} &= P\left(\max\left(\{t_{12}^2\} \cup S'_1\right) < F_{S_2,[R]}\right) \\ &= \int P\left(\max\left(\{t_{12}^2\} \cup S'_1\right) < c\right) g_{2(N-R+1)}(c)dc \\ &= \int_{t_{12}^2}^{\infty} \left[G_{11}\left(\frac{3c - t_1^2}{2(1+h_1^2(\boldsymbol{\theta}))}\right) G_{12}\left(\frac{3c - t_2^2}{2(1+h_2^2(\boldsymbol{\theta}))}\right)\right]^{p-2} g_{2(N-R+1)}(c)dc, \end{aligned}$$

$g_{2(N-R+1)}(\bullet)$ is the PDF of the (N–R+1)th order statistics distribution with the following density function: $g_{2(N-R+1)}(c) = \frac{N!}{(N-R)!(R-1)!} G_2(c)^{N-R}[1-G_2(c)]^{R-1} g_2(c)$, $G_2(\bullet)$ and $g_2(\bullet)$ are the CDF and PDF of the distribution of (13) respectively.

If R is neither too small nor too large, i.e. $R/N \to c$, $0<c<1$, as $N \to \infty$, we can use quantiles to replace the order statistics in order to simplify the calculation [20], i.e., $F_{S_2,[R]} \to G_2^{-1}\left(\frac{N-R+0.5}{N}\right) \equiv Q$. So for a given (t_{12},t_1,t_2), we can approximately replace the integrand P_{t_{12},t_1,t_2} with $I_{\{t_{12}^2 \leq Q\}}(t_{12}) \left[G_{11}\left(\frac{3Q - t_1^2}{2(1+h_1^2(\boldsymbol{\theta}))}\right) G_{12}\left(\frac{3Q - t_2^2}{2(1+h_2^2(\boldsymbol{\theta}))}\right)\right]^{p-2}$, where $I_A(x)$ denotes the indicator function of set A. Simulations (results not shown) illustrate that the approximation of integrand is reasonably accurate for the integration.

Forward Search

Statistics and Asymptotic Distributions

For forward search, first we derive the distributions of test statistics, which will be used to calculate the corresponding statistical power. Here we need to handle the comparison between two models: the model with SNPs 1 and j, j=3, …, p, taking form (4), and the model with SNP $j$taking form (3). Let $F_{1|j}$ be the F statistic measuring the significance of the extra terms in the bigger model over the smaller model [6]. Define $T_{1|j} \equiv \sqrt{F_{1|j}}$. When $b_1+b_3(p_2-q_2) \neq 0$, following the asymptotic result in (5), we can derive

$$T_{1|j} - \mu_{T_{1|j}} \xrightarrow{L} N\left(0, \tau^2_{i|j}\right),$$

$$\mu_{T_{1|j}} = \left(\frac{np_1q_1(b_1 + b_3(p_2 - q_2))^2}{2p_2q_2\left((b_2 + b_3p_1)^2 - 2b_2b_3q_1 + b_3^2q_1^2\right) + \sigma^2} \right)^{1/2}, \quad \textbf{(16)}$$

and the formula for $\tau^2_{T_{1|j}}$ with j=3. Both $\mu_{T_{1|j}}$ and $\tau^2_{T_{1|j}}$ do not depend on the allele frequency p_j. When $b_1+b_3(p_2-q_2)=0$, $T^2_{1|j}$ has a $\frac{1}{2}\chi^2_2$distribution by (7). Similarly we can get the asymptotic distribution of $T_{2|j} \equiv \sqrt{F_{2|j}}$ when comparing the model having SNPs 2 and j in form (4) with the model having SNP j in form (3). The covariance $Cov(T_{1|j},T_{2|j})$ can also be calculated. As an example the formula of $Cov(T_{1|3},T_{2|3})$

Moreover, the statistics $(T_1,T_2,T_{1|j},T_{2|j})'$ involving true SNPs have a multivariate normal distribution:

$$(T_1,T_2,T_{1|j},T_{2|j})' - \boldsymbol{\mu}_{T_1,T_2,T_{1|j},T_{2|j}} \xrightarrow{L} MNV(\mathbf{0}, \boldsymbol{\tau}_{T_1,T_2,T_{1|j},T_{2|j}}). \quad \textbf{(17)}$$

When j=3, the details of the calculation and the formulas for $\boldsymbol{\mu}_{T_1,T_2,T_{1|j},T_{2|j}}$ and $\boldsymbol{\tau}_{T_1,T_2,T_{1|j},T_{2|j}}$

Through result (6), we have proved that T_j and $F_{1|j}$ are asymptotically independent, i.e.

$$Cov(T_j, T_{1|j}) \rightarrow 0, j = 3, \ldots, p. \quad \textbf{(18)}$$

When comparing the model having two incorrect SNPs j and k ($3 \le j < k \le p$) in form (4) with the model having SNP j in form (3), the corresponding F-statistic $F_{k|j}$ has the asymptotic distribution

$$F_{k|j} \xrightarrow{L} \frac{1}{2}\chi^2_2. \quad \textbf{(19)}$$

Based on the result in (7), the proof for (19) with j=3 and k=4 as an example. This distribution is consistent with $F(2, n-4)$ which can be derived with the fixed design matrix and is routinely used for $F_{k|j}$ in the traditional model comparison [6],[12].

Power of Forward Search Procedure

In the forward search procedure, we first apply marginal search to find the most significant SNP among models (3). Based on the selected SNP, we then fit models (4) in the second step to find the SNPs that have strong joint effects, while controlling for R false discoveries. Under power definition (A) for finding the exact true model, we need to calculate the probability of forward search to choose SNP 1 or 2 in the first step, and then pick up the true model in the second step. Define $i^* \equiv \text{argmax}_{i=1,2}\{|T_i|\}$, $S_{i^*} \equiv \{F_{i^*3}, \ldots, F_{i^*p}\}$, as $p \rightarrow \infty$, we can write the power as $P\left(|T_{i^*}| > |T|_{(p-2)} \cap F_{12} \ge F_{S_{i^*},[R]}\right)$

$$= \iiint P\left(|t_{i^*}| > |T|_{(p-2)} \cap t^2_{12} \ge F_{S'_{i^*},[R]}\right) g(t_{12},t_1,t_2) d(t_{12},t_1,t_2)$$

$$\rightarrow \iiint P\left(|t_{i^*}| > |T|_{(p-2)}\right) P\left(t^2_{12} \ge F_{S'_{i^*},[R]}\right) g(t_{12},t_1,t_2) d(t_{12},t_1,t_2)$$

where $g(t_{12},t_1,t_2)$ is the PDF of $(T_{12},T_1,T_2)'$ given in (11), $|T|_{(p-2)} = \max_{j \ge 3}\{|T_j|\}$, $S'_{i^*} = \{\frac{1}{3}t^2_{i^*} + \frac{2}{3}(1 + h^2_{i^*}(\boldsymbol{\theta}))F_{j|i^*}, j=3,\ldots p\}$ by F-statistic decomposition (14), and $P\left(|t_{i^*}| > |T|_{(p-2)}\right) = (1 - 2\Phi(-(|t_1| \vee |t_2|)))^{p-2}$,

$$P(t^2_{12} \ge F_{S'_{i^*},[R]}) = G_{1i^*}(u)^r \sum_{l=0}^{p-2-r} \binom{r+l-1}{l} [1 - G_{1i^*}(u)]^l,$$

where $u = \frac{3t^2_{12} - t^2_{i^*}}{2(1 + h^2_{i^*}(\theta))}$, $h_{i^*}(\boldsymbol{\theta})$ is given in (8) for $i^*=1$, $r=p-2-R+1$, and $G_{1i^*}(\cdot)$ is the CDF of the distribution for $F_{j|i^*}$ given in (15). i^* is fixed for an observed value $(t_1,t_2)'$ of random vector $(T_1,T_2)'$, so it is easy to implement the power calculation with Monte Carlo integration.

Note that $|T|_{(p-2)}$ and $F_{S_{i^*},[R]}$ are asymptotically independent. This is because $corr(|T_j|, F_{j|i^*}) < 1$ for each $j \ge 3$, so with $p \rightarrow \infty$, $P\left(j^* \ne k^* : |T_{j^*}| = |T|_{(p-2)}, F_{k^*|i^*} = F_{S'_{i^*},[R]}\right) \rightarrow 1$. But when $j^* \ne k^*$, $|T_{j^*}|$ and $F_{k^*|i^*}$ are always independent.

When R and p are large, we can simplify the formula of $P(t^2_{12} \ge F_{S'_{i^*},[R]})$ by approximating the Rth largest variable in set $\{F_{j|i^*}, j=3, \ldots, p\}$ with $G^{-1}_{1i^*}\left(1 - \frac{R-0.5}{p-2}\right)$, where $G^{-1}_{1i^*}$ is the quantile function of $F_{j|i^*}$. So we can approximately replace $P(t^2_{12} \ge F_{S'_{i^*},[R]})$ with $I_{\{u > G^{-1}_{1i^*}(1 - \frac{R-0.5}{p-2})\}}(u)$ for calculating the integration.

Under power definition (B), the power of forward model selection method is the sum of P_A: the probability to detect SNP 1 or 2 in the 1st step, and P_B: the probability that step 1 fails but step 2 picks up at least one correct SNP, while controlling for R incorrect models as false positives. Specifically,

$$P_A = P\left((|T_1| \vee |T_2|) > |T|_{(p-2)}\right)$$

$$= \iint (1 - 2\Phi(-|t_1| \vee |t_2|))^{p-2} g(t_1,t_2) dt_1 dt_2,$$

where $g(t_1,t_2)$ is the PDF of joint distribution of $(T_1,T_2)'$ given in (9). Defining $j^* \equiv \text{arg max}_{k \ge 3}\{|T_k|\}$ and $S_{j^*} \equiv \left\{F_{k|j^*}, k \ge 3, k \ne j^*\right\}$, we have $P_B = P\left(\{|T_{j^*}| > (|T_1| \vee |T_2|)\} \cap \left\{(F_{1|j^*} \vee F_{2|j^*}) \ge F_{S_{j^*},[R]}\right\}\right)$.

For each $k \ge 3$, $F_{i|k}$ and T_k are independent, so $F_{i|j^*}$ and T_{j^*} are independent. Given the results in (16) and (19), the distribution of $F_{i|j^*}$ does not depend on j^*. Hence, $F_{i|j^*}$ has the same distribution as $F_{i|j}$, $j=3,\ldots,p$. We then have

$$P_B = \oint P_{t_1t_2} P_{t_{1|j}t_{2|j}} g(t_1,t_2,t_{1|j},t_{2|j})\, d(t_1,t_2,t_{1|j},t_{2|j}),$$

where $g(t_1,t_2,t_{1|j},t_{2|j})$ is the PDF of $(T_1,T_2,T_{1|j},T_{2|j})'$ given in (17), $P_{t_1t_2} = P\left(|T|_{(p-2)} > (|t_1| \vee |t_2|) = 1 - (1 - 2\Phi(-|t_1| \vee |t_2|))\right)^{p-2}$,

$$P_{t_{1|j},t_{2|j}} = P\left(\left(t^2_{1|j} \vee t^2_{2|j}\right) \ge F_{S_j,[R]}\right)$$

$$= G\left(t^2_{1|j} \vee t^2_{2|j}\right)^r \sum_{l=0}^{p-3-r} \binom{r+l-1}{l} \left[1 - G\left(\left(t^2_{1|j} \vee t^2_{2|j}\right)\right)\right]^l,$$

in which $r=p-3-R+1$, and $G(\bullet)$ is the CDF of $F_{k|j}$, $3 \le j < k \le p$, given in (19). We can approximate $F_{S_j,[R]}$ through the quantile function $G^{-1}\left(1 - \frac{R-0.5}{p-3}\right)$ to simplify the calculation of integration.

Calculating Post-Hoc Power with a Given Marginal Model

To demonstrate how to evaluate the power of model selection methods in the empirical analysis, we have applied our approach in a real study example. In this example, the simple regression model on X_1, $\hat{Y}_{i(1)} = \hat{\beta}_{0(1)} + \hat{\beta}_{1(1)} X_{i1}$, is an estimate of marginal model $E(Y_i|X_{i1}) = b_0 + b_2 EX_{i2} + (b_1 + b_3 EX_{i2}) X_{i1}$, based on the full model (2). So the estimator of main effect is $\hat{b}_1 = \hat{\beta}_{1(1)} - b_3 EX_{i2} = \hat{\beta}_{1(1)} - b_3(p_2 - q_2)$. Similarly $\hat{b}_1 = \hat{\beta}_{1(1)} - b_3(p_1 - q_1)$, where $\hat{\beta}_{1(2)}$ is given in the simple regression model on X_2. To estimate the variance of random error, note that $\sigma^2 = Var(Y_i) - Var(b_0 + b_1 X_{i1} + b_2 X_{i2} + b_3 X_{i1} X_{i2})$.

Therefore,

$$\hat{\sigma}^2 = sd(Y)^2 - 2b_1^2 p_1 q_1 - 2b_2^2 p_2 q_2 - 4b_1 b_3 (p_2 - q_2) p_1 q_1 - 4b_2 b_3 (p_1 - q_1) p_2 q_2 - \left[(p_1^2 + q_1^2)(p_2^2 + q_2^2) - (p_1 - q_1)^2 \right] b_3^2$$

With an assumed value of b_3 and the corresponding estimators $\hat{b}_1$, $\hat{b}_2$, and $\hat{\sigma}^2$, we can apply the above calculation to obtain the power of model selection strategies.

ACKNOWLEDGMENTS

We are grateful to Yale University Biomedical High Performance Computing Center for computation support. We thank Dr. Joshua Sampson and Dr. Yedan Zhang for their comments on the paper.

REFERENCES

1. Fan J, Lv J (2008) Sure independence screening for ultra-high dimensional feature space. J R Statist Soc B 70: 849–911.
2. Storey JD, Akey JM, Kruglyak L (2005) Multiple locus linkage analysis of genomewide expression in yeast. PLoS Biolgoy 3(8): 1380–1390. doi:10.1371/journal.pbio.0030267.
3. Brem RB, Storey JD, Whittle J, Kruglyak L (2005) Genetic interactions between polymorphisms that affect gene expression in yeast. Nature 436(7051): 701–703.
4. Marchini J, Donnelly P, Cardon LR (2005) Genome-wide strategies for detecting multiple loci that influence complex diseases. Nat Genet 37(4): 413–417.
5. Evans DM, Marchini J, Morris AP, Cardon LR (2006) Two-stage two-locus models in genome-wide association. PLoS Genet 2(9): e157. doi:10.1371/journal.pgen.0020157.
6. Kutner MH, Nachtsheim CJ, Li W, Neter J (2005) Applied linear statistical models. 5th ed. New York: McGraw-Hill Irwin.
7. Gail MH, Pfeiffer RM, Wheeler W, Pee D (2008) Probability of detecting disease-associated single nucleotide polymorphisms in case-control genome-wide association studies. Biostatistics 9(2): 201.
8. Weedon MN, et al. (2008) Genome-wide association analysis identifies 20 loci that influence adult height. Nat Genet 40: 575–583.
9. Cohen J (1988) Statistical power analysis for the behavioral sciences. Hillsdale, , NJ: Lawrence Erlbaum Association.
10. Benjamini Y, Hochberg Y (1995) Controlling the false discovery rate: A practical and powerful approach to multiple testing. J R Statist Soc B 57: 289–300.
11. Scheffé H (1959) The analysis of variance. New York: John Wiley & Sons Inc.
12. Searle SR (1971) Linear models. New York: John Wiley & Sons Inc.
13. Ambrosius WT, Lange EM, Langefeld CD (2004) Power for genetic association studies with random allele frequencies and genotype distributions. Am J Hum Genet 74(4): 683–693.
14. Efron B (2004) Large-scale simultaneous hypothesis testing: The choice of a null hypothesis. J Am Stat Assoc 99(465): 96–104.
15. Efron B (2007) Correlation and large-scale simultaneous significance testing. J Am Stat Assoc 102(477): 93–103.
16. Gibbs RA, Belmont JW, Hardenbol P, Willis TD, Yu F, et al. (2003) The international HapMap project. Nature 426(6968): 789–796.
17. Ke X, Cardon LR (2003) Efficient selective screening of haplotype tag SNPs. Bioinformatics 19(2): 287–288.
18. Weale ME, Depondt C, Macdonald SJ, Smith A, Lai PS, et al. (2003) Selection and evaluation of tagging SNPs in the neuronal-sodium-channel gene SCN1A: Implications for linkage-disequilibrium gene mapping. Am J Hum Genet 73(3): 551–565.
19. Lehmann EL, Casella G (1998) Theory of point estimation, Second Edition. New York: Springer Verlag.
20. David HA, Nagaraja HN (2003) Order statistics, Third Edition. New York: J. Wiley.

CHAPTER 2 POPULATION STRUCTURE AND EIGENANALYSIS

Nick Patterson, Alkes L. Price, and David Reich

SYNOPSIS

When analyzing genetic data, one often wishes to determine if the samples are from a population that has structure. Can the samples be regarded as randomly chosen from a homogeneous population, or does the data imply that the population is not genetically homogeneous? Patterson, Price, and Reich show that an old method (principal components) together with modern statistics (Tracy–Widom theory) can be combined to yield a fast and effective answer to this question. The technique is simple and practical on the largest datasets, and can be applied both to genetic markers that are biallelic and to markers that are highly polymorphic such as microsatellites. The theory also allows the authors to estimate the data size needed to detect structure if their samples are in fact from two populations that have a given, but small level of differentiation.

INTRODUCTION

A central challenge in analyzing any genetic dataset is to explore whether there is any evidence that the samples in the data are from a population that is structured. Are the individuals from a homogeneous population or from a population containing subgroups that are genetically distinct? Can we find evidence for substructure in the data, and quantify it? This question of detecting and quantifying structure arises in medical genetics, for instance, in case-control studies where uncorrected population structure can induce false positives [1]. It also arises in population genetics, where understanding of the structure may be important to the key scientific issues, especially uncovering the demographic history of the population under study.

We focus on principal components analysis (PCA), which was first introduced to the study of genetic data almost thirty years ago by Cavalli-Sforza [2].

We will use PCA and "eigenanalysis" interchangeably. The latter term focuses attention on the fact that not just the eigenvectors (principal components) are important here, but also the eigenvalues, which underlie our statistical procedures.

PCA has become a standard tool in genetics. In population genetics, we recommend a review paper [3] focusing on the use of "synthetic maps" which use PCA to study genetic geographic variation.

Usually PCA been applied to data at a population level, not to individuals as we do here. Exceptions are [4,5].

In addition to single nucleotide polymorphisms (SNPs) and microsatellites, PCA has been applied to haplotype frequencies [6,7] and the distribution of ALU insertion polymorphisms [8] in order to study population structure. Most of the literature on PCA in genetics is applied, not methodological, and we know of no paper that concentrates as we do here on the statistical significance of the components. Data with hundreds or thousands of individuals and hundreds of thousands of markers are now becoming available, so that small but real effects will be detectable, and it is important to develop rigorous tests for population structure that will be practical, even on the largest datasets. This is our main aim in this paper.

Using some recent results in theoretical statistics, we introduce a formal test statistic for population structure. We

Citation: Patterson N, Price AL, Reich D (2006) Population Structure and Eigenanalysis. PLoS Genet 2(12): e190. doi:10.1371/journal.pgen.0020190

also discuss testing for additional structure after some structure has been found. Finally, we are able to estimate the degree of population differentiation that will be detectable for a given data size.

Our methods work in a broad range of contexts, and can be modified to work with markers in linkage disequilibrium (LD). The methods are also able to find structure in admixed populations such as African Americans—that is, in which individuals inherit ancestry from multiple ancestral populations—as long as the individuals being studied have different proportional contributions from the ancestral populations.

We believe that principal components methods largely fell out of favor with the introduction of the sophisticated cluster-based program STRUCTURE [9,10]. STRUCTURE and similar methods are based on an interpretable population genetics model, whereas principal components seems like a "black box" method. We will discuss how the models underlying the cluster methods, and the PCA technique we will describe, are much closer to each other than they may at first appear to be.

Our implementation of PCA has three major features. 1) It runs extremely quickly on large datasets (within a few hours on datasets with hundreds of thousands of markers and thousands of samples), whereas methods such as STRUCTURE can be impractical. This makes it possible to extract the powerful information about population structure that we will show is present in large datasets. 2) Our PCA framework provides the first formal tests for the presence of population structure in genetic data. 3) The PCA method does not attempt to classify all individuals into discrete populations or linear combinations of populations, which may not always be the correct model for population history. Instead, PCA outputs each individual›s coordinates along axes of variation. An algorithm could in principle be used as a post-processing step to cluster individuals based on their coordinates along these axes, but we have not implemented this.

We note that STRUCTURE is a complex program and has numerous options that add power and flexibility, many of which we cannot match with a PCA approach. Perhaps the central goal of STRUCTURE is to classify individuals into discrete populations, but this is not an object of our method. We think that in the future both cluster-based methods such as STRUCTURE and our PCA methods will have a role in discovering population structure on genetic data, so that, for example, our PCA methods offer a good default for the number of clusters to use in STRUCTURE. In complex situations, such as uncovering structure in populations where all individuals are equal mixtures of ancestral populations, it may remain necessary to use statistical software that explicitly models admixture LD, such as [10–13], which allow estimation of local ancestry at arbitrary points of the genome.

In this study we aim to place PCA as applied to genetic data on a solid statistical footing. We develop a technique to test whether eigenvectors from the analysis are reflecting real structure in the data or are more probably merely noise. Other papers will explore applications to medical genetics [14] and to the uncovering of demographic history. In this paper, our main purpose is to describe and to validate the method, rather than to make novel inferences based on application to real data, which we leave to future work. We show that statistically significant structure is real and interpretable, and also that our methods are not failing to recover real structure that is found by other techniques.

Two important results emerge from this study. First, we show that application of PCA to genetic data is statistically appropriate, and provide a formal set of statistical tests for population structure. Second, we describe a "phase change" phenomenon about the ability to detect structure that emerges from our analysis: for a fixed dataset size, divergence between two populations (as measured, for example, by a statistic like F_{ST}) that is below a threshold is essentially undetectable, but a little above threshold detection will be easy. Based on these results, we are able to give an estimate of how much data will be required to find population structure given a level of genetic divergence such as F_{ST} (as defined by Cavalli-Sforza, [15, p. 26, Equation 3].)

The theory shows that the methods are sensitive, so that on large datasets, population structure will often be detectable. Moreover, the novel result on the phase change is not limited just to PCA, but turns out to reflect a deep property about the ability to discover structure in genetic data. For example, in the paper we present simulations that show the ability to detect structure occurs with the same dataset size when STRUCTURE and PCA are used; that is, the phase change manifests itself in the same place.

The phase change effect was suggested by a recent paper in theoretical statistics [16], which demonstrated the phenomenon for a situation that is mathematically similar to ours. The theory has continued to develop and nearly all we need has now been proved, the most recent paper being [17]. We believe that the applications to genetics still pose some interesting questions for the theorists. While our methods are derived from asymptotic theory (where the datasets are very large), they also seem to work well on small datasets, and we would be interested in seeing a theoretical explanation.

RESULTS

The basic technique is simple. We assume our markers are biallelic, for example, biallelic single nucleotide polymorphisms (SNPs). Regard the data as a large rectangular matrix C, with rows indexed by individuals, and columns indexed by polymorphic markers. For each marker choose a reference and variant allele. We suppose we have n such markers and m individuals. LetC(i,j) be the number of variant alleles for marker j, individual i. (Thus for autosomal data we have C(i,j) is 0,1 or 2.) For now suppose that there is no missing data. From each column we subtract the column means. So set for column j:

$$\mu(j) = \frac{\sum_{i=1}^{m} C(i,j)}{m} \tag{1}$$

and then the corrected entries are:

$$C(i,j) - \mu(j) \tag{2}$$

Set p(j) = μ(j)/2, an estimate of the underlying allele frequency (autosomal data). Then each entry in the resulting matrix is

$$M(i,j) = \frac{C(i,j) - \mu(j)}{\sqrt{p(j)(1 - p(j))}} \quad (3)$$

Equation 3 is a normalization step, which is motivated by the fact that the frequency change of a SNP due to genetic drift occurs at a rate proportional to $\sqrt{p(j)(1 - p(j))}$ per generation. It also normalizes (at least if the data is in Hardy-Weinberg equilibrium) each data column to have the same variance. We note that Nicholson et al. use the same normalization, and motivate it similarly [18].

We verified (unpublished data) that the normalization improves results when using simulated genetic data, and that on real data known structure becomes clearer. (However all the results are just as mathematically valid even without the normalizations.)

The methods also are applicable to data such as microsatellites, where there are more than two alleles at a single site. We use a device of Cavalli-Sforza [2,15], making a "marker" j out of each allele, and then setting C(i,j) to be the number of occurrences of the allele for sample i. We omit the normalization step of Equation 3 for microsatellites, merely subtracting the mean. The normalization has no clear justification for microsatellite data, and results on real data (unpublished) show that it produces worse performance in this case.

An alternative, suggested by a referee, is to use the microsatellite allele length as a continuous variable, and carry out PCA directly after a suitable normalization.

Now we carry out a singular value decomposition on the matrix M. (A standard reference for the numerical methods is [19]. Public domain software is readily available—we used the well-known package LAPACK, http://www.netlib.org/lapack.) We are chiefly interested here in the case that the number of samples is less than the number of markers: m < n. Computationally we will form $X = \frac{1}{n}MM'$ the sample covariance of the columns of M. The resulting matrix is m × m, with a dimension equal to the number of samples in the dataset. We then compute an eigenvector decomposition of X. Eigenvectors corresponding to "large" eigenvalues are exposing nonrandom population structure. This means that a central issue for this paper is what is "large" here, or, more precisely, what is the distribution of the largest eigenvalues of X at random (when there is no population structure)?

The method is fast. In practice, the running time is dominated by the calculation of the matrix product MM′, which for extremely large problems is readily computed on a parallel architecture. On a fast workstation, the matrix product for a dataset of 100 individuals and 100,000 markers takes just four seconds. For data with m individuals and n markers, the work is proportional tom^2n, and thus for a set of 2,000 individuals and 500,000 markers would take about 2.5 hours on the same single processor (see Methods for more details). For many of the problems we have analyzed, reading and storing the data takes longer than the analysis.

Most, though not all, previous applications of PCA to analysis of population structure have taken the data to be a matrix where the rows are indexed by populations not by individuals (e.g., [2,15]). We prefer to consider the larger array where the rows are indexed by individuals. Even when we have population labels, it is useful to examine within-population variation, and we also are often able to find outliers in the data. Furthermore, when population labels are available, we can carry out an analysis to check that the labels do correspond to structure that the eigenanalysis has uncovered.

We note that population labels may be socially constructed. This makes us nervous about employing them in an initial data study. On the other hand, the individual samples certainly do not have any such construct, and even if population labels are available, initial analysis at an individual level allows us to check the meaningfulness of the labels [20].

Cavalli-Sforza [15, pp. 39–42] gives an explanation of why PCA can be expected to reveal population structure. We give a different explanation, oriented towards analysis at the individual level. If $\mathbf{e}^{[1]}$ is the principal eigenvector of the matrix X, this means that the sum of squares

$$S = \sum_k \left(\sum_j \mathrm{e}_j^{[1]} M_{jk} \right)^2 \quad (4)$$

is maximized over all vectors with constant norm. The second eigenvector $\mathbf{e}^{[2]}$ maximizes the same expression with the constraint that $\mathbf{e}^{[1]}$, $\mathbf{e}^{[2]}$ are orthogonal, and so on. Why would we expect this to reveal population structure? Suppose that in our sample, we have just two populations and that each is homogeneous. Choose a vector with coordinates constant and positive for samples from one population, and coordinates constant and negative for samples from the other. Arrange so that the vector coordinates sum to zero. Then, since alleles within a population will tend to agree more than in the sample as a whole, the quantity S of Equation 4will tend to be large. This is exactly what we maximize as a function of the vector **e**. More generally, if we have K distinct populations, there are K − 1 vectors constant on each population, summing to zero and linearly independent. This implies that, if the number of markers is sufficiently large, there will be K − 1 eigenvalues and K − 1 corresponding eigenvectors of our matrix that are significant and meaningful. Vectors orthogonal to these K − 1 vectors are showing within-population variance, and if each population is homogeneous, this is just reflecting sampling noise.

Tracy–Widom Theory

We now turn to some recent theoretical statistics. Consider an m × n matrix M, each entry of which has an independent standard normal random variable. We are interested in the case that m < n.

(A notational issue is that in our genetic data, if m is the number of individuals, then the square matrix for which we calculate eigenvalues has rank m − 1 [we lose a dimension by forcing each column to sum to zero]. We will, for the majority of the paper, write m′ = m − 1 for the number of nonzero eigenvalues. However in this theoretical section, we will assume there are m nonzero eigenvalues.) Let $X = \frac{1}{n}MM'$ X is a W is hart matrix. Let $\{\lambda_i\}_{1 \le i \le m}$ be the eigenvalues of X. The probability density of $(\lambda_1, \ldots \lambda_m)$ is known [21] but not directly relevant to our work here, so we omit the details.

Order the eigenvalues so that $\lambda_1 > \lambda_2 \ldots > \lambda_m$ Johnstone in a key paper [22] showed that suitably normalized, and for m, n, large, the distribution of the largest eigenvalue λ_1 is approximately a distribution discovered by Tracy and Widom [23], which in this paper we call TW. Set

$$\mu(m,n) = \frac{(\sqrt{n-1}+\sqrt{m})^2}{n} \tag{5}$$

$$\sigma(m,n) = \frac{(\sqrt{n-1}+\sqrt{m})}{n}\left(\frac{1}{\sqrt{n-1}}+\frac{1}{\sqrt{m}}\right)^{1/3} \tag{6}$$

Now set

$$x = \frac{\lambda_1 - \mu(m,n)}{\sigma(m,n)} \tag{7}$$

Then the distribution of x is approximately TW.

More precisely, if as m,n $\rightarrow \infty$, n/m $\rightarrow \gamma \geq 1$, then Johnstone proves [22, Theorem 1.1] that xtends to TW in distribution. As we show later (Theorem 2), Johnstone's theorem also holds if in the expression for x in Equation 7, we replace x by:

$$x = \frac{L_1 - \mu(m,n)}{\sigma(m,n)} \tag{8}$$

where

$$L_1 = \frac{m\lambda_1}{\sum_{i=1}^{m}\lambda_i} \tag{9}$$

The only difference here is that the m eigenvalues have been normalized to have sum m.

In [22] Johnstone proved his theorem for the case that n,m $\rightarrow \infty$ with m/n bounded away from 0, but this condition was shown in [23] not to be necessary. Johnstone [22] gives convincing evidence that the fit is good even for values as small as m = 5, n = 20.

We show in Figure 1 a plot of the Tracy–Widom density.

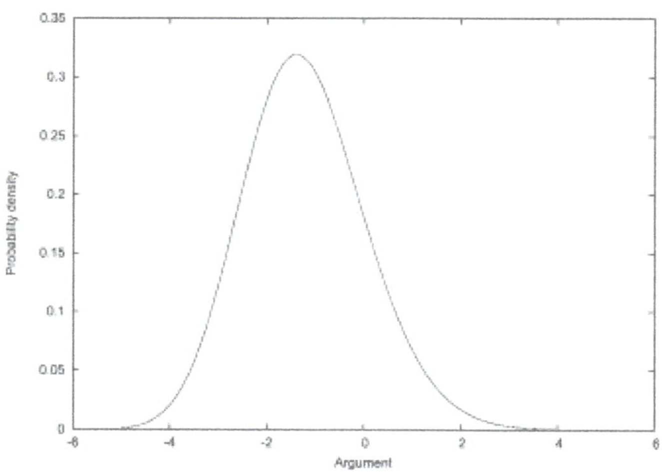

Figure 1: The Tracy–Widom Density Conventional percentile points are: P = 0.05, x = .9794; P = 0.01, x = 2.0236; P = 0.001,x = 3.2730.

The complexity of the TW definition is irrelevant to its application to real data. One computes a statistic, and then looks up a p-value in tables or through a computational interface. This is little different from how one uses (say) a conventional chi-squared test.

One concern with applying this approach to genetic data is that the entries in the matrix M do not have the Gaussian distributions expected for a Wishart matrix; instead, they correspond to the three possible genotypes at each SNP. However it is not critical that the entries in the m × nmatrix M be Gaussian. Soshnikov [25] showed that the same TW limit arose if the cell entries were any distribution with high-order moments no greater than the Gaussian. The matrix X is a sum of n rank 1 matrices, and Soshnikov›s result suggests that the same limit would be obtained from any probability distribution in which the columns of M are independent, isotropic (all directions are equiprobable), and such that the column norms have moments no larger than those for a column of independent Gaussian entries. In all our genetic applications, the column norms are in fact bounded, so we can expect the sample covariance matrices to behave well.

This theory, originally developed for the case of Gaussian matrix entries, thus seemed likely to work well with large genetic biallelic data arrays. The remainder of this paper verifies that this is the case.

Applying Eigenanalysis to Datasets with Linked Markers

For genetic applications we cannot necessarily assume that all our markers are unlinked and thus independent. For instance, in the International Haplotype Map project [26], markers were chosen about 5,000 bases apart (phase 1), or about 1,000 bases apart (phase 2), and so nearby markers will often be in LD. Mathematically this will induce correlation between nearby columns of our matrix M. The effect of this will be that the matrix$X = MM'$should be "Wishart-like," but the nonindependence of the columns will reduce the effective sample size. We will discuss this further (see Correcting for LD) but now introduce a new idea. This adds robustness to our methods, so that minor deviations from the model become of lesser importance.

Suppose we have m individuals. We will analyze X = MM′ as a Wishart matrix. The rank of X will be m − 1 (assuming we have many SNPs compared with m). We will think of the eigenvalues of X as coming from a (m − 1) × (m − 1) W is hart, and write m′ = m − 1.

There are two unknowns that we can regard as parameters to the Wishart: 1) σ^2: the variance of the normal distribution used for the cells of the rectangular matrix M; 2) n′: The number of columns of M.

We want to carefully distinguish here between n, the actual number of columns of our data array, and n′, a theoretical statistical parameter, modeling the approximate Wishart distribution of the square matrix X. We originally fit σ,n′ by maximum likelihood. The likelihood, as a function of the two parameters, has two sufficient statistics, which are $\sum_i \lambda_i$, and $\sum_i \log \lambda_i$. Maximum likelihood did not always work well, in our genetic applications, probably because $\sum_i \log \lambda_i$ is sensitive to small eigenvalues, while we are only interested in large. We recommend a moments estimator:

$$n' = \frac{(m+1)\left(\sum_i \lambda_i\right)^2}{\left((m-1)\sum_i \lambda_i^2\right) - \left(\sum_i \lambda_i\right)^2} \qquad (10)$$

which is justified later. Note that n′ is invariant to scaling of the matrix M as it should be. We estimate σ by:

$$\hat{\sigma}^2 = \frac{\sum_i \lambda_i}{(m-1)n'}$$

A Test for Population Structure

This leads immediately to a formal test for the presence of population structure in a biallelic dataset.

1. Compute the matrix M as in Equations 1, 2 and 3. M has m rows, n columns.
2. Compute X = MM′. X is m × m.
3. Order the eigenvalues of X so that $\lambda_1 > \lambda_2 ... > \lambda_{m'} > 0$ where m′ = m − 1. (On a large dataset X will always have rank m′.)
4. Using the eigenvalues λ_i ($1 \le i \le m'$), estimate n′ from Equation 10.
5. The largest eigenvalue of M is λ_1. Set
$$l = \frac{(m')\lambda_1}{\sum_{i=1}^{m'} \lambda_i}$$
6. Normalize l with Equations 5–7, where the effective number of markers n′ replaces n. This yields a test statistic x = x(M).

Our statistic x(M) is approximately TW-distributed. A p-value can now be computed from tables of the TW distribution. Notice that our statistic is independent of the scaling of the λ_i, and it is convenient to normalize by scaling so that the sum of the eigenvalues (that is the trace of M) ism′. All eigenvalues we report are scaled in this manner.

Simulations to Demonstrate Robustness of the Tests of Significant Structure

We first made a series of simulations in the absence of population structure. (Some additional details are in the Methods section.) Our first set of runs had 100 individuals and 5,000 unlinked SNPs, and the second 200 individuals and 50,000 unlinked SNPs. In each case we ran 1,000 simulations and show in Figure 2A and 2B probability–probability (P–P) plots of the empirical and TW tail areas. The results seem entirely satisfactory, especially for low p-values in the top right of Figures 2A and 2B. For assessment of statistical significance, it is the low p-value range that is relevant. The simulations show more generally that the TW theory is relevant in a genetic context, that the normalizations of Equations 5–7 are appropriate, and that the calculation of the effective marker size has not seriously distorted the TW statistic.

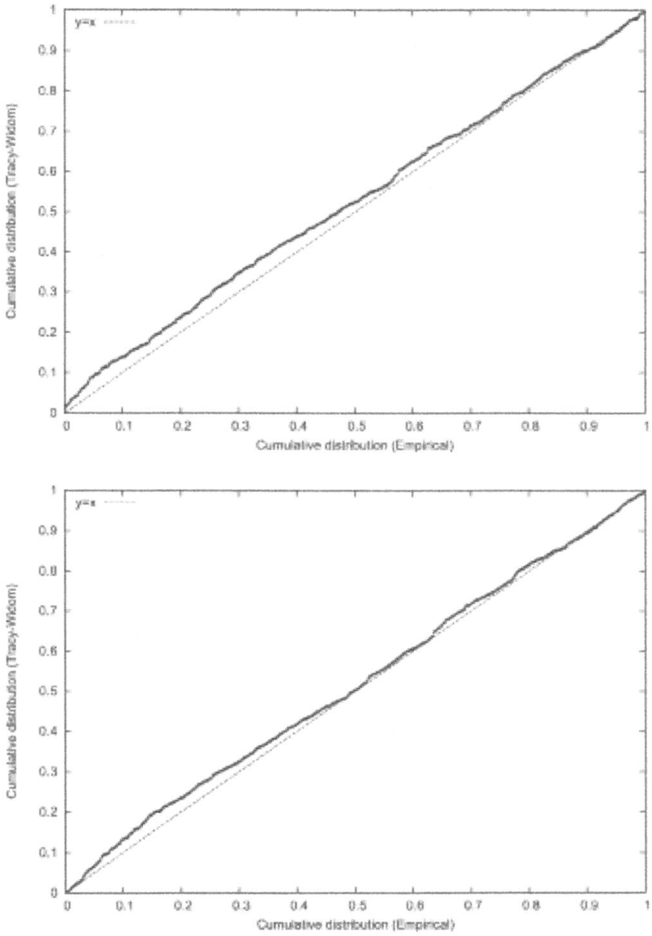

Figure 2: Testing the Fit of the TW Distribution (A) We carried out 1,000 simulations of a panmictic population, where we have a sample size of m = 100 and n = 5,000 unlinked markers. We give a P–P plot of the TW statistic against the theoretical distribution; this shows the empirical cumulative distribution against the theoretical cumulative distribution for a given quantile. If the fit is good, we expect the plot will lie along the line y = x. Interest is primarily at the top right, corresponding to low p-values. (B) P–P plot corresponding to a sample size of m = 200 and n = 50,000 markers. The fit is again excellent, demonstrating the appropriateness of the Johnstone normalization.

Detecting Additional Structure

It is very important to be able to answer the question: Does the data show evidence of additional population structure over and above what has already been detected? The test we propose is extremely simple. If our matrix X has eigenvalues $\lambda_1, \lambda_2, ..., \lambda_k, \lambda_{k+1}, ... \lambda_{m'}$ and we already have declared the top k eigenvalues to be significant, then we simply test $\lambda_{k+1}, ... \lambda_m$ as though X was a (m′ − k) × (m′ − k) Wishart matrix. Johnstone shows [22, Proposition 1.2] that this procedure is conservative, at least for a true Wishart matrix. We tested this by generating data in which there is one eigenvalue that is overwhelmingly significant, and examined the distribution of the second eigenvalue. As shown by the P–P plot of Figure 3, the fit is again very good, especially for small p-values. If an eigenvalue is not significant, then further testing of smaller eigenvalues should not be done.

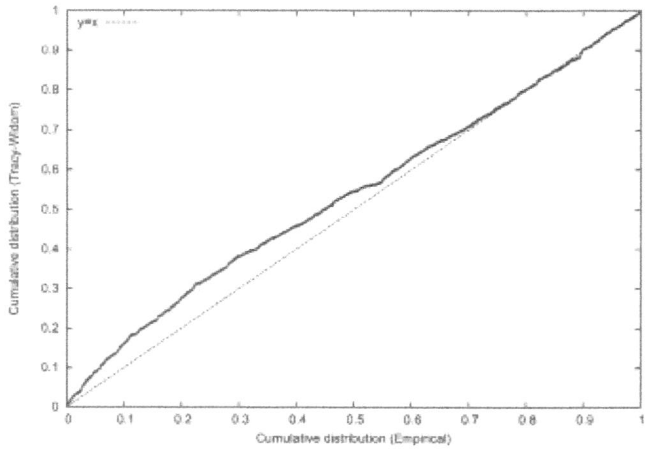

Figure 3: Testing the Fit of the Second Eigenvalue We generated genotype data in which the leading eigenvalue is overwhelmingly significant (F_{ST} = .01, m = 100, n = 5,000) with two equal-sized subpopulations. We show P–P plots for the TW statistic computed from the second eigenvalue. The fit at the high end is excellent.

Cluster Analysis and PCA

There is a much closer relationship between our PCA and a cluster-based analysis than is at first apparent. Consider a model of genetic structure where there are K populations, and fix a marker and variant allele. The populations have diverged from an ancestral population recently. Suppose that the allele frequency of the variant in the ancestral population is P, and in population i is p_i. Conditional on P, assume that $\mathbf{p} = (p_1,p_2,\ldots p_K)$ has mean (P,P,…P) and covariance matrix P(1 − P)B for some matrix B. Much past work in genetics uses this paradigm, with variations on the distribution of B, and on the detailed distribution of **p** conditional on P; for instance, both Nicholson et al. [18] and STRUCTURE [9] in "correlated frequency mode," and in the "F-model" of [10]. The setup here is nearly inevitable if one is considering allele frequencies in populations that have only diverged a small amount. In [18, p. 700] for the case of a diagonal matrix B, it is shown that the diagonal term B_{ii} can be interpreted as the "time on the diffusion timescale" (inversely proportional to effective population size) in which population i has undergone genetic drift.

Suppose we sample (autosomal) genotypes from these K populations. Assume there are M_i samples from population i, and set $M = \sum_{i=1}^{K} M_i$ We suppose that the divergence of each population from a root population, as measured byF_{ST} or equivalently by divergence time on the diffusion timescale, is of order τ, which is small. What are the eigenvalues of the theoretical covariance C of the samples for the marker after our mean adjustment and normalization? Let M become large, while the relative abundance of the samples stays constant across populations. It can be shown (see the mathematical details, Theorem 3) that if B has full rank, then C has K − 1 large eigenvalues that tend to infinity withM, M − K eigenvalues that are 1 + O(τ) and one zero eigenvalue that is a structural zero, arising from the fact that our mean adjusted columns all have zero sum. We are interested in the case that $\tau \ll 1$ while $M \gg 1$.

Thus, natural models of population structure predict that most of the eigenvalues of the theoretical covariance will be "small," nearly equal, and arise from sampling noise, while just a few eigenvalues will be "large," reflecting past demographic events. This is exactly the situation that Johnstone's application of Tracy–Widom theory addresses. We also note that on real data (as we show below), the TW theory works extremely well, which shows that the model will be a reasonable approximation to "truth" in many cases.

Axes of Variation

Thus, we expect that the theoretical covariance matrix (approximated by the sample covariance) will have K − 1 "large" eigenvalues, with the remainder small and reflecting the sampling variance. We call the eigenvectors of the theoretical covariance, corresponding to the large eigenvalues, "axes of variation." These are a theoretical construct, as of course we only observe the sample covariance. Nevertheless, for eigenvectors that are highly significant by our tests, we expect the corresponding eigenvector to correlate well with the true "axis of variation." An analogy here is that we would often think of an allele as having a "true" population frequency in a population, and would regard the frequency of the allele in a sample as an estimator of the true frequency.

As defined, our axes of variation do depend on the relative sample sizes of the underlying populations, so that differences between populations each with a large sample size are upweighted. This is worth remembering when interpreting the results, but does not seem a major impediment to analysis.

A Formal Test Is Appropriate in Our Applications

We do not review in detail older methods for testing for significance. One technique is the "broken stick" model [27,28], used, for instance, in a recent population genetics analysis [5]. In this model, one normalizes the m′ nonzero eigenvalues to sum to 1, then sorts them in decreasing order, and compares the k-th eigenvalue with the expected size of the k-th largest subinterval of the unit interval, partitioned by "breaking" the interval at m′ − 1 uniformly chosen points. This method does not use the number of markers in any way, thus it cannot be making optimum use of the data. In particular for datasets with large numbers of markers, real population structure may go undetected.

We believe that the application of PCA to genetic data—and our way of analyzing the data—provides a natural method of uncovering population structure, for reasons that are subtle; thus, it is useful to spell them out explicitly. In most applications of PCA, the multivariate data has an unknown covariance, and PCA is attempting to choose a subspace on which to project the data that captures most of the relevant information. In many such applications, a formal test for whether the true covariance is the identity matrix makes little sense.

In genetics applications we believe the situation is different. Under standard population genetics assumptions such as a panmictic population, the natural null is that the eigenvalues of the true covariance matrix are equal, a formal test is appropriate, and deviations from the null are likely to be of real scientific and practical significance. To support this, in our experience on real data we take our null very seriously and attempt to explain all statistically significant axes of variation.

Often the explanation is true population structure in the data, but we also often expose errors or difficulties in the data processing. Two examples follow.

In some population genetic data from African populations, the fourth axis of variation showed some San individuals at each end of the axis. This made little genetic sense, and the cause was some related samples that should have been removed from the analysis.

In a medical genetic study, an unexplained axis of variation was statistically correlated with the micro-titer plates on which the genotyping had been carried out. This suggested that the experimental setup was contributing to the evidence for structure, instead of real population differentiation.

In both these cases more careful data preprocessing would have eliminated the problem, but analysis and preparation of large datasets is difficult, and more tools for analysis and error-detection are always of benefit.

ANOVA Statistics Given Labeled Populations

In many practical applications, samples will already be grouped into subpopulations (for instance, in medical genetics there are often two populations: cases and controls). It is natural to want to test if our recovered eigenvectors reflect differences among the labeled subpopulations. We therefore fix some eigenvector, and can regard each individual as associated with the corresponding coordinate of the eigenvector. We want to test if the means of these coordinate values in each subpopulation differ significantly. Our motivation is firstly that this is a powerful check on the validity of our (unsupervised) Tracy–Widom statistics, and secondly that the supervised analysis helps in interpretation of the recovered axes of variation.

The conventional statistic here is an ANOVA F-statistic. (See for instance [29]). We have here a "one-way layout," where we want to test if the group means significantly differ. This amounts to a check on our Tracy–Widom statistic, which we compute ignoring the labels. We also routinely compute an F-statistic for every pair of populations, and each eigenvector (unpublished data). We give three examples of ANOVA analysis on real data. In the first, we look at population data from sub-Saharan Africa, genotyped with 783 microsatellites and 210 biallelic indels in the CEPH–HGDP dataset [30,31]. We group the West African and Bantu speaking populations (Yoruba, Bantu South Africa, and Bantu Kenya) as "Bantu" and also examine samples from San and Mandenka. We show plots of the first two eigenvectors in Figure 4. Table 1 shows the key statistics for this dataset. In Table 1, the ANOVA p-value is obtained from the usual F-statistic, and we apply ANOVA to each of the first three eigenvectors.

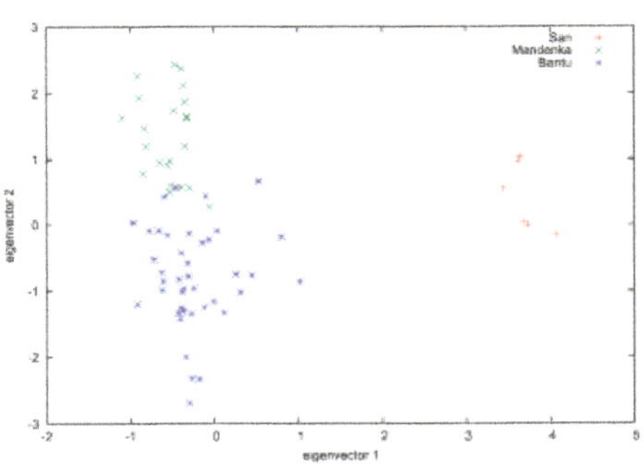

Figure 4: Three African Populations Plots of the first two eigenvectors for some African populations in the CEPH–HGDP dataset [30]. Yoruba and Bantu-speaking populations are genetically quite close and were grouped together. The Mandenka are a West African group speaking a language in the Mande family [15, p. 182]. The eigenanalysis fails to find structure in the Bantu populations, but separation between the Bantu and Mandenka with the second eigenvector is apparent.

Table 1: Statistics from HGDP African Data

Number	Eigenvalue	TW Statistic	TW *p*-Value	ANOVA *p*-Value
1	2.07	46.2	$<10^{-12}$	$<10^{-12}$
2	1.40	6.717	3.08×10^{-7}	$<10^{-12}$
3	1.31	0.380	.108	.74

doi:10.1371/journal.pgen.0020190.t001

There is excellent agreement between the supervised and unsupervised analysis. The lack of significance of the third eigenvector is an indication that no additional structure was apparent within the Bantu.

Our second study took samples from three regions: Northern Thailand, China (Han Chinese), and Japan. The last two population samples were available from the International Hapmap Project [32]. The Thai samples (25 individuals after removing some close relatives and outliers) were collected by J. Seidman and S. Sangwatanaroj as part of a disease study, though here we focus on the population genetics. Our analysis of these data used 40,560 SNPs.

In Figure 5 we plot the first two eigenvectors. Notice that the population separation is clear, but that the natural separation axes are not the eigenvectors. Further, the Thai and Chinese populations appear to show a cline, rather than two discrete clusters grouped around a central point. We suspect that this shows some evidence of genetic admixture, perhaps involving a population in Thailand that is related to the Chinese. (See also Figure 8, which we describe later.) Table 2 shows the eigenvalues, the TW significance, and an ANOVA p-value for the first three eigenvectors. Again there is excellent agreement between the supervised and unsupervised analyses.

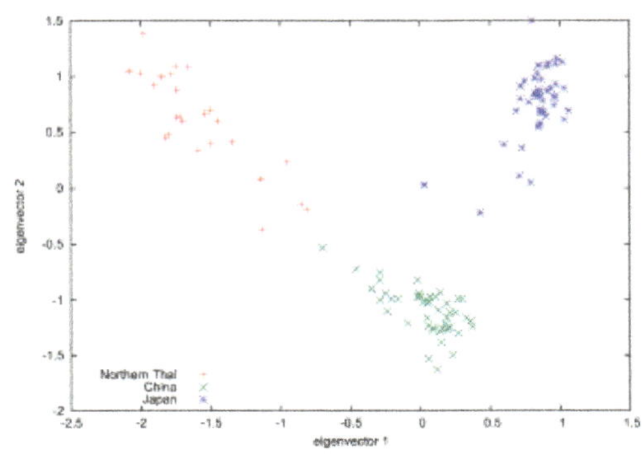

Figure 5: Three East Asian Populations Plots of the first two eigenvectors for a population from Thailand and Chinese and Japanese populations from the International Haplotype Map [32]. The Japanese population is clearly distinguished (though not by either eigenvector separately). The large dispersal of the Thai population, along a line where the Chinese are at an extreme, suggests some gene flow of a Chinese-related population into Thailand. Note the similarity to the simulated data of Figure 8.

Table 2: Statistics from Thai/Chinese/Japanese Data

Number	Eigenvalue	TW Statistic	TW *p*-Value	ANOVA *p*-Value
1	2.21	92.34	$<10^{-12}$	$<10^{-12}$
2	1.47	31.15	$<10^{-12}$	$<10^{-12}$
3	1.23	−1.61	.61	.97

doi:10.1371/journal.pgen.0020190.t002

In the third dataset, which was created and analyzed by Mark Shriver and colleagues [5], we have data from 12 populations. The missing data pattern showed some evidence of population structure, with the missing data concentrated in particular samples, populations, and SNPs. For this reason, we only used markers for analysis for which there was no missing data, and we corrected for LD using our regression technique (see below). The details of the data preprocessing steps are described in Methods. We analyzed samples from 189 individuals on 2,790 SNPs. On this dataset, we find the leading eigenvalue statistics to be as shown in Table 3.

Table 3: Statistics from Shriver Dataset

Number	Eigenvalue	TW Statistic	TW *p*-Value	ANOVA *p*-Value
1	22.36	76.091	$<10^{-12}$	$<10^{-12}$
2	8.20	106.870	$<10^{-12}$	$<10^{-12}$
3	5.09	106.071	$<10^{-12}$	$<10^{-12}$
4	3.81	103.146	$<10^{-12}$	$<10^{-12}$
5	3.33	115.239	$<10^{-12}$	$<10^{-12}$
6	2.09	60.090	$<10^{-12}$	$<10^{-12}$
7	1.89	51.768	$<10^{-12}$	$<10^{-12}$
8	1.44	14.658	$<10^{-12}$	$<10^{-12}$
9	1.30	2.038	.010	1.09×10^{-7}
10	1.27	0.084	.084	0.78

doi:10.1371/journal.pgen.0020190.t003

In all the datasets mentioned above, we have very good agreement between the significance of the TW statistic, which does not use the population labels, and the ANOVA, which does. This verifies that the TW analysis is correctly labeling the eigenvectors as to whether they are reflecting real population structure.

Shriver and colleagues [5], using different principal components methods and broken stick statistical analysis [27,28], recovered four significant components on this dataset. Our analysis has clearly recovered more meaningful structure, providing empirical validation of the power of this approach.

An Estimate for the Data Size Needed for Significance

A recent paper by Baik, Ben Arous, and Péché [16] gives theorems for the asymptotics of the distribution of the largest eigenvalue of a sample covariance matrix when the true covariance matrix has a few eigenvalues greater than 1 and the rest equal to 1. This is the situation in genetic data for which there are just a few meaningful axes of variation. Unfortunately the theorems proved are only for the case of data matrices whose entries are complex numbers, but Baik, Ben Arous, and Péché conjecture that the results hold for real data, too. We state a form of the conjecture, which we call the BBP conjecture, and then provide evidence for its applicability to genetics.

Let l_1 be the lead eigenvalue of the theoretical covariance matrix, with the remainder of the eigenvalues 1. Set $\gamma^2 = n/m$. Let L_1 be the largest eigenvalue of the sample covariance. We will let n, m become large with the ratio n/m tending to a limit.

BBP Conjecture [16]:

(1) If $l_1 < 1 + 1/\gamma$, then as $m,n \to \infty$, L_1, suitably normalized, tends in distribution to the same distribution as when $l_1 = 1$.

(2) If $l_1 > 1 + 1/\gamma$, then as $m,n \to \infty$, the TW statistic becomes unbounded almost surely.

That is, the behavior of L_1 is qualitatively different depending on whether l_1 is greater or less than $1 + 1/\gamma$. This is a phase-change phenomenon, and we will define $1 + 1/\gamma = \frac{\sqrt{m} + \sqrt{n}}{\sqrt{n}}$ as the BBP threshold. This is an asymptotic result, showing that as the data size goes to infinity, the transition of the behavior, as l_1 varies, becomes arbitrarily sharp. The result, as stated above, is proved in [16] for data where the matrix entries are complex numbers, and statement (2) of the conjecture is proved in [17], which demonstrates that the behavior is qualitatively different according to whether l_1 is greater or less than $1 + 1/\gamma$. There seems little doubt as to the truth of statement (1) above. It has been shown (D. Paul, Asymptotic behavior of the leading sample eigenvalues for a spiked covariance model,http://anson.ucdavis.edu/~debashis/techrep/eigenlimit.pdf) that, under the assumptions of statement (1) above, the lead eigenvector of the sample covariance is asymptotically uncorrelated with the lead eigenvector of the theoretical covariance, but we believe that the question of the distribution of the leading eigenvalue is still open.

Consider an example of two samples each of size m/2, diverged from each other at time τ,where unit time is 2N generations, and assume that N is the effective population size. We assume τ is small, from which it follows that

$$F_{ST} \approx \tau$$

We find that

$$l_1 = 1 + m\tau \tag{11}$$

It follows that the BBP threshold is reached when $\tau = \frac{1}{\sqrt{nm}}$

This is interesting by itself:

Define D, the data size, to be the product of the number of samples and number of SNPs genotyped. For two subpopulations of equal sample size, the phase change threshold is reached when $1/F_{ST}$ is equal to the square root of the data size D, independently of the number of individuals and markers, at least when both are large.

At a fixed data size, the expected value of the leading eigenvalue of the data matrix (and the power to detect structure) of course is a continuous function of F_{ST}, but the BBP conjecture suggests that for large data sizes there will only be a small transition region. Above the region, detection of structure will be easy, and below it, impossible. Let us take $nm = 2^{20}$ (about one million genotypes), so that the BBP threshold is $F_{ST} = 2^{-10}$. We let $m = 2^k$ $(k = 5\ldots8)$ and set $n = 2^{20-k}$ so that $nm = 2^{20}$.

Now for each value of m, generate simulated data, varying F_{ST} from 2^{-13} to 2^{-7}. For each simulation, we compute L_1, the TW statistic, and a p-value. We show the TW statistics in Figure 6.

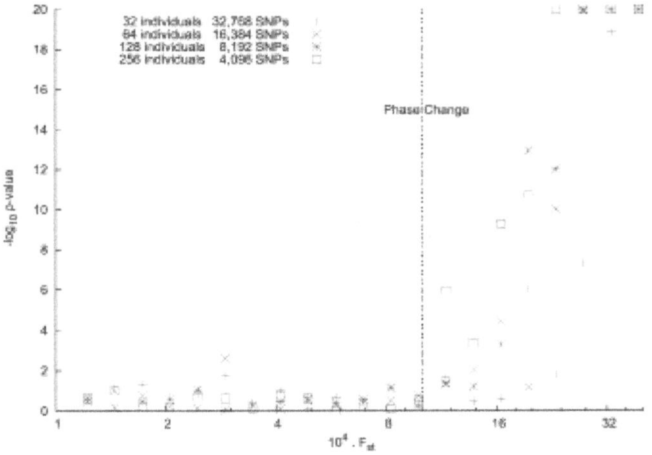

Figure 6: The BBP Phase Change We ran a series of simulations, varying the sample size m and number of markers n but keeping the product at mn = 2^{20}. Thus the predicted phase change threshold is $F_{ST} = 2^{-10}$. We vary F_S and plot the log p-value of the Tracy–Widom statistic. (We clipped $-\log_{10}$ p at 20.) Note that below the threshold there is no statistical significance, while above threshold, we tend to get enormous significance.

The phase change is evident. Further, from [16, p. 1650ff] (also see [17, Equation 1.10]): above the BBP threshold we have that

$$L_1 \to l_1 + \frac{1}{\gamma^2(l_1 - 1)}$$

in probability as m,n → ∞. It then follows that above the BBP threshold, we can expect the TW statistic to be increasing with the number of individuals m if the data size mn is fixed. That is, increasing sample size, rather than marker number, is advantageous for detecting structure above the BBP threshold, but not below it. This effect is clearly visible in Figure 6 (note the behavior of the p-value for m = 256). We summarize:

For two equal size subpopulations, there is a threshold value of F_{ST}, $1/\sqrt{mn}$, below which there will be essentially no evidence of population structure. Above the threshold, the evidence accumulates very rapidly, as we increase the divergence or the data size. Above the threshold for fixed data size mn, the evidence is stronger as we increase m, as long as n ≫ m.

Another implication is that these methods are sensitive. For example, given a 100,000 marker array and a sample size of 1,000, then the BBP threshold for two equal subpopulations, each of size 500, is F_{ST} = .0001. An F_{ST} value of .001 will thus be trivial to detect. To put this into context, we note that a typical value of F_{ST} between human populations in Northern and Southern Europe is about .006 [15]. Thus, we predict: most large genetic datasets with human data will show some detectable population structure.

The BBP phase change is not just a phenomenon of the eigenvector-based analysis we are discussing here. We suspect that at least for biallelic unlinked markers, no methods for detecting structure will do much better than our TW-based techniques. This implies that no method will have any significant success rate if population divergence is below the BBP threshold, while above threshold, reasonable methods will succeed. To test this we made a series of simulations, each with 1,600 biallelic markers and two populations each of size 50. We varied F_{ST} and ran both our eigenanalysis and STRUCTURE. (See Methods for more detail about the simulations and analysis.) We were not successful in using STRUCTURE to produce a higher likelihood for the existence of two clusters rather than one except for the very largestF_{ST} levels. We wanted to place our methods and STRUCTURE on a "level playing field." Our PCA methods return a leading eigenvector, while running STRUCTURE with K = 2 clusters, returns for each individual the probability of belonging to cluster 1. We used a nonparametric idea, applying a probit transform to both the output of both the PCA and of STRUCTURE, and then running an ANOVA analysis, both for PCA and STRUCTURE output. (The probit transform uses order statistics (ranks) to map the observations into points appropriate if the underlying distribution is standard normal. See, for example, [33].) This amounts to carrying out an unsupervised analysis and then checking to see if the recovered "structure" reflects the truth.

Thus, we will compute three p-values: 1) a TW statistic from an unsupervised analysis; 2) an ANOVA p-value (F-statistic) after probit transform of the leading principal component; 3) an ANOVA p-value (F-statistic) after probit transform of the STRUCTURE cluster probabilities.

Table 4 shows the results from a representative set of runs: we show the geometric mean of the p-value in simulations, based on a TW statistic (unsupervised) or a nonparametric ANOVA analysis, both for the eigenanalysis and for STRUCTURE.

Table 4: BBP Phase Change: Eigenanalysis and STRUCTURE

F_{ST}	*P* (TW)	*P* (ANOVA, Eigen)	*P* (ANOVA, STRUCTURE)
0	0.436	0.565	0.432
.000625	0.292	0.188	0.278
.00125	0.312	0.075	0.154
.00250	0.185	5.94×10^{-5}	0.085
.00500	1.19×10^{-6}	$<10^{-12}$	$<10^{-12}$
.01000	$<10^{-12}$	$<10^{-12}$	$<10^{-12}$

We give the geometric mean *P* of *p*-values (20 runs).
___, the expected position of the phase change (F_{ST} = .0025).
doi:10.1371/journal.pgen.0020190.t004

Here the BBP threshold is .0025. Below the threshold nothing interesting is found by the TW unsupervised statistic. Above the threshold, the TW statistic is usually highly significant, and the ANOVA analyses show that the true structure has become apparent. At the threshold wesometimes have recovered significant structure, but it will be hard (usually impossible) to tell if the structure is real or a statistical artifact. Below the threshold, the structure is too weak to be useful. In these runs, at the critical threshold, the eigenanalysis slightly outperformed STRUCTURE. We have not carefully investigated whether we could obtain better results by varying the STRUCTURE parameters.

Summarizing: below the threshold, neither procedure succeeds with reasonable probability, at the threshold success is variable, and above the threshold success is nearly guaranteed.

Admixture

In an admixed population, the expected allele frequency of an individual is a linear mix of the frequencies in the parental populations. Unless the admixture is ancient—in which case the PCA methods will fail as everyone will have the same ancestry proportion—then the mixing weights will vary by individual. Because of the linearity, admixture does not change the axes of variation, or, more exactly, the number of "large" eigenvalues of the covariance is unchanged by adding admixed individuals, if the parental populations are already sampled. Thus, for example, if there are two founding populations, admixed individuals will have coordinates along a line joining the centers of the founding populations.

We generated simulated data, by taking a trifurcation between populations (A,B,D) 100 generations ago. Population C is a recent admixture of A and B. The mixing proportion of A in an individual from C is Beta-distributed B(3.5,1.5) so that the average contribution of populationA in an individual of population C is .7 (see Figure 7). Effective population sizes are 10,000 for each population. We then simulated data for 10,000 unlinked markers (more details are in the Methods section). F_{ST} between any pair of A,B,D is .005. We are attempting to mimic the data of Figure 5, and chose to run our analysis on simulated samples from populations B,C,D, not using samples from A. We expect two significant eigenvalues corresponding to the splits of populations B,C, and D. If population A is included in the analysis, we also get just two significant eigenvalues, as predicted by theory. This is what is observed (unpublished data), with, as predicted, the admixed population not adding to the number of axes of variation (the third eigenvalue is not significant). In Figure 8 we show a plot of the first two eigenvectors. Note the dispersion of population C along a line. This is diagnostic of admixture. The resemblance ofFigures 5 and 8 is striking.

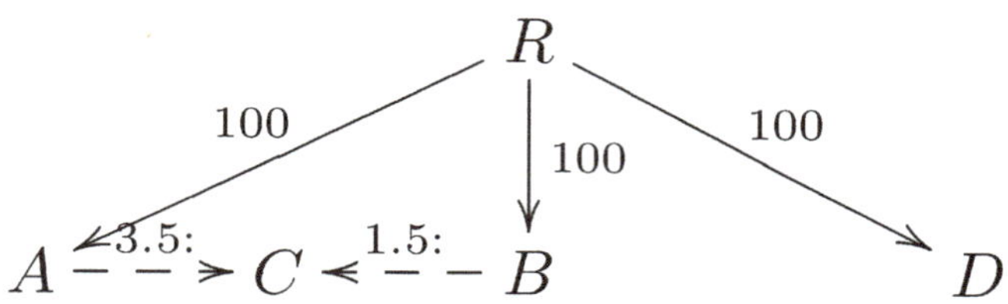

Figure 7: Simulation of an Admixed Population We show a simple demography generating an admixed population. Populations A,B,Dtrifurcated 100 generations ago, while population C is a recent admixture of A and B. Admixture weights for the proportion of population A in population C are Beta-distributed with parameters (3.5,1.5). Effective population sizes are 10,000.

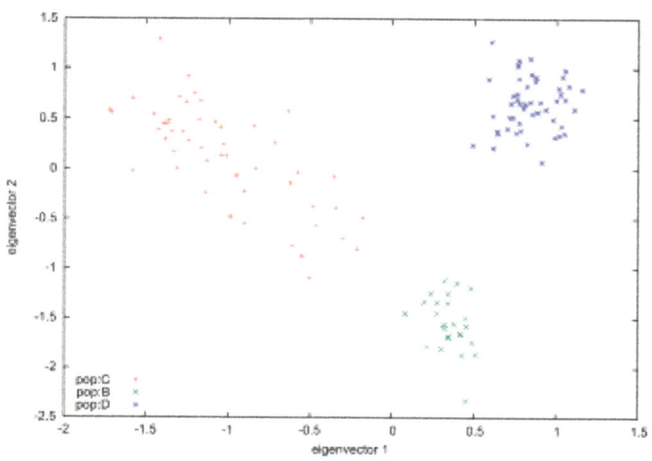

Figure 8: A Plot of a Simulation Involving Admixture (See Main Text for Details) We plot the first two principal components. Population C is a recent admixture of two populations, B and a population not sampled. Note the large dispersion of population C along a line joining the two parental populations. Note the similarity of the simulated data to the real data of Figure 5.

There remain issues to resolve here. Firstly, recent admixture generates large-scale LD which may cause difficulties in a dense dataset as the allele distributions are not independent. These effects may be hard to alleviate with our simple LD correction described below. STRUCTURE [10] allows careful modeling. Secondly, more ancient admixture, especially if the admixed population is genetically now homogeneous, may lead to a causal eigenvalue not very different from the values generated by the sampling noise. Suppose, for example, in our simulation above, we let population C mate panmictically for another 20 generations. Then we will get three clusters for A, B, C that are nearly collinear, but not exactly because of the recent 20-generation divergence, which is reflecting genetic drift unique to that population.

A third issue is that our methods require that divergence is small, and that allele frequencies are divergent primarily because of drift. We attempted to apply our methods to an African-American dataset genotyped on a panel of ancestry-informative markers [34]. The Tracy–Widom theory breaks down here with dozens of "significant" axes that we do not believe have genetic meaning. Perhaps this is to be expected, as on our informative panel F_{ST} is big (.58) and the theory could be expected to perform poorly. In addition our methods are here not dealing adequately with LD caused by large admixture blocks.

This is an issue for our TW techniques, but not for PCA as such. Indeed, on this dataset the correlation of our principal eigenvector with the estimated European ancestry for each individual recovered by the admixture analysis program ANCESTRYMAP [12] is a remarkable .995 (STRUCTURE produces similar results). ANCESTRYMAP has complex modeling of admixture LD, and was also provided with parental allele frequencies, but did no better than the simple PCA. (There is an issue of interpretation here: the leading eigenvector is almost perfectly correlated with ancestry, but to infer actual ancestry proportions an affine transform must be applied, translating and scaling the values. In practice, some parental allele frequencies will be needed to determine the appropriate transform. A similar issue arises with STRUCTURE if parental frequencies are unknown.)

Finally, if "admixture LD" is present, so that in admixed individuals long segments of the genome originate from one founder population, simple PCA methods will not be as powerful as programs such as STRUCTURE [10], ADMIXMAP [11], and ANCESTRYMAP [12], where there is careful modeling of the admixture blocks and the transitions. The power of these methods lies in the fact that genome-wide samples may have similar proportions of inheritance from the ancestral populations, but locally they will inherit either 0, 1, or 2 alleles from each ancestral population. Methods that specifically attempt to assign local ancestries will be able to determine the specific patterns typical of each ancestral population locally. An interesting and challenging problem is to build tools that retain the power of these more complex models on admixed data and that also run rapidly on large datasets.

Correcting for LD

The theory above works well if the markers are independent (that is have no LD), but in practice, and especially with the large genotype arrays that are beginning to be available, this is difficult to ensure. In extreme cases uncorrected LD will seriously distort the eigenvector/eigenvalue structure, making results difficult to interpret. Suppose, for example, that there is a large "block" [35,36] in which markers are in complete LD, and we have genotyped many markers in the block. A large eigenvector of our Wishart matrix X will tend to correlate with the genotype pattern in the block (all markers producing the same pattern). This will distort the eigenvector structure and also the distribution of eigenvalues.

We recommend the following if LD between markers is a concern in the data. Pick a small integer k > 0, corresponding to the number of adjacent markers one uses for adjustment (k = 1 will often suffice). In the data matrix M we will "predict" each column by running a multivariate regression on the k previous columns. We then will analyze the residuals. Concretely: we first form M, as in Equation 2. For each column j

Set:

$$\mathbf{a} = a_s^{[j]}(1 \leq s \leq k)$$

$$R(i,j) = M(i,j) - \sum_{s=1}^{k} a_s^{[j]} M(i,j-s)(1 \leq i \leq m) \tag{12}$$

Choose **a** to minimize

$$\sum_i R^2(i,j)$$

and now calculate X = RR′ instead of MM′. It is first important to check that in the absence of LD the suggested correction does not seriously distort the Tracy–Widom statistic. In Figure 9A and9B we show P–P plots, uncorrected, and with five levels (k = 1…5) of correction. The first figure is with 100 individuals and 5,000 markers, the second with 200 individuals and 50,000 markers. Then in Figure 10A and 10B we analyze a simulated dataset with severe LD. We generate blocks in perfect LD, in which the probability that a block contains L markers is 2^{-L}. We show the corresponding plots. Note that here the uncorrected statistic is distributed quite differently than the Tracy–Widom distribution. Our suggested correction strategy seems to work well, and should be adequate in practice, especially as most large genotype arrays will attempt to avoid high levels of LD. We would recommend that before analyzing a very large dataset with dense genotyping, one should filter the data by removing a marker from every pair of markers that are in tight LD.

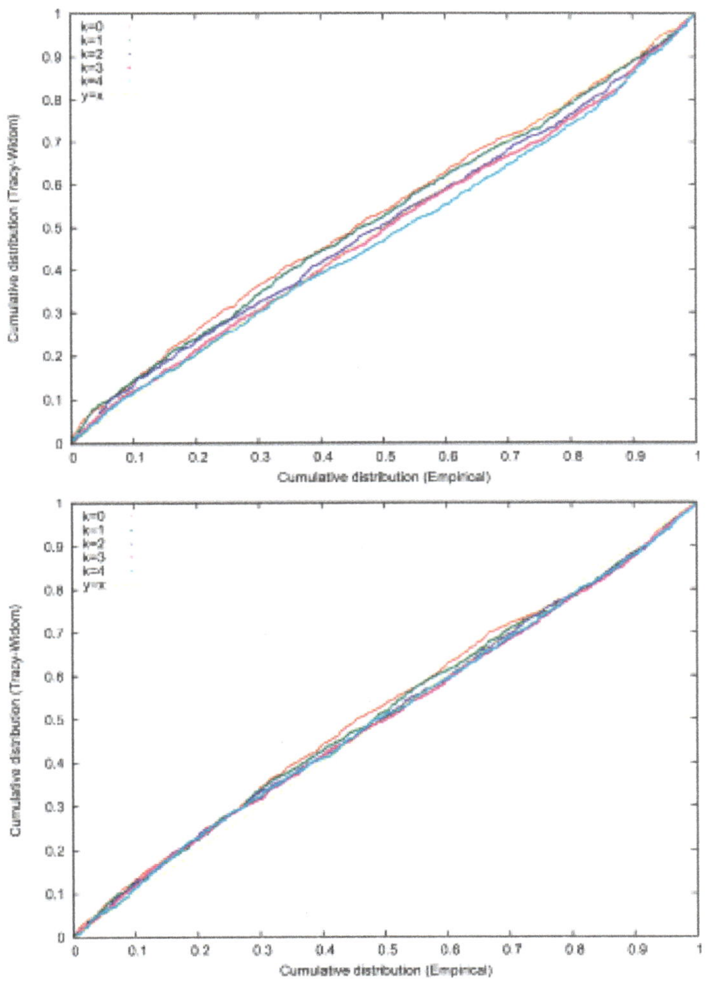

Figure 9: LD Correction with no LD Present P–P plots of the TW statistic, when no LD is present and after varying levels (k) of our LD correction. We first show this (A) for m = 500, n = 5,000, and then (B) for m = 200, n= 50,000. In both cases the LD correction makes little difference to the fit.

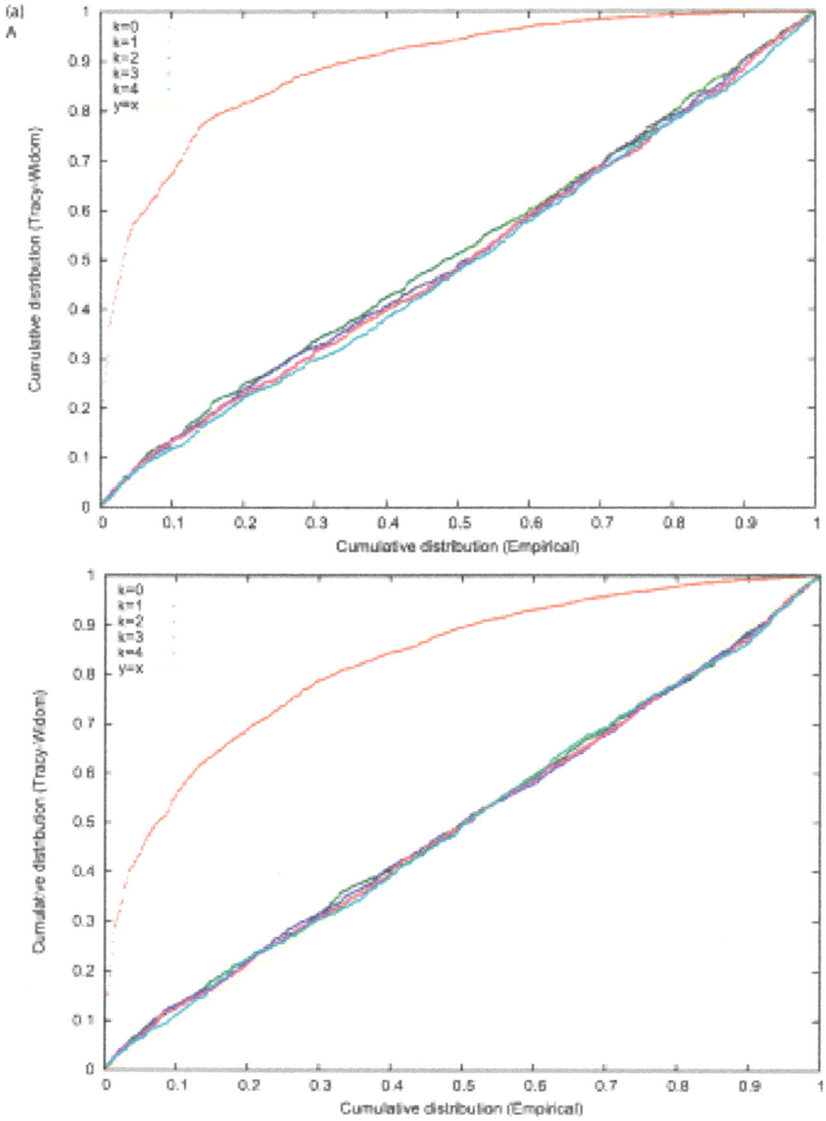

Figure 10: LD Correction with Strong LD (A) Shows P–P plots of the TW statistic (m = 100, n = 5,000) with large blocks of complete LD. Uncorrected, the TW statistic is hopelessly poor, but after correction the fit is again good. Here, we show 1,000 runs with the same data size parameters as inFigure 2A, m = 500, n = 5,000, varying k, the number of columns used to "correct" for LD. The fit is adequate for any nonzero value of k. (B) Shows a similar analysis with m = 200, n = 50,000.

Comparison with STRUCTURE

In the work above on the BBP phase change, we already showed some comparisons between STRUCTURE and our methods. A fair comparison to STRUCTURE is not easy, as the two programs have subtly different purposes and outputs. STRUCTURE attempts to describe the population structure by probabilistic assignment to classes, and we are attempting to determine the statistically significant "axes of variation," which does not necessarily mean the same thing as assigning individuals to classes.

Our impression, confirmed by Table 4, is that when our analysis finds overwhelmingly evident population structure, then STRUCTURE will as well, and when nothing at all is found, STRUCTURE will fail, too. In a problem where the effect is marginal, it may be hard to say which analysis is preferable.

STRUCTURE is a sophisticated program with many features we have not attempted to match. STRUCTURE has an explicit probability model for the data, and this allows extra options and flexibility. It incorporates a range of options for ancestry and for allele frequencies, and has explicit options for modeling microsatellite distributions.

On the other hand, eigenanalysis has advantages over STRUCTURE. First, it is fast and simple, and second, it provides a formal test for the number of significant axes of variation.

One future possibility is to somehow incorporate recovered significant eigenvectors into STRUCTURE—in particular with regard to choosing the number of subpopulations, which is not statistically robust in the STRUCTURE framework. A sensible default for the number of clusters in STRUCTURE is one more than the number of significant eigenvalues under the TW statistic.

Missing Data and Other Problems

The most problematic issue when applying any method to infer population structure is that genotyping may introduce artifacts that induce apparent (but fallacious) population structure.

Missing genotypes by themselves are not the most serious concern. Simply setting M(i,j) = 0 in Equation 3 if marker j is missing for individual i is reasonable if we are testing the null, that there is no structure, and the missing data is "missing at random." Unfortunately "informative missingness" [37,38] is extremely frequent in genetic data. Probably the most common and serious issue is that with current technology, heterozygotes are more difficult to call than homozygotes. Thus, true heterozygotes are more likely to be called as missing. This is discussed in detail in [38], which is recommended as a very useful discussion of the issues, especially as they apply to medical genetics. If DNA quality (or quantity) varies among our samples, then certain individuals may have an unusual amount of missing data, and then appear as outliers in our eigenanalysis—we in fact have seen this in many runs on real data.

Another issue that may produce confounding effects is if data from different populations or geographical areas is handled differently (which may be inevitable, especially in the initial processing); then, in principle, this may induce artifacts that mimic real population structural differences. Even restricting analysis to markers with no missing data, apart from an inevitable power loss, does not necessarily eliminate the problems. After all, if a subset (the missing data) is chosen in a biased way, then the complementary subset must also be biased.

We have no complete solution to these issues, though there is no reason to think that our eigenvector-based methods are more sensitive to the problems than other techniques [9]. One check we do recommend is to generate a test matrix by taking the initial counts C(i,j) to be 0 if the corresponding data is present; otherwise, set C(i,j) = 1. This is equivalent to only focusing on the pattern of missing data. The eigenanalysis on this test matrix will show significant TW statistics if the missing data by itself is showing evidence of population structure. If so, the results should be regarded with some suspicion, especially if the eigenvectors show high correlation to the eigenvectors of the main analysis. We here echo [38] and recommend that the analyst should "control all aspects of source, preparation and genotyping, using the paradigms of blindness and randomization," but, as the reference states, this will not always be possible.

Another possible source of error, where the analyst must be careful, is the inclusion of groups of samples that are closely related. Such a "family" will introduce (quite correctly from an algorithmic point of view) population structure of little genetic relevance, and may confound features of the data of real scientific interest. We found that this occurred in several real datasets that we analyzed with eigenanalysis and in which related individuals were not removed.

DISCUSSION

For many genetic datasets, it is important to try to understand the population structure implied by the data. STRUCTURE [9], since its introduction, has been the tool of choice, especially for small datasets. We think we have provided some evidence that PCA has advantages also, as it is fast, easily implemented, and allows accurate testing of significance of a natural null model.

We can only uncover structure in the samples being analyzed. As pointed out in [39], the sampling strategy can affect the apparent structure. Rosenberg et al. [29] give a detailed discussion of the issue, and of the question of whether clines or clusters are a better description of human genetic variation. However, our "axes of variation" are likely to be relatively robust to this cline/cluster controversy. If there is a genetic cline running across a continent, and we sample two populations at the extremes, then it will appear to the analyst that the two populations form two discrete clusters. However, if the sampling strategy had been more geographically uniform, the cline would be apparent. Nevertheless, the eigenvector reflecting the cline could be expected to be very similar in both cases.

Our methods are conceptually simple, and provide great power, especially on large datasets. We believe they will prove useful both in medical genetics, where population structure may cause spurious disease associations [1,40–43]; and in population genetics, where our statistical methods provide a strong indication of how many axes of variation are meaningful. A parallel paper [14] explores applications to medical genetics.

Mathematical Details

A moments estimator

We justify our estimator of the "effective number of markers."

Theorem 1. Let $\lambda_1, \lambda_2, \ldots \lambda_m$ be eigenvalues of an m × m Wishart matrix MM′, where M is m × n with entries that are Gaussian with mean 0 variance σ^2. Define

$$L_1 = \sum_{i=1}^{m} \lambda_i$$

$$L_2 = \sum_{i=1}^{m} \lambda_i^2$$

If n,σ^2 are unknown, estimates are:

$$\hat{n} = \frac{m(m+2)}{S_2 - m} \tag{13}$$

$$\hat{\sigma}^2 = \frac{S_1}{m\hat{n}} \tag{14}$$

where

$$S_1 = \sum_{i=1}^{m} \lambda_i = L_1 \tag{15}$$

$$S_2 = \frac{m^2 \sum_{i=1}^{m} \lambda_i^2}{S_1^2} = \frac{m^2 L_2}{L_1^2} \tag{16}$$

With these values of n^ and $\hat{\sigma}$, the observed values of L_1 and $2L_2 + L_1^2$ are equal to their expected values.

Note that in this section we define our Wishart as MM′, not $\frac{MM'}{n}$, as n is unknown. This scaling hardly matters in applications, as our procedures are always scale-invariant. That is, we avoid assumptions on the variance of the Gaussian entries of M.

Proof: Let **a** = $(a_1,a_2,\ldots a_m)$ be a random vector uniformly distributed on the unit m-sphere. a_i^2 is Beta (1/2,(m − 1)/2)-distributed, and it follows that

$$E(a_i^2) = \frac{1}{m}$$

$$E(a_i^4) = \frac{3}{m(m+2)}$$

Let

$$s = \sum a_i^2 \lambda_i.$$

Then

$$E(s|\lambda) = \frac{1}{m}\sum_{i=1}^{m} \lambda_i \tag{17}$$

$$E(s^2|\lambda) = \frac{1}{m(m+2)}\left(3\sum_{i}^{m} \lambda_i^2 + \sum_{i \neq j} \lambda_i \lambda_j\right) \tag{18}$$

$$= \frac{1}{m(m+2)}\left(2\sum_{i=1}^{m} \lambda_i^2 + \left(\sum_{i=1}^{m} \lambda_i\right)^2\right) \tag{19}$$

To obtain the distribution of s, unconditioned on λ, we see that we can write s as $s = \mathbf{a}D\mathbf{a}'$where D = diag($\lambda_1, \lambda_2, \ldots \lambda_m$). After an orthogonal transformation

$$s = \mathbf{b}X\mathbf{b}' \tag{20}$$

where X is our Wishart matrix and **b** is uniform (isotropic) on the unit sphere. By properties of the Gaussian distribution, the distribution of s as given by Equation 20 is independent of **b**. We choose **b** to be (1,0,0,…). It follows that s/σ² is distributed as a $\chi^2_{[n]}$ variate so that s = 2σ²Gwhere G is Γ(n/2)-distributed. Thus,

$$E(s) = n\sigma^2 \tag{21}$$

$$E(s^2) = \sigma^4 n(n+2) \tag{22}$$

Comparing Equations 17 and 21, this proves:

$$E\left(\sum_{i=1}^{m} \lambda_i\right) = mn\sigma^2 \tag{23}$$

and comparing Equations 19 and 22, we find:

$$E\left(2\sum_{i=1}^{m} \lambda_i^2 + \left(\sum_{i=1}^{m} \lambda_i\right)^2\right) = m(m+2)n(n+2)\sigma^4 \tag{24}$$

From Equations 23 and 24:

$$\frac{E\left(2\sum_{i=1}^{m} \lambda_i^2 + \left(\sum_{i=1}^{m} \lambda_i\right)^2\right)}{\left(E\left(\sum_{i=1}^{m} \lambda_i\right)\right)^2} = \frac{(m+2)(n+2)}{mn}$$

so that a natural estimator for n is:

$$\hat{n} = \frac{(m+2)\left(\sum_{i=1}^{m} \lambda_i\right)^2}{\left(m\sum_{i=1}^{m} \lambda_i^2\right) - \left(\sum_{i=1}^{m} \lambda_i\right)^2} = \frac{(m+2)L_1^2}{mL_2 - L_1^2} \tag{25}$$

We then obtain as an estimate for σ:

$$\hat{\sigma}^2 = \frac{L_1}{m\hat{n}} \tag{26}$$

If we set: $S_2 = \frac{m^2 L_2}{L_1^2}$ then Equation 25 simplifies to:

$$\hat{n} = \frac{m(m+2)}{S_2 - m} \tag{27}$$

This completes the proof of Theorem 1.

It would be interesting to estimate the standard error for n^ .

We next show that normalizing the eigenvalues of an m × m Wishart to sum to m does not change the asymptotics of the largest eigenvalue. In our data analysis we always normalize the empirical eigenvalues in this way.

Theorem 2. Consider a Wishart matrix X with eigenvalues λ_i, originating from an m × m matrix M whose entries are Gaussian with mean 0 and variance 1. That is, $X = \frac{MM'}{n}$. Let λ_1 be the largest eigenvalue of X. Define$L = \lambda_1$

$$L' = \frac{m\lambda_1}{\sum_{i=1}^{m} \lambda_i} \tag{28}$$

Define τ by

$$\tau = \frac{L - \mu(m,n)}{\sigma(m,n)}$$

$$\tau' = \frac{L' - \mu(m,n)}{\sigma(m,n)}$$

which normalizes L,L′ by the Johnstone normalization of Equation 7 with μ and σ defined as inEquations 5 and 6. Then L and L′ both tend in distribution to the Tracy–Widom distribution as m,n → ∞,n/m → γ > 1. That is, the normalization of Equation 28 does not change the asymptotic distribution of L.

Proof:

Let

$$T = \frac{\sum_i \lambda_i}{m}$$

Then

$$mT = \sum_i \lambda_i = Trace(X) = Trace(MM')/n$$

So

$$T = \frac{\sum_{ij} M_{ij}^2}{mn}$$

Each entry of M is standard normal, and so T has mean 1 and standard deviation

$$u = \frac{\sqrt{2}}{\sqrt{mn}}$$

Let s = σ(m,n) be the scale factor of the Johnstone normalization. Then we can show (we used Maple) that as n → ∞, $\frac{u}{s} \sim \frac{\sqrt{2}}{m^{1/3}}$

Write T = 1 + x so that x has mean 0 and standard deviation u. Thus, x/s → 0 in probability asm → ∞.

$$\tau - \tau' = \frac{L - L/T}{s}$$

$$= \frac{xL}{sT} \tag{29}$$

We now show that this implies that τ − τ′ tends to 0 in probability. From the definition of μ(m,n) inEquation 5, we have μ(m,n) < 4. Pick a constant (say 10) >4. Since as m → ∞, (L − μ(m,n))/σ(m,n) tends to TW in distribution, and σ(m,n) → 0, it follows that P(L > 10) tends to 0 as m → ∞. Similarly, P(T < 1/2) tends to 0. Take > 0. From Equation 29:

$$P(|\tau - \tau'|>\varepsilon) < P(L>10) + P(T < 1/2) + P(x/s > \varepsilon/20) \tag{30}$$

All three probabilities on the right hand side of Equation 30 can be made arbitrarily small for large enough m.

By Johnstone's theorem, τ → TW in distribution, and so τ′ → TW also.

The Spectrum of the Covariance Matrix

We now turn to genetic (genotype count) data, and analyze the theoretical covariance matrix of the data. We concentrate on the covariance of the sample genotypes at a single biallelic marker. Note that in contrast to the results for a Wishart discussed in Theorem 2, we are now interested in a case where there is population structure, which implies dependence between the samples.

Consider sampling a marker from samples belonging to K populations. Suppose the allele has frequency p_i in population i. We sample diploid genotypes, obtaining counts C_j of the variant allele from sample j. We suppose sample j belongs to population i = i(j), and that the sample size for population i is M(i). We discuss the spectrum (eigenvalues) of the covariance matrix of the raw counts C_j. Note that this is for the theoretical covariance not the sample covariance.

We must specify the covariance of the population frequency vector

$$\mathbf{p} = (p_1, p_2, ...p_K)$$

We assume that there is a hidden allele frequency P whose exact distribution will not be important to us, but is diffuse across the unit interval (0,1). Then conditional on P we assume that **p** has mean P(1,1,…,1) and covariance matrix P(1 − P) B where B is independent of P. This is a natural framework, used (filling in details variously) by Balding and Nichols [44], Nicholson et al. [18], and STRUCTURE [9] in the correlated allele mode. For small population divergence, we can take the diagonal entry B_{ii} as the divergence (F_{ST}) between P and p_i. Set$\tau_i = B_{ii}$and assume that all τ_i are of order τ, which is small. Conditional on **p**, then the C_j are independent. C_j has mean p and variance 2p(1 − p) where p = $p_{i(j)}$. This assumes Hardy–Weinberg equilibrium in each of the K populations.

Theorem 3.

With the assumptions above, define

$$C_i^* = C_i - \frac{\sum_{j=1}^{M} C_j}{M}$$

so that C_i^* has mean 0. Let V^* be the covariance matrix of C^* and set

$$\tilde{V} = \frac{V^*}{2P(1-P)}.$$

Conditional on the root frequency P:

1. $\tilde{V}$ does not depend on P.

2. $\tilde{V}$ has an eigenvalue 0 with eigenvector $\frac{(1,1,...,1)}{\sqrt{M}}$.

3. $\tilde{V}$ has for each k (1 ≤ k ≤ K), M(k) − 1 eigenvalues equal to 1 − τ_k. (We will call these the small eigenvalues.)

4. $\tilde{V}$ has K − 1 eigenvectors that span a vector space F^* consisting of vectors **v** of length M whose coordinates are constant on samples from each population, and such that the sum of the coordinates of **v** are 0.

5. If the matrix B (the scaled covariance of the population frequencies **p**) has rank r, then r − 1 of the eigenvalues of $\tilde{V}$ that correspond to eigenvectors in F^* depend on B. (So if B has full rank, all these eigenvalues depend on B.) If we allow each sample size M(k) → ∞, then then all such eigenvalues also → ∞. (We will call the corresponding eigenvalues the large eigenvalues).

Proof:

Let V be the covariance matrix of the counts C. Regard V = ‖ V_{ij} ‖ as a linear operator in the natural way. Write π(i) for the population index of sample i(1 ≤ i ≤ K). We can write V = V_{ij} as D+ W where D is a diagonal matrix with the diagonal element D_{ii} = $d_{\pi(i)}$ and W_{ij} = $q_{\pi(i),\pi(j)}$. So the covariance structure depends only on the population labels of the samples. It follows that the vector space of M long column vectors has an orthogonal decomposition into subspaces invariant under V consisting of: 1) a subspace F of vectors whose coordinates are constant within a population. F has dimension K; 2) subspaces S_i (1 ≤ i ≤ K). Vectors of S_i are zero on samples not belonging to population i, and have coordinate sum 0, which implies that they are orthogonal to F. It now follows that V has K eigenvectors in F, and for each k (1 ≤ i ≤ K), (M(k) − 1 eigenvectors in S_k each of which have the same eigenvalue λ_k. Conditional on **p**, V acts onS_k as $2p_k$(1 − p_k)I where I is the identity matrix. (The factor 2 comes from the two chromosomes sampled for each individual.) Thus,

$$\lambda_k = E(2p_k(1 - p_k)|P)$$

Now

$$E(p_k^2|P) = P^2 + P(1 - P)\tau_k$$

and so the eigenvalues corresponding to eigenvectors of S_k are:

$$\lambda_k = E(2p_k(1 - p_k)|P) = 2P(1 - P)(1 - \tau_k)$$

V^* and V act identically on S_k, the vectors of which have coordinate sum 0, so this proves assertion 3 of Theorem 3. We now consider the action of V on the K-dimensional subspace F. It is convenient to define $m(k) = \sqrt{M(k)}$, a quantity we will need repeatedly. Let for each k ($1 \leq k \leq K$), $\mathbf{f}^{[k]}$ be the vector whose coordinates are 0 except for samples i where $\pi(i) = k$, and where for such samples:

$$\mathbf{f}_i^{[k]} = \frac{1}{m(k)}$$

The vectors $\mathbf{f}^{[k]}$ form an orthonormal basis for F. Write $d_v = \mathbf{f}^{[k]}.C$. Set E to be the diagonal matrix$diag(1 - \tau_1, 1 - \tau_2, ...1 - \tau_K)$ It is easy to calculate that the random variables d_k have, conditional on P, covariance matrix R, where

$$R = (4DBD + 2E)P(1 - P) \tag{31}$$

and D = diag(m(1),m(2),...m(K)). Here E corresponds to sampling noise.

In the main paper we subtract the sample mean from the counts C. So define the M long vector$\mathbf{1} = (1,1,\ldots,1)$. Then

$$\mathbf{1} = \sum_{k=1}^{K} m(k)\mathbf{f}^{[k]} \tag{32}$$

Set $C_j^* = C_j - \frac{1}{M}\sum_{k=1}^{M} C_k$, this is a linear transform T where

$$T(C) = C^* = C - \frac{(\mathbf{1}.C)\mathbf{1}}{M}$$

We are interested in the action of T on F. Write

$$T(\mathbf{f}^{[k]}) = \sum_{l=1}^{K} T_{kl}\mathbf{f}^{[k]}.\mathbf{1}$$

Then from Equation 32, regarding T as a K × K matrix (abusing notation): T = I − Q where I is the identity matrix and

$$Q_{kl} = \frac{m(k)m(l)}{M}$$

Set$d_k = \mathbf{f}^{[k]}.C^*$It now follows from Equation 31 that if R^* is the covariance matrix of the d_k, then

$$R^* = (4TDBDT + 2TET)P(1 - P) \tag{33}$$

This is enough to prove that

$$\tilde{V} = V/2P(1 - P)$$

does not depend on P (assertion 1 of Theorem 3).

Next, $T(\mathbf{1}) - R^*(\mathbf{1}) = \mathbf{0}$, which proves assertion 2 of Theorem 3. The space F^* of vectors Forthogonal to 1 is invariant under V and $\tilde{V}$, thus R^* will have K − 1 eigenvectors of F^*(assertion 4 of Theorem 3). If B has rank K (which will be true except in special cases), thenTDBDT has rank K − 1 and if $M(k) \to \infty$ for each k, then R^* will have K − 1 nonzero eigenvalues which become arbitrarily large. More generally, if B has rank r, then the matrix TDBDT will have rank r − 1, and the r − 1 eigenvalues of R^* that depend on B, again will become arbitrarily large as $M(k) \to \infty$. Note that the matrix TET which arises from sampling noise is bounded. (In factTET is a contraction and has all eigenvalues less than 1.) This completes the proof of Theorem 3. The case in which B does not have full rank occurs if there has been a genetically recent admixture between two or more populations. In this case, even if there are K clearly distinct populations, fewer than K − 1 eigenvalues will become large as the sample size increases.

Definition of the TW Density

For completeness, we define the TW density. Our description is taken from [22].

Let q(x) be the solution of the differential equation:

$$q''(x) = xq(x) + 2q^3(x)$$

with the boundary condition:

$$q(x) \sim Ai(x) \text{ as } x \to \infty$$

and Ai(x) is the Airy function. Then the TW distribution is given by:

$$TW(s) = \exp\left(-\frac{1}{2}\int_s^{\infty} q(x) + (x - s)q^2(x)dx\right) \tag{34}$$

A table of the TW right-tail area, and density, is available on request.

Some Questions in Theoretical Statistics

We believe this work raises some challenges to theoretical statisticians. Our results with genetic simulations would be even more convincing if there were theorems (say for the Wishart case where the data matrix has Gaussian entries) that showed: 1) that using the effective number of markers calculated by Equation 10 instead of the true number of markers does not affect the asymptotics; 2) that the BBP phase change holds for real Wishart matrices as well as for complex; 3) in Figures 2 and 3 the P–P plots show a noticeably better fit at the high end, corresponding to low p-values. Explain!

METHODS

Datasets used.

For the data used in Figure 4, we use the H952 subset of the CEPH–HGDP panel [30,31,45] where some atypical samples and pairs of close relatives have been removed.

For the data used in Figure 5, we use an unpublished sample collected and genotyped by Dr. Jonathan Seidman and Dr. S. Sangwatanaroj. This consisted of 25 samples from Northern Thailand (after removing some individuals who are close relatives of people whose samples we retained) and 45 samples each from China and Japan (data drawn from the International Human Haplotype Map Project [32]). The Northern Thai samples were genotyped using an Affymetrix Xba chip. The dataset analyzed consisted of the overlap between the SNPs successfully genotyped in HapMap and the Affymetrix chip, and included 40,560 SNPs.

For the data of Mark Shriver and colleagues [5], we analyzed only autosomal data where no SNP had any missing data. We removed one individual who was a duplicate, two Burunge and Mbuti samples that represented close relatives of other samples, and nine Nasioi individuals who our data suggest are part of one or two extended families.

Algorithm details.

In the eigenanalysis of the Shriver data, we examine no more than two markers as independent regression variables for each marker we analyze, insisting that any marker that enters the regression be within 100,000 bases of the marker being analyzed. This slightly sharpens the results. Varying these parameters made little difference.

For all STRUCTURE runs, we ran with a burn-in of 10,000 iterations with 20,000 follow-on iterations, and no admixture model was used. Computations were carried out on a cluster of Intel Xeon compute nodes, each node having a 3.06-GHz clock.

For our coalescent simulations, we assumed a phylogenetic tree on the populations, and at each simulated marker, ran the coalescent back in time to the root of the tree. At this point we have a set of ancestors A of the sampled chromosomes. We now assume that the marker is biallelic and that the population frequency f of the variant allele in the ancestral population is distributed uniformly on the unit interval. Sample the frequency f and then choose an allele for each ancestor of A, picking the allele for each ancestor with probability f. Now retain the marker if it is polymorphic in our samples. This process is mathematically equivalent to having a very large outgroup population diverging from the sampled populations at the phylogenetic root, with the population panmictic before any population divergence, and ascertaining by finding heterozygotes in the outgroup. If our simulated samples have n individuals, our procedure yields a sample frequency that is approximately uniform on $(1,2,\ldots,2n-1)$.

For the admixture analysis that created the plot of Figure 8 we had a population C that was admixed with founder populations A and B. For each individual of C, we generated a mixing value x that is Beta-distributed B(3.5,1.5). Now for each marker independently, the individual was assigned to population A with probability x or B with probability $1 - x$.

ACKNOWLEDGMENTS

We are grateful to Alan Edelman for very helpful advice and references to the modern statistical literature and a very useful preprint, and to Plamen Koev for a numerical table of the TW-distribution. We thank Craig Tracy for some important corrections and advice, and Jinho Baik for alerting us to his recent work. The comments of three anonymous referees have greatly improved the manuscript. We thank Jonathan Seidman and Dr. S. Sangwatanaroj for early access to the Thai data. We are grateful to Mark Shriver for giving us access to the data of [5]. We thank Stephen Schaffner for sharing a powerful and flexible coalescent simulator [46] which was helpful for many of our simulations, and Mira Bernstein for catching an important error.

REFERENCES

1. Devlin B, Roeder K (1999) Genomic control for association studies. Biometrics 55: 997–1004.
2. Menozzi P, Piazza A, Cavalli-Sforza L (1978) Synthetic maps of human gene frequencies in Europeans. Science 201: 786–792.
3. Cavalli-Sforza LL, Feldman MW (2003) The application of molecular genetic approaches to the study of human evolution. Nat Genet 33(Supplement): 266–275. Historical article.
4. Chakraborty R, Jin L (1993) A unified approach to study hypervariable polymorphisms: Statistical considerations of determining relatedness and population distances. In: Pena S, Jeffreys A, Epplen J, Chakraborty R, editors. DNA fingerprinting, current state of the science. Basel: Birkhauser. pp. 153–175.
5. Shriver M, Mei R, Parra E, Sonpar V, Halder I, et al. (2005) Large-scale SNP analysis reveals clustered and continuous patterns of human genetic variation. Human Genomics 2: 81–89.
6. Capelli C, Redhead N, Romano V, Cali F, Lefranc G, et al. (2006) Population structure in the Mediterranean basin: A Y chromosome perspective. Ann Hum Genet 70: 207–225.
7. Lovell A, Moreau C, Yotova V, Xiao F, Bourgeois S, et al. (2005) Ethiopia: Between Sub-Saharan Africa and western Eurasia. Ann Hum Genet 69: 275–287.
8. Stoneking M, Fontius JJ, Clifford SL, Soodyall H, Arcot SS, et al. (1997) Alu insertion polymorphisms and human evolution: Evidence for a larger population size in Africa. Genome Res 7: 1061–1071.
9. Pritchard J, Stephens M, Donnelly P (2000) Inference of population structure using multilocus genotype data. Genetics 155: 945–959.
10. Falush D, Stephens M, Pritchard J (2003) Inference of population structure using multilocus genotype data: Linked loci, and correlated allele frequencies. Genetics 164: 1567–1587.
11. Hoggart C, Shriver M, Kittles R, Clayton D, McKeigue P (2004) Design and analysis of admixture mapping studies. Am J Hum Genet 74: 965–978.
12. Patterson N, et al. (2004) Methods for high-density admixture mapping of disease genes. Am J Hum Genet 74: 979–1000.
13. Montana G, Pritchard J (2004) Statistical tests for admixture mapping with case-control and cases-only data. Am J Hum Genet 75: 771–789.
14. Price A, Patterson N, Plenge R, Weinblatt M, Shadick N, et al. (2006) Principal components analysis corrects for stratification in genome-wide association studies. Nat Genet 38: 904–909.
15. Cavalli-Sforza L, Menozzi P, Piazza A (1994) The history and geography of human genes. Princeton: Princeton University Press. 428 p.
16. Baik J, Ben Arous G, Péché S (2005) Phase transition of the largest eigenvalue for nonnull complex sample covariance matrices. Ann Probability 33: 1643–1697.
17. Baik J, Silverstein J (2006) Eigenvalues of large sample covariance matrices of spiked population models. J Multivariate Anal 97: 1643–1697.
18. Nicholson G, Smith A, Jonsson F, Gustaffson O, Stefansson K, et al. (2002) Assessing population differentiation and isolation from single-nucleotide

polymorphism data. JRSS(B) 64: 695–715.

19. Golub G, Van Loan C (1996) Matrix computations. 3rd edition. Baltimore: Johns Hopkins.
20. Bowcock AM, Ruiz-Linares A, Tomfohrde J, Minch E, Kidd JR, et al. (1994) High resolution of human evolutionary trees with polymorphic microsatellites. Nature 368: 455–457.
21. Wilks S (1962) Mathematical statistics. New York: Wiley.
22. Johnstone I (2001) On the distribution of the largest eigenvalue in principal components analysis. Ann Stat 29: 295–327.
23. Tracy C, Widom H (1994) Level-spacing distributions and the Airy kernel. Commun Math Phys 159: 151–174.
24. El Karoui N (2003) On the largest eigenvalue of Wishart matrices with identity covariance when p/n → ∞. Available at http://www.citebase.org/fulltext?format=application%2Fpdf&identifier=oai%3AarXiv.org%3Amath%2F0309355. Accessed 15 November 2006.
25. Soshnikov A (2002) A note on universality of the distribution of the largest eigenvalues in certain sample covariance matrices. J Stat Physics 108: 1033–1056.
26. Altshuler D, Brooks LD, Chakravarti A, Collins FS, Daly MJ, et al. (2005) A haplotype map of the human genome. Nature 437: 1299–1320.
27. Macarthur R (1957) On the relative abundance of bird species. Proc Natl Acad Sci U S A 43: 293–295.
28. Pielou E (1975) Ecological diversity. New York: Wiley.
29. Searle J (1971) Linear models. New York: Wiley.
30. Ramachandran S, Deshpande O, Roseman CC, Rosenberg NA, Feldman MW, et al. (2005) Support from the relationship of genetic and geographic distance in human populations for a serial founder effect originating in Africa. Proc Natl Acad Sci 102: 15942–15947.
31. Rosenberg N, Mahajan S, Ramachandran S, Zhao C, Pritchard J, et al. (2005) Clines, clusters, and the effect of study design on the inference of human population structure. PLoS Genet 1(6): e70..
32. Gibbs R, et al. (2004) The International Hapmap Project. Nature 426: 789–796.
33. Finney DJ (1971) Probit analysis. 3rd edition. Cambridge (United Kingdom): Cambridge University Press.
34. Smith M, Patterson N, Lautenberger L, Truelove A, McDonald G, et al. (2004) High-density admixture map for disease gene discovery in African Americans. Am J Hum Genet 74: 1001–1013.
35. Daly M, Rioux J, Schaffner S, Hudson T, Lander E (2001) High-resolution haplotype structure in the human genome. Nat Genet 29: 229–232.
36. Patil N, Berno AJ, Hinds DA, Barrett WA, Doshi JM, et al. (2001) Blocks of limited haplotype diversity revealed by high-resolution scanning of human Chromosome 21. Science 294: 1719–1723.
37. Allen A, Rathouz P, Satten GA (2003) Informative missingness in genetic association studies: Case-parent designs. Am J Hum Genet 72: 671–680.
38. Clayton DG, Walker NM, Smyth DJ, Pask R, Cooper JD, et al. (2005) Population structure, differential bias and genomic control in a large-scale, case-control association study. Nat Genet 37: 1243–1246.
39. Serre D, Pääbo S (2004) Evidence for gradients of human genetic diversity within and among continents. Genome Res 14: 1679–1685.
40. Spielman R, McGinnis R, Weiss S, Ewens W (1993) Transmission test for linkage disequilibrium: The insulin gene region and insulin-dependent diabetes mellitus (IDDM). Am J Hum Genet 52: 506–516.
41. Freedman M, Reich D, Penney K, Macdonald G, et al. (2004) Assessing the impact of population stratification on genetic association studies. Nat Genet 36: 388–393.
42. Marchini J, Cardon L, Phillips M, Donnelly P (2004) The effects of human population structure on large genetic association studies. Nat Genet 36: 512–517.
43. Helgason A, Yngvadottir B, Hrafnkelsson B, Gulcher J, Stefansson K (2005) An Icelandic example of the impact of population structure on association studies. Nat Genet 37: 90–95.
44. Balding DJ, Nichols RA (1995) A method for quantifying differentiation between populations at multi-allelic loci and its implications for investigating identity and paternity. Genetica 96: 3–12.
45. Rosenberg N (2006) Standardized subsets of the HGDP–CEPH human genome diversity cell line panel, accounting for atypical and duplicated samples and pairs of close relatives. Ann Hum Gen 70(Part 6): 841–847.
46. Schaffner S, Foo C, Gabriel S, Reich D, Daly M, et al. (2005) Calibrating a coalescent simulation of human genome sequence variation. Genome Res 15: 1576–1583.

CHAPTER 3 STATISTICAL MODELLING OF TRANSCRIPT PROFILES OF DIFFERENTIALLY REGULATED GENES

Daniel C Eastwood, Andrew Mead†, Martin J Sergeant and Kerry S Burton

BACKGROUND

Various statistical approaches have been specifically developed to summarise the vast quantities of data that are produced in microarray studies [1, 2, 3], employing analysis of variance (ANOVA), clustering and network modelling. Analysis of variance (ANOVA) has been used to identify those gene expression responses that are most affected by different treatments, often taking account of particular forms of treatment structure, such as the correlations between sample times in a time-course study [4]. Approaches for clustering genes with similar responses range from simple methods for observed data, the calculation of correlations between genes [5], through to clustering based on linear [6] or polynomial regression [7] or spline models [8]. Network models are used to reconstruct transcription factor activity [9] or infer regulatory networks [10], assuming a particular mechanistic model for the behaviour of each regulation function based on observed microarray gene expression data.

This paper aims to use standard statistical non-linear regression models to enhance the biological interpretation of individual gene expression profiles. Such regression models provide accessible methods to describe the shape of each gene expression profile as a function of time, thus providing an insight into the underlying processes rather than simply identifying significant differences. For example, non-linear models can be used to identify the time of a particular event in a gene expression profile, such as the time of rapid up- or down-regulation. Similarly, modelling transcript changes using parametric equations that allow biological interpretation can further allow the comparison or clustering of the shapes of the expression profiles based on biological interpretable parameters. Such non-linear regression techniques are commonly used in agronomic studies to describe responses to a range of quantitative input variables, but are not commonly used in the examination of gene expression data.

The initial model system used to investigate the potential of statistical parametric, non-linear regression approaches for gene profiling was fungal morphogenesis with data provided by quantitative reverse transcriptase PCR (qRT-PCR) which provides a more precise method than either Northern analysis or microarrays [11]. This system encompasses a range of growth forms from vegetative mycelium to multicellular organs which enable the fungus to respond to changes in nutrition and environment, and undergo pathogenesis or reproduction. The fruiting bodies of the basidiomycete fungus Agaricus bisporus, the cultivated mushroom, are ideal for studying fungal morphogenesis as they are macroscopic, the tissues are clearly de-lineated (stipe, caps and gills) and the initiation of fruiting body morphogenesis is controlled environmentally. Differential screening and targeted gene cloning procedures have identified genes up-regulated post-harvest in A. bisporus fruiting bodies, based on Northern analysis [12, 13, 14]. Genes have also been identified which are expressed in developing fruiting bodies of several other fungi, includingLentinula edodes [15], Pleurotus ostreatus [16], Flammulina velutipes [17] and Coprinus cinereus(Coprinopsis cinerea) [18, 19].

This study investigated how expression profiles, generated from qRT-PCR data of differentially regulated genes in A. bisporus fruiting bodies, could be statistically modelled both to estimate the time of up-regulation and determine

Citation: Daniel C Eastwood, Andrew Mead, Martin J Sergeant and Kerry S Burton, Statistical modelling of transcript profiles of differentially regulated genes, DOI: 10.1186/1471-2199-9-66.

similar temporal expression patterns. The five genes chosen for profiling are functionally distinct, and therefore unlikely to have obvious common regulatory mechanisms: they are cruciform DNA binding protein, cytochrome P450II, β (1–6) glucan synthase, glucuronyl hydrolase and riboflavin aldehyde-forming enzyme [12, 20]. Whilst being functionally distinct, these genes were expected to show broadly similar patterns of expression following harvest, allowing the fitting of a single model form to all five responses. This enables the comparison of the profiles via biologically interpretable parameters rather than simply clustering genes based on the observed data. To determine the time when transcription first increased for each gene, transcript levels of each gene were examined at 3 h intervals for 24 h. Transcript levels were also measured at 24 hour intervals over 5 days. These profiles were modelled to provide directly interpretable parameter values, offering an insight into the regulation of the genes. Spatial control of gene expression was also assessed by comparing transcription in tissues of the harvested mushroom during the first 48 hours post-harvest storage.

Furthermore, this study has applied these regression modelling approaches to publicly-available microarray data sets from published studies, to identify groups of genes showing similar regulatory patterns. The potential application of this approach to fully exploit the large quantities of high-throughout data was discussed.

RESULTS

The qRT-PCR-derived data were initially assessed to ensure suitability for further study. Standard curves show that the PCR reactions were operating at close to 100% efficiency. Melting curve analyses showed that in all cases a single product was obtained showing that the specificity of the reaction was high. The PCR control treatments showed no evidence of DNA contamination or active reverse transcription after the 85°C treatment (data not shown).

Comparison of methods of measuring gene expression in A. bisporus

Gene transcript levels were obtained by qRT-PCR and Northern analysis from the same RNA extracts obtained from the mushroom tissues. These data were then compared by calculating correlation coefficients and fitting simple linear regression relationships for Northern analysis response as a function of the qRT-PCR response, for each gene separately within each of the three experiments. Northern analysis responses increased with increasing values of the qRT-PCR response, and in most cases linear regression lines fitted well. However, the Northern analysis response appears to reach an upper threshold at high values of the qRT-PCR response, e.g. for cruciform DNA-binding enzyme and glucuronyl hydrolase (0–5d and tissues experiments), and β(1–6) glucan synthase (tissues experiment). Exponential regression curves were then fitted to the responses and for ten of the 15 data sets these curves provided a better fit than the simple linear regression models, with the curvature of the response suggesting asymptotic regression, for example, glucuronyl hydrolase, 0–5d experiment (Figure 1).

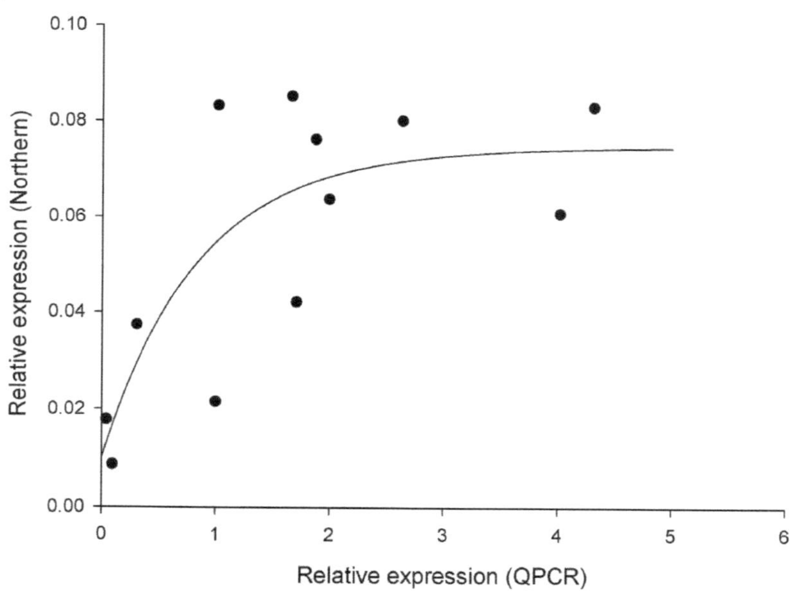

Figure 1 Example showing the saturation of Northern-derived signal. Exponential regression curve showing the relationship between the Northern analysis response (y axis) and the qRT-PCR response (x axis) for glucuronyl hydrolase during 5 days post-harvest storage. Fitted equation is $y = 0.0746 - 0.0646 * 0.309^x$, $R^2 = 52.5\%$.

Transcription in the first 24 hours (A. bisporus)

The different expression patterns for each gene over the first 24 hours following harvest, as obtained using qRT-PCR, are shown in Figure 2. During this period, transcript levels increased significantly, by approximately 10 fold or more, for all genes except riboflavin aldehyde-forming enzyme (less than 2 fold). Transcript levels of cruciform DNA-binding protein increased shortly after harvest to very high levels, while for cytochrome P450II and glucuronyl hydrolase the profiles showed an initial period of little change followed by increases in transcript levels (approx. 12 and 18 h after harvest respectively). In contrast the transcript levels of β(1–6) glucan synthase increased continuously during the first 24 hours post-harvest, with a notable sudden increase at about 9 h.

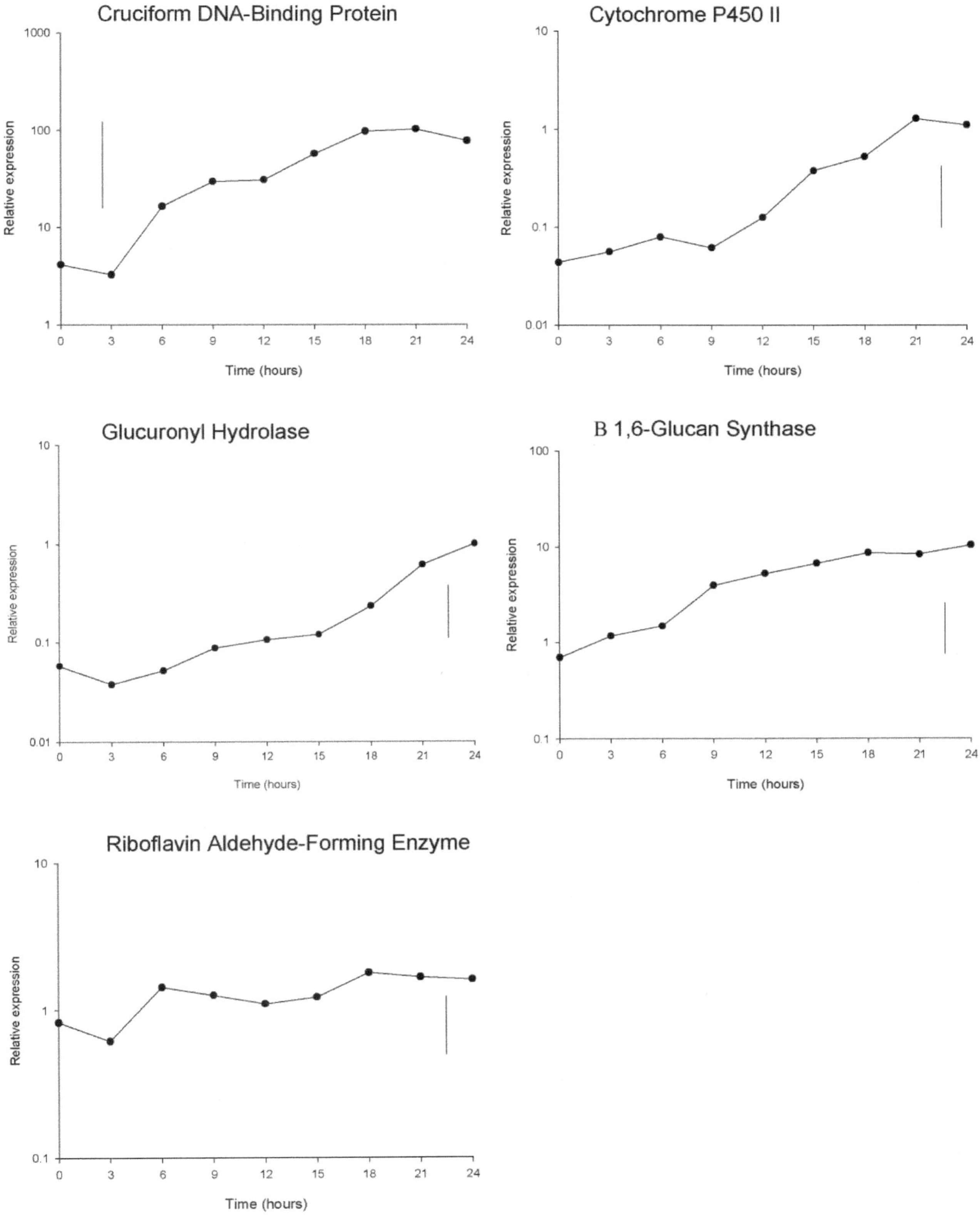

Figure 2 Gene expression during the first 24 hours post-harvest sampling at 3 hourly intervals. Mean qRT-PCR (log_{10}-transformed) measurements of gene expression of the 5 selected genes during the first 24 hours post-harvest storage, sampling at 3 hourly intervals. Vertical lines show LSD (5%, 16d.f.) for comparing means at different times, as calculated from the residual mean square obtained from the ANOVA.

'Split-line' or 'broken-stick' analysis was used to model the transcription profile data from the first 24 hours to estimate the time at which an initial increase in transcription occurred. The model was applied successfully to the transcript data for cytochrome P450II and glucuronyl hydrolase, with these data sets each described by two separate linear regression line segments, the first line having a slope of zero (Figure3). More precise estimates of when transcription first increased were determined in these analysis as 13.5 hours (+/- 2.1 hours (95% confidence interval)) for cytochrome P450II (Figure 3A) and 16.5 hours (+/- 2.1 hours (95% confidence interval)) for glucuronyl hydrolase (Figure 3B). This analytical approach was not successful in describing the transcription profiles of cruciform DNA-binding protein and β(1–6) glucan synthase, as there were insufficient early time points to establish an initial baseline response (line with zero slope). Transcripts of riboflavin aldehyde-forming enzyme showed no clear upward trend in the first 24 hours, and so the 'broken-stick' analysis approach was again not successful.

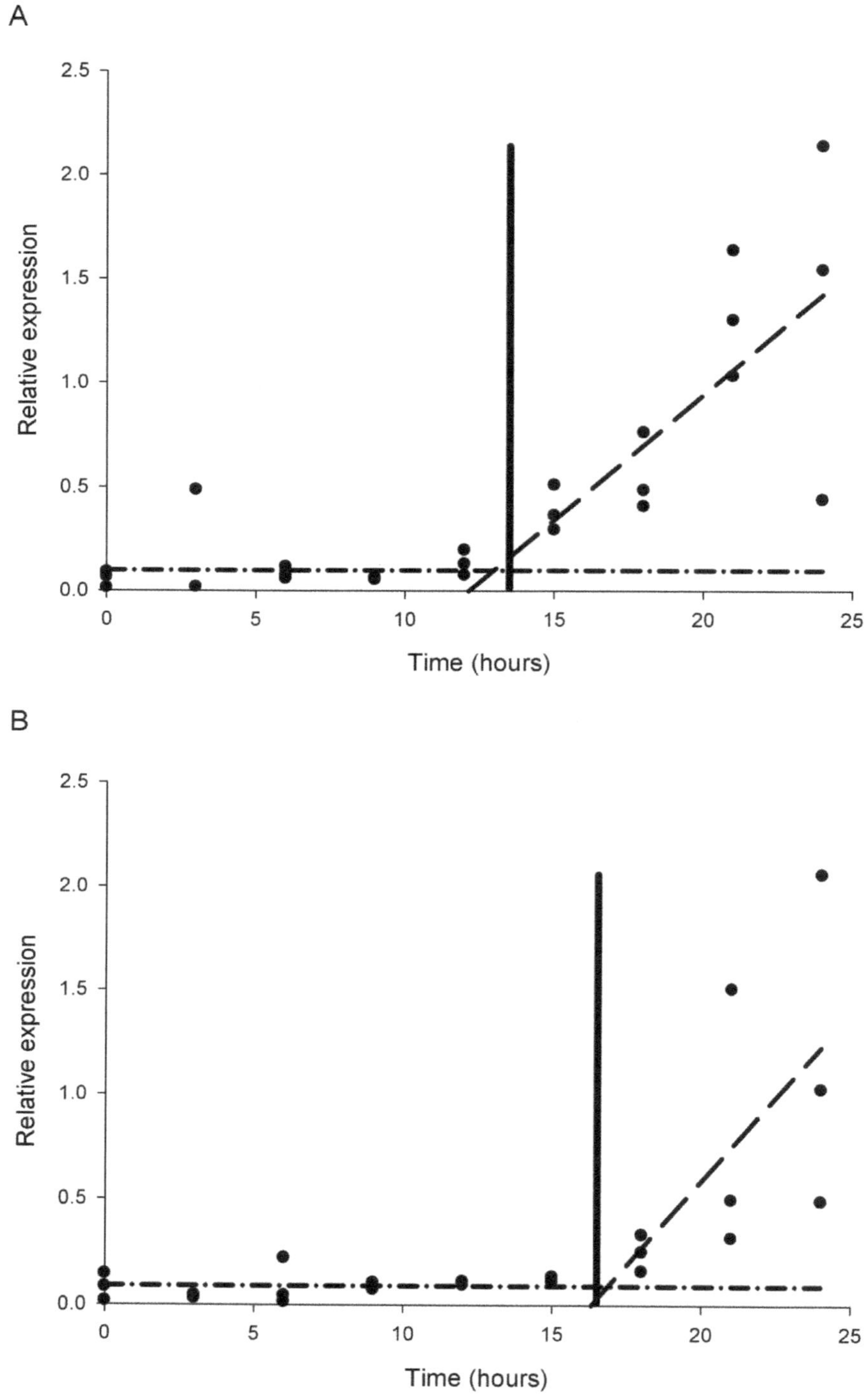

Figure 3 Broken-stick analysis showing the point of increased transcription. A) cytochrome P450II (CYPII) at 13.5 hours (+/- 2.13 hours) and B) glucuronyl hydrolase (GHYD) at 16.5 hours (+/- 2.05 hours) in A. bisporus fruiting bodies over the first 24 hours following harvest, sampling at 3 hourly intervals.

Transcription profiling over 5 days post-harvest (A. bisporus)

The 5-day transcript profiles, as obtained using qRT-PCR, showed an initial increase in transcript levels for all five genes for 1–2 days, followed by a plateau or a decline (Figure 4). The extent of increase in transcript levels over the first two days ranged from 668 fold for cruciform DNA-binding protein, to 47 fold for riboflavin aldehyde-forming enzyme and 36 fold for glucuronyl hydrolase. Gene expression over five days storage, as measured using qRT-PCR, was modelled as a function of storage time by non-linear regression analysis of $\log_{10}$-transformed data using a critical exponential curve (Equation 1: $y(t) = A + (B + Ct)R^t + \varepsilon$). This curve was selected in preference over either the simpler single exponential curve or more complex double exponential curve, based both on the shape of the response, and a formal comparison of the goodness of fit of each model. This was achieved by comparing each more complex model to the simpler alternative (the critical exponential can be considered a simpler alternative to the double exponential, and the single exponential a simpler alternative to the critical exponential). The improvement in fit was assessed using an F-test to identify the significance of the ratio of the change in residual variance between models to the residual variance for the more complex model.

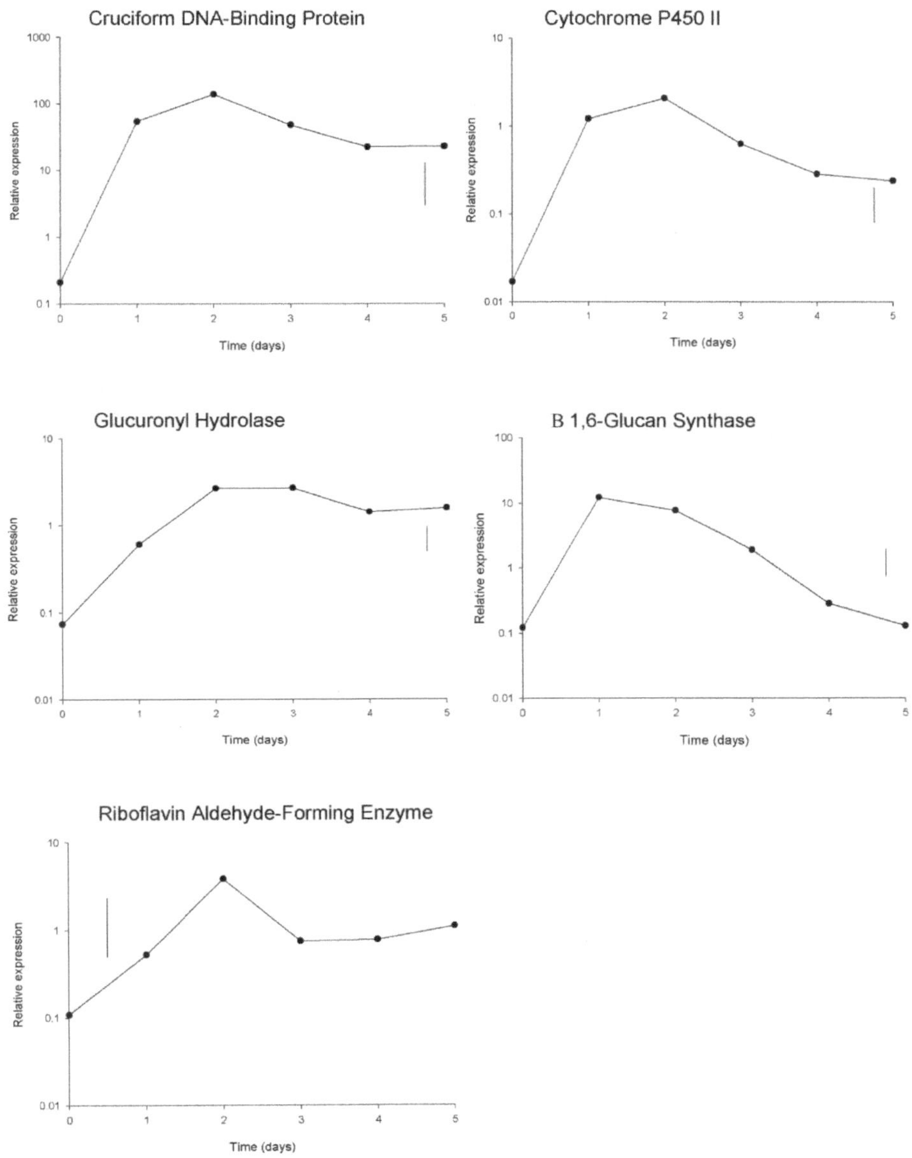

Figure 4 Gene expression over 5 days post-harvest development. Mean qRT-PCR ($\log_{10}$-transformed) measurements of gene expression of the 5 selected genes during 5 days post-harvest storage, sampling at 24 hour intervals. Vertical lines show LSD (5%, 10d.f.) for comparing means at different times, as calculated from the residual mean square obtained from the ANOVA.

For all genes, there was a significant improvement in the fit when choosing the critical exponential rather than the single exponential, but no significant improvement when choosing the double exponential over the critical exponential (data not shown). Simultaneous fitting of the critical exponential curve to the data for all five genes allowed a comparison of the fitted parameters, and hence the detection of degrees of commonality between the patterns of expression for the genes. This analysis identified that there was no significant improvement to the fit when allowing parameter R (related to the curvature of the response) to be different for the five genes, and so this parameter could be constrained to be the same. However, constraining the other three parameters to be the same across all five genes resulted in significantly worse fits, though for some pairs of genes the fitted (and derived) parameters did suggest some similarities (Table1). The different parameters (both fitted and derived) can be interpreted in terms of particular features of the shape of the response. The size of parameter C indicates the magnitude of the decline from the maximum expression response, whilst the ratio of B over C is related to the time to the maximum response. ParameterA measures the asymptotic response level after lengthy storage, A + B is the response at time t = 0, and the maximum response is dependent on all four parameters, obtained by inserting the time of maximum response into the critical exponential equation (Equation 1).

The analysis identified three distinct regulatory patterns (Figure 5). Cruciform DNA-binding protein and cytochrome P450II were identified as having similar shaped curves (similar values of C) and similar times of peak transcript levels (similar ratios of B over C), despite large differences in transcript magnitudes during this five-day period (different values of both A and A+B). Similarly, the transcript profiles of glucuronyl hydrolase and riboflavin aldehyde-forming enzyme shared a common curve shape (similar values of C) and similar transcript values for both the initial and asymptotic parts of the curve (similar values of both A andA+B). The time of maximum transcript level of each of these genes was later than for the other genes examined (larger ratios of B over C). The 5 day β(1–6) glucan synthase profile had a different curve shape with the earliest peak of transcript level (smallest ratio of B over C) followed by a rapid decline (largest value of C, smallest value of A).

Table 1 Critical exponential curve models for the transcription patterns of the 5 genes during long-term A. bisporus fruitbody post-harvest storage.

	Fitted parameters			Derived descriptors			
	A	B	C	A+B	-B/C	Time of maximum response (days)	Maximum response
CBP	1.886	-3.426	7.801	-1.540	0.439	1.814	1.753
CYP II	-2.572	-1.500	7.350	-4.072	0.204	1.579	0.633
GHYD	0.348	-3.049	2.125	-2.701	1.435	2.810	0.727
GSYN	-3.592	1.473	11.350	-2.119	-0.130	1.245	2.717
RAFE	-0.423	-1.896	2.585	-2.319	0.733	2.108	0.344

Fitted parameters for five genes (CBP = cruciform DNA-binding protein, CYP II = cytochrome P450II, GHYD = glucuronyl hydrolase, GSYN = β (1–6) glucan synthase, and RAFE = riboflavin aldehyde-forming enzyme) with parameter R constrained to be common across all five genes (R = 0.4832 (s.e. = 0.0288)). Additional descriptors of response shape derived from the fitted parameters.

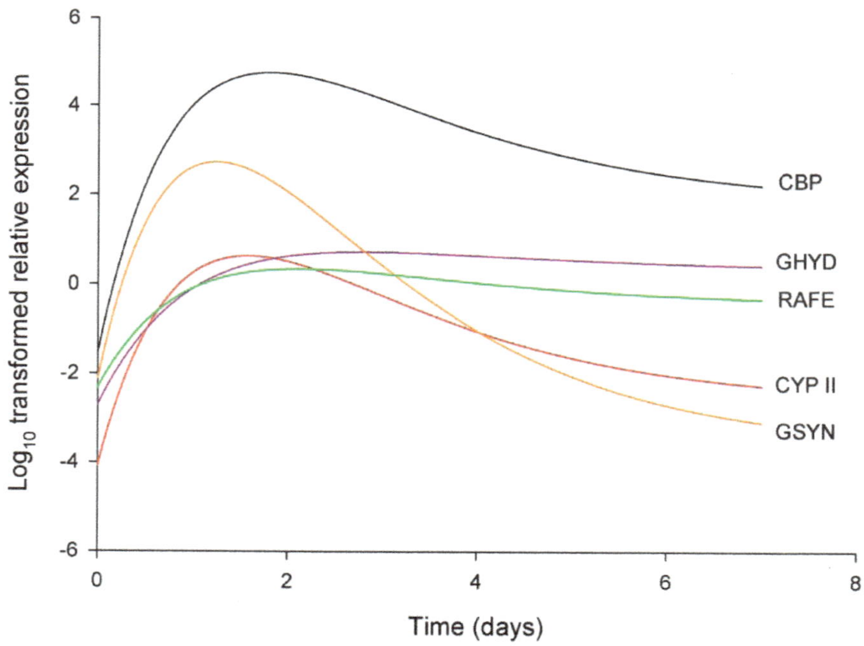

Figure 5 Critical exponential curve models for transcription patterns during 5 days post-harvest development. Sampling was conducted at 24 hour intervals. Models for $\log_{10}$-transformed qRT-PCR gene expression as given by Equation 1 with fitted

parameters as given in Table 1. CBP (black line) = cruciform DNA-binding protein, CYPII (red line) = cytochrome P450II, GHYD (blue line) = glucuronyl hydrolase, GSYN (orange line) = β (1–6) glucan synthase, and RAFE (green line) = riboflavin aldehyde-forming enzyme.

Transcript expression between tissues (A. bisporus)

Transcript levels of each gene were measured in stipe, cap and gill tissues of harvested mushrooms over 2 days storage, using qRT-PCR (Figure 6). Differences in transcript levels, between tissues, between storage times and due to the interaction of these two factors, were assessed using ANOVA. Average transcript levels of cruciform DNA-binding protein, cytochrome P450II, glucuronyl hydrolase and β (1–6) glucan synthase in stipe and cap tissues were similar and significantly higher than in the gills. For riboflavin aldehyde-forming enzyme, transcript levels were significantly higher in the stipe tissue compared with the cap or gills, which had similar levels. Despite differences in transcript levels observed between the tissues, all genes showed an increased level of expression in all tissues from day 0 to 2.

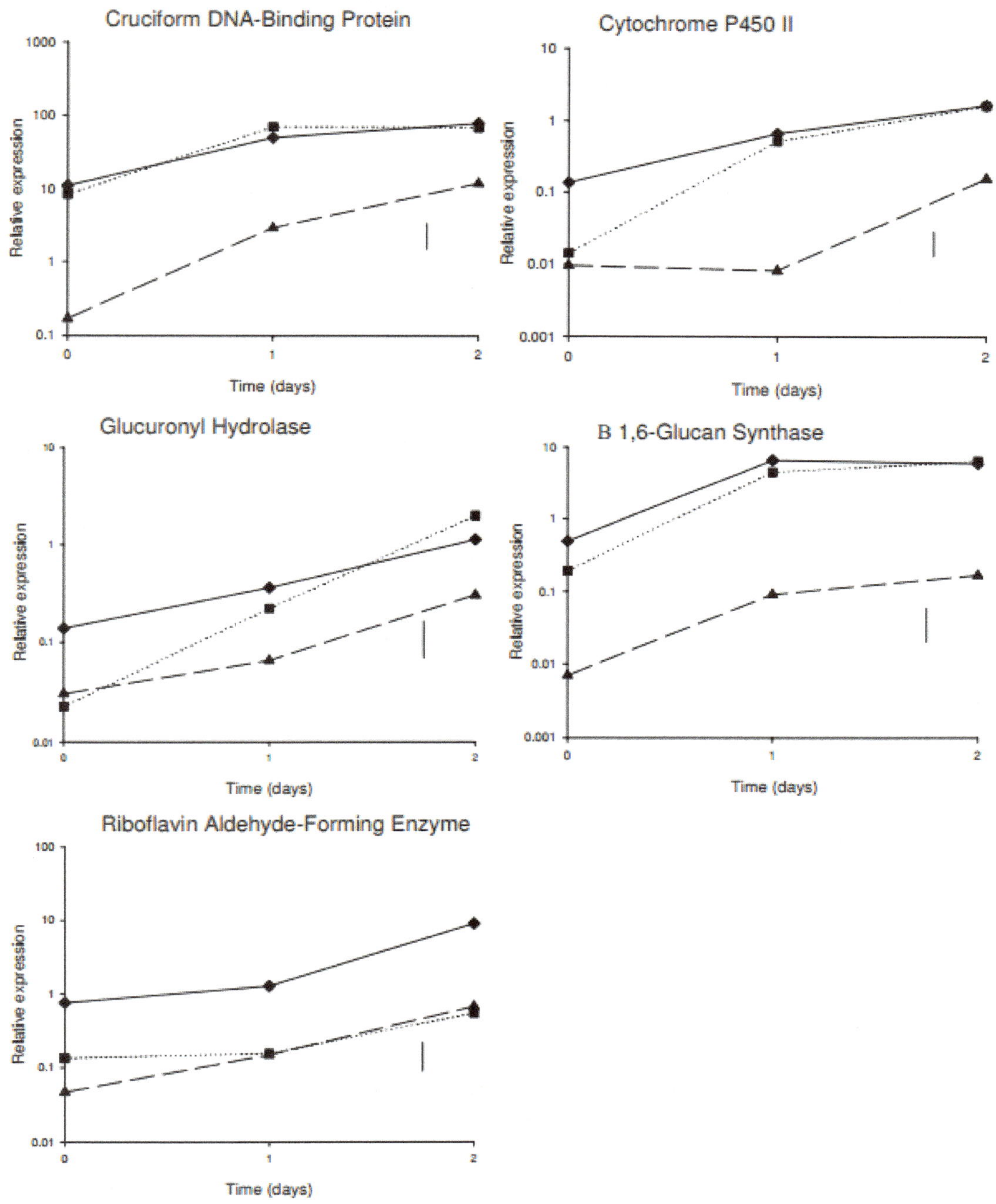

Figure 6 Gene expression in stipe, cap and gill tissues post-harvest. Mean qRT-PCR (log_{10}-transformed) measurements of gene expression of the 5 selected genes at 24 hour intervals post-harvest for 2 days, where mushrooms were dissected into stipe (◆), cap (■) and gill (▲) tissue. Vertical lines show LSD (5%, 16d.f.) for comparing means for different combinations of time and tissue, as calculated from the residual mean square obtained from the ANOVA.

Application of regression approaches to microarray datasets (E. coli and R. norvegicus)

Regression analyses were applied to time course profiles obtained from two published microarray datasets [21, 22]. Gene responses of E. coli to treatment with paraquat [21] were analysed by fitting an exponential function. From over 10,000 features on the microarray the profiles for 11% were described well by the exponential function, with significance levels of $p < 0.05$; 2% of the gene profiles fitted with significance levels of $p < 0.001$ (Figure 7).

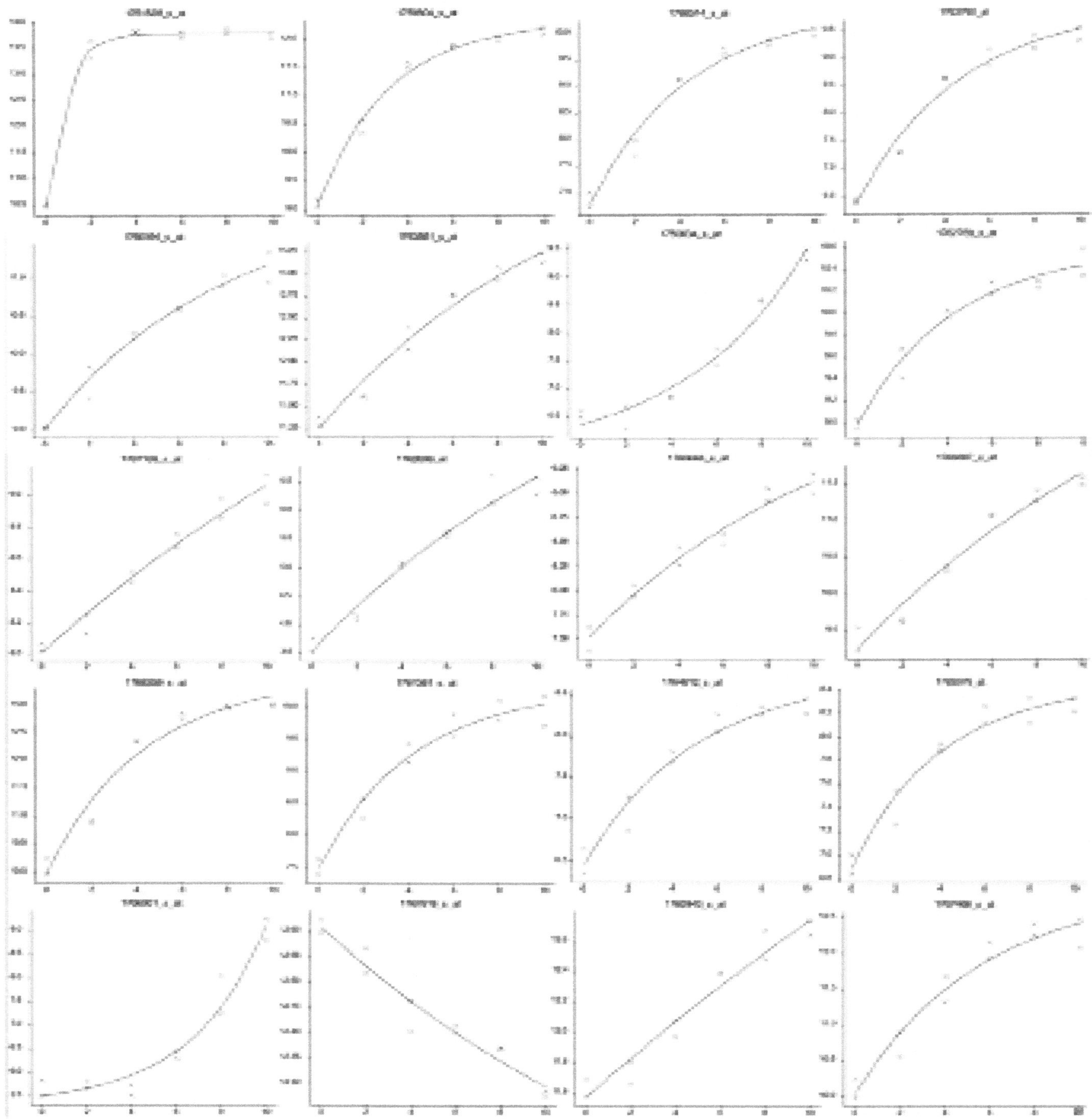

Figure 7 Gene expression profiles from E. coli microarray study. Fitted exponential curves for the 20 best fitting profiles together with observed data. Horizontal axis is time in minutes, vertical axis is log (base 2) expression value.

The critical exponential function was fitted to the gene time-course responses in the rat liver tissue to the corticosteroid, methylprednisolone, [22]. The R. norvegicus microarray (Affymetrix GeneChips Rat Genome U34A) consisted of 7000 full length sequences and over 1000 expressed sequence tagged clusters. From over 8000 features on the microarray, the profiles for over 25% were described well by the critical exponential ($p < 0.05$), with over 9% with significant levels of $p < 0.001$ (Figure 8).

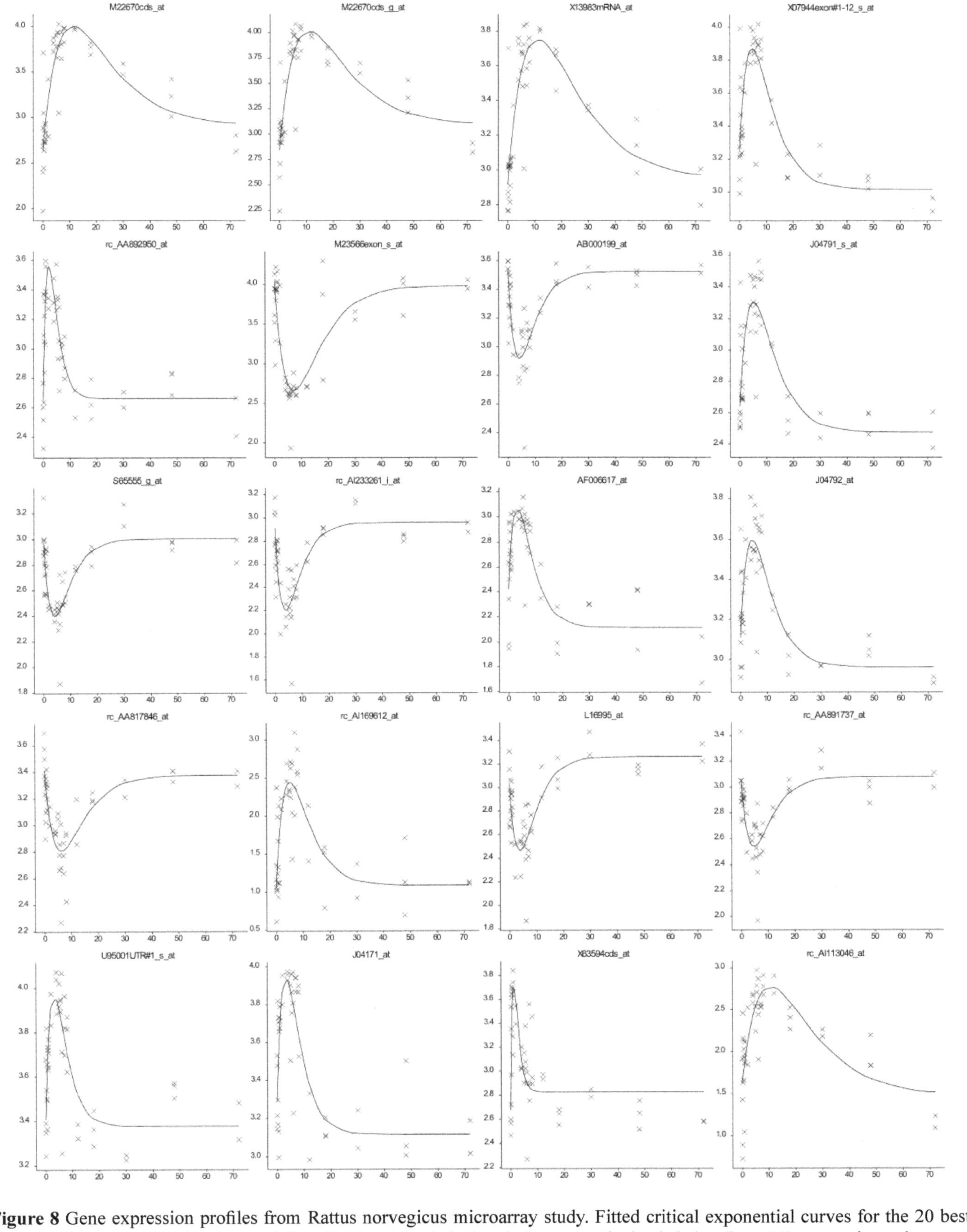

Figure 8 Gene expression profiles from Rattus norvegicus microarray study. Fitted critical exponential curves for the 20 best fitting profiles together with observed data. Horizontal axis is time in hours, vertical axis is log (base 10) expression value.

For both studies the chosen functions allow the description of a number of distinct forms of response. The fitted responses for the 20 most significant fits from each study demonstrate the variety of profiles that can be described by each of these models (Figures 7 and 8).

Discussion

Gene expression studies were conducted to investigate the benefit of applying statistical regression approaches to the fitting of mathematical models for the analysis of transcriptional data. In this study these approaches have been developed using precisely measured transcript levels for a small number of genes and application of the approaches has been further demonstrated for microarray datasets. As microarray technologies continue to be developed, the variability of gene expression data from such technologies will be reduced, leading to the widespread application of the regression modelling techniques developed in this study, thus allowing the comparative analysis of larger numbers of gene expression profiles. A range of statistical regression techniques, both linear and non-linear, are readily available. The selection of appropriate techniques is critically dependent on the specific question being addressed and the data that are collected.

For A. bisporus, the increases in transcript levels in the first 24 hours following harvest are largely due to transcription rather than losses due to mRNA turnover. ‹Split-line or ‹broken-stick› regression analysis was used to calculate the time when transcription was initiated, at 13.5 h post-harvest for cytochrome P450II and 16.5 h post-harvest for glucuronyl hydrolase. The novel application of this approach to transcript profiling demonstrates the potential value of this simple mathematical model which has been used previously in such diverse applications as estimating the thresholds for patch size in ecological studies [23], humidity levels in plant pathogen germination experiments [24] and the mineral density of bones [25]. Successful application of the ‹split-line› or ‹broken-stick› model for cruciform DNA-binding protein and β (1–6) glucan synthase would require more sampling points to be made in the first 6 hours to provide sufficient time points to allow the fitting of the baseline response, zero-slope line, and hence allow estimation of the time of initial transcription. For the riboflavin aldehyde-forming enzyme further data are needed beyond 24 hours (but still at 3-hour intervals) to allow estimation of the second linear regression segment, and to again allow calculation of the time of initial transcription.

The time of increased transcription for at least 4 of the 5 tested genes occurs at different times in the first 24 hours post-harvest. This suggests that the response of the mushroom to harvest is not under the control of a single regulatory pathway, such as the signal transduction pathways described for fungal oxidative and osmotic stress responses [26]. The controlling events in the mushroom are likely to be affected by a range of stimuli, such as stress, nutrient limitation, continued maturation and spore formation, which might illicit both primary or immediate responses, and secondary responses. Here we observed increased transcription first of cruciform DNA-binding protein (approximately 3–6 h), followed by β (1–6) glucan synthase (approximately 9 h), cytochrome P450II (13.5 h), glucuronyl hydrolase (16.5 h) and riboflavin aldehyde-forming enzyme (> 24 h). Cruciform DNA-binding protein and β (1–6) glucan synthase may be part of a primary response, while cytochrome P450II, glucuronyl hydrolase and riboflavin aldehyde-forming enzyme are from a secondary response or caused by a later stimulus.

Statistical regression modelling showed similar expression patterns for two A. bisporus genes, glucuronyl hydrolase and riboflavin aldehyde-forming enzyme, the latter of which is known to be up-regulated during the development of the non-harvested mushroom [20]. Further study is required to determine whether the common pattern observed between the genes post-harvest is also observed in the morphogenesis of the non-harvested fruiting body. The pattern of β (1–6) glucan synthase gene expression during 5 days storage was different from the other genes studied, with transcript levels falling greatly after 2 d following an initial increase in gene expression. The gene has been hypothesised to be involved in cell wall synthesis [12]. The initial increase in gene expression coincides with the period when hyphae in the cap and stipe elongate, i.e. in the first 2 days post-harvest, a process for which cell wall synthesis is important. Similarly, the reduction in expression after day 2 coincides with the cessation of cell wall synthesis following the full extension of the cap [27, 28].

The fitted critical exponential models for the 5-day profiles of cruciform DNA-binding protein and cytochrome P450II had similar shapes, whilst the times of initial transcriptional increase for these two genes, as determined by split-line regressions, were markedly different (3–6 h and 13.5 h respectively). This apparent paradox illustrates the importance of considering transcript responses over a number of different time-scales. The precise function of cruciform DNA-binding protein is not known, however, it is unlikely to be involved in recombination as transcript levels are low in the gill tissue where meiosis occurs. In other organisms, proteins with similar cruciform DNA-binding activity (i.e. HMG proteins) cause the increased and decreased transcription of genes [29, 30]. It is possible that the early and abundant transcription of cruciform DNA-binding protein in A. bisporus fruiting bodies acts to regulate the expression of other genes.

The spatial transcript levels were different between tissues and for all genes were significantly lower in the gill tissue, indicating a physiological difference from the stipe and cap. The gills are actively growing, respiring and producing spores via meiosis. They are a nutrient ‹sink› and are therefore physiologically different from the stipe and cap tissues, which export nutrients and are subject to stress from cell damage. However the increased respiration in gill tissue [31, 28] may result in increased ribosomal, and therefore 18S rRNA, levels, to which transcript levels from qRT-PCR are normalised, so the quantitative differences between gills and stipe/cap tissues may be influenced by this. While pairs of genes showed similar patterns of response when described using the critical exponential model, the spatial distribution of transcripts between different tissues varied in some cases. For example, cytochrome P450II and cruciform DNA-binding protein showed similar overall patterns, but cytochrome P450II showed a delayed initial increase in transcription in the gill tissue. Further and more detailed studies of the expression of these genes in the separate tissues are needed to understand the potentially different regulatory mechanisms acting in each tissue.

The use of a statistical non-linear regression approach to model the gene expression profiles over an extended period offers the opportunity to compare the shapes of the response curves between genes. The critical exponential curve, selected by the observed response shapes and goodness of fit, can be explained in terms of the combination of two processes, in this case RNA synthesis and degradation. A more complex model for such a situation would be the double exponential curve, which is a natural function for a two-timescale process. The critical exponential is the degenerate case of this model and occurs when two processes in a system have the same timescale. In this case, however, there was no evidence for choosing the more complex model. Choice of an appropriate model can be important, but many common non-linear models are based on functional forms derived from observed biological processes. Increased gene transcription is responsible for the initial rapid increase in transcript levels between days 0 to 2. Transcript levels continue to rise until a maximum is reached, followed by a decline towards a steady level, possibly as a consequence of a balance between transcription and degradation (transcript turnover). The critical exponential model was successful in identifying genes with quantitatively similar patterns of response, which could not have been predicted from their putative protein functions. This approach, therefore, offers a new method by which a large number of genes could be classified according to their initial transcription regulation and subsequent turnover.

Our approach to first model and then cluster allows more genes to be considered and potentially a greater insight to understand the system. The application of this approach to a microarray dataset allows the screening of genes to identify responses that can be described by a particular mathematical function. Thus each gene profile is reduced from noisy observations to a smaller set of biologically-interpretable parameters. In the analysis of the microarray datasets, different shapes of profiles fitted by the exponential or critical exponential functions can be identified (Figures 7 &8), allowing the grouping of genes based on the parameter values. Eliminating the inherent variability in the data through the regression modelling approach allows a more precise comparison of gene profiles and thus improved clustering. For example, the 9% of R. norvegicus genes identified that followed the critical exponential curve at the $p < 0.001$ level represents approx 720 genes compared with the 200 genes identified and modelled by Jin et al (2003) [22]. The groupings of genes then generated by the improved clustering propose hypotheses of regulatory association between genes. For example, the aim of the E. coli microarray study was to identify those genes co-regulated with the main regulatory gene, sox S, which was demonstrated to have an exponential-type response following the application of paraquat [21]. By using an initial regression analysis to identify the subset of genes that can be described by an exponential function, subsequent cluster analyses can focus on this subset of genes with similar, but not identical (see Figure 7), shapes of expression profiles. The fitted exponential function parameters for this gene subset could then be used to better identify those genes most closely co-regulated with sox S. Whilst our study demonstrates the application of a regression modelling approach to describe gene expression profiles, this approach can be expanded to fully exploit microarray datasets. Application of a wider range of functional forms (for example including functions with similar shapes but also some temporal variation or time delays) offers the potential to develop regulatory networks based on relationships between the shapes of expression profiles as captured by the fitted parameters. Further interpretation of the parameters, alongside knowledge of gene function, might allow the identification of the stimuli driving the observed gene expression responses.

Compared with standard clustering for gene profiles of microarray data, the statistical regression modelling of mathematical functions to describe these profiles eliminates the inherent variability in the data and allows the direct comparison of profile shapes.

CONCLUSION

This study has illustrated how the use of standard statistical modelling approaches (analysis of variances (ANOVA), linear regression modelling, non-linear regression modelling) commonly used in plant, microbial and ecological sciences, can be used to aid and extend the interpretation of gene expression profiles obtained from qRT-PCR. These approaches have been applied to model profiles of larger numbers of genes obtained from expression microarray studies, and could be further applied to other high-throughput "-omic" technologies. A wide range of statistical approaches have been specifically developed to analyse the vast quantities of data generated in microarray-based studies [32], assessing both similarities and differences between genes and between treatments. Similarly a number of approaches have been developed to generate mathematical models for assumed networks of gene pathways (based on simple mathematical assumptions) [33, 34].

However, there appears to have been little statistical consideration for the detailed modelling of individual gene expression profiles. The statistical regression modelling approaches applied in this study allow the estimation of parameters which succinctly describe the shapes of gene expression profiles. These parameter estimates (or combinations of them) can then be related directly to the processes stimulating and driving the expression of these genes. Comparison of the parameters and expression profiles for a set of genes could then indicate that a sub-set of these genes are co-regulated, with the potential to hypothesise a common regulatory mechanism. Hence, consideration of a wide range of non-linear regression models could provide building blocks for the development of more biologically realistic models of gene expression profiles.

METHODS

Agaricus bisporus strain A15 (Sylvan, UK) was used throughout the study. Mushrooms were grown on composted wheat straw according to commercial practice at the Warwick HRI BioConversion Unit. Mushrooms were harvested at morphogenetic stage 2 [31] and were either frozen immediately under liquid nitrogen, termed time 0, or stored for a specified period in a controlled environment, 18°C and 95–95% relative humidity, before freezing under liquid nitrogen. Stored mushrooms were sampled for gene expression profiling over i) 0 to 24 hour time course post-harvest (three hourly intervals), ii) 0 to 5 day time course following harvest (24 hourly intervals), and iii) 0 to 48 hours post-harvest (24 hour intervals), with mushrooms dissected into stipe, cap and gill tissues. Three replicate mushrooms were taken for each sampling point and frozen samples were stored at -80°C.

RNA isolation

RNA was isolated from mushroom tissues according to established phenol/chloroform extraction protocols [35]. Absorbance measurement at 260 nm and 280 nm were used to assess RNA concentration and purity. RNA integrity was determined with formaldehyde agarose gel electrophoresis [36]. For experiments involving reverse transcriptase, RNA samples were treated with RQ1 RNAse-free DNAse enzyme (Promega, Southampton, UK) according to manufacturer's instructions

Quantitative RT-PCR (qRT-PCR)

Transcript levels were determined using the ABI Prism 7900 HT sequence detector (TaqMan™) and SYBR®Green fluorescent reporter dye. Reverse transcription was carried out using the Thermoscript™ RT-PCR system (Invitrogen, Life Technologies, Paisley, UK) in 20 µl volumes containing 50 ngµl^{-1} random hexamers, 1 µg total RNA, 1 µl Thermoscript reverse transcriptase (15 U µl^{-1}), 4 µl 5× Thermoscript™ buffer, 1 µl 0.1 M DTT and 1 µl RNaseOUT™ (40 U µl^{-1}). Reactions were carried out at 25°C for 10 minutes, followed by 50 minutes at 50°C and terminated at 85°C for 5 minutes. Each cDNA sample was treated with RNAse H according to manufacturer's instructions and diluted to 100 µl final volume. cDNA samples were taken from three replicate mushrooms per time point.

PCR reactions were performed in 15 µl volumes consisting of 1 µM of each primer, 20 ng of cDNA sample and 7.5 µl of 2× SYBR® Green PCR Mix (Applied Biosystems, Warrington, UK). All sample and standard reactions were carried out in triplicate. PCR cycling conditions consisted of one cycle of 50°C for 2 min and 95°C for 10 min followed by 40 cycles 95°C 15 sec and 60°C for 1 min. This was followed by a dissociation step of 95°C for 15 sec, 60°C for 15 sec and increase to 95°C with a 2% ramp rate. The dissociation step was used for melting curve analysis in order to detect primer dimers and non-specific products in the reaction. Standard curves were generated for each gene using cDNA (0.625 ngµl^{-1} to 20 ngµl^{-1}) from a whole 2-day stored mushroom, which contains large amounts of target transcripts. The primer sets used (Table 2) were designed from cDNA sequence information for each gene [12] using the Primer Express® software version 2.0 Applied Biosystems, Warrington, UK).

Table 2 Oligonucleotides used in the qPCR for the selected Agaricus bisporus genes

Gene	Oligonucleotide	Amplicon length (bp)
Cruciform DNA-binding protein	Forward: 5'-CGCTGGTGAAGCTGAGAACA-3'	74
	Reverse: 5'- CAGCGATTTGGTCCGTCATA-3'	
Cytochrome P450II	Forward: 5'-GCCGATATTTGCTCTGAATGC-3'	75
	Reverse: 5'- GCGCAGGCTTGATATCGAA-3'	
β (1–6) Glucan synthase	Forward: 5'-TCAATCTTCTTGATGCTCATTGC-3'	70
	Reverse: 5'- TGCGCAAACAACCTATTCC-3'	
Glucuronyl hydrolase	Forward: 5'-TGATGGAATTGTACCATGGGATT-3'	74
	Reverse: 5'- AGCGATAGTTGCTGCTGAAGAA-3'	
Riboflavin aldehyde-forming enzyme	Forward: 5'-CGGCAGCGGAGACCATT-3'	65
	Reverse: 5'- TGACTTTCACGTATTTGCTTTGT-3'	
18S rRNA	Forward: 5'-ACAACGAGACCTTAACCTGCTAA-3'	78
	Reverse: 5'- GACGCTGACAGTCCCTCTAAGAA-3'	

Data analysis utilised the ABI PRISM sequence detector® software (SDS) (version 2.0) to determine the cycle threshold of each sample (Ct-Target) which was normalised to the cycle threshold of the 18S rRNA qRT-PCR product (Ct-Control) for the same sample [37, 38]. The ΔCt equation ($\Delta Ct = 2^{(CtControl-CtTarget)}$) was used to calculate the amount of each target transcript relative to the amount of 18S rRNA.

The control treatments were (a) water control using sterilised diethylpyrocarbonate (DEPC)-treated water in the place of the cDNA sample to detect environmental DNA contamination and primer-based artefacts (b) DNAse-treated RNA to assess for contaminating DNA in the RNA samples, and (c) the absence of primers during the reverse transcription step, but present during PCR, to detect contaminating DNA and the possibility of active reverse transcriptase present during PCR.

Northern hybridisation analysis

Total RNA, ~10 µg, from each sample was separated by formaldehyde agarose gel electrophoresis and immobilised onto nylon membranes as per established protocols [35]. Hybridisation was carried out using randomly primed [α-^{32}P]

dCTP probes and post-hybridisation washes carried out using established protocols [35]. To produce the probes, phagemid clones containing the cDNAs were restricted with Hin dIII and Bam HI and fragments separated by agarose gel electrophoresis, excised and purified using the Qiagen gel purification protocol. Purified fragments were used as templates for random priming incorporating [α-^{32}P] dCTP (Redi prime kit, Amersham Pharmacia Biotech., Buckinghamshire, UK). Agaricus bisporus 28S rRNA gene was used as a loading control as described previously [12, 39]. Hybridisation intensity of each gene-specific probe used in Northern analysis was determined using scanning densitometry (Personal Densitometer SI, Molecular Dynamics, CA, USA). Transcript levels for each gene were calculated relative to the hybridisation intensity recorded for the 28S rRNA gene probe for each sample tested. Northern analysis was performed on total RNA from two replicate mushrooms per time sample or time × tissue sample for transcripts of each gene examined.

Statistical analysis

Comparisons of the transcript levels, as determined by Northern analysis scanning densitometry and qRT-PCR, were made for each gene by calculating correlation coefficients, and by fitting linear and exponential regression responses to explain the Northern analysis measurements in terms of those from the qRT-PCR. Within each experiment, two replicate Northern analysis measurements were paired with the qRT-PCR values obtained from the same replicate mushroom RNA extracts (note that for one replicate of each sampling point within each experiment no Northern analysis measurement was obtained).

Quantitative RT-PCR data of transcription levels for each gene were analysed using analysis of variance (ANOVA) for each experiment (0–24 h, 0–5d and 0–48 h between different tissues) separately. Three replicate mushrooms were assayed at each time or for each tissue-by-time combination. Prior to analysis, the data were subjected to a logarithm (base 10) transformation to satisfy the ANOVA assumption of homogeneity of variance. The significance of the overall treatment effects (time only in two experiments, time, tissue and the interaction between these factors in the third) was assessed using an F-test, and the significance of differences between individual treatment means was assessed by comparison with appropriate standard errors of differences (SEDs). Treatment differences noted in the text are significant at the 5% level unless stated otherwise.

For the qRT-PCR data only, regression analyses were used to model the gene expression changes over time. 'Split-line' or 'broken-stick' regression analysis of transcription levels from 0–24 h was applied to estimate the time when the up-regulation of each gene commenced. The 'broken-stick' model consists of two linear regression segments fitted to distinct subsets of the data, with separate estimates of slope and intercept for each segment. In this case the first line segment was constrained to have a slope of zero. A sequence of models was fitted to the data for each gene, splitting the data set into two parts (time $\leq$ xhours: time > x hours, for each of the observed values of x). The best model for each gene was chosen as the one with the minimum sum of residual sums of squares for the two regressions. The time point where the two lines crossed was postulated as the time when increased gene transcription began. The long-term gene transcript profiles (0–5d) were modelled using the critical exponential curve (Equation 1), fitted to the $\log_{10}$-transformed data.

$$y(t) = A + (B + Ct)R^{t} + \varepsilon \qquad (1)$$

where A, B, C and R are parameters, y is the gene expression response ($\log_{10}$ transformed), t is storage time, and ε represents the errors, assumed to follow a Normal distribution with mean zero and a constant variance. This form of curve was selected following an initial graphing of the responses, as it can be used to describe a rapidly increasing phase followed by a decline or plateau, and after assessment of how well it fitted the observed data compared with both the simpler exponential model and the more complex double exponential model. The parameters of this non-linear response can be interpreted in terms of a postulated mechanism driving the observed gene expression responses, in this case potentially quantifying the relationship between transcript synthesis and degradation. The fitted parameters, and hence the shapes of the fitted curves, were compared between genes using a parallel curves analysis, either constraining each parameter to be the same across all five genes, or allowing variation in the values taken by each parameter between genes. This analysis provides a basis for comparing a sequence of possible models, and assessment of the change in residual variance between models allows the most appropriate model for the observed data to be determined.

Application of regression modelling to microarray datasets

The regression modelling approach was applied to publicly-available microarray datasets from different organisms (E. coli and R. norvegicus), previously published [21, 22]. The datasets were selected as having an appropriate time course with a fixed time point at which a treatment was applied generating an expression response, with evidence that gene profiles could be described by a standard response function. For the E. coli study [21] the master regulatory gene sox S demonstrated an exponential-type response to the application of paraquat. To identify all genes with a similar exponential shape of response, an exponential function was fitted using the regression modelling approach to all gene expression profiles from this microarray study, and the significance of each fit was determined. Similarly, a number of genes from R. norvegicus liver tissue treated with corticosteroid displayed profiles appearing to follow the same critical exponential curve as fitted to the A. bisporus data (Equation 1) [22]. The critical exponential function was thus fitted to all genes in this dataset to determine the proportion of gene profiles that were adequately described by this function.

DECLARATIONS

Acknowledgements

Funding was provided by the UK Government Department for Food and Rural Affairs (DEFRA) project HH2116SMU.

Authors' contributions

DCE participated in the design of the study, prepared all samples, carried out molecular genetic studies and drafted the manuscript. AM carried out statistical analysis and helped draft the manuscript. MJS participated in the design of the study and aided in molecular genetic studies. KSB conceived of the study, participated in its design and helped to draft the manuscript.

REFERENCES

1. Dopazo J, Zanders E, Dragoni I, Amphlett G, Falciani F: Methods and approaches in the analysis of gene expression data. J Immunol Methods 2001, 250(1–2):93-112. 10.1016/S0022-1759(01)00307-6..
2. Tamames J, Clark D, Herrero J, Dopazo J, Blaschke C, Fernandez JM, Oliveros JC, Valencia A: Bioinformatics methods for the analysis of expression arrays: data clustering and information extraction. J Biotechnol 2002, 98: 269-283. 10.1016/S0168-1656(02)00137-2..
3. Reimers M: Statistical analysis of microarray data. Addict Biol 2005, 10: 23-35. 10.1080/13556210412331327795..
4. Tai YC, Speed TP: A multivariate empirical Bayes statistic for replicated microarray time course data. Ann Stat 2006,34(6):2387-2412. 10.1214/009053606000000759..
5. Manfield IW, Jen CH, Pinney JW, Michalopoulos I, Bradford JR, Gilmartin PM, Westhead DR: Arabidopsis Co-expression Tool (ACT): web server tools for microarray-based gene expression analysis. Nucleic Acids Res 2006, 34:504-509. 10.1093/nar/gkl204..
6. Persson S, Wei H, Milne J, Page GR, Somerville CR: Identification of genes required for cellulose synthesis by regression analysis of public microarray data sets. Proc Natl Acad Sci USA 2005, 102(24):8633-8638. 10.1073/pnas.0503392102..
7. Conesa A, Neuda MJ, Ferrer A, Talön M: maSigPro: A method to identify significantly differential expression profiles in time-course microarray experiments. Bioinformatics 2006, 22(9):1096-1102. 10.1093/bioinformatics/btl056..
8. Heard NA, Holmes CC, Stephens DA: A quantitative study of gene regulation involved in the immune response of Anopheline mosquitoes: An application of Bayesian hierarchical clustering of curves. J Am Stat Assoc 2006,101(473):18-29. 10.1198/016214505000000187..
9. Kahnin R, Vinciotti V, Mersinias V, Smith CP, Wit P: Statistical reconstruction of transcription factor activity using Michaelis-Menten kinetics. Biometrics 2007, 63(3):816-823. 10.1111/j.1541-0420.2007.00757.x..
10. Nachman I, Regev A, Friedman N: Inferring quantitative models of regulatory networks from expression data. Bioinformatics 2004, 20(suppl 1):i248-i256. 10.1093/bioinformatics/bth941..
11. Liss B: Improved quantitative real-time RT-PCR for expression profiling of individual cells. Nucleic Acids Res 2002,30(17):89-98. 10.1093/nar/gnf088..
12. Eastwood DC, Kingsnorth CS, Jones HJ, Burton KS: Genes with increased transcript levels following harvest of the sporophore of Agaricus bisporus have multiple physiological roles. Mycol Res 2001, 105(10):1223-123. 10.1016/S0953-7562(08)61993-0..
13. Kingsnorth CS, Eastwood DC, Burton KS: Cloning and post-harvest expression of serine proteinase transcripts in the cultivated mushroom Agaricus bisporus . Fungal Gen Biol 2001, 32: 135-144. 10.1006/fgbi.2001.1257..
14. Wagemaker MJM, Eastwood DC, Wellboren W, Burton KS, Drift C, Jetten MSM, Van Griensven LJLD, Op Den Camp HJM: Argininosuccinate synthetase and argininosuccinate lyase: two ornithine cycle enzymes from Agaricus bisporus . Mycol Res 2007, 111: 493-502. 10.1016/j.mycres.2007.01.016..
15. Miyazaki Y, Nakamura M, Babasaki K: Molecular cloning of developmentally specific genes by representational difference analysis during fruiting body formation in the basidiomycete Lentinula edodes . Fungal Gen Biol 2005, 42:493-505. 10.1016/j.fgb.2005.03.003..
16. Lee S-H, Kim B-G, Kim K-J, Lee J-S, Yun D-W, Hahn J-H, Kim G-H, Lee K-H, Suh D-S, Kwon S-T, Lee C-S, Yoo Y-B:Comparative analysis of sequences expressed during liquid-cultured mycelia and fruit body stages of Pleurotus ostreatus . Fungal Gen Biol 2002, 35: 115-134. 10.1006/fgbi.2001.1310..
17. Yamada M, Sakuraba S, Shibata K, Taguchi G, Inatomi S, Okazaki M, Shimosaka M: Isolation and analysis of genes specifically expressed during fruiting body development in the basidiomycete Flammulina velutipes by fluorescence differential display. FEMS Microbiol Lett 2006, 254: 165-172. 10.1111/j.1574-6968.2005.00023.x..
18. Kues U: Life history and developmental processes in the basidiomycete Coprinus cinereus . Microbiol Mol Biol Rev2000, 64(2):316-353. 10.1128/MMBR.64.2.316-353.2000..
19. Kamada T: Molecular genetics of sexual development in the mushroom Coprinus cinereus . BioEssays 2002, 24: 449-459. 10.1002/bies.10083..
20. Sreenivasaprasad S, Eastwood DC, Browning N, Lewis SMJ, Burton KS: Differential expression of a putative riboflavin-aldehyde-forming enzyme (raf) gene during development and post-harvest storage and in different tissue of the sporophore in Agaricus bisporus . Appl Microbiol Biotechnol 2006, 70: 470-476. 10.1007/s00253-005-0084-9..
21. Blanchard JL, Wholey W-Y, Conlon EM, Pomposiello PJ: Rapid changes in gene expression dynamics in response to superoxide reveal SoxRS-dependent and independent transcriptional networks. PLoS ONE 2007, 2(11):e1186. 10.1371/journal.pone.0001186..
22. Jin JY, Almon RR, Dubois DC, Jusko J: Modelling of corticosteroid pharmacogenomics in rat liver using gene microarrays. J Pharmacol Exp Ther 2003, 307: 93-109. 10.1124/jpet.103.053256..
23. Bascampte J, Rodriguez MA: Habitat patchiness and plant species richness. Ecol Lett 2001, 4: 417-420. 10.1046/j.1461-0248.2001.00242.x..
24. Carroll JE, Wilcox WF: Effects of humidity on the development of grapevine powdery mildew. Phytopathology 2003,93: 1137-1144. 10.1094/

PHYTO.2003.93.9.1137..

25. Price RI, Walters MJ, Retallack RW, Henderson NK, Kerr D, Henzell S, Dhaliwal S, Prince RL: Impact of the analysis of a bone density reference range on determination of the T-score. J Clin Densitom 2003, 6(1):51-62. 10.1385/JCD:6:1:51..

26. Ikner A, Shiozaki K: Yeast signalling pathways in oxidative stress response. Mutat Res-Fund Mol Mech Mutagen 2005,569(1–2):13-27. 10.1016/j.mrfmmm.2004.09.006..

27. Umar MH, van Griensven LJLD: Morphological studies on the life span, development stages, senescence and death of fruiting bodies of Agaricus bisporus . Mycol Res 1997, 101: 1409-1422. 10.1017/S0953756297005212..

28. Braaksma A, van Doorn AA, Kieft H, van Aelist AC: Morphometric analysis of ageing mushrooms (Agaricus bisporus) during post-harvest development. Postharvest Biol Technol 1998, 13: 71-79. 10.1016/S0925-5214(97)00069-0..

29. Ge H, Roeder RG: The high-mobility group protein HMG1 can reversibly inhibit class-II gene-transcription by interaction with the TATA-binding protein. J Biol Chem 1994, 269(25):17136-17140.PubMed

30. Stros M, Ozaki T, Bacikova A, Kageyama H, Nakagawara A: HMGB1 and HMGB2 cell-specifically down-regulate the p53-and p-73-dependant sequence-specific transactivation from the human Bax gene promoter. J Biol Chem 2002,277(9):7157-7164. 10.1074/jbc.M110233200..

31. Hammond JBW, Nichols R: Changes in respiration and carbohydrates during the post-harvest storage of mushrooms (Agaricus bisporus). J Sci Food Agric 1975, 26: 835-842. 10.1002/jsfa.2740260615..

32. Stekel D: Microarray Bioinformatics. Cambridge University Press, Cambridge, UK; 2003..

33. Rangel C, Angus J, Ghahramani Z, Lioumi M, Sotheran E, Gaiba A, Wild DL, Falciani F: Modelling T-cell activation using gene expression profiling and state-space models. Bioinformatics 2004, 20(9):1361-1372. 10.1093/bioinformatics/bth093..

34. Beal MJ, Falciani F, Ghahramani Z, Rangel C, Wild DL: A Bayesian approach to reconstructing genetic regulatory networks with hiddenfactors. Bioinformatics 2005, 21(3):349-356. 10.1093/bioinformatics/bti014..

35. Sambrook J, Russell DW: Molecular cloning: a laboratory manual. 3rd edition. Cold Spring Harbor Laboratory Press, Cold Spring Harbor, NY; 2001.

36. Rosen KM, Villa-Komaroff L: An alternative method for the visualization of RNA in formaldehyde agarose gels. Focus1993, 12(2):23-24.

37. Goidin D, Mamessier A, Statquet M.-J, Schmitt D, Berthier-Vergnes O: Ribosomal 18S RNA prevails over Glyceraldehyde-3-phosphate dehydrogenase and β-actin genes as internal standards for quantitative comparison of mRNA levels in invasive and noninvasive human melanoma cell subpopulations. Anal Biochem 2000, 295(1):17-21. 10.1006/abio.2001.5171..

38. Lekanne Deprez RH, Fijnvandraat AC, Ruijter JM, Moorman AFM: Sensitivity and accuracy of quantitative real-time polymerase chain reaction using SYBR green I depends on cDNA synthesis conditions. Anal Biochem 2002,307(1):63-69. 10.1016/S0003-2697(02)00021-0..

39. de Groot PWJ, Schaap PJ, van Griensven LJLD, Visser J: Isolation of developmentally regulated genes from the edible mushroom Agaricus bisporus . Microbiology 1997, 143: 1993-2001..

CHAPTER 4

LESSONS FROM DWARF8 ON THE STRENGTHS AND WEAKNESSES OF STRUCTURED ASSOCIATION MAPPING

Sara J. Larsson, Alexander E. Lipka, Edward S. Buckler

INTRODUCTION

Association mapping, which was developed as a necessity for large-scale human studies, is commonly used in conjunction with family (linkage) mapping in plant and animal genetic studies. The application of association mapping for plants was originally assessed in Thornsberry J.M. (2001) [1] with Buckler as senior author. It was concluded that association mapping offers higher resolution than linkage mapping due to quicker linkage disequilibrium (LD) decay, that structured association mapping is crucial for controlling false positives arising from population structure, and that Dwarf8 (d8) (RefGen_v2 position: Chr. 1; 266,094,769–266,097,836 bp) is associated with flowering time. This initial study has been cited extensively, and has been the basis of several reanalyses of d8. New data and statistical tools give us the opportunity to reevaluate this locus. Results show that the d8 associations reported by Thornsberry et al. (2001) are likely false positives (i.e., spurious associations), which resulted from insufficient correction of population structure. Indeed, the application of association mapping to animal and plant studies has been very successful, culminating in many important findings [2]–[10]. In this light, the Thornsberry et al (2001) study has attracted a lot of interest to the area and led to more studies and the development of techniques to control for population structure and familial relatedness. When the phenotype is strongly correlated with population structure (e.g., flowering time), it is often difficult to obtain statistically significant results when the models used include covariates accounting for population structure. This leads to uncertainty when determining which associated sites are causative. Thus, linkage mapping is a valuable complementary approach in these situations, and in maize, large-scale connected mapping populations issued from diverse founders have been developed [11], [12] in order to conduct joint linkage-association analyses [10], [13], [14].

A major issue with association studies is false positives. In particular, indirect associations that are not causal will not be eliminated by increasing the sample size or the number of markers [15]. The main sources of such false positives are linkage between causal and noncausal sites, more than one causal site, and epistasis. These indirect associations are not randomly distributed throughout the genome and are less common than false positives arising from population structure. This makes them more difficult to control for than false positives arising from population structure.

The identification of a statistically significant association between a genotypic marker and a trait is considered to be proof of linkage between the phenotype and a casual site. This assumption is true for random mating populations with fast LD decay [16]. However, it is important to consider that population structure is typically present in association panels and it has an impact on the results. Population structure exists among all species in forms such as colonies, ethnic groups, and other subdivisions based on selection or geography. Typically, population structure leads to spurious associations between markers and the trait [17].

The ability to account for population structure in a given data set is influenced by the population size, the number of markers, the level of admixture, and the divergence in allele frequency between the subpopulations [18]. One commonly used method for controlling population structure is structured association

Citation: Larsson SJ, Lipka AE, Buckler ES (2013) Lessons from Dwarf8 on the Strengths and Weaknesses of Structured Association Mapping. PLoS Genet 9(2): e1003246. doi:10.1371/journal.pgen.1003246

(SA), which relies on randomly selected markers from the genome to estimate population structure. This estimate is then incorporated into the association analysis [16], [18], [19]. Another methodology for controlling population structure is to conduct a principal component analysis (PCA) [20], [21]. This approach summarizes the variation observed across all markers into a smaller number of underlying component variables. One interpretation of these principal components relates them to separate, unobserved subpopulations from which the individuals in the data set originate. The loadings (i.e., coefficient values) of the individuals for each principal component describe their relationship to the subpopulations. Both SA and PCA are limited to correcting for spurious associations by clustering on a global level of genetic variation. Thereby, they do not adequately capture the relatedness between individuals.

Correcting for population structure is not sufficient to eliminate all false positives. Therefore, the unified mixed linear model (MLM; also called the Q+K model) [22] was developed to further reduce the false positive rate by controlling for both population structure and cryptic familial relatedness. This approach uses a mixed model framework that has traditionally been used by animal geneticists [23], [24]. Specifically, covariates accounting for population structure are included as fixed effects (Q), and the individuals in the association panel are included as random effects. A kinship matrix (K) is calculated to estimate the variance-covariance between the individuals. Typically, the covariates used in the unified MLM are either principal components of the markers or covariates from SA approaches (e.g., STRUCTURE [17]). The advantages of the MLM are that it crosses the boundary between family-based and population-based samples. However, not all associations that are eliminated will be false. If a polymorphism is perfectly correlated with population structure, it is not possible to differentiate between true and false positives.

The initial study by Thornsberry et al. (2001) identified nine polymorphisms within d8 [25] that were associated with variation in flowering time in an association panel consisting of 92 diverse inbred lines. The most significant site was an 18 bp deletion (RefGen_v2 position: Chr. 1; 266,094,529 bp) in the promoter region. A 6 bp indel (RefGen_v2 position: Chr. 1; 266,095,483) was also identified. This allele is over-represented in Northern Flint lines and is located near a Src Homology 2-like domain, which is an important binding domain within this class of transcription factors. The initial association analysis was performed using logistic regression analyses, accounting for population structure. Population structure was estimated as a modification of SA using STRUCTURE software [18] with k=3.

Using a general linear model (GLM) without population structure, Andersen et al. (2005) obtained similar results for six of the nine d8 polymorphisms identified by Thornsberry et al. (2001). However, when including population structure in the model, (using STRUCTURE with both k=2 and k=3 subpopulations), it was found that the association results were overestimated. Each subpopulation was also analyzed separately, and a spurious association was still detectable [26].

Camus-Kulandaivelu et al. (2006) examined the association between d8 and flowering time using a panel of 375 inbred lines (including the 92 from the initial study) as well as a panel consisting of 275 traditional landraces from American and European origins [27]. Population structure was estimated using STRUCTURE, and association analysis was performed using both GLM and logistic regression. Their analysis revealed that the 6 bp indel at 266,095,483 bp (identified in Thornsberry et al., 2001) was spuriously associated with flowering time when covariates accounting for population structure were not included. In contrast, no association between d8 and flowering time was detected in the inbred panel when accounting for population structure. However, this spurious association was still detectable in the traditional landraces panel, including Andean material that has no relationship to the Northern Flint material.

The d8 gene produces a signaling factor involved in the gibberellin pathway. Gibberellins are types of endogenous plant growth regulators [28]. Maize d8 and wheat Rht-B1/Rht-D1 have been shown to be orthologous of the GAI gene [25]. Mutants of d8 have severe height phenotypes due to alterations of the DELLA domain. In maize, these are dominant, gain-of-function mutations, suggesting that d8 is a negative regulator. Conversely, recessive mutants of the GAI gene in Arabidopsis result in loss-of-function, specifically in polypeptides truncated upstream of the SH2-like domain. As a consequence, the gene product does not function as a negative regulator, resulting in normal height phenotypes [1].

Two evolutionary processes have likely impacted the d8 locus. First, the associated allele, specifically the 6 bp indel reported in Thornsberry et al. (2001), is related with Northern Flint maize. Maize originated from southern Mexico, where there are long growing seasons and high temperatures. As maize agriculture expanded from Mexico through the Southwestern United States to the Eastern United States (with its shorter growing season and lower temperatures), a severe bottleneck occurred in maize diversity, resulting in the Northern Flint subpopulation[29]. The bottleneck created extensive long range LD in this subpopulation. Northern Flints were substantially isolated from all other maize subpopulations [29] until the introduction of the Southern Dents in the 1600s [30].

Additionally, the d8 locus is located only 347,057 bp from the tb1 (teosinte branched1) locus (RefGen_v2 position: Chr. 1; 265,745,979–265,747,712 bp), which is one of the key genes involved in maize domestication [31]. The tb1 locus lost much of its diversity during the domestication process [31], [32]. The original d8 study [1] identified evidence of purifying selection with substantial diversity loss; however, there was little LD identified in the region between d8 and tb1. Although unconfirmed, some Northern Flint allied germplasm (e.g. sweet corn, P39) have a morphology that looks like the undomesticated tb1 phenotype. It is likely that the region around d8 and tb1 has been through a bottleneck with multiple selective sweeps, resulting in complex extended haplotypes.

Most of the loci controlling flowering time in maize have been identified through QTL studies. Of these, only d8 and vegetative to generative transition 1 (vgt1) have been confirmed with association and fine mapping [33]. Located on chromosome 8, vgt1 is arguably the most important flowering time locus in maize. It contains an APETALA2-like gene, ZmRap2.7, which is controlled by an enhancer region about 70 kb upstream [33]. The association between vgt1and flowering time is supported by a study conducted in the maize nested association mapping (NAM) population, where a major QTL was identified in this region [11]. This study also detected an allelic series at this QTL, suggesting that more than one causative allele is present. One of these alleles is from northern germplasm and is in linkage with a MITE whose association with early flowering time was confirmed in the NAM population [11]. Although the lack of the vgt1 early flowering allele did not completely explain the late flowering time, a SNP identified in the ZmRap2.7 gene showed association with the late flowering effect [11].

An association study by Ducrocq et al. (2008) [34] reported P-values for vgt1 association several magnitudes lower that those obtained by Salvi et al. (2007) [33]. Both studies accounted for population structure. Compared to Salvi et al. (2007) [33], Ducrocq et al. (2008) used a more genetically diverse and larger association panel, including a higher number of lines from Northern Flint and European germplasm [34]. In the case of d8, the association between the site and the trait becomes less significant, and even undetectable, when increasing the number of lines examined. This supports no association between the 6 bp indel in d8 and flowering time in maize. Including d8 in the model when performing association mapping for flowering time does not change the result for the SNPs in vgt1 [34]. This indicates that there is no interaction between the two loci.

The purpose of this study was to reanalyze the work of Thornsberry et al. (2001) utilizing some of the latest association mapping methodologies and data sets. This study compared association results from various statistical approaches using a maize diversity panel and the NAM population [11], [12]. Single nucleotide polymorphisms (SNPs) and insertions/deletions (indels) from recent genotyping efforts (e.g., HapMap sequencing from Gore et al. 2009 [35]and Chia et al. 2012 [36]) were used to evaluate these various approaches and the d8association.

RESULTS

Association Study

The results from the Thornsberry et al. (2001) study showed significant association at both the 18 bp deletion (266,094,829 bp) in the promoter region and the 6 bp indel (266,095,483 bp). Our reanalysis of the two sites using the Q model and a significantly larger association panel (consisting of 282 lines) resulted in less significant associations at both loci (Table 1). By increasing the number of lines we are able to obtain a larger sample size within each of the subpopulations and thus, more accurately estimate the underlying population structure (i.e., Q).

Sampling has a larger effect on some sites than others. The 6 bp indel is more significantly associated with flowering time in the smaller population (92 lines) than it is in the 282 association panel analyzed with MLM (K model) without controlling for population structure, but controlling for familial relatedness. The site is, in fact, carried by Northern Flint lines, which are underrepresented in the smaller population. The results for the 282 association panel suggest that the GLM (Q) approach overestimates the association. In contrast, the MLM (Q+K) approach, which accounts for both population structure and relatedness between individuals, gives a moderately significant association between the 6 bp indel (P-value=0.0127) and flowering time variation (Table 1).

Table 1. Association between polymorphisms at the d8 **locus and variation in flowering time in the 92 and 282 association panel, and association between polymorphisms in the region between** d8 **and** tb1 **(**d8/tb1) and variation in flowering time in the 282 line association panel.

	SNP	Population	Naïve Model[a]	K[b]	Q[c]	Q+K[d]
			p-value	p-value	p-value	p-value
d8	18 bp	282	0.0775	0.3996	0.8422	0.3676
		92	7.95×10^{-4}**	0.1585	0.0021*	0.0847
	3 bp	282	2.32×10^{-5}**	0.5759	0.0077*	0.8697
		92	0.1649	0.1411	0.3143	0.2403
	6 bp	282	9.70×10^{-6}**	0.0142*	0.0018*	0.0127*
		92	2.51×10^{-5}**	3.23×10^{-4}**	0.0012*	0.0017*
d8/tb1	36	282	0.0017*	0.309	0.005*	0.062
	72	282	0.003*	0.3123	0.0259*	0.062
	174	282	5.38×10^{-5}**	0.1354	0.0084*	0.046*
	287	282	5.38×10^{-5}**	0.1357	0.0084*	0.046*

[a]A general linear model not controlling for population structure.
[b]A mixed linear model controlling for kinship but not population structure.
[c]A general linear model controlling for population structure ($k=5$).
[d]A mixed linear model controlling for both population structure ($k=5$) and kinship.

The proportion of the genetic variation explained by the different models varies significantly. In this study, the best models are the Q+K and K models (the latter being a MLM that only includes familial relatedness between individuals as random effects) because they explain the highest amount of the genetic variance (Table 2). The reason for the minimal difference between the two models is that K most likely controls for the majority of the relatedness between individuals.

Table 2. Genetic variance explained by respective model used for the association study.

Model	SNP	R^2 Model
Naïve	none	0.000
	6 bp	0.084
	18 bp	0.022
Q	none	0.446
	6 bp	0.461
	18 bp	0.456
K	none	0.898
	6 bp	0.916
	18 bp	0.917
Q+K	none	0.898
	6 bp	0.914
	18 bp	0.914

This study confirms the weak association between the 6 bp indel in d8 and flowering time analyzed using both GLM and MLM approaches (Table 1). However, the association is not as significant as previously reported by Thornsberry et al. in 2001. Additionally, the GLM and MLM analyses of the 282 association panel imply there is no association between the 18 bp deletion in d8 and flowering time (Table 1). The initial study by Thornsberry et al. (2001) found this site to be the most significant. Our results from the Q+K and K models yielded a more significant P-value for the 92 association panel than the 282 association panel.

We also sequenced a 3 bp indel (266,097,198 bp), which is present in tropical late-flowering lines when we examined sequences available at NCBI. However, new genotypic data for the 282 association panel suggest that there is no association between this site and variation in flowering time in maize (Table 1).

Our study confirms the results presented by Camus-Kulandaivelu et al. (2008) [37], that there are regions between d8 and tb1 associated with variation in flowering time (Table 1) (Figures S3 and S4). However, these sites are moderately significant at α=0.05 when using the K and Q+K models. Association mapping of d8 on other traits results in a number of weak associations with other traits, in addition to flowering time (e.g., plant height, ear height, and node number) (Table 3). All the associations are in the same range of significance as flowering time. No clear pattern can be observed between correlation among traits except for what can be expected (e.g., the high correlation between days to silk and days to anthesis) (Figure 1). Collectively, these results undermine the conclusion that d8 is of more importance for flowering time than any of the other traits.

	TasselBranchLength	#OfNodesRootToEar	#OfEars	#OFNodesTasselToEar	#OfBraceRootsNodes	PlantHeight	EarHeight	MiddelLeafAngel	DaysToAnthesis
TasselBranchLength									
#OfNodesRootToEar	0.30								
#OfEars	0.11	0.29							
#OFNodesTasselToEar	0.20	0.55	0.11						
#OfBraceRootsNodes	0.34	0.65	0.14	0.53					
PlantHeight	0.32	0.68	0.22	0.51	0.54				
EarHeight	0.36	0.83	0.29	0.57	0.57	0.88			
MiddelLeafAngel	0.21	0.47	0.06	0.39	0.37	0.46	0.46		
DaysToAnthesis	0.38	0.79	0.22	0.62	0.61	0.62	0.73	0.47	
DaysToSilk	0.38	0.78	0.20	0.63	0.61	0.60	0.71	0.44	0.99

Figure 1. Pearson correlation coefficient between multiple traits.

No clear pattern can be observed between correlation between traits and its association to the 6 bp and 18 bp deletions in d8.

Table 3. Results from association study between polymorphisms within d8 **and a range of traits using MLM (Q+K).**

	P-value		
	6 bp	**18 bp**	**3 bp**
Days to Silk	0.0013		
Days to Tassel	0.0014		
Number of Ears		0.0469	
Number of Nodes Tassel to Ear		0.0473	0.0083
Middle Leaf Angle	0.0072		
Number of Nodes Ear to Roots	0.0185		
Ear Height	0.0207		
Cob Color	0.0343		
Plant Height	0.0478		
Number of Brace Root Nodes			0.0035
Tassel Branch Length			0.0171

From a genome-wide perspective, there were a large number of sites with a similar degree of association (from the MLM approach) with flowering time as d8 (Figure 2A). The contrasting results from the various models fitted at the SNPs in the genomic regions surrounding d8 andtb1 are illustrated in Figure 2B and 2C. In particular, the GLM model overestimated the significance of the results in comparison to the Q+K and K models. GWAS of flowering time detected SNPs within d8 that have a weak statistically significant association at α=0.05 (Figure 2C).

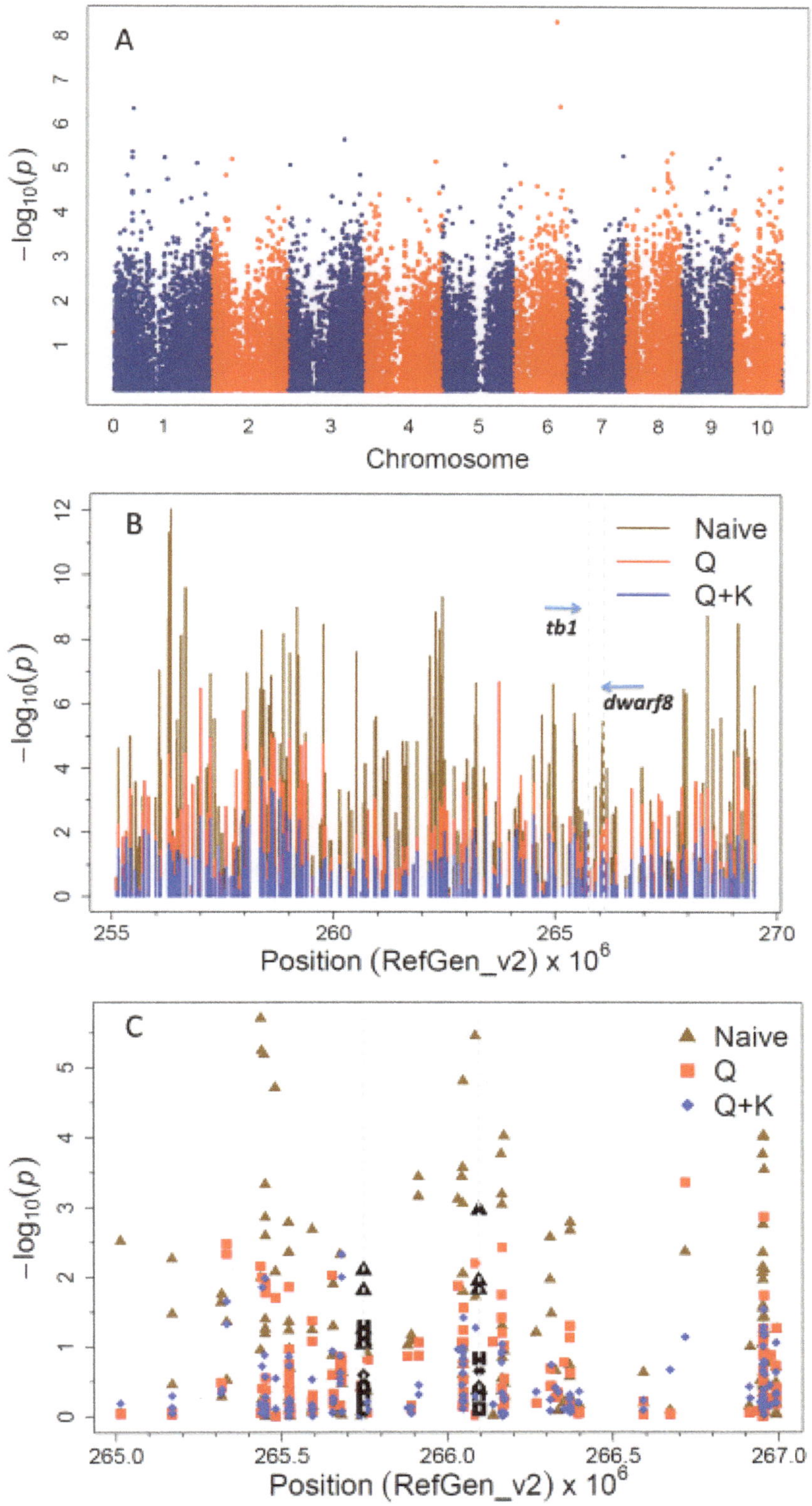

Figure 2. Genome-wide association results for flowering time.

A. GWAS results for flowering time (days to silking) in the 282 association panel using genotyping by sequencing (GBS) and 55k SNPs. The Q+K mixed linear model was fitted at each SNP to account for population structure (Q) and kinship (K). Genome-wide association results using the naïve model and Q model in Figures S1 and S2. B. GWAS results for flowering time (days to silking) using three models in the chromosomal region surrounding tb1 (Chr. 1; 265,745,979–265,747,712 bp) and d8 (Chr. 1; 266,094,769–266,097,836 bp). All GBS and 55K SNPs between 255 Mb and 270 Mb on Chr. 1 are included in the figure. Brown lines indicate results from naïve model, red lines indicate results from Q model, and blue lines indicate results from Q+K model. C. GWAS results for flowering time (days to silking) using three models in the chromosomal region surrounding tb1 (Chr. 1; 265,745,979–265,747,712 bp) and d8 (Chr. 1; 266,094,769–266,097,836 bp). All GBS and

55K SNPs between 265 Mb and 267 Mb on Chr. 1 are included in the figure. Black markers on the right are significant SNPs located within d8. Black markers on the left are significant SNPs located within tb1. Triangles indicate results from naïve model, squares indicate results from Q model, and diamonds indicate results from Q+K model.

Linkage Mapping

Linkage mapping of flowering time in the NAM population detected a number of QTL. A small QTL (P-value=0.0127) colocalized with d8 (RefGen_v2 position: Chr. 1; 269,321,476–269,322,794 bp), supporting the association identified by association mapping (Figure 3). In the initial study by Thornsberry et al. (2001), the effect of d8 was estimated to be between 7–10 days. The d8 polymorphism should be in three of the mapping families, and modest effects are seen in the right direction for all three, but the estimated effect is always less than half a day.

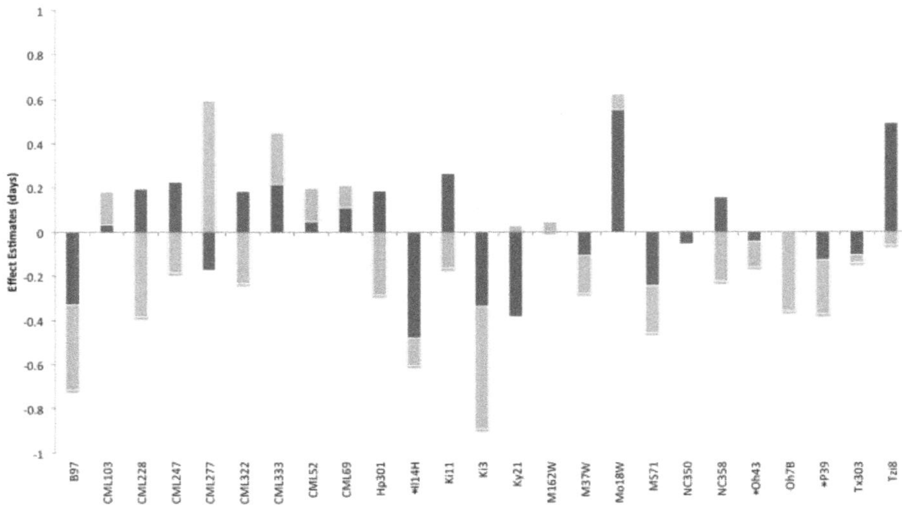

Figure 3. Effect estimates in days for NAM subpopulations carrying QTL in the region of d8, p-value<0.05.

Light gray bar shows QTL effect estimate at marker position 116 (RefGen_v2 position: Chr. 1; 231,701,106–231,703,173 bp) (137.6 cM) on the NAM map. Dark gray bar shows QTL effect estimate at marker position 155 (181.3 cM). d8 is located closest to marker 135 (RefGen_v2 position: Chr. 1; 269,321,476–269,322,794 bp), (RefGen_v2 position: Chr. 1; 286,977,415–287,063,457 bp), (162.2 cM). * indicates taxa with the 6 bp deletion in d8.

Additionally, many of the subfamilies appear to have other QTL along this section of chromosome 1 (RefGen_v2 position: Chr. 1; 231,701,106–231,703,173 bp and Chr. 1; 286,977,415–287,063,457 bp), but the favored positions are millions of base pairs away. It is quite possible that the mapping position of these joint linkage QTL could be synthetic, but there is little to no support for a QTL in this exact region.

A GWAS in the NAM population for flowering time using 26.5 million segregating SNPs was performed [35], [36]. This approach in the NAM population offers in-depth power and resolution because it utilizes both historic and recent recombination. No significant sites were identified in the region of d8 (Figure S5). This supports the result that d8 is not associated with flowering time.

Haplotype Structure

Hapmap data [35], [36] suggest extended haplotypes for Northern Flint lines in the region ofd8. Data show modest F_{st} between temperate and tropical subpopulations. However, there could potentially be differences in diversity between these two groups and Northern Flint lines. Hapmap data are only available for a few Northern Flint lines, which limits these studies.

GBS SNPs were used to examine the range of LD decay within the different subpopulations (Northern Flint, stiff stalk, non-stiff stalk, and tropical) of the 282 association panel. Extended LD is observed for the Northern Flint lines compared to the other subpopulations. Likewise, the stiff stalk lines, which were only founded from 16 inbred lines, also show a pattern of extended haplotypes, although not as extreme as the Northern Flints (Figure 4). The extended haplotype pattern in the Northern Flints make it difficult to control for false positives and to identify the causative SNP using association mapping.

White dot indicates median R^2 for each bin. This graph shows that there is more extended LD in Northern Flint than in other subpopulations.

The 6 bp indel in d8 is carried by Northern Flint lines. When we examine the LD between the 6 bp indel and the 13,815 high coverage GBS SNPs on chromosome 1 (Figure 5), an extended area around the 6 bp exhibits fairly high values of R^2. This is additional evidence that extended haplotypes exist in the Northern Flint lines in the d8 region.

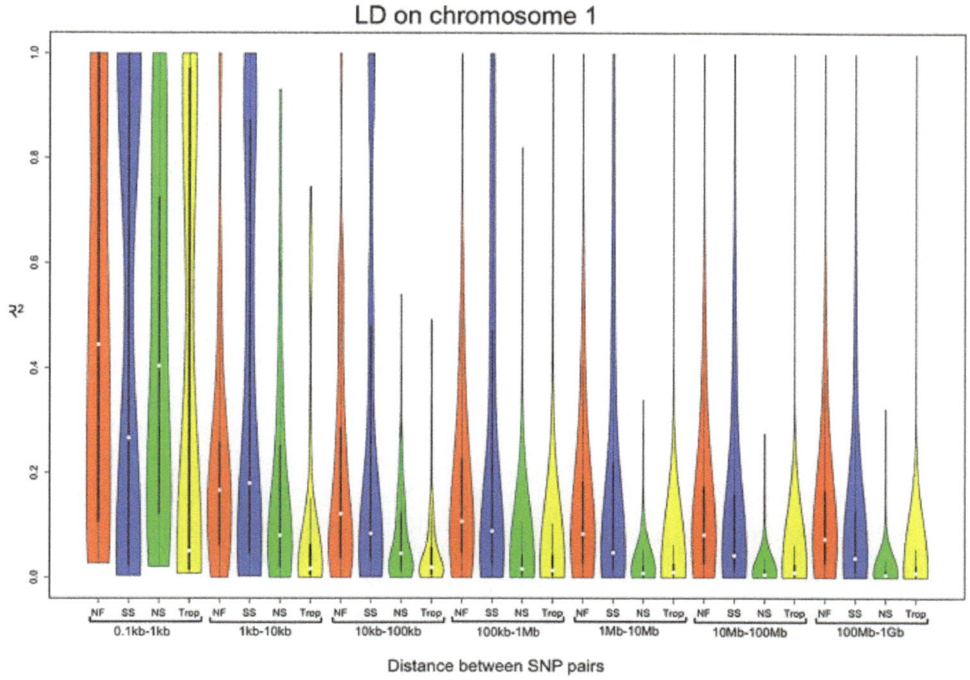

Figure 4. LD on chromosome 1 for the subpopulations, Northern Flint (red), stiff stalk (blue), non-stiff stalk (green), tropical (yellow), of the 282 association panel.

In fact, there are two regions with high LD at 20 Mbp and 0.9 Mbp away, which contain previously identified domestication gene candidates (i.e., GRMZM2G034217 RefGen_v2 position: chr. 1 246,720,001–247,030,000, a mitochondrial transcription termination factor) [38]. In contrast, LD between the MITE in vgt1and the 7,539 GBS SNPs on chromosome 8 (Figure S6) show sites with high R^2 values close to the position of the MITE, but LD decays much more rapidly. To test for two-way interaction between the 6 bp and 18 bp indels and the MITE, a series of mixed models including two-way interaction terms were fitted. The most significant interaction was between the 18 bp indel and the MITE (P-value 0.0418). However, this association is not likely to be statistically significant after controlling for the multiple testing problem across the entire genome.

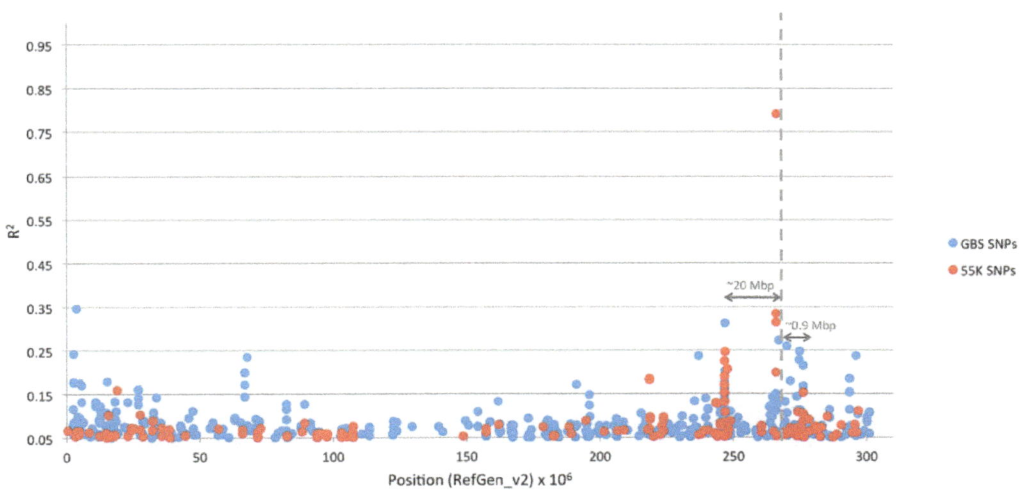

Figure 5. R^2 **between the 6 bp indel in** d8 **and all the other sites on chromosome 1.**

Blue dots indicate results from 13,815 GBS SNPs present in 200 or more of the 282 lines. Red dots indicate results from 7,695 55K SNPs present in 200 or more of the 282 lines.

DISCUSSION

Association Study

The results underscore the importance of properly accounting for population structure in association studies. The analysis in Thornsberry et al. (2001) divided their 92 association panel into three subpopulations. This subdivision did not fully account for population structure, and thus, the effect of the d8 allele carried by Northern Flint lines was overestimated. In contrast, our study accounted for population structure using both k=3 (stiff stalk, non-stiff stalk, and tropical) and k=5 (stiff stalk, non-stiff stalk, tropical, sweet corn, and popcorn) subpopulations. This was important for sites such as the 6 bp indel within d8, which is present at a higher frequency in Northern Flint lines (which includes sweet corn), and this signature of population structure was unaccounted for when k=3 was used.

Of all the models tested, the Q+K model [22] was the most suitable approach for analyzing the 282 association panel because it controls for both population structure and cryptic familial relatedness. It is especially important to control for the latter with traits such as flowering time, which is highly correlated with population structure. Additionally, the Q+K model is beneficial for association studies because Q and K capture different types of long range LD [22], [39].

In general mixed models sufficiently account for population structure and familial relatedness. In contrast, false positives arising from other sources, although rare, are typically unaccounted for in association studies. For example, spurious associations could arise from markers that are in long-range LD with causative polymorphisms. Additionally, causative polymorphisms for one trait may not necessarily be causal for another highly correlated trait (and, hence a spurious association), but will be statistically associated with both traits. Finally, when a trait is controlled by multiple loci in LD, it is likely that the site with the largest effect is an indirect association. One reason for this result arises from differing minor allele frequencies among the causal sites. All three of these types of false positives do not occur randomly across the genome and thus, they are more challenging to eliminate. Haplotype-based association studies is one approach for addressing many of these issues. Nevertheless, multiple sites, selection for multiple traits, and population structure result in spurious associations and these need to be accounted for when performing association studies.

Contrast with Linkage Mapping

Association mapping is limited when the trait analyzed is correlated with population structure. However, linkage mapping can overcome this problem by crossing individuals with known relatedness, spurious associations can be broken.

In this study, we were able to detect a small QTL at the general location of d8. However the favored QTL locations are on both sides of d8: RefGen_v2 position Chr. 1; 231,703,173–287,063,457. Association results suggest that the majority of the QTL effects detected aroundd8 are from rare extended haplotypes that include other linked QTLs. Another possible explanation for the weakness of the QTLs detected is the population sampled. The associated haplotype is present only in Northern Flint lines, which are underrepresented in the population.

Haplotype Structure

Flowering time is strongly correlated with population structure. Our study showed that d8 had a very small effect on flowering time. One possible explanation for this result is that d8 is associated with another trait that was selected along with flowering time (e.g., cold tolerance). This hypothesis is supported by the extended haplotype pattern observed in Northern Flint lines as well as the associations that are detected with traits like plant height and node number. Northern Flint lines are underrepresented in both the 282 association panel and the NAM population, and it is difficult to scrutinize associations with low allele frequencies. Northern Flint lines have been shown to be distinctive compared to other subpopulations, especially in regions like d8 and tb1, which have been under selection pressure.

Consistent with the findings of previous studies on the d8 locus, we observed a strong correlation between d8 and population structure. Thus, the functional site of d8 is not likely to be involved in flowering time. Indeed, d8 and tb1 are strong integrators in plant signals that are adjacent to each other on chromosome 1. However, our results demonstrated that these signals are a signature of population structure instead of true biological signals. The extended LD in the Northern Flint lines around d8 supports the hypothesis that this gene is regulated in a similar manner as tb1 and vgt1. For both tb1 and vgt1, cis-acting regulatory sites located more than 50 kb from the actual genes have been shown to be the functional regions and not the genes themselves [31], [33], [40].

Signatures of selection on d8 have been observed in teosinte [41]. Because apical dominance (tb1) and gibberellin signaling (d8) have both played key roles for domestication phenotypes, it is likely that the genomic region surrounding d8 and tb1 has been under selection since early maize domestication. Northern Flint lines differ from Corn Belt dent lines in a number of traits such as leaf angle, plant height, and cold tolerance. Thus, the long range LD block around d8could be a signature of selection from the development of Northern Flint lines that happens to be associated with one of these traits distinguishing Northern Flint from Corn Belt dent. Consequently, it has been possible to detect a weak association between flowering time andd8 because of the correlation between flowering time and the Northern Flint specific traits due to population structure. Using this rationale, it may be possible to detect associations between the d8 locus and phenotypes such as carbon allocation and harvest index, when considering the differences in the usage of Northern Flints (sweet corn and silage) and Corn Belt dent.

CONCLUSION

The basic d8 associations identified in Thornsberry et al. (2001) have been replicated by other independent groups [26], [27], but population structure has always remained a consistent issue. This reanalysis using SNPs within and near d8 suggests that these associations are either incorrect or vastly overestimated. This work implemented more powerful statistical approaches, germplasm resources, and whole genome sequencing data, enabling a more thorough understanding of this locus.

This analysis underscores the importance of controlling for population structure. All three previously published studies on the d8 locus illustrate how naïve association results overestimated effect sizes. In our study, we used the unified MLM to control for both population structure and relatedness between individuals, which are more accurate in effect estimation and give a truer level of significance. Even in species with rapid LD decay, like maize, it is possible to have subpopulations that can exhibit LD many orders of magnitude greater than the average length. This long range LD resulted in the extended haplotype lengths observed in Northern Flint lines for the genomic region surrounding d8. Northern Flint lines are underrepresented in the association panel, which makes it difficult to accurately account for the population structure of this subpopulation. Another issue is the strong correlations between traits. It is very likely that in the case of d8 there has been selection for other correlated traits, such as cold tolerance. Because of the correlation between the population structure and flowering time, we can detect a weak association between flowering time and d8, but d8 does not actually have an effect on time of flowering. Genes like d8 have been targets of strong selection and, as such, are among the hardest to identify in GWAS and accurately estimate their effect size. NAM-like linkage populations with bi-parental crosses in a reference design to minimize population structure may be necessary for dissecting the most structured traits.

Although our results strongly suggest that the previously reported association between d8 and flowering time is an artifact of population structure, further research on this complex locus is warranted. The long range LD present at d8 for Northern Flint lines is a signature of selection, and it is important to determine the traits that are regulated by this gene. By applying the appropriate statistical models, we have shown that flowering time is not one of these traits.

MATERIALS AND METHODS

Germplasm

The association panel consists of 282 diverse maize lines that have been previously described[42]. These lines can be subdivided into five major subpopulations, namely stiff stalk, non-stiff stalk, tropical or semitropical lines (related to the non-stiff stalk lines), sweet corn and popcorn. The association panel includes the 25 founder lines of the NAM population. The maize NAM population consists of 5,000 RILs (Recombinant Inbred Lines) derived from crossing B73 with 25 diverse maize inbred lines, and then selfing for 5 generations [43].

Phenotypic Data

Phenotypic data were collected from the NAM population and the 282 association panel, grown in eight environments including Ithaca, NY, Clayton, NC, Champaign, IL, and Colombia, MO, during the summers of 2006 and 2007. Flowering time was measured separately for female flowers (number of days-to-silk) and male flowers (days-to-anthesis) from the day of planting. The flowering date was defined as the day when the anthers or silk were visible on 50% of all plants within a row.

Sequencing Data

DNA sequence data were obtained for d8 from Thornsberry et al. (2001), available at NCBI. Primers were designed for PCR amplification of gene fragments of interest from the 282 lines in the association panel.

Each PCR product was cleaned by treating the samples with Exonuclease (ExoI) and Shrimp Alkaline Phosphatase (SAP) and incubated at 37°C for 3 min followed by 80°C for 10 min. The samples were prepared for sequencing using a mixture with a total volume of 10 μl containing 0.7 μl forward primer, 0.7 μl reverse primer (5 pmol/μl), 0.5 μl Big Dye terminator, 1.7 μl 5× sequencing buffer, 7.1 μl distilled water and the PCR product. The thermal cycler was set on the following program: Initial denaturation at 96°C for 4 min, followed by 30 cycles at 96°C for 10 sec, 50°C for 5 sec and 60°C 4 min, with a final, incubation at 10°C. Sanger(3730XL) DNA sequencing was performed using an Applied Biosystems Automated 3730 DNA Analyzer. The software BioLign alignment and multiple contig editor with codon code phred-phrap analysis was used for alignment using consensus sequence contigs and sequence quality scores.

The alignments from NCBI were also used to reanalyze the results published in the initial study by Thornsberry et al. (2001).

To obtain sequence data for the region between d8 and tb1, the same protocol was used as described above. However, primer sequences were obtained from Camus-Kulandaivelu et al. (2008)

STATISTICAL ANALYSIS

Field spatial correction.

Best linear unbiased predictions (BLUPs) of the lines in the 282 association panel and the NAM population were the same as those reported in Buckler et al. (2009). These were obtained from a random effects model fitted in ASREML version 2.0 software [44] that accounts for spatial correlation and field effects.

Association mapping—candidate gene study.

TASSEL (Trait Analysis by aSSociation, Evaluation, and Linkage) was used for data processing analysis [45], and results were confirmed by using SAS [46]. Association between polymorphisms and phenotypes were evaluated using General Linear Model (GLM) and Mixed Linear Model (MLM) by incorporating phenotypic and genotypic data, population structure (Q) and kinship matrix (K).

Population structure was predicted using a Bayesian approach that estimates the relationship between subpopulations by grouping genotypic correlations at unlinked markers within the population with the software STRUCTURE [18] as described in [42]. This approach uses the proportion of an individual's genome that originated from each subpopulation to estimate the genetic background matrix (Q).

In MLM, the familial relatedness between the individuals is taken into consideration through a kinship matrix. This model corrects for spurious associations arising from population structure and familial relatedness [47]. In this study we used marker-based kinship, which was determined on the basis of the definition that random pairs of inbreds are unrelated. Kinship was calculated using the software package SPAGeDi [48]. It has been suggested that marker based kinship is more appropriate for association studies than kinship based on pedigree records [19], [40]. The same set of markers was used to create the population structure and kinship matrix. The GLM approach in this study for phenotype, **y**, is: $y = X\beta + \varepsilon$ **(1)**Where, the **Xβ** term represents the fixed effects, including genotypes and population structure, Q, and ε is a vector of residual effects following a multivariate normal distribution with mean 0 and variance-covariance matrix $\sigma^2_\varepsilon I$. The naïve model is the same as GLM without the population structure effect.

The MLM approach in this study is the same model as used by Yu et al., 2006.

Mixed model, for phenotype, **y**, is: $y = X\beta + Z\mu + \varepsilon$ **(2)**Where, the **Xβ** term represents the fixed effects, including genotypes and population structure, Q, and the **Zμ** term represents random line effects, including the matrix of kinship coefficients, K, and vector of polygene background effects. ε is a vector of residual effects following a multivariate normal distribution with mean 0 and variance-covariance matrix $\sigma^2_\varepsilon I$.

Genome-wide association study.

Genome-wide association studies (GWAS) were carried out in the 282 association panel using 51,741 SNPs obtained from the Illumina MaizeSNP50 BeadChip and 591,552 SNPs from the genotyping by sequencing (GBS) protocol [49]. Three different approaches that take into account varying degrees of population structure and familial relatedness were undertaken. The first approach, called the naïve approach, uses a model similar to the one presented inEquation (1), except that the Q matrix representing population structure is not included among the fixed effects. The next approach is the GLM approach, which uses the model in Equation (1), with the first five principal components (PCs) of the non-industry subset of the Illumina MaizeSNP50 BeadChip SNPs (34,368 SNPs) included as fixed effects to represent population structure. The final approach is the MLM approach, with the aforementioned first five PCs representing population structure, and a kinship matrix calculated from the non-industry subset of these SNPs for the variance-covariance matrix of the random line effects. This kinship matrix is calculated using the method of [50]. In each approach, these models are fitted to each SNP. After all SNPs with minor allele frequencies (MAFs) less than 0.05 are removed from the analysis, the Benjamini-Hochberg [51] procedure adjusts for the multiple testing problem by controlling the false discovery rate (FDR) at 0.05. This phase of the anlaysis was conducted using the genome association and prediction integrated tool (GAPIT) package in the R programming language [52].

Joint-Linkage Mapping.

Joint Linkage Mapping of BLUPs for the phenotype across environments was performed using the proc GLMSelect in SAS, as described in Buckler et al. (2009) [11]. BLUPs were calculated for each phenotype and used together with imputed genetic marker intervals and stepwise regression to identify QTLs. Missing marker data were imputed by utilizing genetic distance between missing and flanking markers. A permutation procedure was implemented to obtain empirical α=0.05 thresholds for including and excluding terms in the joint linkage model [53].

Linkage Disequilibrium.

To calculate the linkage disequilibrium between the SNPs within d8, tested in this association study, against the rest of the genome the LD function SitebyAll in the TASSEL software was used [45]. For genotypic data, the Illumina MaizeSNP50 Beadchip was used, as well as 458k GBS (Genotyping by Sequencing) SNPs [49].

SUPPORTING INFORMATION

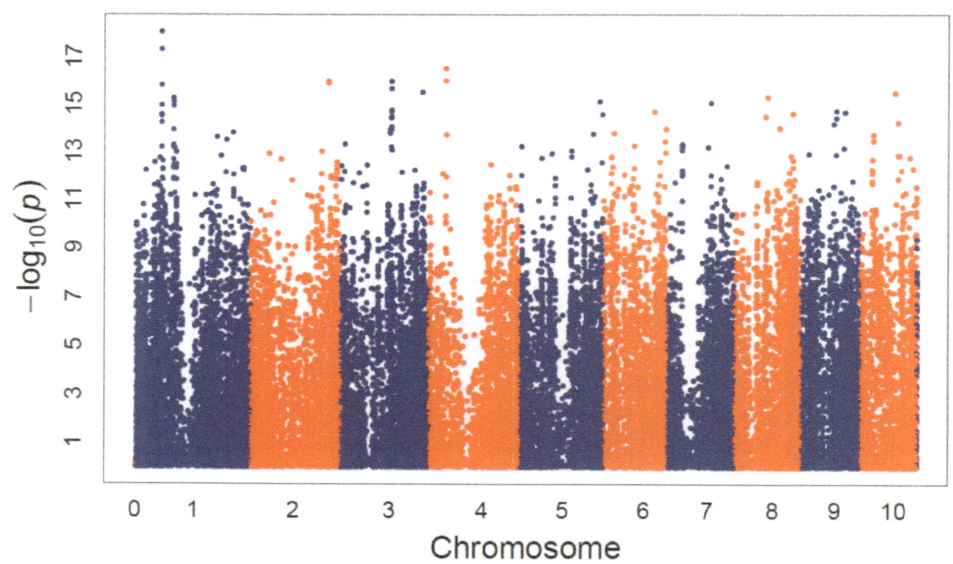

Figure S1.

Genome-wide association results for flowering time (days to silking) in the 282 association panel using genotyping by sequencing (GBS) and 55k SNPs. The naïve model, which does not account for population structure, was fitted at each SNP.

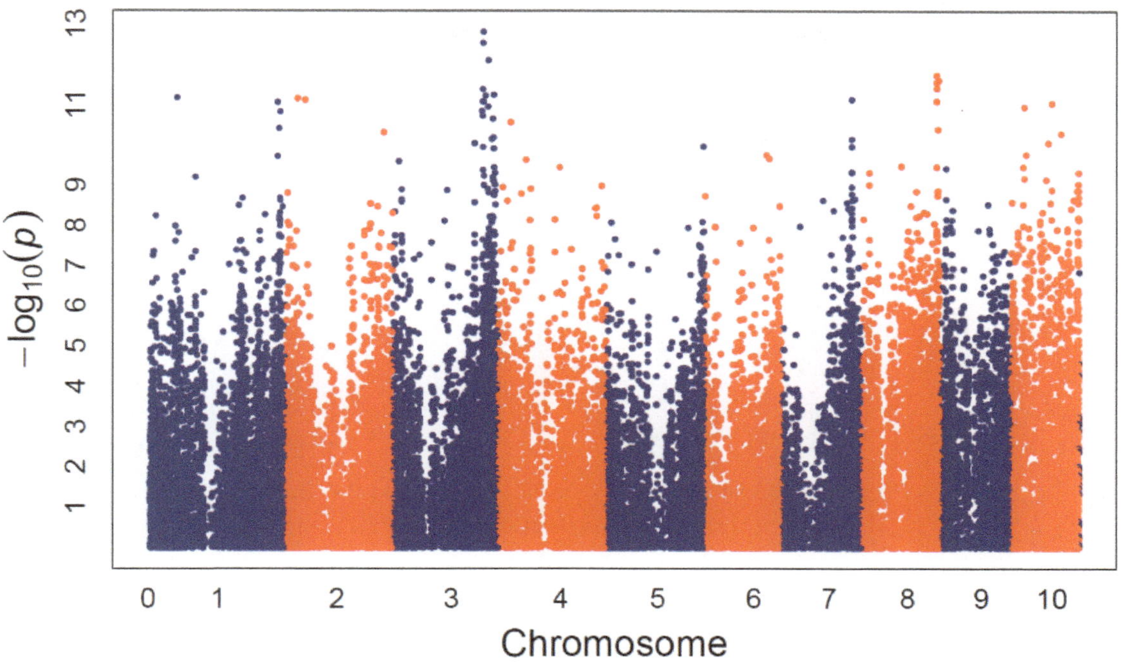

Figure S2.

Genome-wide association results for flowering time (days to silking) in the 282 association panel using genotyping by sequencing (GBS) and 55k SNPs. The Q model was fitted at each SNP to account for population structure (Q).

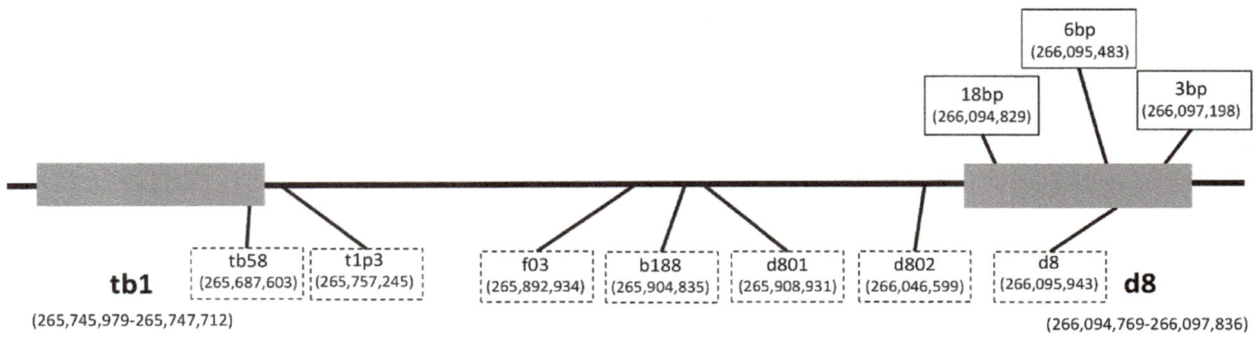

Figure S3.

Physical positions of tb1 and d8 on RefGen_v2. Positions of SNPs are obtained by blasting primer sequences using www.maizesequence.org and are approximate. Sites above the line in solid black boxes are evaluated in this study. Sites below the line in dashed boxes are from the study by Camus-Kulandaivelu et al. (2008).

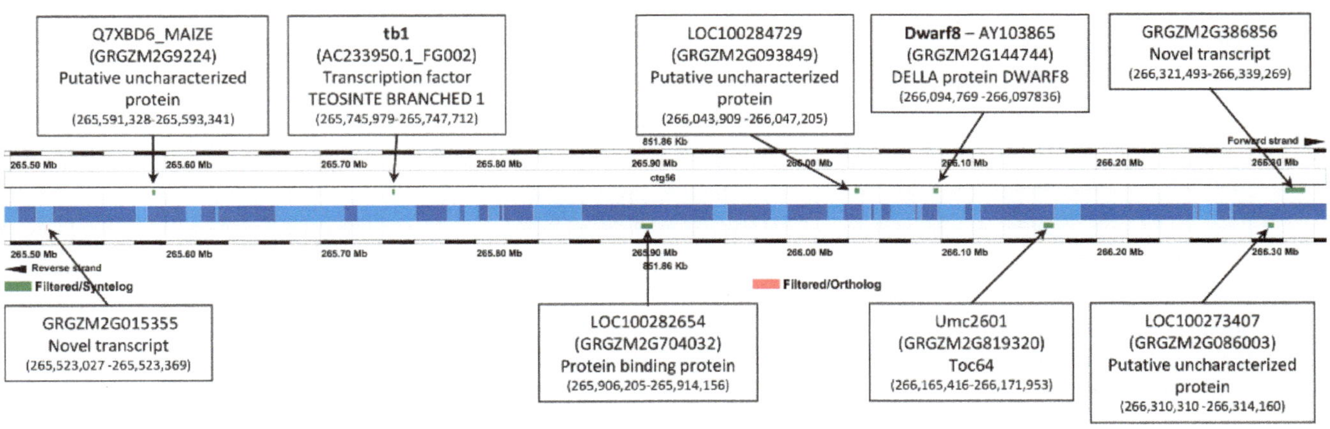

Figure S4.

The region around tb1 and d8 on chromosome 1 (265,495,979–266,347,836 RefGen_v2), and all identified gene transcripts available at www.maizesequence.org. There are no other obvious candidate genes for flowering time in the region.

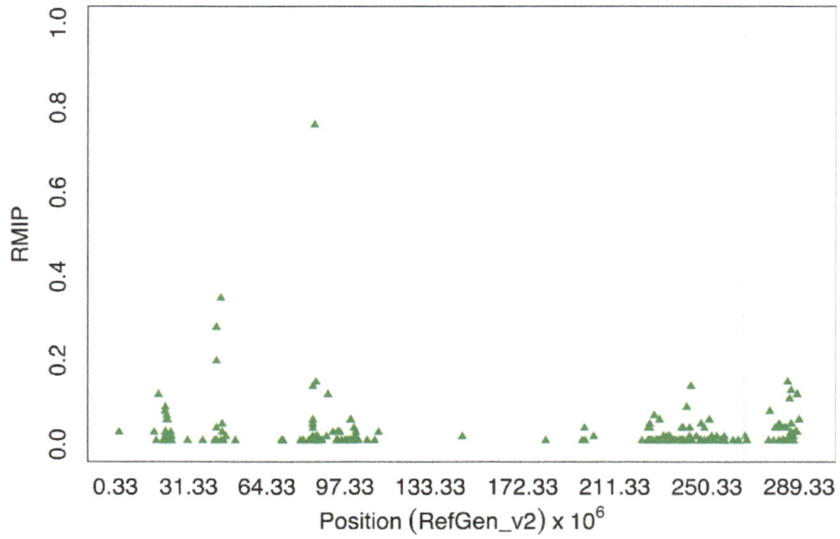

Figure S5.

Genome-wide association results for flowering time (days to silking) in the NAM population using maize HapMapv1 and HapMapv2 SNPs. There are no significant sites identified in the region of d8 (indicated by the gray line).

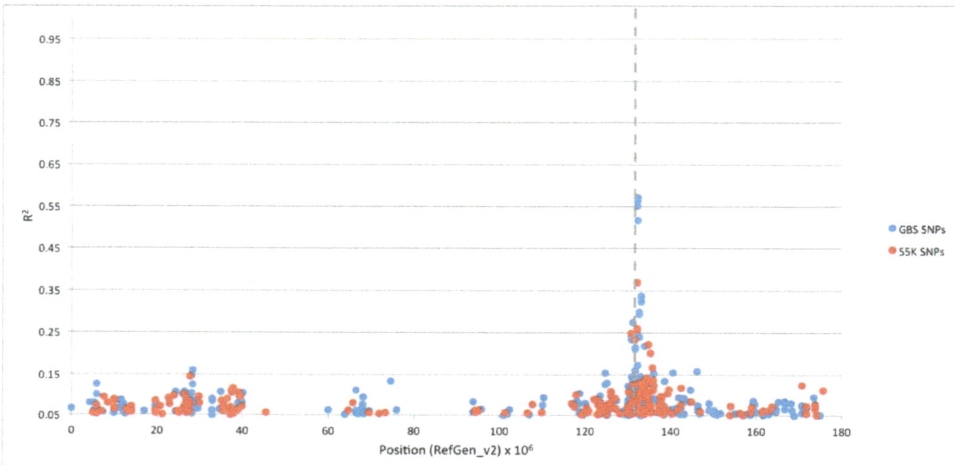

Figure S6.

R^2 between MITE in vgt1 and all the other sites on chromosome 8. Blue dots indicate results from 7,539 GBS SNPs present in 200 or more of the 282 lines. Red dots indicate results from 4,197 55K SNPs present in 200 or more of the 282 lines.

ACKNOWLEDGMENTS

The authors would like to thank Denise Costich and Sara Miller for their review and edits of the manuscript. We also thank past and present members of the Maize Diversity Project for their assistance in phenotypic data collection.

Author Contributions

Conceived and designed the experiments: SJL ESB. Performed the experiments: SJL ESB. Analyzed the data: SJL ESB AEL. Contributed reagents/materials/analysis tools: SJL ESB. Wrote the paper: SJL ESB AEL.

REFERENCES

1. Thornsberry JM, Goodman MM, Doebley J, Kresovich S, Nielsen D, et al. (2001) Dwarf8 polymorphisms associate with variation in flowering time. Nat Genet 28: 286–289. doi: 10. 1038/90135
2. Wilson LM, Whitt SR, Ibanez AM, Rocheford TR, Goodman MM, et al. (2004) Dissection of Maize Kernel Composition and Starch Production by Candidate Gene Association. Plant Cell 16: 2719–2733. doi: 10. 1105/tpc. 104. 025700
3. Breseghello F, Sorrells ME (2006) Association mapping of kernel size and milling quality in wheat (Triticum aestivum L.) cultivars. Genetics 172: 1165–1177. doi: 10. 1534/genetics. 105. 044586
4. Beló A, Zheng P, Luck S, Shen B, Meyer DJ, et al. (2008) Whole genome scan detects an allelic variant of fad2 associated with increased oleic acid levels in maize. Molecular Genet Genomics 279: 1–10. doi: 10. 1007/s00438-007-0289-y
5. González-Martínez SC, Huber D, Ersoz E, Davis JM, Neale DB (2008) Association genetics in Pinus taeda L.

II. Carbon isotope discrimination. Heredity 101: 19–26. doi: 10. 1038/hdy. 2008. 21

6. Harjes CE, Rocheford TR, Bai L, Brutnell TP, Kandianis CB, et al. (2008) Natural genetic variation in lycopene epsilon cyclase tapped for maize biofortification. Science (New York, NY) 319: 330–333. doi: 10. 1126/science. 1150255

7. Atwell S, Huang YS, Vilhjálmsson BJ, Willems G, Horton M, et al. (2010) Genome-wide association study of 107 phenotypes in Arabidopsis thaliana inbred lines. Nature 465: 627–631. doi: 10. 1038/nature08800

8. Yan J, Kandianis CB, Harjes CE, Bai L, Kim E-H, et al. (2010) Rare genetic variation at Zea mays crtRB1 increases beta-carotene in maize grain. Nat Genet 42: 322–327. doi: 10. 1038/ng. 551

9. Kump KL, Bradbury PJ, Wisser RJ, Buckler ES, Belcher AR, et al. (2011) Genome-wide association study of quantitative resistance to southern leaf blight in the maize nested association mapping population. Nat Genet 43: 163–168. doi: 10. 1038/ng. 747

10. Tian F, Bradbury PJ, Brown PJ, Hung H, Sun Q, et al. (2011) Genome-wide association study of leaf architecture in the maize nested association mapping population. Nat Genet 43: 159–162. doi: 10. 1038/ng. 746

11. Buckler ES, Holland JB, Bradbury PJ, Acharya CB, Brown PJ, et al. (2009) The genetic architecture of maize flowering time. Science (New York, NY) 325: 714–718. doi: 10. 1126/science. 1174276

12. McMullen MD, Kresovich S, Villeda HS, Bradbury P, Li H, et al. (2009) Genetic properties of the maize nested association mapping population. Science (New York, NY) 325: 737–740. doi: 10. 1126/science. 1174320

13. Bergelson J, Roux F (2010) Towards identifying genes underlying ecologically relevant traits in Arabidopsis thaliana. Nat Rev Genet 11: 867–879. doi: 10. 1038/nrg2896

14. Li H, Bradbury P, Ersoz E, Buckler ES, Wang J (2011) Joint QTL linkage mapping for multiple-cross mating design sharing one common parent. PLoS ONE 6: e17573 doi:10. 1371/journal. pone. 0017573.

15. Platt A, Vilhjálmsson BJ, Nordborg M (2010) Conditions under which genome-wide association studies will be positively misleading. Genetics 186: 1045–1052. doi: 10. 1534/genetics. 110. 121665

16. Pritchard JK, Rosenberg NA (1999) Use of unlinked genetic markers to detect population stratification in association studies. Am J Hum Genet 65: 220–228. doi: 10. 1086/302449

17. Pritchard JK, Stephens M, Rosenberg NA, Donnelly P (2000) Association mapping in structured populations. Am J Hum Genet 67: 170–181. doi: 10. 1086/302959

18. Pritchard JK, Stephens M, Donnelly P (2000) Inference of population structure using multilocus genotype data. Genetics 155: 945–959.

19. Falush D, Stephens M, Pritchard JK (2003) Inference of population structure using multilocus genotype data: linked loci and correlated allele frequencies. Genetics 164: 1567–1587.

20. Price AL, Patterson NJ, Plenge RM, Weinblatt ME, Shadick NA, et al. (2006) Principal components analysis corrects for stratification in genome-wide association studies. Nat Genet 38: 904–909. doi: 10. 1038/ng1847

21. Kang HM, Zaitlen NA, Wade CM, Kirby A, Heckerman D, et al. (2008) Efficient control of population structure in model organism association mapping. Genetics 178: 1709–1723. doi: 10. 1534/genetics. 107. 080101

22. Yu J, Pressoir G, Briggs WH, Bi IV, Yamasaki M, et al. (2006) A unified mixed-model method for association mapping that accounts for multiple levels of relatedness. Nat Genet 38: 203–208. doi: 10. 1038/ng1702

23. Henderson CR (1984) Applications of linear models in animal breeding. Guelph: University of Guelph.

24. George AW, Visscher PM, Haley CS (2000) Mapping quantitative trait loci in complex pedigrees: a two-step variance component approach. Genetics 156: 2081–2092.

25. Peng J, Richards DE, Hartley NM, Murphy GP, Devos KM, et al. (1999) "Green revolution" genes encode mutant gibberellin response modulators. Nature 400: 256–261.

26. Andersen JR, Schrag T, Melchinger AE, Zein I, Lübberstedt T (2005) Validation of Dwarf8 polymorphisms associated with flowering time in elite European inbred lines of maize (Zea mays L.). Theor Appl Genet 111: 206–217. doi: 10. 1007/s00122-005-1996-6

27. Camus-Kulandaivelu L, Veyrieras J-B, Madur D, Combes V, Fourmann M, et al. (2006) Maize adaptation to temperate climate: relationship between population structure and polymorphism in the Dwarf8 gene. Genetics 172: 2449–2463. doi: 10. 1534/genetics. 105. 048603

28. Harberd NP, King KE, Carol P, Cowling RJ, Peng J, et al. (1998) Gibberellin: inhibitor of an inhibitor of…? BioEssays 20: 1001–1008. doi: 10. 1002/(sici)1521-1878(199812)20:12<1001::aid-bies6>3. 0. co;2-o

29. Doebley JF, Goodman MM, Stuber CW (1986) Exceptional Genetic Divergence of Northern Flint Corn. Am J Bot 73: 64–69. doi: 10. 2307/2444278

30. Doebley J, Wendel JD, Smith JSC, Stuber CW, Goodman MM (1988) The origin of cornbelt maize: The isozyme evidence. Econ Bot 42: 120–131. doi: 10. 1007/bf02859042

31. Studer A, Zhao Q, Ross-Ibarra J, Doebley J (2011) Identification of a functional transposon insertion in the maize domestication gene tb1. Nat Genet 43: 1160–1163. doi: 10. 1038/ng. 942

32. Wang R-L, Stec A, Hey J, Lukens L, Doebley J (1999) The limits of selection during maize domestication. Nature 398: 236–239. doi: 10. 1038/18435

33. Salvi S, Sponza G, Morgante M, Tomes D, Niu X, et al. (2007) Conserved noncoding genomic sequences associated with a flowering-time quantitative trait locus in maize. Proc Natl Acad Sci U S A 104: 11376–11381. doi: 10. 1073/pnas. 0704145104

34. Ducrocq S, Madur D, Veyrieras J-B, Camus-Kulandaivelu L, Kloiber-Maitz M, et al. (2008) Key impact of Vgt1 on flowering time adaptation in maize: evidence from association mapping and ecogeographical information. Genetics 178: 2433–2437. doi: 10. 1534/genetics. 107. 084830

35. Gore MA, Chia J-M, Elshire RJ, Sun Q, Ersoz ES, et al. (2009) A first-generation haplotype map of maize. Science (New York, NY) 326: 1115–1117. doi: 10. 1126/science. 1177837

36. Chia J-M, Song C, Bradbury PJ, Costich D, De Leon N, et al. (2012) Maize HapMap2 identifies extant variation from a genome in flux. Nat Genet 44: 803–807. doi: 10. 1038/ng. 2313

37. Camus-Kulandaivelu L, Chevin L-M, Tollon-Cordet C, Charcosset A, Manicacci D, et al. (2008) Patterns of molecular evolution associated with two selective sweeps in the Tb1-Dwarf8 region in maize. Genetics 180: 1107–1121. doi: 10. 1534/genetics. 108. 088849

38. Hufford MB, Xu X, Van Heerwaarden J, Pyhäjärvi T, Chia J-M, et al. (2012) Comparative population genomics of maize domestication and improvement. Nat Genet 44: 808–811. doi: 10. 1038/ng. 2309

39. Zhao K, Aranzana MJ, Kim S, Lister C, Shindo C, et al. (2007) An Arabidopsis example of association mapping in structured samples. PLoS Genet 3: e4 doi:10. 1371/journal. pgen. 0030004.

40. Clark RM, Linton E, Messing J, Doebley JF (2004) Pattern of diversity in the genomic region near the maize domestication gene tb1. Proc Natl Acad Sci U S A 101: 700–707. doi: 10. 1073/pnas. 2237049100

41. Tenaillon MI, U'Ren J, Tenaillon O, Gaut BS (2004) Selection versus demography: a multilocus investigation of the domestication process in maize. Mol Biol Evol 21: 1214–1225. doi: 10. 1093/molbev/msh102

42. Flint-Garcia SA, Thuillet A-C, Yu J, Pressoir G, Romero SM, et al. (2005) Maize association population: a high-resolution platform for quantitative trait locus dissection. Plant J 44: 1054–1064. doi: 10. 1111/j. 1365-313x. 2005. 02591. x

43. Yu J, Holland JB, McMullen MD, Buckler ES (2008) Genetic design and statistical power of nested association mapping in maize. Genetics 178: 539–551. doi: 10. 1534/genetics. 107. 074245

44. Gilmour AR, Gogel BJ, Cullis BR, Thompson R (2005) ASReml User Guide.

45. Bradbury PJ, Zhang Z, Kroon DE, Casstevens TM, Ramdoss Y, et al. (2007) TASSEL: software for association mapping of complex traits in diverse samples. Bioinformatics 23: 2633–2635. doi: 10. 1093/bioinformatics/btm308

46. SAS Institute (2004) SAS/STAT user's guide. Version 9. 2. SAS Inst. , Cary, NC

47. Stich B, Möhring J, Piepho H-P, Heckenberger M, Buckler ES, et al. (2008) Comparison of mixed-model approaches for association mapping. Genetics 178: 1745–1754. doi: 10. 1534/genetics. 107. 079707

48. Hardy OJ, Vekemans X (2002) spagedi: a versatile computer program to analyse spatial genetic structure at the individual or population levels. Mol Ecol Notes 2: 618–620. doi: 10. 1046/j. 1471-8286. 2002. 00305. x

49. Elshire RJ, Glaubitz JC, Sun Q, Poland JA, Kawamoto K, et al. (2011) A robust, simple genotyping-by-sequencing (GBS) approach for high diversity species. PLoS ONE 6: e19379 doi:10. 1371/journal. pone. 0019379.

50. Loiselle BA, Sork VL, Nason J, Graham C (1995) Spatial Genetic Structure of a Tropical Understory Shrub, Psychotria officinalis (Rubiaceae). Am J Bot 82: 1420–1425. doi: 10. 2307/2445869

51. Benjamini Y, Hochberg Y (1995) Controlling the False Discovery Rate: A Practical and Powerful Approach to Multiple Testing. J R Stat Soc 57: 289–300.

52. Lipka AE, Tian F, Wang Q, Peiffer J, Li M, et al. (2012) GAPIT: Genome Association and Prediction Integrated Tool. Bioinformatics 1–2. doi: 10. 1093/bioinformatics/bts444

53. Churchill GA, Doerge RW (1994) Empirical threshold values for quantitative trait mapping. Genetics 138: 963–971.

CHAPTER 5

FROM QTL TO QTN: CANDIDATE GENE SET APPROACH AND A CASE STUDY IN PORCINE IGF1-FOXO PATHWAY

Minghui Wang, Qishan Wang, Yuchun Pan

INTRODUCTION

The function of any biological process is determined by both its composition and its structure. The genetic architecture that links quantitative traits operates under the same conditions, wherein both gene identities as well as relationships amongst genes determine the phenotype. Over the past two decades, the candidate gene approach and linkage disequilibrium analysis have been used to discover QTGs (Quantitative trait genes) and QTNs (Quantitative Trait Nucleotide). The candidate gene approach is based on a prior knowledge including the physiological mechanisms described in other studies [1], for example, the estrogen receptor (ESR) gene [2]. Linkage disequilibrium analysis based on well-characterized populations has driven QTL (quantitative trait locus, a fragment of DNA covering one or several genes) mapping nearly to completion for almost all major livestock species. This approach exploits crosses of reference strains or individuals related through a known pedigree. Up to now, a huge amount of information has been accumulated and deposited in Animal QTLdb(http://www.animalgenome.org/QTLdb/[3]), a valuable resource which is freely available for further mining.

In order to make use of the previous QTL mapping results, we proposed a complementary, alternative approach, named candidate gene set approach (CGSA), to identify QTG and QTN in a specific set of related genes such as regulatory networks, pathways, etc. The CGSA was designed to decrease false discoveries by considering a functional set and thus improve statistical power. The performance of the proposed approach was assessed by simulation based on 820 hydrid pigs and demonstrated by a real example of growth traits of 111 hydrid pigs.

Citation: Wang M, Wang Q, Pan Y (2013) From QTL to QTN: Candidate Gene Set Approach and a Case Study in Porcine IGF1-FoxO Pathway. PLoS ONE 8(1): e53452. doi:10.1371/journal.pone.0053452

MATERIALS AND METHODS

Candidate Gene Set Approach

Defining candidate gene set.

Gene set, as the name suggests, is a group of genes, which are functionally or structurally related to each other. There are many possible sources used for defining gene set, including gene ontology annotations [4], KEGG pathways [5], Molecular Signatures Database (MSigDB)[6], co-expression genes from microarray analysis, etc. They may even be chromosome regions covered by related QTL. The sources above are not an exhaustive list, but give a good idea on the types of analyses that can be done using the methods we described in this study. Parts of the gene sets can be selected as candidate gene sets based on some prior information for further analyses.

For animals (livestock) with a poor annotation of genes, we can define candidate gene set by comparative genomics, namely identifying orthologous genes in livestock by Blast searching, because researches on model animals have produced a huge amount of information. When such search indicates a livestock gene with unknown mapping data, the genes adjacent to the target gene in the query, can be similarly searched in the livestock genome in order to infer the location of livestock gene based on synteny. Recently, our group have developed a functional annotation platform called SNPpath for animals (livestock) SNP [7], and it can provide functional annotations of livestock SNP markers from several commercial platforms and dbSNP database. The web server may be particularly beneficial for the analysis of combining SNP association analysis with the CGSA.

Mapping genes to QTL.

As mentioned above, by fine design of experiments, QTL mapping has obtained a huge amount of information, including QTL location (chromosome, location, and location span), flanking markers, peak markers, test statistics, QTL effects and traits. For example, up to June of 2012, there were 6,818 QTLs that represent 585 different traits for pig [3]. If a gene within the candidate gene set can be mapped to the confidence interval of QTL that have some physiological relevance to the trait, it will be reasonably considered as primary candidate QTGs [8], especially, overlapping with multiple QTL of interest. Some QTL in the pig QTLdb have very large confidence interval, so we suggest that research should set a limitation of confidence interval by considering overlapping with multiple QTL of interest. We have successfully written a Perl script to relatively locate genes within the interval of the QTL.

Predicting potential SNPs.

Though a few thousand of SNPs in animal are currently available, which comes from commercial array or annotation database like dbSNP, the SNP density in animal is much lower than that in human. The low SNP density might limit the power of identifying genes involved in the traits of interest. The ongoing genome sequencing project and the releasing of the genome draft assembly of animal have provided the opportunity to compare and detect SNP candidates using alignment algorithms [9]. Kerstens (2009) successfully used this strategy to mine novel SNPs of pig using whole genome shotgun dataset generated by the Danish-Chinese Pig Genome Sequencing Initiative [10]. Therefore, we could perform similar pipeline to identify candidate SNPs.

SNP genotyping.

The predicted candidate SNPs as well as SNPs from commercial array and annotation database need to be genotyped in a panel of target population for association studies. Owing to advances in the area of molecular genetics and improvements in genotyping technology, a large number of SNP genotyping techniques were used to type allele-specific products for SNPs of interest followed by genotype determination. In addition to high cost in genotyping and stringent requirements for accuracy, the throughput has been a critical factor in many farm animals studying with large sample populations. Therefore, in most cases, we need to make a reasonable compromise between throughput and cost. For instance, typing SNP candidates overlapped with QTLs or that in all members of gene set is determined by cost to some extent.

Association test.

The CGSA method makes an attempt to answer the following questions: First, whether is there the association between genetic variation and phenotypic variation in the gene set level? Second, if the gene set is significantly associated with some traits, which SNPs or combinations play a key role?

To answer the two questions, we first used the following Mixed Liner Model (MLM) to perform our CGSA on each measured trait.

The matrix format of this model is that: $\mathbf{y}=\mathbf{Xb}+\mathbf{Z}_1\mathbf{a}+\mathbf{Z}_2\mathbf{d}+\mathbf{Z}_3\mathbf{h}_{\mathbf{AA}}+\mathbf{Z}_4\mathbf{h}_{\mathbf{AD}}+\mathbf{Z}_5\mathbf{h}_{\mathbf{DD}}+\mathbf{e}$,where **b** is a vector of fixed effects, **a** is vector of random additive genetic effects of candidate gene set, **d** is vector of random dominance effect of candidate gene set, and $\mathbf{h}_{\mathbf{AA}}$, $\mathbf{h}_{\mathbf{AD}}$ and $\mathbf{h}_{\mathbf{DD}}$ represent the interaction effects of additive-by-additive (AA), additive-by-dominance (AD) and dominance-by-dominance (DD) respectively. $\mathbf{X}$, $\mathbf{Z}_1$, $\mathbf{Z}_2$, $\mathbf{Z}_3$, $\mathbf{Z}_4$ and $\mathbf{Z}_5$ are the corresponding design matrix.

It is assumed that.

$$\mathbf{a} \sim MVN(0, \mathbf{A}\sigma_a^2)$$

$$\mathbf{d} \sim MVN(0, \mathbf{D}\sigma_d^2)$$

$$\mathbf{h}_{\mathbf{AA}} \sim MVN(0, \mathbf{H}_{\mathbf{AA}}\sigma_{AA}^2)$$

$$\mathbf{h}_{\mathbf{AD}} \sim MVN(0, \mathbf{H}_{\mathbf{AD}}\sigma_{AD}^2)$$

$$\mathbf{h}_{\mathbf{DD}} \sim MVN(0, \mathbf{H}_{\mathbf{DD}}\sigma_{DD}^2)$$

$$\mathbf{e} \sim MVN(0, \mathbf{I}\sigma_e^2)$$

MVN represents multivariate normal distribution, **A** and **D** represent the corresponding additive (dominance) effect relationship matrix in candidate gene set level, respectively. The matrices can be estimated by the SNPs in select candidate gene set using the software of PLINK [11]. The PLINK estimates the probability of sharing 0, 1, or 2 alleles IBD (Identiy by Descent) for two subjects. The elements of A matrix can be expressed as $\mathrm{P(IBD=2)}+0.5*\mathrm{P(IBD=1)}$and the elements of D matrix can be calculated as $\mathrm{P(IBD=2)}$ [11]. The corresponding epistatic variation effect relationship matrix could obtain by the Hadamard products of the A and D matrices [12]. The likelihood ratio test could be used to test the significance of the additive effects, dominance effect and epistatic effect for the candidate gene set.

Second, if the candidate gene set is significantly associated with some traits, the single SNP general linear model or multiple higher order interaction models such as MB-MDR method can be further used to study the genetic mechanism. MB-MDR method proposed by Calle et al.[13] not only assesses joint significance of multiple higher order interaction models at once, but also facilitates distinguishing between epistatic effects and contributing main effects to the multilocus signal via the 'MB' part in MB-MDR [14].

SIMULATIONS

Simulation data.

We compared the statistical power between our CGSA and the traditional candidate gene approach across a variety of heritabilities in a real experimental genotype data and simulated phenotype data produced by R program. The pig dataset was collected from 820 commercial female pigs. There were 51,385 SNPs scored on these individuals [15]. SNP markers were aligned to the corresponding Ensemble gene IDs (the Sus scrofa Build 9.2 downloaded from UCSC genome browser). The genes including 50 kb flanking regions (upstream and downstream of gene), were used for the assignment of SNPs to genes. The 57 SNPs mapped to 17 genes in the insulin and insulin growth factor-1/FoxO (IGF1-FoxO) signal pathway were used in the simulation procedure.

Simulation procedure.

Two simulation experiments were conducted to assess the performance of our method. In the first simulation experiment, only additive genetic effects were simulated. Fifteen SNPs was randomly sampled from the IGF1/FoxO signal pathway as causal QTNs for the simulated traits. The distribution of these QTN effects was assumed as a normal distribution with mean of 0 and variance of 1. Phenotypes were calculated as the sum of additive effect and the random residual effect. The total additive effect was the sum of additive effects across all QTNs and the residual variance was computed as $V_e = V_a(1\text{-}h_2)/h_2$, where V_a is the empirical additive genetic variance and h_2 is the heritability. A residual error was assumed as a normal distribution with mean of 0 and variance of V_e. Five levels of heritability were analyzed (h_2=0, 0.05, 0.1, 0.25 and 0.5) in this simulation experiment.

In the second simulation experiment, additive effects, dominance effects and epistatic effects were simulated simultaneous. Thirteen SNPs from the IGF1/FoxO signal transduction pathway were assumed as causal QTNs for the simulated traits. All the main effects and the effects of interaction (epistatic effects) of the makers with their positions. Three paired SNPs were simulated as interacting QTN effect. It is assumed that the effects of paired SNPs were seen only if an individual is heterozygous at both QTNs. The simulated additive genetic variance and total genetic variance for the true 820 commercial female pigs were 6.05 and 9.01 respectively. The residual variance was set as 10. The power was calculated as the proportion of QTNs detected or the significant pathway with Type I error rate 0.01. A total of 1000 replications were conducted for each method. The R program written by the authors based on GAPIT software was used to perform analysis for the two simulation experiments[16].

ANALYSIS OF REAL DATA

Ethics statements

Prior approval by the Institutional Animal Care and Use Committee of Shanghai Jiao Tong University (Contract 2009-0068) was given for all experimental procedures involving animals in the present study.

Experimental design and procedure.

The 111 Duroc ×Landrace ×Yorkshire (DLY) hybrid pigs were phenotyped on daily feed intake and body weight. All pigs were fed the same corn-soybeanmill based ration during the feeding period. Pigs were automatically weighed on their way to feeding using OSBORNE FIRE system. Feed intake and body weight (BW) were measured several times a day, which were then arithmetically averaged to one value for further analysis. If some measurements were missing, the remaining measurements were used and treated as a daily measurement. For generating variables representing BW changes from born to 100 kg and further analysis of the BW data, individual measurements were first smoothed using S-shaped logistic curves. In this study, we mainly focus on the corresponding timing intervals from birth to 30 kg (BW 30), from 30 to 60 kg (BW 60), from 60 to 100 kg (BW 100), average daily gain (ADG) and total feed intake (DFI). The heritability of BW 30, BW 60, BW 100, ADG and DFI are 0.39, 0.35, 0.34, 0.37 and 0.15 separately in present population.

Defining candidate gene set

To make use of the results from the related experiments of model organisms, we defined the gene sets based on our previous work, which presents the transcriptomic profile during skeletal muscle regeneration using time-course expression data and motif scanning information [17]. Our study recovered some signaling pathways involved in the regulation of muscle differentiation, and the IGF1/FoxO signal transduction pathway was selected to define a gene set for the current study.

Predicting potential SNP positions and SNP genotyping.

Two data sources were used to predict SNP positions, one from the commercial array annotations (Illumina PorcineSNP60 BeadChip), and the other from the NCBI Trace repository. The identification of novel SNPs was performed by a 2-step process for the NCBI Trace repository. First, the shotgun sequences were assigned to a reference sequence (member form gene set) by clustering based on their sequence similarity. Secondly, the sequences within cluster were aligned to search for potential SNPs. A total of 111 genomic DNA samples from DLY hybrid pigs comprising 58 females and 53 castrates, were genotyped by SNaPshot method. The primer sequences for analysis of 23 identified SNPs.

Association test

The mixed linear model is as following, $y_{ijk} = \mu + s_i + p_j + a_k + d_k + e_{ijk}$, where y_{ijk} is the phenotypic value of each trait, $\mu$is the overall mean for each trait, s_i is the fixed gender effect (i=1,2), $p_j$is fixed sire effect (j=1,2,3), a_k and d_k are the pathway additive effect and dominance effect of the kth individual,$e_{ijk}$is the random residual effect. The additive and dominance genetic relationship matrix was estimated based on the TagSNPs in select candidate signaling pathway using the software of PLINK [11]. Then ASReml was used to estimate the pathway effects and test the significance level by the likelihood ratio test [18]. In this case study, we can take full advantage of the opportunities provided by MB-MDR model to study simultaneously the association of a group of genetic variants in predefined gene set, which can help us to holistically unravel the complex genetic structure of the studied trait and to gain insight into the biological processes and mechanisms.

RESULTS

Simulation Results

For the first simulation experiment, generally, along all the levels of heritability investigated, as heritability increases, the statistical power of both methods increased as expected (Figure 1). Our CGSA performed higher statistical power over the traditional candidate gene approach across all kinds of heritabilities. The differences among these methods varied along the level of heritabilities. Figure 1 showed that the differences among the methods with mid-level and low-level of heritability were greater than the one with high heritability. For the second experiment, the statistical power of our CGSA and candidate gene approach. Compared to the traditional candidate gene approach, the CGSA performed the significantly higher statistical power for both additive effect and dominance effects and similar statistical power for epistatic effect in the present simulation scenario.

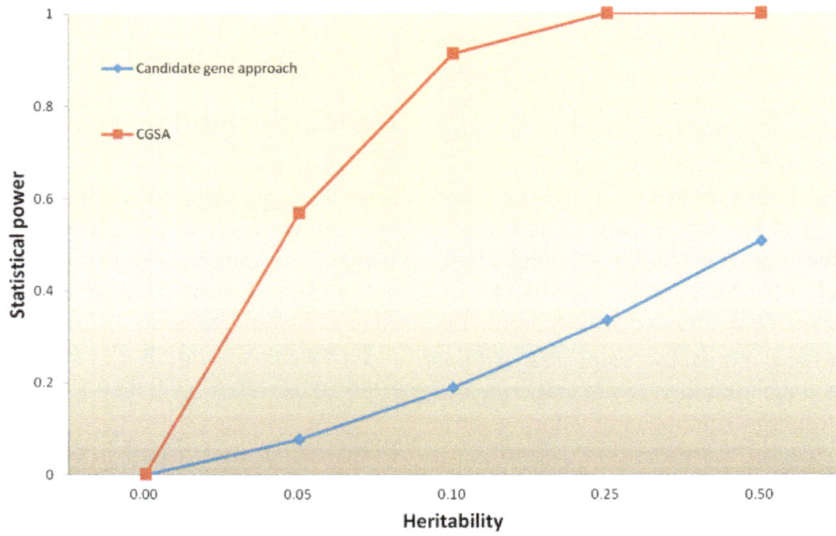

Figure 1. Statistical powers between CGSA and candidate gene approach under different heritability levels.

The power was examined on a trait simulated from 15 causative mutations (QTNs). A total of 1000 replications were conducted for each method. The heritability of the trait varied from 0 to 0.5. The differences between our CGSA and candidate gene set approach with mid-level and low-level of heritability were greater than the one with high heritability.

Real Data Results

There were 28 murine genes in the IGF1/FoxO signal transduction pathway, and a simple scheme of IGF1/FoxO pathway components is shown in Figure 2 (modified from [19]). These 28 genes have been aligned to the pig chromosomes to identify orthologous genes using BLASTn program [20] from the blastall tool [21] with default parameters. We identify many pig orthologs of the murine genes and the compared results are shown in **Table 1**. However, the chromosomal locations for 4 genes (INS2, IRS2, PIK3CA and PIK3CB) are still unknown.

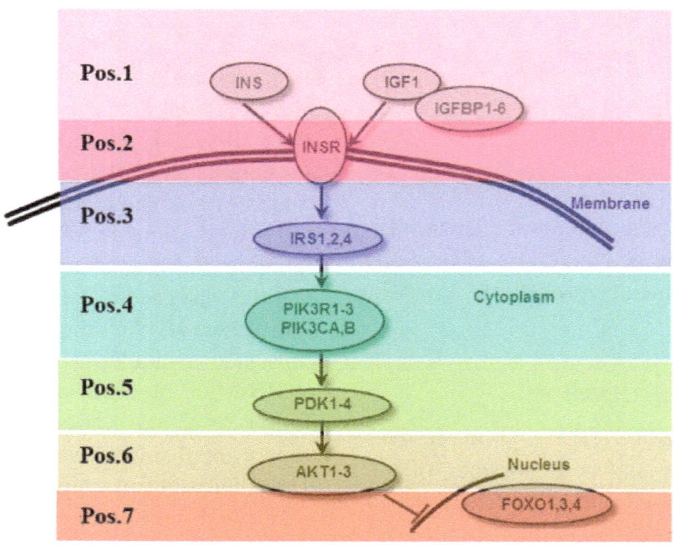

Figure 2. An illustration of the IGF1/FoxO pathway genes.

Arrows indicate the direction of signal transduction. The numbers on the left side represent the position of the IGF1/FoxO pathway genes.

Table 1. The comparison of orthologs members between pig and murine IGF1/FoxO pathway.

Ensemble No (mouse)	Mouse gene name	Mouse chr.	Mouse genome position	Ensemble No (pig)	Pig gene name	Pig chr by blast	Pig genome Position
ENSMUSG00000020053	Igf1	10	87321010-87399792	ENSSSCG00000000857	IGF1	5	77082628-77154428
ENSMUSG00000020429	Igfbp1	11	7097785-7102549	ENSSSCG00000016728	IGFBP1	18	48650114-48654870
ENSMUSG00000039323	Igfbp2	1	72871077-72899048	*	IGFBP2	15	112022157-112022652
ENSMUSG00000020427	Igfbp3	11	7106089-7113926	ENSSSCG00000016729	IGFBP3	18	48778107-48782267
ENSMUSG00000017493	Igfbp4	11	98902558-98913969	ENSSSCG00000017472	IGFBP4	12	19797073-19811336
ENSMUSG00000026185	Igfbp5	1	72904506-72921458	ENSSSCG00000016178	IGFBP5	15	112017411-112019845
ENSMUSG00000023046	Igfbp6	15	101974793-101979942	ENSSSCG00000000255	IGFBP6	5	16854964-16855290
ENSMUSG00000000215	Ins2	7	149864561-149885415	/	/	/	/
ENSMUSG00000005534	Insr	8	3150922-3279617	*	INSR	2	50637472-50720384
ENSMUSG00000055980	Irs1	1	82229676-82287991	ENSSSCG00000016242	IRS1	15	120872701-120981690
ENSMUSG00000038894	Irs2	8	10986980-11008458	/	/	/	/
ENSMUSG00000054667	Irs4	X	138145541-138159806	ENSSSCG00000012577	IRS4	X	88228629-88230746
ENSMUSG00000041417	Pik3r1	13	102450716-102538172	ENSSSCG00000016958	PIK3R1	16	44114529-44120792
ENSMUSG00000031834	Pik3r2	8	73292075-73300612	ENSSSCG00000013900	PIK3R2	2	62387523-62399642
ENSMUSG00000028698	Pik3r3	4	115894223-115975661	ENSSSCG00000003909	PIK3R3	6	118327752-118488382
ENSMUSG00000027665	Pik3ca	3	32296593-32367408	/	/	/	/
ENSMUSG00000032462	Pik3cb	9	98938821-99041040	/	/	/	/
ENSMUSG00000006494	Pdk1	2	71711281-71741915	ENSSSCG00000015958	PDK1	15	73606993-73615575
ENSMUSG00000038967	Pdk2	11	94887572-94902668	*	PDK2	12	24797209-24801353
ENSMUSG00000035232	Pdk3	X	91009946-91077540	ENSSSCG00000012181	PDK3	X	19401655-19471675
ENSMUSG00000019577	Pdk4	6	5433351-5446309	ENSSSCG00000015334	PDK4	9	70465829-70477355
ENSMUSG00000001729	Akt1	12	113892032-113913095	ENSSSCG00000003194	AKT1	6	38477164-38484612
ENSMUSG00000004056	Akt2	7	28376571-28425845	ENSSSCG00000002989	AKT2	6	33533100-33560034
ENSMUSG00000019699	Akt3	1	178950204-179188334	ENSSSCG00000010872	AKT3	10	16162075-16280499
ENSMUSG00000044167	Foxo1	3	52072259-52154031	ENSSSCG00000009370	FOXO1	11	15075341-15085340
ENSMUSG00000048756	Foxo3	10	41901647-41996561	ENSSSCG00000004387	FOXO3	1	78223324-78349962
ENSMUSG00000042903	Foxo4	X	98449867-98456212	ENSSSCG00000012399	FOXO4	X	56862227-56867783
ENSMUSG00000052135	Foxo6	4	119939684-119959954	ENSSSCG00000009371	FOXO6	11	15207819-15208487

Each of the genes that were mapped on the pig genome has been co-localized with published QTL from pigQTLdb. The genes identified as being co-localized with a QTL. FOXO1 gene has been co-localized with 22 QTL, FOXO3 gene with 48 QTL, FOXO6 gene with 32 QTL, IGFBP6 gene with 27 QTL, and PDK3 gene with 4 QTL. Only the results for the FOXO3 gene are detailed here (**Table 2**). We found that many traits were closely associated with growth and development traits, for example, average daily gain (QTL_id 5680, 329 and 5928) and feed intake (QTL_id 871). Each locus (QTL_id) corresponded to one publication.

Table 2. Co-localization of QTL map from Pig QTLdb and candidate gene (FOXO3) from IGF1/FoxO pathway.

QTL_ID	QTL_symbol	Trait_name	QTL_start	QTL_end
3793	BFT	Average backfat thickness	52423837	166525431
5670	BFT	Average backfat thickness	3320998	144078329
5680	ADG	Average daily gain (10 weeks-slaughter)	3320998	193909568
329	ADG	Average daily gain (25–90 kg)	32980500	109360545
5928	ADG	Average daily gain (on weaning)	52423837	86769928
45	LUMBF	Backfat at last lumbar	73990528	154961837
3794	LRIBF	backfat at last rib	52423837	166525431
5674	LRIBF	backfat at last rib	7302766	163511869
651	BFTR	Backfat at rump	43291013	144078329
3795	10RIBBFT	Backfat at tenth rib7	52423837	158592899
5672	10RIBBFT	Backfat at tenth rib	26500027	86769928
5679	BYLEAN	Belly meat content	7302766	163511869
2845	BELLYWT	Belly weight	51386391	139615854
5931	WWT	Body weight (weaning)	52423837	86769928
4260	CD2L	CD2-positive leukocyte number	24598042	144803085
4261	CD4L	CD4-positive leukocyte number	24598042	144803085
5669	cond	Conductivity 24 hours postmortem (ham)	52423837	166525431
5668	cond	Conductivity 24 hours postmortem (loin)	52423837	118433791
6366	CREAT	Creatinine level	33269805	126505160
8885	EAREA	Ear area	43291013	109360545
8886	EAREA	Ear area	43291013	109360545
8853	EARWT	Ear weight	43291013	109360545
8854	EARWT	Ear weight	43291013	109360545
5678	ECLC	Estimated carcass lean content	7302766	163511869
5676	FATAREA	Fat area	11402561	144078329
5677	FP	Fat ratio (percentage)	7302766	163511869
871	FEEDIN	Feed Intake	26957266	91781628
8908	FSCOREF	feet score (front)	32980500	108464751
860	HEADWT	Head weight	26957266	91781628
5420	HCT	hematocrit	33269805	126505160
8910	LSCOREH	leg score (hind)	32980500	108464751
872	LIVWT	Liver weight	26957266	91781628
3796	LMA	Loin muscle area	52423837	158592899
5468	LYMPH	Lymphocyte number	33269805	126505160
2930	MARB	Marbling	52423837	91781628
4019	MARB	Marbling	27710381	179573387
78	MARB	Marbling	73990528	86769928
5667	COLORO	Meat color OPTO QTL	52423837	163511869
5664	pH	pH for Longissmus Dorsi	52423837	118433791
5666	pH	pH for Longissmus Dorsi	52423837	118433791
5665	pH	pH for Semimembranosus	52423837	118433791
6380	BPOTASS	Potassium level	33269805	126505160
9658	PRRSVAB	PRRSV antibody titer	26500027	144251236
5675	SIDEF	Side fat	26500027	86769928
5671	SHOUFATD	Subcutaneous fat depth at shoulder	3320998	163511869
6481	TNUM	Teat number	43291013	109360545
79	TOTLIP	Total lipid	24598042	129115585
611	WBC	White blood cell counts	32980500	108464751

At last, 23 single nucleotide polymorphisms (SNPs) in 9 genes (IGF1, IGFBP1, INSR, IRS1,PIK3R3, PDK3, PDK4, AKT3 and FOXO3) were identified in the IGF1/FoxO pathway, and 11 of which were predicted novel SNPs. Using this approach, 13 SNPs were determined to be polymorphic in our panel, three of which were novel SNPs (S14, S18 and S28 in **Table S3**). The allelic and genotypic frequencies, as well as the concrete distribution in this population were determined by SNaPshot method. Analysis of the same site using PCR-RFLP generated similar results to those of the SnaPshot analysis (data not shown). Our study showed that the SNaPshot method can reliably replace sequencing and RFLP testing, particularly in cases in which no restriction endonuclease recognizes the polymorphic site being analyzed. Moreover, the same results can be achieved in a shorter time by SNaPshot analysis for small or medium output.

Using both our MLM model and the likelihood ratio test, we tested the significance of the additive effect and dominance in IGF1-FoxO pathway level on each of the 5 measured traits. Our results showed that the IGF1-FoxO pathway significantly associated with BW100 (0.007) and ADG (0.010). No significant dominance effect was found in the present study.

For further identifing which SNP (or combinations of SNPs) plays a key role(s) in the IGF1-FoxO pathway, we performed single-SNP association analysis and interaction models analysis. The single SNP association analysis was initiated using linear regression with adjustment for gender and pedigree. Of the 13 SNPs analyzed, 4 SNPs (AS3, AS6, AS9 and AS10) were showing the strong association with BW100 and ADG. Overall, most of SNP associations were moderate in single SNP analysis, suggesting that there appeared to be multiple weak associations in the studied pathway. These SNPs may therefore interact with each other to exert their effect.

In order to complement pathway-based analysis and provide additional insights into the genetic architecture of studied traits, a generalized multifactor dimensionality reduction method was used to determine the relationship between interacted SNPs (combined effect) and studied traits. Several interactions were shown to be significant: a two-SNP interaction model (AS3 and S14) and a three-SNP interaction (AS6, AS9 and S18) were related BW100 as well as a two-SNP interaction (AS10 and S28) and a three-SNP interaction (AS6, AS9 and S18) involved to ADG was found. Our study indicates that the susceptibility SNPs identified by single SNP analysis might independently and/or in a combined manner influence studied trait. Overall, we can identify many SNPs of moderate effect that influence studied traits though interaction, and most of the SNPs found have been reported in the literature as functional elements correlated with the model animals' growth [22], [23], [24].

DISCUSSION

Over the past decade, researchers have made great progresses in identifying economical relevance factors (genes, QTLs and SNPs) contributing to trait variation. SNPs have been the markers of choice in recent years, due to their high stability, density and the highly automated way in which SNPs are detected. Various statistical models and techniques have been developed and applied in order to make inferences about the general population using studied samples as well as relate the genotype information to observable/measurable phenotypes [25]. Our approach is different from traditional candidate gene strategies, which identify sets of SNPs/variants showing allele frequency and genotypic concordance among subjects. Parts of the traditional strategies based on the linkage disequilibrium between markers mainly consider haplotypes [26], [27], but is restricted to areas of high LD (haplotype blocks). In addition, clustering and principal components were also used to group markers based on LD [28], [29]. Unlike these, our CGSA approach can be considered as an improvement of traditional candidate gene approach. We group markers based on functional considerations, which we believe is in better concordance with the goal of identifying variation that is associated with phenotype.

In order to improved statistical power, several similar candidate pathway approaches [30], [31]were published to deal with some of the same issues as our study. However, our study was conducted differently in a variety of ways. First, our method can make full use of the large scale study results performed on model animals (human, mouse) which have provided the potential to define candidate gene sets to identify the complex processes involved in the phenotype. Second, our approach takes full advantage of previously reported QTL, candidate gene sets that lie within the region of the QTL, and that have physiological relevance to the trait (considered as primary candidates for the QTL), particularly within multiple overlapping QTL of interest. Third, most of existing candidate pathway approaches [30] use multiple regression models to test the significance, but our method allows us to test whether a set of genes are associated with a trait of interest based on MLM framework which could eliminate false positives effectively both in candidate gene association study and GWAS [32], [33].

Using our approach, we succeed in identifying combined effect members in our predefined set, which is associated with several economical traits in pigs. The increase in power when compared to single-marker approaches based on the joint reduction of false positives and false negatives. Reducing false negatives comes from the fact that moderately strong signals can be combined into a stronger signal, whereas, these members might be ignored by strong global significance in single SNP analysis. Reducing false positives is because of our method based on MLM framework which could eliminate false positives effectively [32], [33]. In the present case study, 2 SNPs associated with the BW 30, 1 SNP with BW 60 in single-marker approach were excluded in case of false positives because our gene set approach didn't indicate the significant association in the pathway level. In the present case study, no significant dominance effect was found because sample size is relatively too small. So, the real results cannot demonstrate the advantage of the new approach. Our group is trying to apply our approach to other dataset with large sample size to verify the relevant conclusions furtherly.

Finally, the results from this approach offer a clearer picture on the functional relevance of the discoveries. The significant SNPs found using this approach warrant further experimental exploration. Especially, SNPs from FoxO3, which were not only significant in single SNP analysis, but also in combined effect analysis. This FoxO3 gene was overlapped with multiple QTLs (48 QTLs) of pigs' growth and development traits, and was reported to be related to muscle growth abundantly [34], [35], [36]. The validation experiments would be more or less complex depending on the nature of the trait (mono- or polygenic). As biotechnology and genetic transformation techniques advance, we will be able to demonstrate experimentally whether specific SNPs truly determine variation in a particular trait.

It has become clear that gene sets rather than individual gene are essential in understanding carcinoma [37], [38]. One drawback of this approach, however, is the reliance of prior assumptions that genes identified in the QTL regions are well annotated, the explicitly recording from KEGG and so on. If not, we may overlook or miss some genes or SNPs involved in the phenotype for incompleteness of annotation and complex biological process.

CONCLUSIONS

We have proposed a novel approach for determining specific genes and their SNPs that are associated with studied traits in the gene set level. The simulation results demonstrated that our CGSA performed higher statistical power over the traditional candidate gene approach. We also used this approach to study the relationship between IGF1-FoxO pathway and growth and development traits of pig. The results suggested that genetic variations in the IGF1-FoxO pathway modulate the growth and development in pigs. The CGSA is flexible to be extended to model complex genetic structures and can be applied by other gene sets. Computer programs (R and perl source code) are available at http://klab.sjtu.edu.cn/CGSA.

ACKNOWLEDGMENTS

The authors are grateful to Dr Bin Fan for providing genotype data of 820 commercial female pigs.

Author Contributions

Conceived and designed the experiments: YP QW. Performed the experiments: MW QW. Analyzed the data: QW MW. Contributed reagents/materials/analysis tools: QW MW YP. Wrote the paper: QW MW YP.

REFERENCES

1. Rothschild M, Soller M (1997) Candidate gene analysis to detect genes controlling traits of economic importance in domestic livestock. Probe 8: 13–20.
2. Short TH, Rothschild MF, Southwood OI, McLaren DG, de Vries A, et al. (1997) Effect of the estrogen receptor locus on reproduction and production traits in four commercial pig lines. J Anim Sci 75: 3138–3142.
3. Hu ZL, Fritz ER, Reecy JM (2007) AnimalQTLdb: a livestock QTL database tool set for positional QTL information mining and beyond. Nucleic Acids Res 35: D604–609. doi: 10. 1093/nar/gkl946
4. Ashburner M, Ball CA, Blake JA, Botstein D, Butler H, et al. (2000) Gene ontology: tool for the unification of biology. The Gene Ontology Consortium. Nat Genet 25: 25–29.
5. Kanehisa M, Goto S (2000) KEGG: kyoto encyclopedia of genes and genomes. Nucleic Acids Res 28: 27–30. doi: 10. 1093/nar/28. 1. 27
6. Subramanian A, Tamayo P, Mootha VK, Mukherjee S, Ebert BL, et al. (2005) Gene set enrichment analysis: a knowledge-based approach for interpreting genome-wide expression profiles. Proc Natl Acad Sci U S A 102: 15545–15550. doi: 10. 1073/pnas. 0506580102
7. Wang Q, Wamg M, Yang Y, Pan Y (2011) SNPpath: Characterizing cattle SNPs by enriched pathway terms. Animal Science Journal 83: 279–283. doi: 10. 1111/j. 1740-0929. 2011. 00952. x
8. Ron M, Israeli G, Seroussi E, Weller JI, Gregg JP, et al. (2007) Combining mouse mammary gland gene expression and comparative mapping for the identification of candidate genes for QTL of milk production traits in cattle. BMC Genomics 8: 183. doi: 10. 1186/1471-2164-8-183
9. Myers EW, Miller W (1988) Optimal alignments in linear space. Comput Appl Biosci 4: 11–17. doi: 10. 1093/bioinformatics/4. 1. 11
10. Wernersson R, Schierup MH, Jorgensen FG, Gorodkin J, Panitz F, et al. (2005) Pigs in sequence space: a 0. 66X coverage pig genome survey based on shotgun sequencing. BMC Genomics 6: 70.
11. Purcell S, Neale B, Todd-Brown K, Thomas L, Ferreira MAR, et al. (2007) PLINK: a tool set for whole-genome association and population-based linkage analyses. The American Journal of Human Genetics 81: 559–575. doi: 10. 1086/519795
12. Henderson C (1985) Best linear unbiased prediction of nonadditive genetic merits in noninbred populations. Journal of animal science 60: 111–117.
13. Calle ML, Urrea V, Malats N, Van Steen K (2010) mbmdr: an R package for exploring gene-gene interactions associated with binary or quantitative traits. Bioinformatics 26: 2198–2199. doi: 10. 1093/bioinformatics/btq352
14. Mahachie John JM, Van Lishout F, Van Steen K (2011) Model-Based Multifactor Dimensionality Reduction to detect epistasis for quantitative traits in the presence of error-free and noisy data. Eur J Hum Genet 19: 696–703. doi: 10. 1038/ejhg. 2011. 17
15. Fan B, Onteru SK, Du ZQ, Garrick DJ, Stalder KJ, et al. (2011) Genome-wide association study identifies loci for body composition and structural soundness traits in pigs. PloS one 6: e14726. doi: 10. 1371/journal. pone. 0014726
16. Lipka AE, Tian F, Wang Q, Peiffer J, Li M, et al. (2012) GAPIT: genome association and prediction integrated tool. Bioinformatics 28: 2397–2399. doi: 10. 1093/bioinformatics/bts444
17. Wang M, Wang Q, Zhang X, Yang Y, Zhao H, et al. (2011) Uncovering the transcriptional circuitry in skeletal muscle regeneration. Mamm Genome 22: 272–281. doi: 10. 1007/s00335-011-9322-x
18. Gilmour A, Gogel B, Cullis B, Thompson R, Butler D, et al. . (2009) ASReml user guide release 3. 0. VSNi website. Available: http://www. vsni. co. uk/software/asreml. Accessed 2012 Apr 3.
19. Taniguchi CM, Emanuelli B, Kahn CR (2006) Critical nodes in signalling pathways: insights into insulin action. Nature Reviews Molecular Cell Biology 7: 85–96. doi: 10. 1038/nrm1837
20. Altschul SF, Gish W, Miller W, Myers EW, Lipman DJ (1990) Basic local alignment search tool. J Mol Biol 215: 403–410. doi: 10. 1016/s0022-2836(05)80360-2
21. Altschul SF, Madden TL, Schaffer AA, Zhang J, Zhang Z, et al. (1997) Gapped BLAST and PSI-BLAST: a new generation of protein database search programs. Nucleic Acids Res 25: 3389–3402. doi: 10. 1093/nar/25. 17. 3389
22. Soroceanu L, Kharbanda S, Chen R, Soriano RH, Aldape K, et al. (2007) Identification of IGF2 signaling through phosphoinositide-3-kinase regulatory subunit 3 as a growth-promoting axis in glioblastoma. Proceedings of the National Academy of Sciences 104: 3466–3471. doi: 10. 1073/pnas. 0611271104
23. Schiaffino S, Mammucari C (2011) Regulation of skeletal muscle growth by the IGF1-Akt/PKB pathway: insights from genetic models. Skelet Muscle 1: 4. doi: 10. 1186/2044-5040-1-4
24. Williamson DL, Raue U, Slivka DR, Trappe S (2010) Resistance exercise, skeletal muscle FOXO3A, and

85-year-old women. J Gerontol A Biol Sci Med Sci 65: 335–343. doi: 10. 1093/gerona/glq005

25. Liang Y, Kelemen A (2006) Associating phenotypes with molecular events: recent statistical advances and challenges underpinning microarray experiments. Funct Integr Genomics 6: 1–13. doi: 10. 1007/s10142-005-0006-z
26. Ginja C, Telo da Gama L, Penedo MC (2009) Y chromosome haplotype analysis in Portuguese cattle breeds using SNPs and STRs. J Hered 100: 148–157. doi: 10. 1093/jhered/esn080
27. Meidtner K, Schwarzenbacher H, Scharfe M, Severitt S, Blocker H, et al. (2009) Haplotypes of the porcine peroxisome proliferator-activated receptor delta gene are associated with backfat thickness. BMC Genet 10: 76. doi: 10. 1186/1471-2156-10-76
28. Durrant C, Zondervan KT, Cardon LR, Hunt S, Deloukas P, et al. (2004) Linkage disequilibrium mapping via cladistic analysis of single-nucleotide polymorphism haplotypes. Am J Hum Genet 75: 35–43. doi: 10. 1086/422174
29. Gauderman WJ, Murcray C, Gilliland F, Conti DV (2007) Testing association between disease and multiple SNPs in a candidate gene. Genetic epidemiology 31: 383–395. doi: 10. 1002/gepi. 20219
30. Lesnick TG, Papapetropoulos S, Mash DC, Ffrench-Mullen J, Shehadeh L, et al. (2007) A genomic pathway approach to a complex disease: axon guidance and Parkinson disease. PLoS genetics 3: e98. doi: 10. 1371/journal. pgen. 0030098
31. García-Gámez E, Reverter A, Whan V, McWilliam SM, Arranz JJ, et al. (2011) Using Regulatory and Epistatic Networks to Extend the Findings of a Genome Scan: Identifying the Gene Drivers of Pigmentation in Merino Sheep. PloS one 6: e21158. doi: 10. 1371/journal. pone. 0021158
32. Zhang Z, Ersoz E, Lai CQ, Todhunter RJ, Tiwari HK, et al. (2010) Mixed linear model approach adapted for genome-wide association studies. Nature genetics 42: 355–360. doi: 10. 1038/ng. 546
33. Yu J, Pressoir G, Briggs WH, Bi IV, Yamasaki M, et al. (2005) A unified mixed-model method for association mapping that accounts for multiple levels of relatedness. Nature genetics 38: 203–208. doi: 10. 1038/ng1702
34. Hribal ML, Nakae J, Kitamura T, Shutter JR, Accili D (2003) Regulation of insulin-like growth factor-dependent myoblast differentiation by Foxo forkhead transcription factors. J Cell Biol 162: 535–541. doi: 10. 1083/jcb. 200212107
35. Mammucari C, Milan G, Romanello V, Masiero E, Rudolf R, et al. (2007) FoxO3 controls autophagy in skeletal muscle in vivo. Cell Metab 6: 458–471. doi: 10. 1016/j. cmet. 2007. 11. 001
36. Dentice M, Marsili A, Ambrosio R, Guardiola O, Sibilio A, et al. (2010) The FoxO3/type 2 deiodinase pathway is required for normal mouse myogenesis and muscle regeneration. The Journal of clinical investigation 120: 4021–4030. doi: 10. 1172/jci43670
37. Wood LD, Parsons DW, Jones S, Lin J, Sjo blom T, et al. (2007) The genomic landscapes of human breast and colorectal cancers. Science 318: 1108–1113.
38. Vogelstein B, Kinzler KW (2004) Cancer genes and the pathways they control. Nature medicine 10: 789–799. doi: 10. 1038/nm1087

CHAPTER 6

INFERENCE OF POPULATION SPLITS AND MIXTURES FROM GENOME-WIDE ALLELE FREQUENCY DATA

Joseph K. Pickrell, Jonathan K. Pritchard

INTRODUCTION

The extant populations in a species result from an often-complex demographic history, involving population splits, gene flow, and changes in population size. It has long been recognized that genetic data can be used to learn about this history [1]–[3]. In humans, early approaches to inferring history from genetics were limited to using a relatively small number of blood group or other protein polymorphisms [1], [4]–[6]. These types of studies were then superseded by analyses of DNA markers, which have progressed from single marker studies [3] to studies involving hundreds of thousands of markers [7]. It is now feasible to collect genome-wide genetic data in any species; to a large extent it is no longer the data collection, but rather the statistical models used for analysis, that limit the historical insight possible.

There are many statistical approaches to demographic inference from genetic data. One approach is to develop an explicit population genetic model for the history of a set of populations, framed in terms of the effective population sizes of the populations, the times of population splits, the times of demographic events (such as population bottlenecks), and other relevant parameters. The values of these parameters can then be learned from the data using a variety of techniques, often involving simulation [8]–[16]. These approaches have the advantage of allowing flexible modeling of a wide variety of demographic scenarios, but the disadvantage that they can only be applied to one or a few populations at a time. Another type of approach to learning about population history uses methods that summarize the major components of genetic variation in a sample by clustering or principal components analysis [17]–[20]. Although these methods do not model history explicitly, the inferred components can often be interpreted *post hoc* as representing historical populations, and individuals or populations that are mixtures of different components as evidence of admixture between these populations (e.g., [17], [21]–[23]). However, these methods are not directly informative about history; indeed, the relationship between the major components of genetic variation and true underlying demography is not always intuitive [24]–[26].

A different class of approaches focuses on the relationships between populations, by representing a set of populations as a bifurcating tree [1], [27]–[32]. In these models, the details of the demographic histories of the population are absorbed into the branch lengths of the tree [1], [33]. This approach has the advantage of being applicable to large numbers of populations; however, a major caveat when modeling the history of populations as a tree is that gene flow violates the assumptions of the model [2], [34], [35]. It is often difficult to know, *a priori*, how well the history fits a simple bifurcating tree. Explicit tests for the violation of a tree model have been developed [35]–[40]. These tests have been used, most notably, to infer the existence of gene flow between modern and archaic humans [39], [41], [42], as well as between diverged modern human populations [37], [43], [44]. In this paper, we present a unified statistical framework for building population trees and testing for the presence of gene flow between diverged populations. In this framework, the relationship between populations is represented as a graph, allowing us to model both population splits and gene flow. Graph-based models are of growing interest in phylogenetics [45], [46], but have been

Citation: Pickrell JK, Pritchard JK (2012) Inference of Population Splits and Mixtures from Genome-Wide Allele Frequency Data. PLoS Genet 8(11): e1002967. doi:10.1371/journal.pgen.1002967

rarely used in population genetics (with some exceptions [37], [40], [47]).

Results

The starting point for our model was first proposed by Cavalli-Sforza and Edwards [1], and we draw additionally on related models by Nicholson et al. [33] and Coop et al. [48]. Our goal is to provide a statistical framework for inferring population networks that is motivated by an explicit population genetic model, but sufficiently abstract to be computationally feasible for genome-wide data from many populations (say, 10–100). Our primary aim is to represent the topology of relationships between populations, rather than the precise times of demographic events. Our approach to this problem is to first build a maximum likelihood tree of populations. We then identify populations that are poor fits to the tree model, and model migration events involving these populations. Below, we first describe this approach in an idealized setting, and then describe the modifications necessary for implementation in practice.

Model

In the most simple case, consider a single SNP, and let the allele frequency of one of the alleles at this SNP in an ancestral population be x_A. (We use a lowercase x to denote that this is a parameter rather than a random variable. We initially consider distributions conditional on x_A). Now consider a descendant population B. We model X_B, the allele frequency of the SNP in population B, as

$$X_B = x_A + \varepsilon_B \quad (1)$$

With

$$\epsilon_B \sim N(0, c_B x_A[1 - x_A]) \quad (2)$$

where c_B is a factor that reflects the amount of genetic drift that has occurred between the ancestral population and B. This Gaussian model was first introduced by Cavalli-Sforza and Edwards [1], and the motivation for this model is outlined in Nicholson et al. [33], if the amount of genetic drift between the two populations is small (at most on a timescale of the same order as the effective population size), then the diffusion approximation to a Wright-Fisher model of genetic drift leads to Equation 2 with $c_B \approx \frac{t}{2N_e}$, where t is the number of generations separating the two populations, and N_e is the effective population size [33]. We do not model the boundaries of the allele frequencies at zero and one, nor do we consider new mutations. This means that this model will be most accurate for alleles that were at intermediate frequency in the ancestral population. Now consider a descendant population of B; let us call this population C, and the allele frequency in the population X_C. Using the same model:

$$X_C = X_B + \epsilon_C \quad (3)$$

$$= x_A + \epsilon_B + \epsilon_C \quad (4)$$

Where

$$\epsilon_C \sim N(0, c_C X_B[1 - X_B]). \quad (5)$$

We can write down the expectation and variance of X_C as:

$$E[X_C] = E[x_A + \epsilon_B + \epsilon_C] \quad (6)$$

$$= x_A \quad (7)$$

and:

$$Var(X_C) = Var(x_A + \epsilon_B + \epsilon_C) \quad (8)$$

$$= Var(\epsilon_B) + Var(\epsilon_C) + 2Cov(\epsilon_B, \epsilon_C). \quad (9)$$

We then assume that the amount of genetic drift between all the populations is small. This implies that $X_B[1 - X_B]$ is well-approximated by $x_A[1 - x_A]$ in Equation 5, and hence the amount of genetic drift between A and B is approximately independent of the amount of genetic drift between B and C [35]. With these simplifications:

$$Var(X_C) \approx Var(\epsilon_B) + Var(\epsilon_C) \quad (10)$$

$$\approx (c_B + c_C) x_A [1 - x_A]. \quad (11)$$

We thus have a model for X_C, conditional on

$$x_A: X_C \sim N(x_A, (c_B + c_C) x_A [1 - x_A]). \quad (12)$$

Multiple populations

Now consider a set of four populations, all related to an ancestral population by a tree, as depicted in Figure 1A. Let the allele frequencies in the four populations be denoted X_1, X_2, X_3, and X_4, respectively, and the vector of all four frequencies be $\vec{X}$. We want to write down a joint distribution for $\vec{X}$ given the tree. We start by writing down the covariance between any two populations with respect to the ancestral allele frequency (i.e. $Cov(X_i, X_j) = E[(X_i - x_A)(X_j - x_A)]$). This is simply the variance of the common ancestor of the two populations:

$$Cov(X_1, X_2) = c_2 x_A [1 - x_A] \quad (13)$$

$$Cov(X_3, X_4) = c_1 x_A [1 - x_A] \quad (14)$$

$$Cov(X_1, X_3) = 0 \quad (15)$$

and so on (Figure 1B).

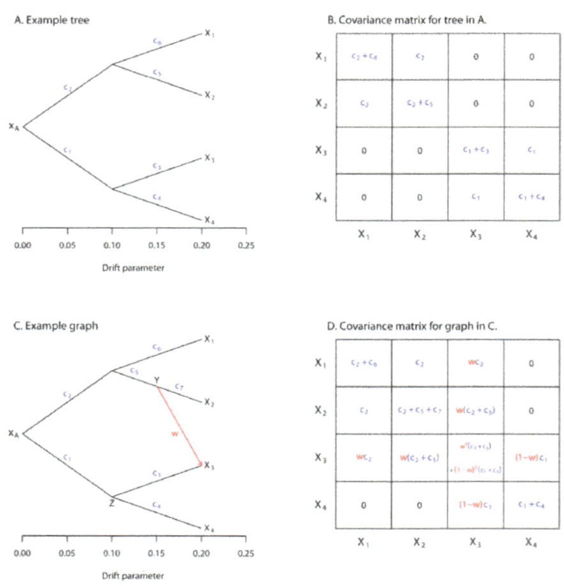

Figure 1. Simple examples.

A. An example tree. B. The covariance matrix implied by the tree structure in A. Note that the covariance here is with respect to the allele frequency at the root, and that each entry has been divided by $x_A[1-x_A]$ to simplify the presentation. C. An example graph. The migration edge is colored red. Parental populations for population 3 are labeled Y and Z; see the main text for details. D. The covariance matrix implied by the graph in C; again, each entry has been divided by $x_A[1-x_A]$. The migration terms are in red, and the non-migration terms are in blue.

Let us use $\mathbf{V}$ to denote the variance-covariance matrix of allele frequencies between populations implied by the tree. Now, if we knew the value of x_A, we could model $\vec{X}$ as:

$$\vec{X} \sim MVN(\vec{x}_A, V) \quad (16)$$

where $\vec{x}_A = [x_A, x_A, x_A, x_A]$ and MVN denotes the multivariate normal distribution. The covariance matrix $\mathbf{V}$ is distinct from the sample covariance matrix; we return to this distinction later. This multivariate normal model was proposed by [28]. Additionally, a multivariate normal model was used by Coop et al. [48] and Weir and Hill [49], although these authors did not explicitly model the variance-covariance matrix in terms of a tree.

Modeling migration.

To extend this framework to include migration, we allow populations to have ancestry from multiple parental populations [35], [40]. The contribution of each parental population is weighted; if we assume admixture occurs in a single generation, these weights are related to the fraction of alleles in the descendant population that originated in each parental population. Consider population 3 in Figure 1C (recall that the allele frequency in this population is X_3). We have labeled the two parental populations Y and Z; let the allele frequencies in these populations be X_Y and X_Z, respectively. We model

X_3 as

$$X_3 = wX_Y + (1-w)(X_Z + \varepsilon_3) \quad (17)$$

where $\epsilon_3 \sim N(0, c_3 x_A[1-x_A])$. Note that there is some question as to how to weight ϵ_3, the genetic drift specific to population 3. In reality, it comes from three sources: drift since Y but before the population mixture, drift since Z but before the population mixture, and drift since the mixture. These three components should have weights w, $1-w$, and 1, respectively. However, the three components are not all separately identifiable. For ease of computation, we estimate only a single drift parameter in this situation, and weight it by $1-w$ (Figure S1).

Additionally, there is a choice of whether the edge from Z or the edge from Y should be considered the "migration" edge; these two possibilities not identifiable in the model. In practice, we set the edge with the largest weight as the non-migration edge, and the other edge (or edges) as the "migration" edge(s).

With these simplifications, the variance of X_3 can be written in the mixture case as

$$Var(X_3) = Var(wX_Y + (1-w)(X_Z + \epsilon_3)) \quad (18)$$

$$= w^2 Var(X_Y) + (1-w)^2[Var(X_Z) + Var(\epsilon_3)] + 2w(1-w)Cov(X_Y, X_Z) \quad (19)$$

We can now consider multiple populations related by a graph instead of a tree (Figure 1C). The variance-covariance matrix $\mathbf{V}$ can be filled in as before, but now including terms for migration (Figure 1D). This model can be written in terms of a directed acyclic graph (the lack of cycles follows from the fact that no population can contribute genetic material to its own ancestor), where the c parameters correspond to edge lengths. For subsets of up to four populations, this model is closely related to the "$f-$ statistics" used as tests for treeness by Reich et al. [37] .

Normalization.

As described above, $\mathbf{V}$ depends on the ancestral allele frequency x_A. This means that the true variance-covariance matrix will differ by a scaling factor between SNPs with different values of x_A. In much work on this type of model, investigators have normalized allele frequencies to account for this. One potential normalization is the arcsine square-root transformation [1]. However, a drawback to this normalization is that it is non-linear; the expected value of the allele frequency in the descendant populations is no longer x_A, but pushed towards the boundaries, which could induce spurious correlations between the most drifted populations [50]. Another plausible transformation would be to scale all allele frequencies by $\hat{\mu}(1-\hat{\mu})$, where $\hat{\mu}$ is the mean allele frequency across populations [19], [33]. Both of these transformations increase the influence of polymorphisms that were rare in the ancestral population. However, these are precisely the loci where the approximation of our model to a true population genetics model is most likely to break down. For these reasons, we choose to work directly with untransformed allele frequencies.

Properties of the sample covariance.

In practice, the multivariate normal model in Equation 16 is impractical because we do not know the ancestral values of allele frequencies, but instead only the values in sampled descendant populations. This means that $\mathbf{V}$ cannot be estimated directly from data. However, consider instead the *sample* covariance matrix $\mathbf{W}$, where $\mathbf{W}_{ij} = E[(X_i - \hat{\mu})(X_j - \hat{\mu})]$, where $\hat{\mu} = \frac{\sum_{i=1}^{m} X_i}{m}$, m is the number of populations, and X_i and X_j are the sample allele frequencies in populations i and j. $\mathbf{W}$ is closely related to $\mathbf{V}$ as follows:

$$\mathbf{W}_{ij} = E[(X_i - \hat{\mu})(X_j - \hat{\mu})] \quad (20)$$

$$= E[(X_i - x_A - \hat{\mu} + x_A)(X_j - x_A - \hat{\mu} + x_A)] \quad (21)$$

$$= E[(X_i - x_A)(X_j - x_A) - (X_i - x_A)(\hat{\mu} - x_A) - (X_j - x_A)(\hat{\mu} - x_A) + (\hat{\mu} - x_A)^2] \quad (22)$$

$$= \mathbf{V}_{ij} - \frac{1}{m}\sum_{k=1}^{m} V_{ik} - \frac{1}{m}\sum_{k=1}^{m} V_{jk} + \frac{1}{m^2}\sum_{k=1}^{m}\sum_{k'=1}^{m} V_{kk'}.$$

(23)

In the following section, we will describe how we perform inference based on the sample covariance matrix $\hat{\mathbf{W}}$.

Estimation from finite samples and many SNPs.

Now assume that we have genotyped n SNPs in each of m populations. Our goal is to use these data to estimate the population history graph G: that is, G is a rooted, directed, acyclic graph with specified branch lengths and mixture weights, as described above. Let the sample allele frequency at SNP k in population i be $\hat{X}_{ik}$. We can estimate the sample covariance matrix $\hat{\mathbf{W}}$:

$$\hat{\mathbf{W}}_{ij} = \frac{\sum_{k=1}^{n} [(\hat{X}_{ik} - \hat{\mu}_k)(\hat{X}_{jk} - \hat{\mu}_k)]}{n} \quad \textbf{(24)}$$

where $\hat{\mu}_k = \frac{1}{m}\sum_{i=1}^{m} \hat{X}_{ik}$. The fact that in practice we have finite samples from each population and a finite number of SNPs has two effects on this matrix. First, sampling leads to a biased estimation of the terms on the diagonal, since sampling can be thought of as adding an amount of "drift" to each population (as well as smaller effects on the off-diagonal terms). Additionally, it leads to some uncertainty in all terms. To account for the biased diagonal terms, in practice we calculate a corrected version of $\hat{\mathbf{W}}$ that removes this bias . To account for uncertainty in the values of this matrix, we use a block resampling approach (see below). Finally, with multiple SNPs, we are working with SNPs with many different values of x_A. In this case, the $x_A[1 - x_A]$ terms described above can be thought of as $\overline{x_A[1 - x_A]}$; i.e., the mean across SNPs of $x_A[1 - x_A]$.

We now want to write down a likelihood for $\hat{\mathbf{W}}$ given G (which in turn implies the expected sample covariance matrix $\mathbf{W}$). One possibility would be to use the Wishart distribution, since the sample covariance matrix of multivariate normal random variables has this form. However, computation of the Wishart density involves computationally-intensive matrix inversion, so we took an alternative approach. Consider the observed covariance between populations i and j, $\hat{\mathbf{W}}_{ij}$. If we had a large number of independent genomic regions and estimated this quantity separately in each independent region, the sampling distribution would be approximately normal with mean $\hat{\mathbf{W}}_{ij}$ (by appeal to the central limit theorem). We thus model $\hat{\mathbf{W}}_{ij}$ as:

$$\hat{\mathbf{W}}_{ij} \sim N(\hat{\mathbf{W}}_{ij}, \sigma_{ij}^2) \quad \textbf{(25)}$$

where σ_{ij} is the standard error in the estimation of $\hat{\mathbf{W}}_{ij}$. Because the allele frequencies at nearby SNPs are correlated (i.e., there is linkage disequilibrium), a naive estimate of σ_{ij} that treated each SNP as independent would be too small. We instead take a resampling approach to estimate σ_{ij}. We split the genome into p blocks, such that there are K SNPs per block (with K chosen so that the block sizes are larger than blocks of linkage disequilibrium) [36]. (If Kdoes not divide evenly into n, we discard the remaining SNPs.) We then calculate $\hat{\mathbf{W}}$ separately in each block. Let $\hat{\mathbf{W}}_{ijk}$ be the sample covariance between two populations i and $j$in block k. Now

$$\hat{\mathbf{W}}_{ij} = \frac{\sum_{k=1}^{p} \hat{\mathbf{W}}_{ijk}}{p} \quad \textbf{(26)}$$

And

$$\hat{\sigma}_{ij} = \sqrt{\frac{\sum_{k=1}^{p} (\hat{\mathbf{W}}_{ijk} - \hat{\mathbf{W}}_{ij})^2}{p(p-1)}}. \quad \textbf{(27)}$$

If we take each pair of populations in turn, we can write down a composite likelihood for $\hat{\mathbf{W}}$:

$$L(\hat{\mathbf{W}}|\mathbf{W}) = \prod_{i=1}^{m}\prod_{j=i}^{m} N(\hat{\mathbf{W}}_{ij}|G, \hat{\sigma}_{ij}^2) \quad \textbf{(28)}$$

where $N(\hat{\mathbf{W}}_{ij}|G, \sigma_{ij}^2)$ is a Gaussian density with mean $\mathbf{W}_{ij}$ (computed from G by Equation 23) and variance σ_{ij}^2 evaluated at $\hat{\mathbf{W}}_{ij}$.

Measuring model fit.

Finally, we wanted to define measures for how well the model fits the data. First, we define the matrix of residuals in this model, R. These quantities are useful for visualization and fitting:

$$\mathbf{R} = \hat{\mathbf{W}} - \mathbf{W}. \quad \textbf{(29)}$$

Positive residuals indicate pairs of populations where the model underestimates the observed covariance, and thus populations where the fit might be improved by adding additional edges. Negative residuals indicate pairs of populations where the model overestimates the observed covariance; these are a necessary outcome of having positive residuals, but can also sometimes be interpreted as populations that are forced too close together due to unmodeled migration elsewhere in the graph. These residuals can be used to define a measure of the fraction of the variance in $\hat{\mathbf{W}}$ that is explained by $\mathbf{W}$. Let us call this fraction f:

$$f = 1 - \frac{\sum_{i=1}^{m}\sum_{j=i+1}^{m} (\mathbf{R}_{ij} - \bar{\mathbf{R}})^2}{\sum_{i=1}^{m}\sum_{j=i+1}^{m} (\hat{\mathbf{W}}_{ij} - \bar{\hat{\mathbf{W}}})^2} \quad \textbf{(30)}$$

where $\bar{\mathbf{R}} = \frac{\sum_{i=1}^{m}\sum_{j=i+1}^{m} \mathbf{R}_{ij}}{m(m-1)/2}$ and $\bar{\hat{\mathbf{W}}} = \frac{\sum_{i=1}^{m}\sum_{j=i+1}^{m} \hat{\mathbf{W}}_{ij}}{m(m-1)/2}$. This quantity approximates the fraction of the variance in relatedness between populations that is accounted for by the model.

Implementation.

We implemented an algorithm, called *TreeMix*, that searches for the graph that maximizes the composite likelihood in Equation 28. A search that enumerates all graphs is infeasible unless $m$is very small, so to simplify the search we make the assumption that the history of the sampled populations is approximately tree-like. We thus start by searching for the maximum likelihood tree, taking an algorithmic approach similar to Felsenstein [30].

After building the tree, we fix the position of the root. (In the tree model the position of the root is not identifiable, as the evolution of allele frequencies along the tree is reversible under the Gaussian model when drift is assumed to be small. In a graph model, though the position of the root is partially identifiable, in all applications we assume that the position of the root is fixed using prior information about known outgroups). We then calculate the residual covariance matrix, $\mathbf{R}$, and add migration edges in a directed matter. First, we find the M pairs of populations with the maximum residuals. We then attempt adding a migration edge between populations in the vicinity of each of the M population pairs. For each attempted graph (or tree) topology, we optimize the branch lengths and migration edge weights (Methods).

After finding the single migration edge that most increases the likelihood, we attempt a series of local changes to the graph structure (Methods). We then iterate over this procedure to add additional migration edges. In principle, migration edges could be added until they are no longer statistically significant (see the following paragraph). In our experience, however, we prefer to stop adding migration events well before this point so that the resulting graph remains interpretable.

Significance testing

After building the maximum likelihood graph, we would like to quantify our uncertainty in the resulting graph structure. In particular, we would like to quantify our confidence in individual migration events. However, because the likelihood in Equation 28 is a composite likelihood, it cannot be used directly for formal tests for significance. Instead, we take a resampling approach to test the support for individual migration edges.

Consider a given migration edge, with corresponding weight w. We wish to calculate a p-value for this weight (under the null hypothesis that $w = 0$, and for a fixed graph structure). To do this, we use the Wald statistic $\frac{\hat{w}}{se(\hat{w})}$, where $se(\hat{w})$ is the standard error in the estimate of the weight, which is distributed $N(0,1)$ under the null. To obtain the standard error, recall that we have split the genome into P independent blocks. We use the jackknife estimates of both $\hat{w}$ and the standard error in $\hat{w}$ (where we jackknife over blocks). Let i index blocks, and $\hat{w}_{\cdot i}$ be the estimated weight computed using all blocks *except* i. Then:

$$\hat{w} = \frac{\sum_{i=1}^{p} \hat{w}_{\cdot i}}{p} \quad (31)$$

$$se(\hat{w}) = \sqrt{\left(\frac{p-1}{p}\right) \sum_{i=1}^{p} (\hat{w}_{\cdot i} - \hat{w})^2} \quad (32)$$

This allows us to calculate a p-value for the migration edge. There are a number of complications to the interpretation of this p-value. First, there is the issue of multiple testing– there are at least $2m-2$ edges in the graph (recall that m is the number of populations), and thus around $4m^2$ possible migration events. More importantly, the p-value is generated under a heavily parameterized model: we are comparing a fixed graph structure with a migration event to that same graph without the migration event. A "significant" p-value simply indicates that the hypothesized migration event significantly improves the fit to the data; this does not account for the possibility of errors in the graph structure, or indicate that the particular migration event tested is the correct one (rather than a migration event between a different pair of populations). For this reason, we treat the precise p-value generated by this procedure with caution, and use additional, less-parameterized methods like three- and four-population tests [37] to test the robustness of the inference.

SIMULATIONS

We tested the performance of the *TreeMix* method in simulations. We generated coalescent simulations from several histories; the basic structure was a set of 20 populations produced by a serial bottleneck model like that used by DeGiorgio et al. [51] to model human history (Figure 2A). The parameters of the simulations were chosen to be reasonable for non-African human populations; we used an effective population size of 10,000, and a history where all 20 populations share a common ancestor 2000 generations in the past. Each individual simulation involved 400 regions of approximately 500 kb each, and thus recapitulated many aspects of real data, including hundreds of thousands of loci and the presence of linkage disequilibrium.

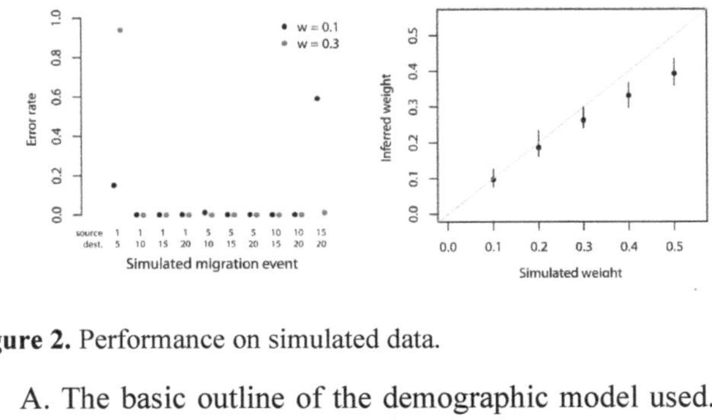

Figure 2. Performance on simulated data.

A. The basic outline of the demographic model used. B. Trees inferred by *TreeMix*. We simulated 100 independent data sets, under the demographic model in A., and inferred the tree. All simulations gave the same topology; plotted are the mean branch lengths. C. Performance in the presence of migration. We added migration events to the tree in A. and inferred the structure of the graph. Each point represents the error rate over 100 independent simulations, defined as the fraction of simulations where the inferred graph topology does not perfectly match the simulated topology. On the x-axis we show the populations involved in the simulated migration event; e.g., if the source population is 1 and the destination population is 10, this is a migration event from population 1 to population 10, as labeled in A. D. Admixture weight estimation. We simulated admixture events with different weights from population 1 to population 10, and inferred the weight. Each point is the mean across 100 simulations, and the bar represents the range.

Tree simulations.

First, we tested the performance of the algorithm on truly tree-like data. We generated 100 independent simulations of 20 chromosomes from each population using the above demographic model without migration, and inferred population trees. The inferred trees perfectly matched the simulated model in all cases (Figure 2B, Figure S2), and the fitted tree model accounted for an average of 99.8% of the variance in $\hat{\mathbf{W}}$. To test the effect of SNP ascertainment, we then inferred trees using only SNPs that were polymorphic in one of the populations (either population 1 or population 20); this ascertainment scheme did not decrease accuracy of the inferred topology, though it did alter the inferred branch lengths (Figure S3).

We used these simulations without migration to test the calibration of our p-values for migration events. For each simulation, after building the maximum likelihood tree, we introduced a migration event between two random populations and tested it for significance. As expected if the p-values are properly calibrated, their distribution is approximately uniform (Figure S4).

Finally, we performed tree simulations in a situation where fixed differences and new mutations (rather than shared polymorphisms inherited from a common ancestor) were common between the populations; in this context the population genetic interpretation of the model breaks down. We performed simulations where all the true branch lengths were 50 times longer than in the original model, corresponding to a history where the 20 populations share a common ancestor approximately 100,000 generations in the past. Again, we see no errors in the topology of the inferred trees (Figures S5, S6). In this situation, the covariances between closely-related populations tend to be slightly underestimated; in more extreme situations this could lead to spurious inferences of migration (Figures S5, S6). However, overall, these simulations suggest that the model will still be useful even in situations where the population genetic interpretation is not strictly correct.

Simulations with migration.

We then introduced migration events into our simulations. We generated simulations under the same model described above; however, we now simulated an admixture event approximately 100 generations before the present where one population receives a fraction of its ancestry (either 10% or 30%) from one of the other populations. We tried ten different pairwise combinations of populations, and generated 100 simulations for each pair. For each simulation, we ran *TreeMix* and allowed it to infer a migration event. We then judged the error rate of the algorithm as the fraction of times the inferred topology of the graph was not exactly correct (this is a conservative estimate of the error rate, in that inferred graph topologies that are very close to the truth are counted as errors). In general, *TreeMix* was able to correctly infer the graph structure in these simulations (Figure 2C). However, accuracy dropped considerably when migration was between closely related populations without outgroups present in the data (these are populations 1 and 20 in the model; Figure 2C). The major types of errors produced in the simulations were incorrectly inferred directions of migration arrows and inference of admixture in populations related to the truly admixed population (Figure S7).

We next asked whether the mixture "weights" inferred in the model can be interpreted as admixture proportions. To do this, we simulated admixture events of varying proportion between the first and tenth population in the serial bottleneck model described above, set the graph to the true topology, and estimated the mixture weight. The weights are indeed correlated with the true ancestry fraction, but underestimate relatively high admixture proportions in these simulations (Figure 2D). The precise bias in the estimation of this parameter will depend, in real data, on largely unknowable parameters .

Application to humans

To test the performance of the *TreeMix* model with real data, we applied it to humans, whose genetic history has been studied extensively [7], [21], [52], [53]. We applied the model to a dataset consisting of about 125,000 SNPs ascertained by low-coverage genome sequencing in a single Yoruban individual and then genotyped in 55 modern and archaic human populations [54]. In all that follows, we excluded the two Oceanian populations because they gave inconsistent results across datasets. We believe this difficulty results from the fact that these populations contain ancestry from multiple sources, making the graph estimation somewhat unstable when they are included (Figure S12). We first built the tree of all 53 remaining populations (Figure 3A). This tree largely recapitulates the known relationships among population groups [7], and explains 98.8% of the variance in relatedness between populations (though this is high, it is less than the 99.8% observed in the simulations of a true tree model). We examined the residuals of the model›s fit to identify aspects of ancestry not captured by the tree (Figure 3B). A number of known admixed populations stand out: in particular, these include the Mozabite and Middle Eastern populations.

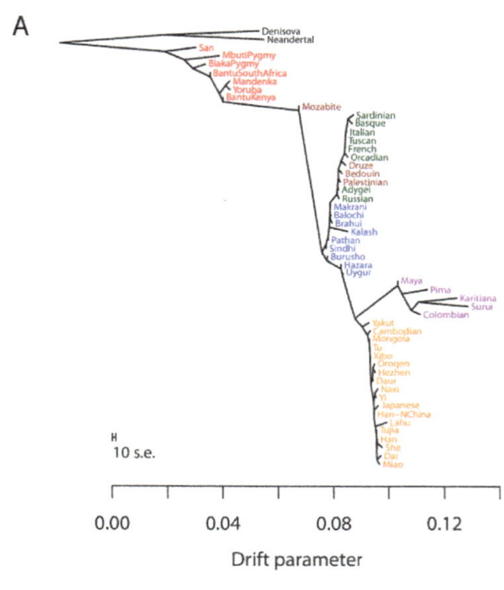

B

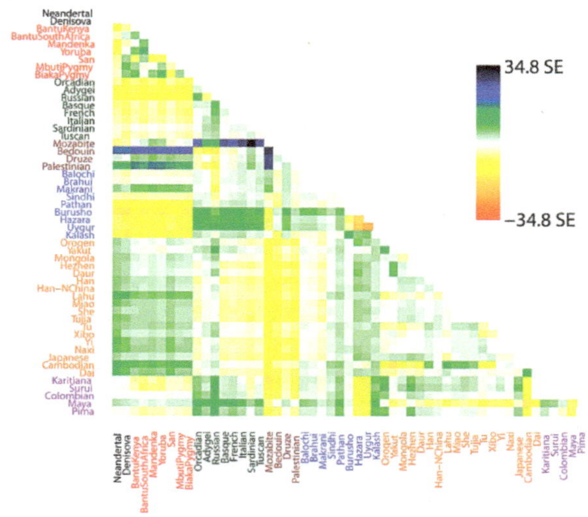

Figure 3. Inferred human tree.

A. Maximum likelihood tree. Plotted is the maximum-likelihood tree. Populations are colored according to geographic location (black: archaic humans, red: Africa, brown: Middle East, green: Europe, blue: Central Asia, purple: America, orange: East Asia). The scale bar shows ten times the average standard error of the entries in the sample covariance matrix ($\hat{\mathbf{W}}$). For analysis including Oceania, see Figures S11 and S12. B. Residual fit. Plotted is the residual fit from the maximum likelihood tree in A. We divided the residual covariance between each pair of populations i and j by the average standard error across all pairs. We then plot in each cell $[i,j]$ this scaled residual. Colors are described in the palette on the right. Residuals above zero represent populations that are more closely related to each other in the data than in the best-fit tree, and thus are candidates for admixture events.

We then sequentially added migration events to the tree. In Figure 4, we show the inferred graph with ten migration edges; p-values for all reported migration edges are less than 1×10^{-30} (we show the graph with the maximum likelihood over several independent runs of *TreeMix* with random orders of input populations). This graph model explains 99.8% of the variance in relatedness between populations. As expected from examination of Figure 3B, the migration events recapitulate many known events in human history. We infer that the Mozabite are the result of admixture between an African and a Middle Eastern population (with about 33% of their ancestry from Africa), and that Middle Eastern populations also have African ancestry (Palestinians and Bedouins: $w = 13\%$ from Africa; Druze: $w = 6\%$). This is consistent with previously reported admixture proportions from these populations [43], [55]. Additionally, we identify the known European ancestry in the Maya ($w = 12\%$) [21], and infer that the Uyghur and Hazara populations are the result of admixture between west Eurasian and East Asian populations ($w = 46\%$ and 47% from west Eurasia, respectively) [20], [21], [56].

Plotted is the structure of the graph inferred by *TreeMix* for human populations, allowing ten migration events. Migration arrows are colored according to their weight. Horizontal branch lengths are proportional to the amount of genetic drift that has occurred on the branch. The scale bar shows ten times the average standard error of the entries in the sample covariance matrix ($\hat{\mathbf{W}}$). The residual fit from this graph is shown in Figure S9. Admixture from Neandertals to non-African populations is only apparent when considering subsets of the data (see Discussion and Figure S15).

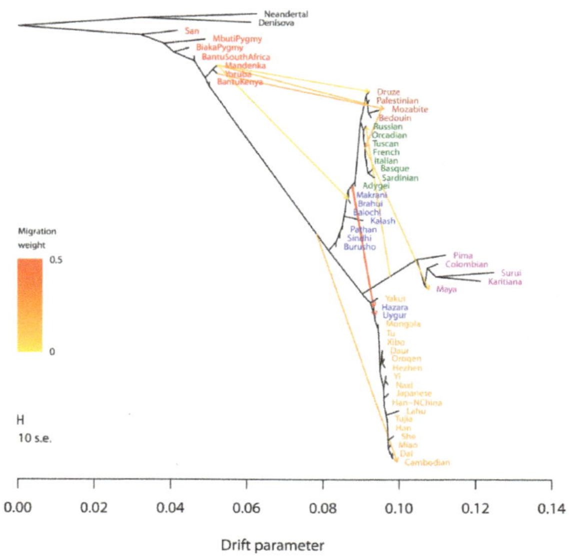

Figure 4. Inferred human tree with mixture events.

Several additional migration events in the human data have not been previously examined in detail, but are consistent with previous clustering analysis of these populations [7], [20], [21]. These include migration from Africa to the Makrani and Brahui in Central Asia ($w = 5\%$) and from a population related to East Asians and Native Americans (which we interpret as likely Siberian) to Russia ($w = 11\%$).

Two inferred edges were unexpected. First, perhaps the most surprising inference is that Cambodians trace about 16% of their ancestry to a population equally related to both Europeans and other East Asians (while the remaining 84% of their ancestry is related to other southeast Asians). This is partially consistent with clustering analyses, which indicate shared ancestry between Cambodians and central Asian populations [7]. To confirm that the Cambodians are admixed, we turned to less parameterized models. The predicted admixture event implies that allele frequencies in Cambodia are more similar to those in African populations than would be expected based on their East Asian ancestry. To test this, we used three-population tests [37]. We tested the trees [African, [Cambodian,Dai]] for evidence of admixture in the Cambodians (Methods). When using any African population, there is strong evidence of admixture (when using Yoruba, $Z = -7.0$ [$p = 1 \times 10^{-12}$]; when using Mandenka, $Z = -7.3$ [$p = 1 \times 10^{-12}$]; when using San, $Z = -4.8$ [$p = 8 \times 10^{-7}$]). We conclude that the Cambodian population is the result of an admixture event involving a southeast Asian population related to the Dai and a Eurasian population only distantly related to those present in these data.

Finally, we infer an admixture edge from the Middle East (a population related to the Mozabite, a Berber population from northern Africa) to southern European populations ($w = 22\%$). This migration edge is the one edge that is not consistent across independent runs of *TreeMix* on these data (Figure S8).

In particular, an alternative graph (albeit with lower likelihood) places the Mozabite as an admixture between southern Europe and Africa (rather than the Middle East and Africa), and does not include an edge from the middle East to southern Europe. We thus hesitate to interpret this result, except to note that the relationship between northern African, the Middle East, and southern Europe involves complex patterns of gene flow that merit further investigation [43], [57].

To test the robustness of our results to SNP ascertainment, we additionally ran *TreeMix* on the same set of populations using a set of SNPs ascertained in a single French individual. The inferred graph was nearly identical (Figure S10). Additionally, as noted above, different random input orders for the populations gave very similar results (Figure S8). We conclude from this that the model is able to consistently and accurately infer the major mixture events in the history of a species. This approach is computationally efficient: building the tree took around five minutes on a standard desktop computer (with a processor speed of 3.1 GHz), and adding ten migration events to the tree took about four and a half hours (the major computational cost is in the iterative estimation of migration weights).

Application to dogs

While human populations have been extensively studied, we next applied the model to dogs, a species where considerably less is known about population history. In particular, we applied the model to a dataset consisting of about 60,000 SNPs genotyped in 82 dog breeds or wild canids [58]. As for humans, we first inferred the maximum likelihood tree (Figure 5A). The differences in history between dogs and humans are striking: there are long terminal branches leading to each dog breed in the inferred tree (Figure 5A, recall that the terminal branch lengths account for sample size). This is consistent with the known strong bottlenecks in the establishment of dog breeds [23]. However, examining the residuals from the model revealed a number of populations that do not fit a strict tree model (Figure 5B); indeed, the tree model explained 94.7% of the variance in relatedness between breeds, somewhat less than between human populations.

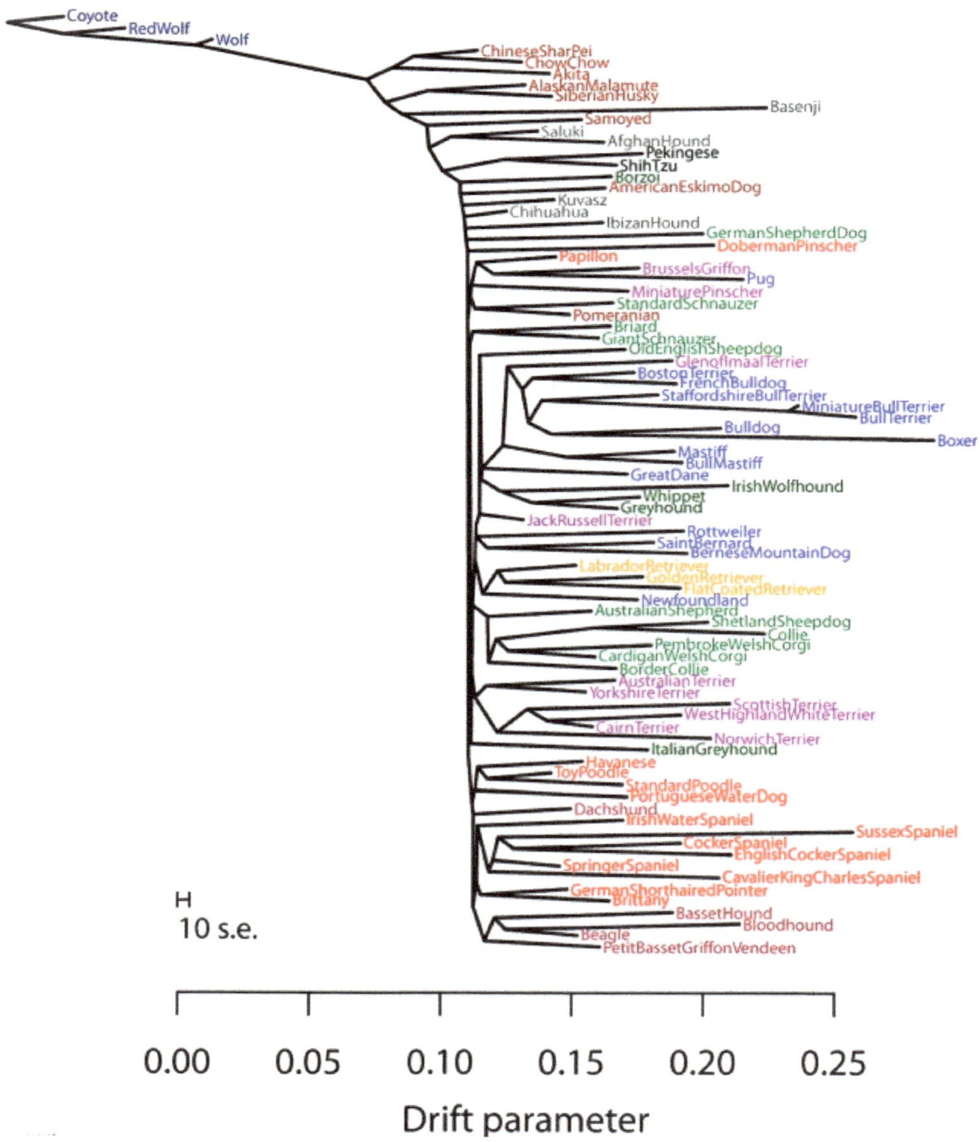

(A)

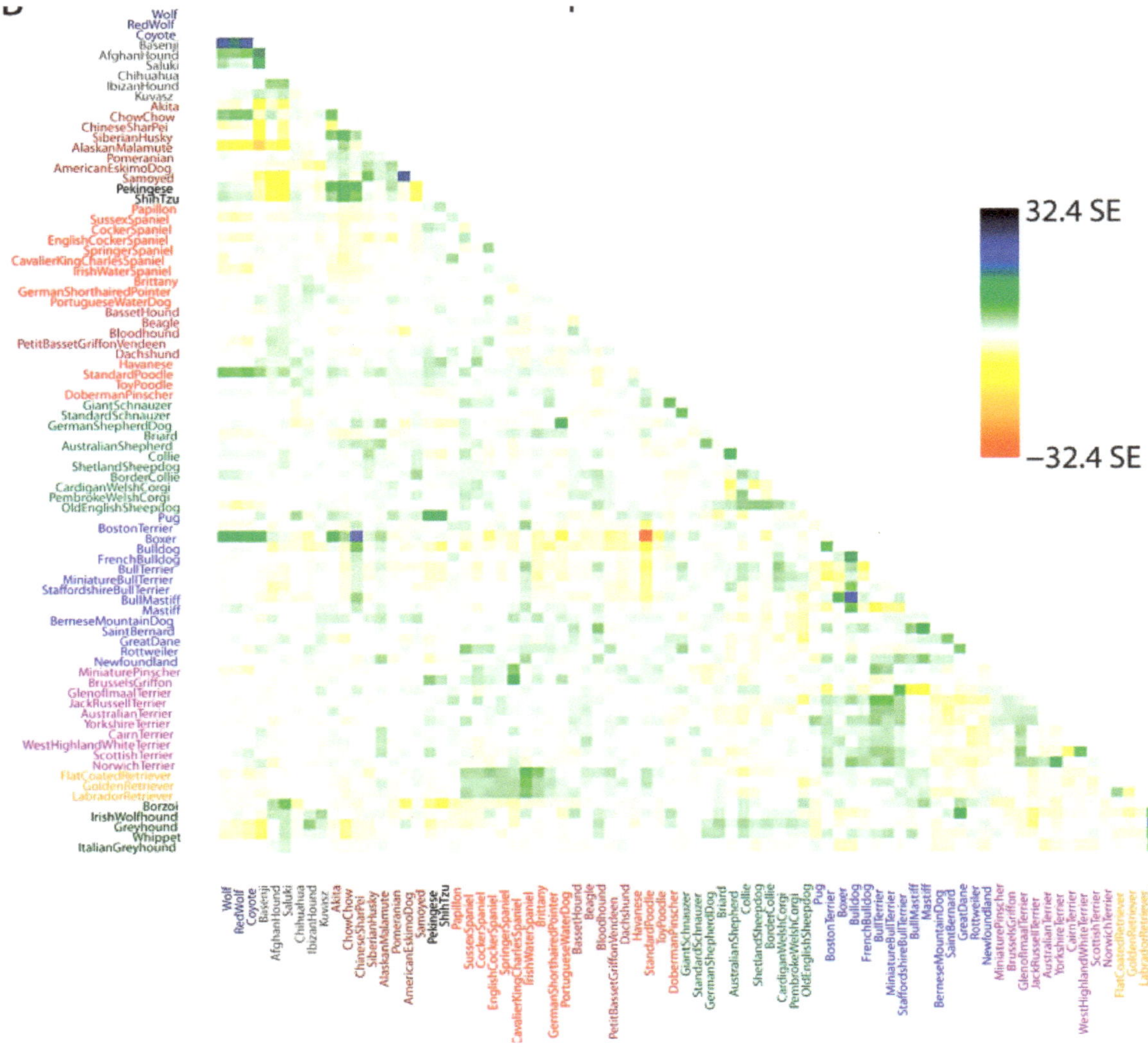

(B)

Figure 5. Inferred dog tree.

A. Maximum likelihood tree. Populations are colored according to breed type. Dark blue: wild canids, grey: ancient breeds, brown: spitz breeds, black: toy dogs, red: spaniels, maroon: scent hounds, dark red: working dogs, light green: herding dogs, light blue: mastiff-like dogs, purple: small terriers, orange: retrievers, dark green: sight hounds. The scale bar shows ten times the average standard error of the entries in the sample covariance matrix ($\hat{\mathbf{W}}$). B. Residual fit. Plotted is the residual fit from the maximum likelihood tree in A. We divided the residual covariance between each pair of populations i and j by the average standard error across all pairs. We then plot in each cell $[i,j]$ this scaled residual. Colors are described in the palette on the right.

We sequentially added migration events to the tree in Figure 5A. In Figure 6, we show the inferred graph with ten migration events, which explains 96.8% of the variance in relatedness between breeds (which suggests that additional events exist in the data). In the following paragraphs, we describe some of these events. Plotted is the structure of the graph inferred by *TreeMix* for dog populations, allowing ten migration events. Migration arrows are colored according to their weight. The scale bar shows ten times the average standard error of the entries in the sample covariance matrix ($\hat{\mathbf{W}}$). See the main text for discussion. The residual fit from this graph is presented in Figure S13.

We infer that the bull mastiff is the result of an admixture event between bulldogs and mastiffs. This is a known event [59]; we estimate the admixture proportions as 33% bulldog and 67% mastiff. We further examined this event using four-population tests for treeness. As expected given the known history, the tree [[boxer,bulldog],[mastiff,bull mastiff]] fails the four-population test ($Z = 3.5$, $p = 0.002$), while replacing the bull mastiff with other related breeds that we do not predict to be involved in the admixture event results in trees that pass this test. For example, the tree [[boxer,bulldog],[mastiff,Bost on terrier]] passes the four-population test with $Z = -0.3$.

The most visually apparent residuals in Figure 5B are accounted for in the graph by an admixture event from the grey wolf into the basenji, an ancient African breed of dog ($w = 25\%$). Such a high mixture fraction is consistent with previous clustering analyses of these data [23], [60]. We again sought to confirm this signal in a less-parameterized model. We tested the four-population tree [[wolf,ancient breed],[basenji, Afghan hound]] with various "ancient" dog breeds. We could not find a tree that passed the four-population test (with Akita as the ancient breed, $Z = 11.7, p < 1 \times 10^{-30}$; with Alaskan Malamute, $Z = 13.0, p < 1 \times 10^{-30}$), confirming the presence of gene flow in these trees. Replacing the basenji with the saluki in these analyses resulted in trees that pass the four-population test (for example, the tree [[wolf, Akita],[Afghan hound, saluki]] passes with $Z = -0.03, p = 0.51$). Though we cannot have complete confidence in the precise migration events, these results are consistent with admixture between gray wolves and the basenji.

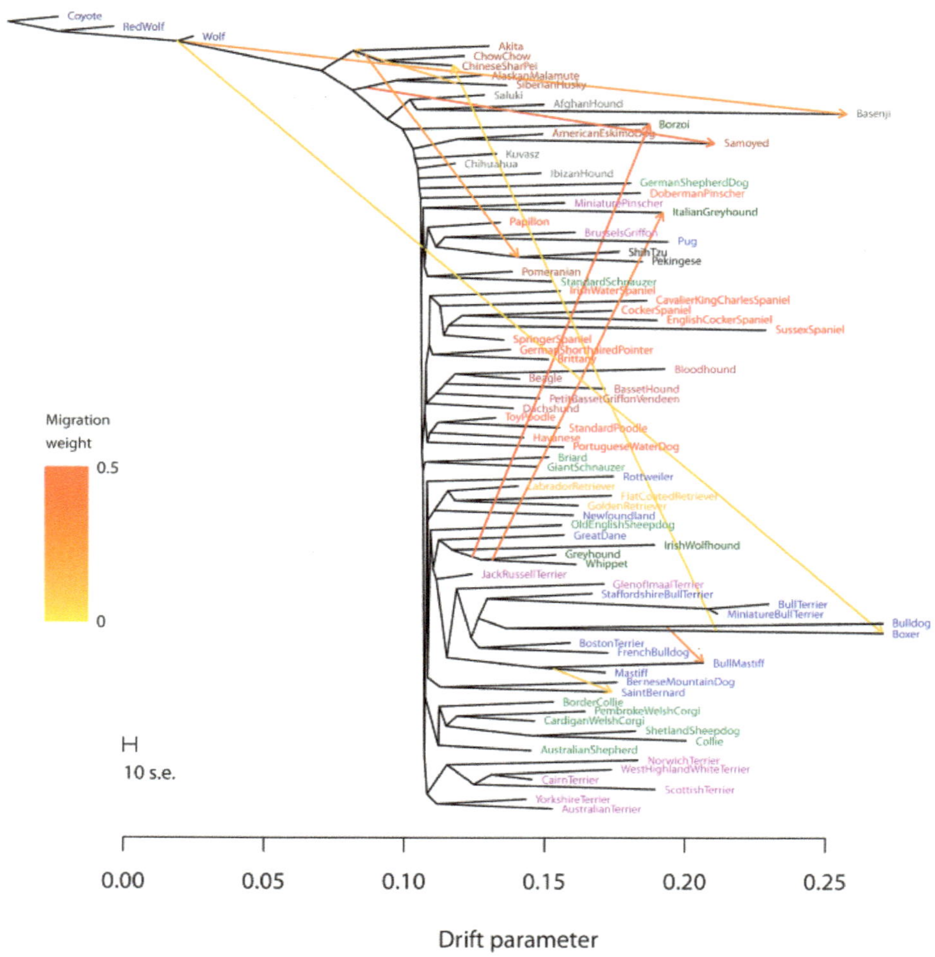

Figure 6. Inferred dog graph.

Another breed that stands out in this analysis is the boxer (Note that many of the SNPs used in this study were ascertained using a boxer individual, so we may have increased power to identify migration events involving this breed). We infer a significant genetic contribution from wolves to the boxer ($w = 8\%$), and migration between the boxer and the Chinese shar-pei, a distantly-related ancient breed ($w = 8\%$). To further examine these events, we again turned to four-population tests. To evaluate the wolf mixture, we tested the tree [[wolf, ancient breed],[boxer, bulldog]]. We did not find a tree that passed the four-population test (with Akita as the ancient breed, $Z = 3.1, p = 0.001$; with Afghan Hound, $Z = 3.4, p = 0.0003$). Replacing the Boxer with the Mastiff in these analyses led to trees that passed the four-population test (for example, with Akita as the ancient breed, $Z = 0.3, p = 0.38$). To evaluate the gene flow from the Boxer to the Chinese shar-pei, we tested the tree [[Chinese shar-pei, Akita],[boxer, bulldog]]; this tree fails the four-population test ($Z = 3.0, p = 0.001$), while the tree [[Chow Chow, Akita],[boxer,bulldog]] passes ($Z = -0.48, p = 0.3$).

Previous analyses of these data have noted that the "toy breeds" of dog cluster together Vonholdt:2010uq. We find that the Chinese toy breeds (the Pekingese and the Shi Tzu) result from admixture between a population related to ancient East Asian dog breeds and a modern population related to the Brussels griffon and the pug ($w = 28\%$ from the East Asian breeds). To confirm the presence of gene flow, we tested four-population trees of the form [[Asian toy breed, Akita/Chow Chow],[Pug,mastiff]]. These trees fail, with varying levels of significance, ranging from [[Chow Chow, Shi Tzu],[Pug, mastiff]] ($Z = -2.7, p = 0.003$) to [[Akita, Pekingese],[Pug, mastiff]] ($Z = -4.7, p = 1 \times 10^{-6}$).

Finally, we noticed that two of the sighthounds (the Borzoi and the Italian greyhound) do not cluster with the other sight hounds in the tree, namely greyhound, whippet and Irish wolfhound (Figure 5A); however, they do show evidence of having sighthound admixture in the graph (Figure 6). These are the borzoi (which appear to be admixed between an ancient or spitz-breed dog, with 47% ancestry from the sighthounds) and the Italian Greyhound (which appears to be admixed with a toy breed, with 34% ancestry from the sighthounds). This is consistent with the known phenotypic characteristics of these dogs; the borzoi is considered a saluki-like breed, and the Italian greyhound is phenotypically a small version of a greyhound [59].

Overall, we conclude that there has been considerable gene flow between dog breeds over the course of domestication; there are many additional migration events that merit further examination.

DISCUSSION

In this paper, we have developed a unified model for inferring patterns of population splits and mixtures from genome-wide allele frequency data. We have shown that this model is accurate in simulations, largely recapitulates the known relationships between well-studied human populations, and is able to identify new relationships between populations in both humans and dogs.

The *TreeMix* model can be thought of as a complement to methods for the identification of population structure [18]–[20]. These latter methods are powerful tools for clustering together individuals into relatively homogenous populations (and to identify individuals that are genetic outliers in their population) [18]–[20]. However, once population structure in a species has been identified, these methods are not well-suited for describing *how* it arose, and are only indirectly informative about the historical relationships between different populations. The model developed in this paper is designed to more directly address these historical questions.

Modeling assumptions

There are a number of assumptions, both implicit and explicit, in the interpretation of the *TreeMix* model. First, we have motivated the model in terms of inferring the historical splits and mixtures of populations. However, a given covariance structure of allele frequencies between populations can be a consequence of either a non-equilibrium demography (population splits and mixtures) or an equilibrium demography (populations at long-term stasis with a fixed migration structure) [2]. For the species analyzed in this paper, population equilibrium over the entire species range is not a tenable hypothesis; however, some subsets of populations may be at equilibrium, and there may be species where this alternative historical interpretation of the model is plausible.

We have also modeled migration between populations as occurring at single, instantaneous time points. This is, of course, a dramatic simplification of the migration process. This model will work best when gene flow between populations is restricted to a relatively short time period. Situations of continuous migration violate this assumption and lead to unclear results (Figure S14). The relevance of this assumption will depend on the species and the populations considered. In humans, the relevance of continuous versus discrete mixture events is an open question–some aspects of genetic variation appear compatible with continuous migration [61], while other aspects do not [37]. Indeed, both sorts of models are likely relevant at different time scales [62]. We also rely on the implicit assumption that the history of the species being analyzed is largely tree-like. We have made this assumption to simplify the search for the maximum likelihood graph; additionally, we speculate that in graphs with complex structure, there will be many graphs that lead to identical covariance matrices, and thus several different histories will be compatible with the data. That said, improvements to the search algorithm could allow the assumption of approximate treeness to be somewhat relaxed. Currently, if the number of admixed populations is large relative to the number of unadmixed populations, this assumption breaks down. For example, in the human data, note that we see no evidence of the documented gene flow from Neandertals to all non-African populations [39] (Figure 3B). The reason for this is that the large number of populations with admixture can be accommodated in the tree by allowing the branch from Neandertals to Africans to be slightly underestimated (additionally, by using SNPs ascertained in Africa, we have selected against sites that are informative about Neandertal ancestry). If only a single non-African population is included in the analysis, the relationship between Neandertals and the non-African population is clearer (Figure S15).

CONCLUSIONS

A number of extensions to the sort of model described here are of potential interest. First, the historical relationships between populations could be useful as null demographic models for the detection of natural selection [48], [63], [64]. Second, in a given individual, the best-fit graph relating the individual to other populations may change along a chromosome; this sort of information could be of use in local ancestry inference. Finally, we have not used the information about demographic history present in linkage disequilibrium; approaches that explicitly use this information may provide additional power to detect migration events and estimate their timing, at an additional computational cost [20], [53], [65].

METHODS

Graph estimation

As described in the Results, we developed an algorithm called *TreeMix* that uses the composite likelihood in Equation 28 to search for the maximum likelihood graph. Estimation involves two major steps. First, for a given graph topology, we need to find the maximum likelihood branch lengths and migration weights. Second, we need to search the space of possible graphs. First consider a given graph topology. We iterate between optimizing the branch lengths and weights. If the edge weights are known, the observed entries of the covariance matrix can be written down as an overdetermined system of linear equations (as in Equations 13–15). We solve this system by non-negative least squares [66]. Though the least squares solution is the maximum composite likelihood solution in the case where all entries of the covariance matrix have equal variance, it is not strictly the maximum likelihood solution in cases with unequal variances. The algorithm could be extended to unequal variances using a weighted least squares approach, but we have not implemented this. We then do a golden section search for the optimal weight (between zero and one) on each migration edge [67]. At each step in the golden section search, we update the branch lengths. We optimize the weight of each migration edge in turn, and iterate over migration edges until convergence.

To search the space of possible graphs, we take a hill-climbing approach. We start by finding a local optimum tree, taking an algorithmic approach similar to Felsenstein [30]. We randomly select three populations, optimize the branch lengths for all three possible trees, and choose the best (in terms of the composite likelihood) tree. Then, we add the remaining populations one by one in a random order. To add a population, we try attaching it to all branches of the current tree, optimizing the branch lengths for each one as described above, and find the most likely spot. We then perform a round of local rearrangements (i.e., nearest-neighbor interchanges [50]) around each internal node, keeping the resulting tree only if it increases the likelihood.

After adding all populations, we calculate the residual covariance matrix, R. We then add migration edges in a directed matter. First, we find the M pairs of populations with the maximum residuals (these are the pairs of populations with the worst fit under the model). In the results reported, $M = 4$. We define a "neighborhood" around each population of a pair as the tips within a distance of E edges of the focal population. In applications above, we use $E = 3$. This defines a set of pairs of populations that either have a poor fit, or are located in the graph near populations with a poor fit. We take each of these pairs in turn. For each pair, we identify the set of nodes in the path from each member of the pair to the root of the graph. This gives us two sets of nodes. We take all pairwise combinations of nodes in each set, and look at residuals between the populations that are the descendants of each node. If all of the residuals are positive, we add a migration edge between the two nodes and estimate its maximum likelihood weight. We then keep only the single edge that most increases the likelihood of the graph. After adding a migration edge, we attempt nearest-neighbor interchanges at the source and destination of the migration event, attempt changing the source and destination of all migration events, and attempt changing the direction of all migration arrows. Once we have reached the local maximum by this method, we attempt nearest-neighbor interchanges at all internal nodes. We iterate over this procedure for a predetermined number of migration edges. We then test the migration edges for significance as described.

The *TreeMix* source code is available at http://treemix.googlecode.com.

Three- and four-population tests of treeness

We implemented three- and four-population tests as described in Reich et al. [37]. For the relationship between the $f-$ statistics and the covariance model underlying *TreeMix*. For the three-population test, we estimated f_3 as in Reich et al. [37], and tested whether is it less than zero. We report the Z-score for this test. To obtain a standard error on the estimate of f_3, we used a block jackknife similar to Reich et al. [37]. However, Reich et al. [37] split the genome into blocks based on distance (with variable numbers of SNPs per block); we split the genome into blocks of K SNPs (and thus the blocks will be of variable size).

For the four-population test for treeness, we calculate the f_4 statistic as in Reich et al. [37], and test whether it is different than zero. Again, we report a Z-score for this test. Standard errors for the f_4 statistic were obtained as for the f_3 statistic.

Human data

The human data we used were downloaded from http://www.cephb.fr/en/hgdp/ on August 16th, 2011 (the data set labeled Harvard HGDP-CEPH genotypes). They consist of several panels of SNPs ascertained from low-coverage genome sequencing of single individual from different populations and then genotyped in the Human Genome Diversity Panel [54]. Additionally, at each site, a single sequencing read from the Denisova and Neandertal genome sequencing projects was sampled and the allele reported. These data have the property that they allow for complete control of the ascertainment strategy, and allow us to test the robustness of inference to different ascertainment schemes. For the main analyses, we used the panel of autosomal SNPs ascertained in a single Yoruban individual; there are 124,115 such sites. For some analyses, we also used the panel of autosomal SNPs ascertained in a single French individual; there are 111,970 such sites. For all analyses with *TreeMix*, we used a window size ($-K$) of 500; this corresponds to a window size of approximately 10 Mb. For all *TreeMix* analyses, we set the Neandertal and Denisova samples as the outgroups.

Since we have only a single allele from the Neandertal and Denisova populations, we cannot calculate heterozygosity in these populations for unbiased estimation of the covariance matrix (see). To account for this, we simply chose a relatively low level of heterozygosity and assigned it to both populations. In the Yoruba ascertained SNPs, we used a heterozygosity of 0.13, and for the French ascertained SNPs, we used a heterozygosity of 0.2. In practice, this only affected the lengths of the terminal branches to Neandertal and Denisova; running *TreeMix* with a heterozygosity of zero in both populations resulted in the same graph topologies (not shown).

Dog data

Allele counts for the dog breeds and wild canids reported in Boyko et al. Boyko:2010fk were downloaded from http://genome-mirror.bscb.cornell.edu/ on July 30, 2011. These data consist of counts of reference and alternate alleles at 61,468 sites in 85 dog breeds and wild canids. We removed the Jackal and Scottish Deerhound for having relatively high amounts of missing data, and the village dogs because it is unclear if they represent a coherent population. We also removed all SNPs on the X chromosome. This left us with 60,615 SNPs in 82 populations. We ran *TreeMix* with a window size ($-K$) of 500. This corresponds to a window size of approximately 20 Mb. For all *TreeMix* analyses, we set the coyote as the outgroup.

The ascertainment scheme used for SNP discovery in dogs was complicated [68]. The largest set of SNPs were ascertained by virtue of being different between the boxer and poodle assemblies. This should lead to an overestimation of the distance between the boxer and the poodle in our analysis. Indeed, in Figure 5B, a considerable negative residual between the boxer and poodle is visible. Another set of SNPs were ascertained by being heterozygous within a boxer individual, and a third set were ascertained by comparison between a boxer and wild canids. These latter SNPs should lead to an overestimation of the distance between the boxer and the wolf in our analysis (as we see for the poodle); in fact, we infer migration between the boxer and the wolf. This ascertainment issue may have led us to underestimate the amount of gene flow in the comparison.

Simulations

All simulations were performed using *ms* [69]. When running *TreeMix* on simulations without ascertainment, we used a window size of 5000 SNPs; for simulations with ascertainment we used windows of 1000 SNPs. Consensus trees were generated using SumTrees v.3.1.0 [70].

Supporting Information

A graph with a mixture event. Capital letters represent nodes, branch length parameters are in blue, and weight parameters are in red.

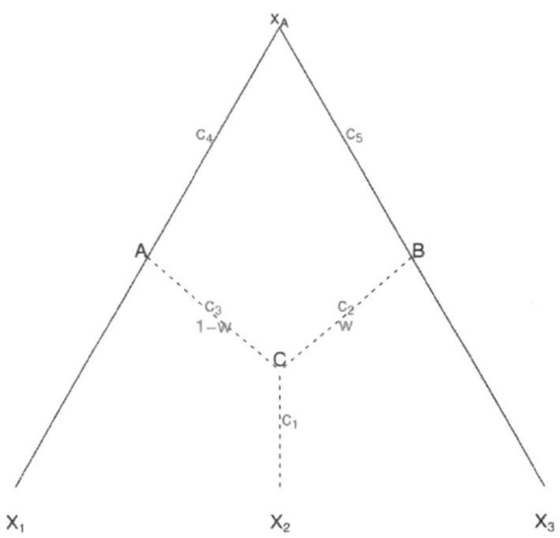

Figure S1.

A graph with a mixture event. Capital letters represent nodes, branch length parameters are in blue, and weight parameters are in red.

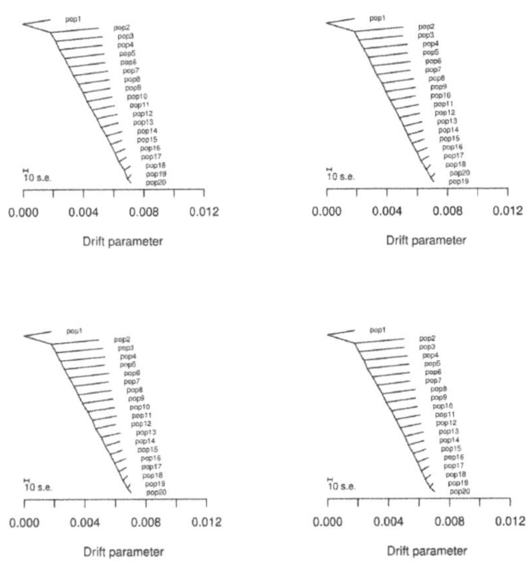

Figure S2.

Replicates of inferred trees from simulated data. We generated tree-like data using the topology in Figure 2A in the main text. In Figure 2B in the main text, we show the inferred tree with mean branch lengths. In this figure, we show four representative individual trees.

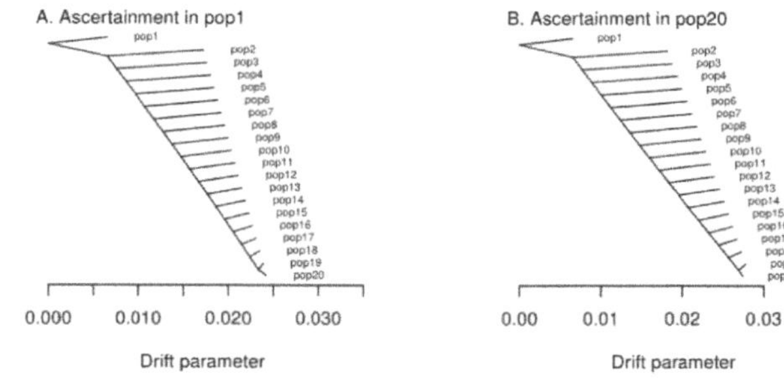

Figure S3.

Inferred trees on ascertained data. We generated tree-like data using the topology in Figure 2Ain the main text. We then used only the SNPs that were polymorphic in either population 1 (A.) or population 20 (B.) to infer the trees. The correct topology was obtained in all 100 simulations; the branch lengths in each figure are the mean across all simulations.

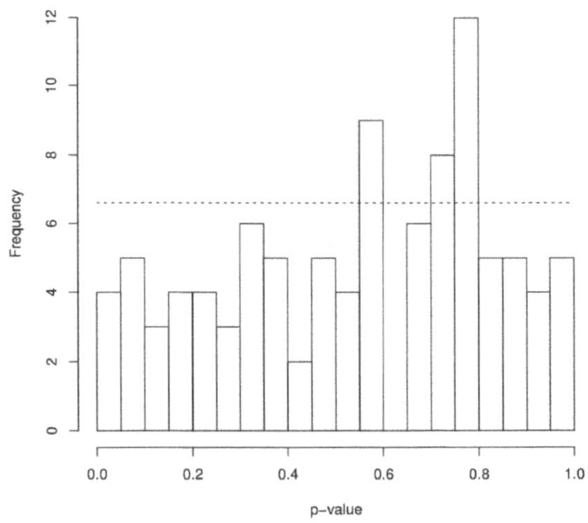

Figure S4.

Histogram of p-values for migration in simulated data. We generated 100 tree-like datasets using the topology in Figure 2A in the main text. We then randomly chose two populations (without replacement), added a migration edge between the two populations, and tested for significance using the procedure described in the main text. Plotted is the histogram of p-values for the significance test. If the p-values are properly calibrated, this distribution should be uniform (dotted line). Though the distribution is not completely uniform, there is no skew towards low p-values.

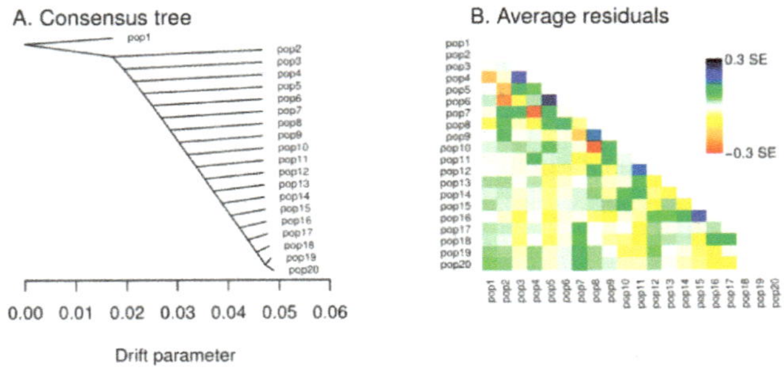

Figure S5.

Consensus tree in simulations with long branches. We generated 100 tree-like datasets using the topology in Figure 2A in the main text, multiplying all branch lengths by 50. We then inferred the maximum likelihood tree. A. Plotted are the mean branch lengths from the simulations. All simulations resulted in the same inferred topology. B. In each simulation, we scaled the residuals by the average standard error, then averaged these scaled residuals across simulations. Plotted are the mean scaled residuals across the 100 simulations. The most extreme residuals are not large (around 0.3 standard errors), but tend to be present between closely related populations.

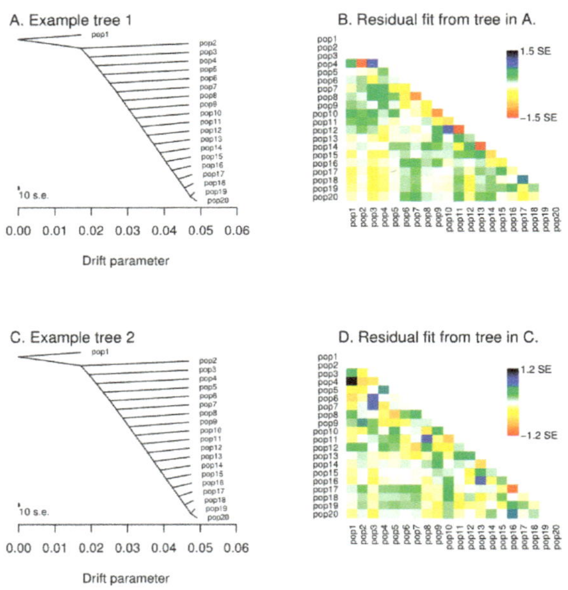

Figure S6.

Example trees from simulations with long branches. We generated 100 tree-like datasets using the topology in Figure 2A in the main text, multiplying all branch lengths by 50. We then inferred the maximum likelihood tree. In Figure S5, we show the average inferred tree. Here, we show two representative trees (A. and C. and the residuals corresponding to each tree (B. and D.).

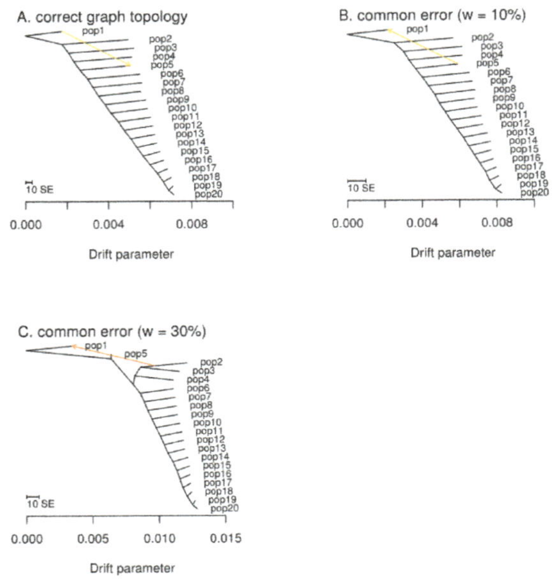

Figure S7.

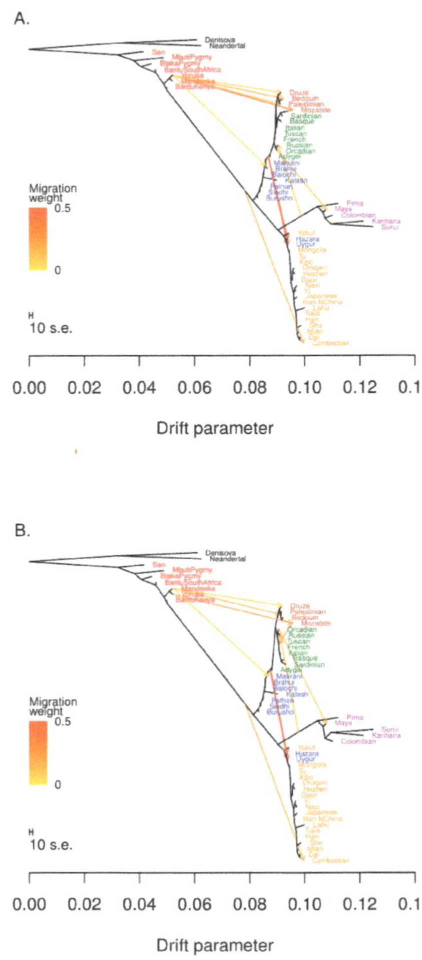

Figure S8.

Representative errors in simulations. We examined the simulations in which *TreeMix* did not reach the correct answer.

A. The correct topology for the simulations presented in the other panels. B. A representative example of an incorrect topology inferred from the simulations of a migration event with weight 10% from population 1 to population 5 (this topology accounted for all observed errors). C. A representative example of an incorrect topology inferred from the simulations of a migration event with weight 30% from population 1 to population 5 (this topology accounted for 95% of all errors).

Replicate graphs inferred in the human data. These graphs were generated in an identical manner as Figure 4 in the main text, but using different random input orders for populations during tree-building. All random input orders gave very similar results.

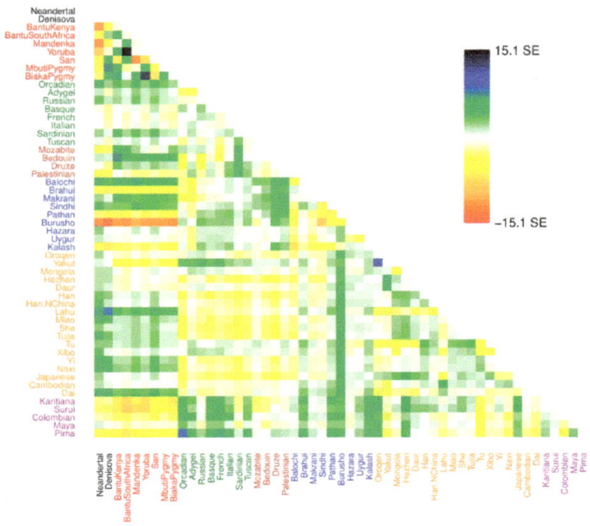

Figure S9.

Residual fit from graph of human data presented in the main text. Plotted are the residuals from the fit of the graph presented in Figure 4 in the main text.

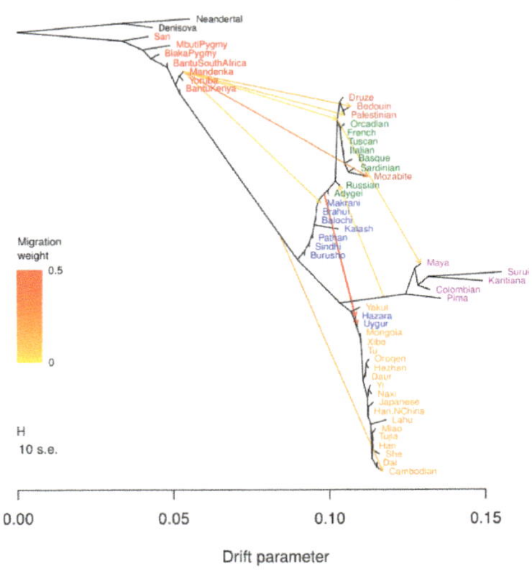

Figure S10.

Graph inferred from SNPs ascertained in a single French individual. The graph was generated in an identical manner as Figure 4 in the main text, but using a panel of SNPs ascertained in a single French, rather than a single Yoruban, individual. The inferred graph is extremely similar to that in Figure 4. The one major difference is that, in this graph, the Mozabite appear as an admixture of a Sardinian population rather than a Middle Eastern population; this configuration is seen in some runs of *TreeMix* on the Yoruba-ascertained data (Figure S8A).

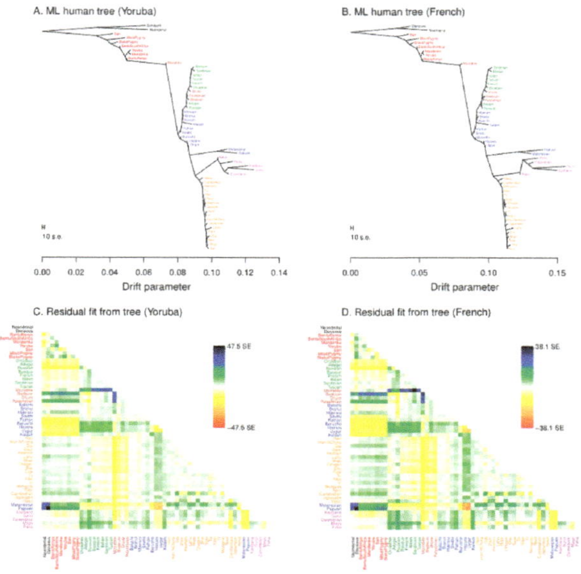

Figure S11.

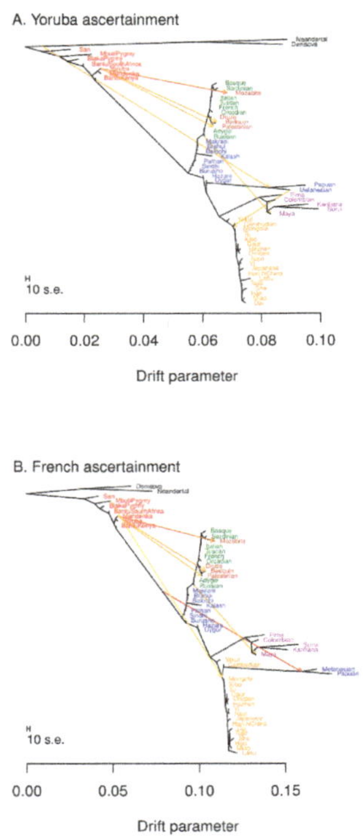

Figure S12.

Trees inferred using the human data including the Oceanians. We show the maximum likelihood trees and residuals for the human data including the Oceanian populations, plotted in the same manner as in Figure 3 in the main text. Trees were inferred using the panel of SNPs ascertained in a single Yoruban individual (A. and C.) and the panel of SNPs ascertained in a single French individual (B. and D.).

Graphs inferred using the human data including the Oceanians. We show the maximum likelihood graphs for the human data including the Oceanian populations, plotted in the same manner as in Figure 4 in the main text. Six migration edges were inferred in each graph. Graphs were inferred using the panel of SNPs ascertained in a single Yoruban individual (A.) and the panel of SNPs ascertained in a single French individual (B.)..

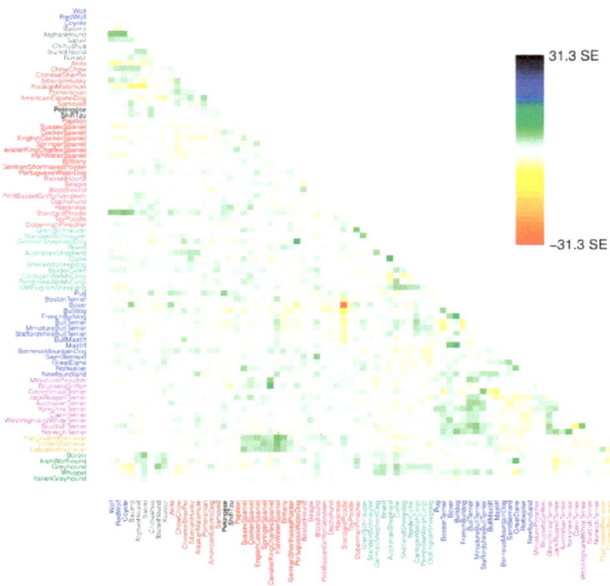

Figure S13.

Residual fit from graph of dog data presented in the main text. Plotted are the residuals from the fit of the graph presented in Figure 6 in the main text.

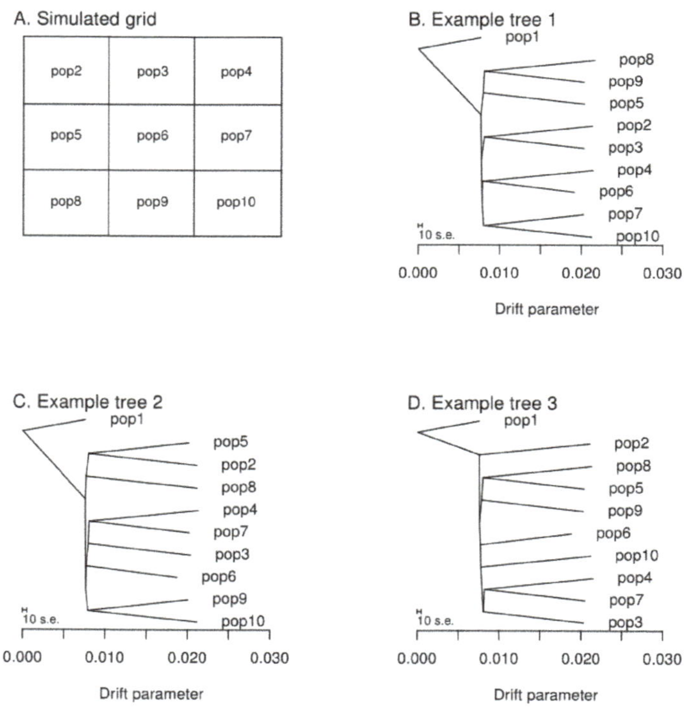

Figure S14.

TreeMix run on populations with continuous migration. We simulated a set of populations on a lattice, where each population has constant gene flow at a rate of $4Nm = 0.1$ with neighboring populations. All populations split from an outgroup 16,400 generations in the past. The configuration of the lattice is presented in A. (population 1 is the outgroup). *TreeMix* inferred no consistent tree structure. Three representative trees are presented in B.-D.

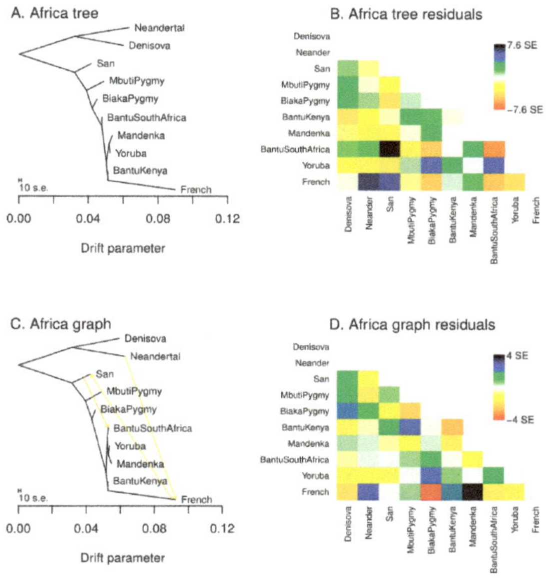

Figure S15.

TreeMix run on human data using only a single non-African population. We inferred the maximum likelihood tree (A.) using only the African populations and one non-African population (French), using SNPs identified in a single Yoruban individual. In examining the residuals (B.), a relationship between the French and the Neandertal is clear. We then inferred three migration events (C.), where we do see that the French contain some Neandertal ancestry ($w = 1.2\%$). Residual fit for this graph is shown in D.

ACKNOWLEDGMENTS

We thank three anonymous reviewers, David Reich, Nick Patterson, Graham Coop, Peter Ralph, Daniel Falush, and Daniel Lawson for helpful comments and suggestions.

Author Contributions

Conceived and designed the experiments: JK Pickrell, JK Pritchard. Analyzed the data: JK Pickrell. Contributed reagents/materials/analysis tools: JK Pickrell. Wrote the paper: JK Pickrell, JK Pritchard.

REFERENCES

1. Cavalli-Sforza LL, Edwards AW (1967) Phylogenetic analysis. Models and estimation proce-dures. Am J Hum Genet 19: 233–57.
2. Felsenstein J (1982) How can we infer geography and history from gene frequencies? J Theor Biol 96: 9–20. doi: 10. 1016/0022-5193(82)90152-7
3. Cann RL, Stoneking M, Wilson AC (1987) Mitochondrial DNA and human evolution. Nature 325: 31–6. doi: 10. 1038/325031a0
4. Nei M, Roychoudhury AK (1974) Genic variation within and between the three major races of man, Caucasoids, Negroids, and Mongoloids. Am J Hum Genet 26: 421–43.
5. Nei M, Roychoudhury AK (1993) Evolutionary relationships of human populations on a global scale. Mol Biol Evol 10: 927–43.
6. Cavalli-Sforza LL, Piazza A, Menozzi P, Mountain J (1988) Reconstruction of human evolution: bringing together genetic, archaeological, and linguistic data. Proc Natl Acad Sci U S A 85: 6002–6. doi: 10. 1073/pnas. 85. 16. 6002
7. Li JZ, Absher DM, Tang H, Southwick AM, Casto AM, et al. (2008) Worldwide human rela-tionships inferred from genome-wide patterns of variation. Science 319: 1100–1104. doi: 10. 1126/science. 1153717
8. Pritchard JK, Seielstad MT, Perez-Lezaun A, Feldman MW (1999) Population growth of human Y chromosomes: a study of Y chromosome microsatellites. Mol Biol Evol 16: 1791–8. doi: 10. 1093/oxfordjournals. molbev. a026091
9. Beaumont MA, Zhang W, Balding DJ (2002) Approximate Bayesian computation in popula-tion genetics. Genetics 162: 2025–35.
10. Schaffner SF, Foo C, Gabriel S, Reich D, Daly MJ, et al. (2005) Calibrating a coalescent simulation of human genome sequence variation. Genome Res 15: 1576–1583. doi: 10. 1101/gr. 3709305
11. Gutenkunst RN, Hernandez RD, Williamson SH, Bustamante CD (2009) Inferring the joint demographic history of multiple populations from multidimensional SNP frequency data. PLoS Genet 5: e1000695 doi:10. 1371/journal. pgen. 1000695.
12. Hey J, Nielsen R (2004) Multilocus methods for estimating population sizes, migration rates and divergence time, with applications to the divergence of Drosophila pseudoobscura and D. persimilis. Genetics 167: 747–60. doi: 10. 1534/genetics. 103. 024182
13. Beerli P, Felsenstein J (1999) Maximum-likelihood estimation of migration rates and effective population numbers in two populations using a coalescent approach. Genetics 152: 763–73.
14. Becquet C, Przeworski M (2007) A new approach to estimate parameters of speciation models with application to apes. Genome Res 17: 1505–19. doi: 10. 1101/gr. 6409707
15. Kubatko LS (2009) Identifying hybridization events in the presence of coalescence via model selection. Syst Biol 58: 478–88.
16. Gronau I, Hubisz MJ, Gulko B, Danko CG, Siepel A (2011) Bayesian inference of ancient human demography from individual genome sequences. Nat Genet 43: 1031–4. doi: 10. 1038/ng. 937
17. Menozzi P, Piazza A, Cavalli-Sforza L (1978) Synthetic maps of human gene frequencies in Europeans. Science

201: 786–92. doi: 10. 1126/science. 356262

18. Pritchard JK, Stephens M, Donnelly P (2000) Inference of population structure using multi-locus genotype data. Genetics 155: 945–59.
19. Patterson N, Price AL, Reich D (2006) Population structure and eigenanalysis. PLoS Genet 2: e190 doi:10. 1371/journal. pgen. 0020190.
20. Lawson DJ, Hellenthal G, Myers S, Falush D (2012) Inference of Population Structure using Dense Haplotype Data. PLoS Genet 8: e1002453 doi:10. 1371/journal. pgen. 1002453.
21. Rosenberg NA, Pritchard JK, Weber JL, Cann HM, Kidd KK, et al. (2002) Genetic structure of human populations. Science 298: 2381–2385. doi: 10. 1126/ science. 1078311
22. Liti G, Carter DM, Moses AM, Warringer J, Parts L, et al. (2009) Population genomics of domestic and wild yeasts. Nature 458: 337–41. doi: 10. 1038/nature07743
23. vonHoldt BM, Pollinger JP, Lohmueller KE, Han E, Parker HG, et al. (2010) Genome-wide SNP and haplotype analyses reveal a rich history underlying dog domestication. Nature 464: 898–902. doi: 10. 1038/ nature08837
24. François O, Currat M, Ray N, Han E, Excoffier L, et al. (2010) Principal component analysis under population genetic models of range expansion and admixture. Mol Biol Evol 27: 1257–68. doi: 10. 1093/molbev/msq010
25. McVean G (2009) A genealogical interpretation of principal components analysis. PLoS Genet 5: e1000686 doi:10. 1371/journal. pgen. 1000686.
26. Novembre J, Stephens M (2008) Interpreting principal component analyses of spatial popula-tion genetic variation. Nat Genet 40: 646–9. doi: 10. 1038/ng. 139
27. Saitou N, Nei M (1987) The neighbor-joining method: a new method for reconstructing phy-logenetic trees. Mol Biol Evol 4: 406–25.
28. Felsenstein J (1973) Maximum-likelihood estimation of evolutionary trees from continuous characters. Am J Hum Genet 25: 471–92.
29. RoyChoudhury A, Felsenstein J, Thompson EA (2008) A two-stage pruning algorithm for likelihood computation for a population tree. Genetics 180: 1095–105. doi: 10. 1534/genetics. 107. 085753
30. Felsenstein J (1981) Evolutionary trees from gene frequencies and quantitative characters: finding maximum likelihood estimates. Evolution 35: 1229–1242. doi: 10. 2307/2408134
31. Sirén J, Marttinen P, Corander J (2011) Reconstructing population histories from single nu-cleotide polymorphism data. Mol Biol Evol 28: 673–83. doi: 10. 1093/molbev/msq236
32. Nielsen R, Mountain JL, Huelsenbeck JP, Slatkin M (1998) Maximum-likelihood estimation of population divergence times and population phylogeny in models without mutation. Evolution 52: 669–677. doi: 10. 2307/2411262
33. Nicholson G, Smith AV, Jónsson F, Gústafsson Ó, Stefánsson K, et al. (2002) Assessing Pop-ulation Differentiation and Isolation from Single-Nucleotide Polymorphism Data. Journal of the Royal Statistical Society Series B (Statistical Methodology) 64: 695–715. doi: 10. 1111/1467-9868. 00357
34. Cavalli-Sforza LL (1973) Analytic review: some current problems of human population genet-ics. Am J Hum Genet 25: 82–104.
35. Cavalli-Sforza LL, Piazza A (1975) Analysis of evolution: evolutionary rates, independence and treeness. Theor Popul Biol 8: 127–65. doi: 10. 1016/0040-5809(75)90029-5
36. Keinan A, Mullikin JC, Patterson N, Reich D (2007) Measurement of the human allele fre-quency spectrum demonstrates greater genetic drift in East Asians than in Europeans. Nat Genet 39: 1251–5. doi: 10. 1038/ ng2116
37. Reich D, Thangaraj K, Patterson N, Price AL, Singh L (2009) Reconstructing Indian popula-tion history. Nature 461: 489–94. doi: 10. 1038/nature08365
38. Durand EY, Patterson N, Reich D, Slatkin M (2011) Testing for Ancient Admixture between Closely Related Populations. Mol Biol Evol 28: 2239–52. doi: 10. 1093/ molbev/msr048
39. Green RE, Krause J, Briggs AW, Maricic T, Stenzel U, et al. (2010) A draft sequence of the Neandertal genome. Science 328: 710–22. doi: 10. 1126/science. 1188021
40. Lathrop GM (1982) Evolutionary trees and admixture: phylogenetic inference when some populations are hybridized. Ann Hum Genet 46: 245–55. doi: 10. 1111/j. 1469-1809. 1982. tb00716. x
41. Reich D, Green RE, Kircher M, Krause J, Patterson N, et al. (2010) Genetic history of an archaic hominin group from Denisova Cave in Siberia. Nature 468: 1053–60. doi: 10. 1038/nature09710
42. Reich D, Patterson N, Kircher M, Delfin F, Nandineni MR, et al. (2011) Denisova admixture and the first modern human dispersals into Southeast Asia and Oceania. Am J Hum Genet 89: 516–28. doi: 10. 1016/j. ajhg. 2011. 09. 005
43. Moorjani P, Patterson N, Hirschhorn JN, Keinan A, Hao L, et al. (2011) The history of African gene flow into Southern Europeans, Levantines, and Jews. PLoS Genet 7: e1001373 doi:10. 1371/journal. pgen. 1001373. .
44. Rasmussen M, Guo X, Wang Y, Lohmueller KE, Rasmussen S, et al. (2011) An Aboriginal Australian genome reveals separate human dispersals into Asia. Science 334: 94–8. doi: 10. 1126/science. 1211177
45. Huson D, Rupp R, Scornavacca C (2010) Phylogenetic Networks. Concepts, Algorithms and Applications. Cambridge University Press.
46. Huson DH, Bryant D (2006) Application of phylogenetic networks in evolutionary studies. Mol Biol Evol 23: 254–67.
47. Dyer RJ, Nason JD (2004) Population Graphs: the graph theoretic shape of genetic structure. Mol Ecol 13: 1713–27. doi: 10. 1111/j. 1365-294x. 2004. 02177. x
48. Coop G, Witonsky D, Di Rienzo A, Pritchard JK (2010) Using environmental correlations to identify loci

underlying local adaptation. Genetics 185: 1411–23. doi: 10. 1534/genetics. 110. 114819

49. Weir BS, Hill WG (2002) Estimating F-statistics. Annu Rev Genet 36: 721–50. doi: 10. 1146/annurev. genet. 36. 050802. 093940
50. Felsenstein J (2003) Inferring Phylogenies. Sinauer Associates, 2nd edition.
51. DeGiorgio M, Jakobsson M, Rosenberg NA (2009) Out of Africa: modern humanorigins special feature: explaining worldwide patterns of human genetic variation using a coalescent- based serial founder model of migration outward from Africa. Proc Natl Acad Sci U S A 106: 16057–62. doi: 10. 1073/pnas. 0903341106
52. Jakobsson M, Scholz SW, Scheet P, Gibbs JR, VanLiere JM, et al. (2008) Genotype, haplotype and copy-number variation in worldwide human populations. Nature 451: 998–1003. doi: 10. 1038/nature06742
53. Hellenthal G, Auton A, Falush D (2008) Inferring human colonization history using a copying model. PLoS Genet 4: e1000078 doi:10. 1371/journal. pgen. 1000078. .
54. Patterson N, Moorjani P, Luo Y, Mallick S, Rohland N, et al. (2012) Ancient admixture. Genetics In Press. doi: 10. 1534/genetics. 112. 145037
55. Price AL, Tandon A, Patterson N, Barnes KC, Rafaels N, et al. (2009) Sensitive detection of chromosomal segments of distinct ancestry in admixed populations. PLoS Genet 5: e1000519 doi:10. 1371/journal. pgen. 1000519. .
56. Xu S, Huang W, Qian J, Jin L (2008) Analysis of genomic admixture in Uyghur and its implication in mapping strategy. Am J Hum Genet 82: 883–94. doi: 10. 1016/j. ajhg. 2008. 01. 017
57. Henn BM, Botigué LR, Gravel S, Wang W, Brisbin A, et al. (2012) Genomic ancestry of North Africans supports back-to-Africa migrations. PLoS Genet 8: e1002397 doi:10. 1371/journal. pgen. 1002397. .
58. Boyko AR, Quignon P, Li L, Schoenebeck JJ, Degenhardt JD, et al. (2010) A simple genetic architecture underlies morphological variation in dogs. PLoS Biol 8: e1000451 doi:10. 1371/journal. pbio. 1000451. .
59. American Kennel Club (2006) The complete dog book. Ballantine Books.
60. Parker HG, Kim LV, Sutter NB, Carlson S, Lorentzen TD, et al. (2004) Genetic structure of the purebred domestic dog. Science 304: 1160–4. doi: 10. 1126/ science. 1097406
61. Novembre J, Johnson T, Bryc K, Kutalik Z, Boyko AR, et al. (2008) Genes mirror geography within Europe. Nature 456: 98–101. doi: 10. 1038/nature07331
62. Novembre J, Ramachandran S (2011) Perspectives on human population structure at the cusp of the sequencing era. Annu Rev Genomics Hum Genet 12: 245–74. doi: 10. 1146/annurev-genom-090810-183123
63. Bhatia G, Patterson N, Pasaniuc B, Zaitlen N, Genovese G, et al. (2011) Genome-wide com-parison of African-ancestry populations from CARe and other cohorts reveals signals of natural selection. Am J Hum Genet 89: 368–81. doi: 10. 1016/j. ajhg. 2011. 07. 025
64. Bonhomme M, Chevalet C, Servin B, Boitard S, Abdallah J, et al. (2010) Detecting selection in population trees: the Lewontin and Krakauer test extended. Genetics 186: 241–62. doi: 10. 1534/genetics. 110. 117275
65. Myers S, Hellenthal G, Lawson D, Busby G, Leslie S, et al. . (2011). LD patterns in dense variation data reveal information about the history of human populations worldwide. URL http://www. ichg2011. org/cgi-bin/ichg11s?&sort=ptimes&sbutton=Detail&absno=21708&sid=806980.
66. Lawson CL, Hanson RJ (1995) Solving least squares problems. Philadelphia, PA: Society for Industrial Mathematics, 3rd edition.
67. Press WH, Teukolsky SA, Vetterling WT, Flannery BP (1992) Numerical recipes in C (2nd ed.): the art of scientific computing. New York, NY, USA: Cambridge University Press.
68. Lindblad-Toh K, Wade CM, Mikkelsen TS, Karlsson EK, Jaffe DB, et al. (2005) Genome sequence, comparative analysis and haplotype structure of the domestic dog. Nature 438: 803–19.
69. Hudson RR (2002) Generating samples under a Wright-Fisher neutral model of genetic varia-tion. Bioinformatics 18: 337–8. doi: 10. 1093/bioinformatics/18. 2. 337
70. Sukumaran J, Holder MT (2010) DendroPy: a Python library for phylogenetic computing. Bioinformatics 26: 1569–71. doi: 10. 1093/bioinformatics/btq228

CHAPTER 7

BIAS CHARACTERIZATION IN PROBABILISTIC GENOTYPE DATA AND IMPROVED SIGNAL DETECTION WITH MULTIPLE IMPUTATION

Cameron Palmer, Itsik Pe'er

INTRODUCTION

Genome-wide association studies (GWAS) have become a primary tool to elucidate the correlations between SNP genotypes and complex phenotypes in large cohorts. Association studies initially assumed the existence of genotype calls: for each sample at each assayed variant, either reference allele homozygote, heterozygote, or alternate allele homozygote. As such, methods developed for analyzing GWAS assumed the existence of such perfect-confidence genotype data. The association study design and related analysis methods have remained in force even as the field has transitioned into the sequencing era and more complete data have become available. In all situations, due to technical and financial limitations, association studies only partially assay the set of common variants in any organism. The variants included on a SNP array typically only include a small fraction of the total pool of variants present, and even sequenced variants are called incompletely and inconsistently. Furthermore, due to the low magnitude of effect of most trait-associated variants, studies prioritize sample size via multisite meta-analysis, involving genetic samples assayed on different technologies. This study design results in a complicated missingness pattern across the entire conceptual set of common variants in a sample. Yet due to shared linkage disequilibrium between different samples, this missingness can be overcome with the addition of external reference data.

Genotype imputation probabilistically estimates unknown genotypes for a study sample by leveraging external reference haplotypes ascertained at a superset of SNPs [1]. Genotype calls and genotype probabilities are fundamentally different. Genotype calls are considered certain data and, under the traditional additive model, may be represented as an integer count of a reference allele present for each study individual. Direct extension of these simple models to probabilistic data is not possible, as the models are not capable of representing the additional variance component introduced by uncertainty. This is critical to understanding the traditional challenge in analyzing imputed genotype data: existing methods are not directly compatible with uncertain data, so probabilistic genotypes must be projected to a lower-dimensional approximation resembling genotypes, with a concomitant loss of information and introduction of bias.

Three primary methods have been developed for the handling of uncertain data in genetic association studies. For the first method, and at one extreme, probabilities may be converted to call-like integral counts by choosing the class with the largest probability. This paradigm requires no additional modification of the analysis method for genotype calls, but all meaningful information about uncertainty is lost. For the second method, in some situations, genotype probabilities may be converted into expected counts of the reference allele: the "allelic dosage." This strategy attempts to maintain some of the uncertainty of the genotype estimate by allowing non-integral values: for example, when the heterozygote and reference allele homozygote classes are equiprobable and the alternate allele homozygote has 0 probability, a sample is considered to have 1.5 alleles. Unfortunately, this strategy is only useful when the underlying algorithm extends to nonintegral data (for example, a generalized linear model with continuous predictor); furthermore, there is no rigorous proof of the degree

Citation: Palmer C, Pe'er I (2016) Bias Characterization in Probabilistic Genotype Data and Improved Signal Detection with Multiple Imputation. PLoS Genet 12(6): e1006091. doi:10.1371/journal.pgen.1006091

of bias or information loss incurred using this method. Finally, as a last method, the algorithm may be modified to directly operate on probabilities [2]. This option attempts to include all uncertainty information at the cost of additional work creating a new algorithm. In practice, this type of custom algorithm design is limited to simple GLM methods; other studies in the field creating more complex statistical models for association studies do not undertake this additional work [3–8].

In the statistics literature, Multiple Imputation (MI; distinct from genotype imputation; [9]) is the rigorous method of conducting analysis on probabilistic estimates of uncertain data. The details of MI are discussed in Methods. Briefly, a small number of complete datasets are randomly drawn according to the probability data. These datasets are then analyzed using any standard analysis technique that generates a normally-distributed effect estimate β and standard error estimate s. Importantly, MI is not a method of estimating hidden data, but rather a method of handling existing estimates. The performance of MI, and indeed of all imputed data analysis methods, is reliant on the quality of the underlying genotype imputation. Imputation accuracy, the agreement between predicted and true genotype, tends to vary across both imputation "quality," as estimated by most imputation software, and minor allele frequency. The extent of this variable performance has not, to our knowledge, been rigorously assessed.

In this study, we seek to rigorously evaluate this variable genotype imputation performance. We show a significant deviation between genotype probabilities generated by imputation, and empirical probabilities estimated at the same sites. This failure of probability consistency is an important confounding effect in imputed data analysis. We show that Multiple Imputation matches or improves upon performance of existing imputed data analysis regimes by better prioritizing true positive associations, while additionally being straightforwardly extensible to future analysis algorithms.

RESULTS

Imputation Accuracy

We compared the allelic dosage (Methods) to the "true" genotype count based on masked genotype data. Fig 1 shows the fraction error between allelic dosage from imputation and masked genotype, stratified by genotype class, allele frequency, and reported imputation quality metric (hereafter called "r^2"). We observe that a single quality metric r^2 masks significant deviations in mean quality between different genotype classes and different allele frequencies. For imputed SNPs reported to be of high quality ($r^2 > 0.9$, left panel; top 40% of GWAS-used SNPs, S1 and S2 Figs), and with sufficiently high minor allele frequency, imputation is indeed well-behaved: variants with minor allele frequency above 0.3 have less than 3% discordance with similar performance across genotype classes. However, SNPs of lesser imputation quality ($0.8 \leq r^2 \leq 0.9$, right panel; approximately 18% of GWAS-used SNPs,S1 and S2 Figs) or low minor allele frequency are inconsistently imputed. Minor allele homozygotes and heterozygotes in particular are subject to highly inflated error rates. While differences across the SNP strata are observed with both IMPUTE2 and minimac3 imputations, the magnitudes observed are distinct (S3 Fig). Equivalent results are observed when evaluating performance by fraction of best-guess genotypes from imputation not matching masked genotypes (S4 Fig).

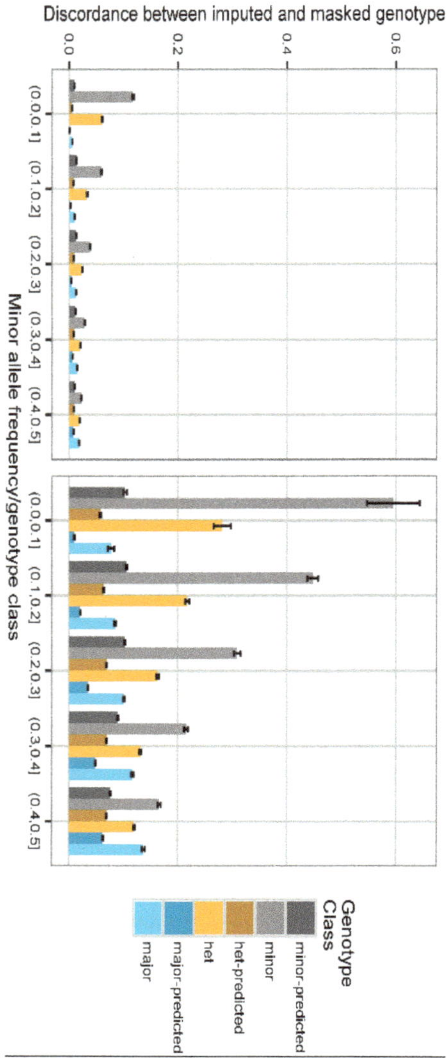

Figure 1. Relationship between quality of estimated allelic dosage from IMPUTE2 imputation and predictors of imputation quality.

Data are estimated from 10% of the original chip (59808 SNPs) masked from imputation. Discordance of predicted allelic dosage (y axis) is the fraction difference between dosage computed from imputation probabilities and dosage based on masked genotype data: for example, if the true genotype is reference homozygote and the allelic dosage from imputation is 1.4, the discordance is $\frac{|2-1.4|}{2} = 0.3$. Left panel: imputation quality greater than 0.9; right panel: quality between 0.8 and 0.9. Clusters correspond to minor allele frequencies of 10%; individual bars represent quality stratified by masked genotype. "Predicted" bars correspond to expected concordance assuming independence of individual haplotypes. Error bars represent 95% confidence intervals of mean discordance estimate.

Imputation Probability Consistency

We next examined the imputation probabilities themselves, to evaluate whether probabilities generated by imputation software correspond to the empirical probability of observing a genotype at a particular site. Results for this comparison for

IMPUTE2 probabilities are shown in Fig 2, across strata of reported quality and predicted call probability. The empirical accuracy significantly deviates from the predicted, and much more so with decreasing r^2; S5 Fig shows similar plots comparing the effect of decreasing minor allele frequency on this distortion, and show weaker but significant changes with decreasing frequency. Of note, the heterozygote genotype class behaves in a distinct but complementary fashion relative to the two homozygote classes.

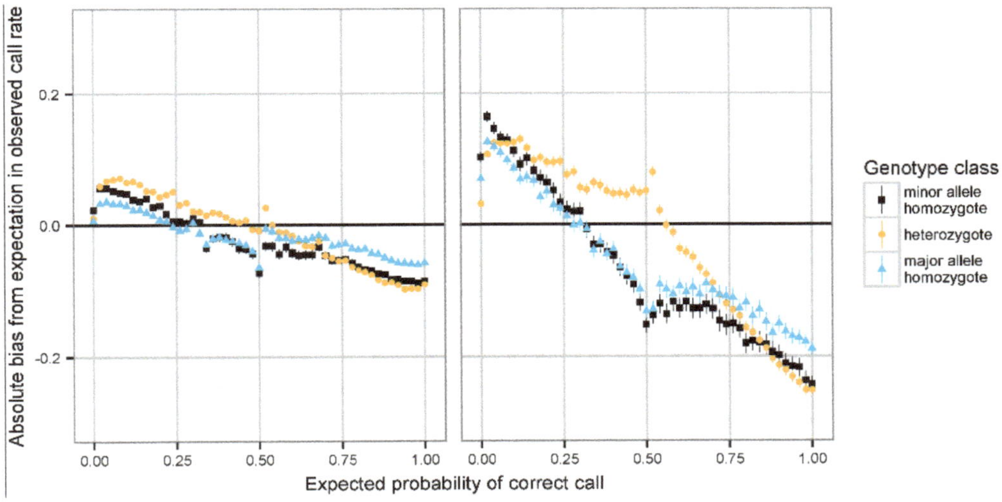

Figure 2. Evaluation of the consistency of probability scores from IMPUTE2 imputation.

Data are estimated from 10% of the original chip (59808 SNPs) masked from imputation. x-axis: 0.02-width bins of imputation probabilities; y-axis: mean deviation between expected and observed accuracy. Data series correspond to results stratified by genotype class. Left panel: IMPUTE2 info metric greater than 0.9; right panel: info metric between 0.8 and 0.9. Error bars represent 95% confidence intervals around mean consistency estimate.

These results are distinguishable between imputation programs: the effect is much stronger in the IMPUTE2 imputation. The most substantial difference between the two programs is IMPUTE2's use of sequential imputation windows to improve performance through parallelization, with potential accuracy tradeoffs, yet we have observed no differences caused by modifying this parameter. We note that differences in imputation performance under different conditions have been observed extensively and unpredictably (see, among many, [10–14]). Our observations are consistent with intermittent observations of MACH-family algorithms nominally outperforming IMPUTE-family algorithms in some cases, yet the precise reason(s) for these differences between similar software has never, to our knowledge, been demonstrated.

Signal Enrichment with Multiple Imputation

We next sought to evaluate whether the ability to prioritize verified trait-associated SNPs in an association study ranking was detectably different using MI or other existing algorithms. We considered 73 replicated loci from a large (N = 339224 individuals) GWAS for BMI [15]. As expected with our modest sample size of 2802, we have little power to detect the majority of these variants at genome-wide significance $5 \cdot 10^{-8}$.

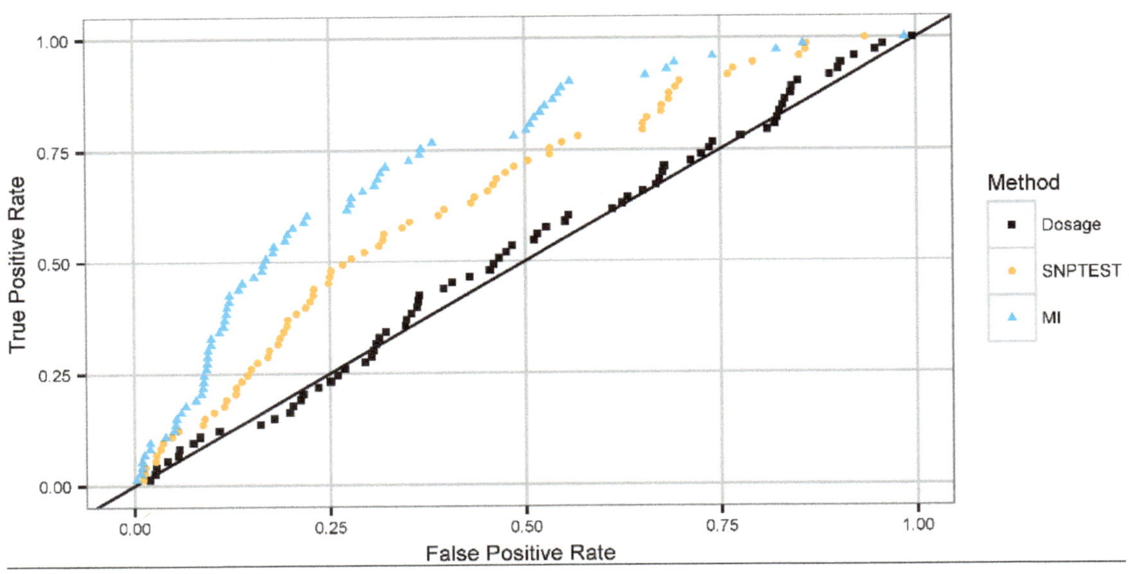

Figure 3. Receiver operating characteristic curves for Health ABC BMI association with IMPUTE2 imputation.

Nevertheless, if the variants are associated with the trait at all, one expects the variants to be relatively better ranked in the final list of variants than variants chosen at random from the study. We conducted a BMI genome-wide association study in Health ABC, as discussed in Methods. Using these SNP association results, we computed the rank percentile of each published variant, comparing these results for two existing imputed data analysis algorithms and MI.

We evaluated the receiver operating characteristic curves for PLINK dosage, SNPTEST score, and MI (Fig 3). MI significantly outperforms all other methods (one-tailed DeLong test $p < 2 \cdot 10^{-16}$). We repeat this analysis with a height GWAS in NFBC66 (Methods), and find a similar significant improvement in signal detection by MI compared to other methods (one-tailed DeLong test $p < 0.0003764$). We conclude from this analysis that significant information loss may occur when uncertainty is incompletely handled in imputed data analysis. There is no evidence in this comparison that Multiple Imputation is inferior to other methods. True positive associations are 73 established BMI variants from [15]. Tracks correspond to uncertainty handling methods: allelic dosage, score test, MI on imputed probabilities.

Changes in Null Distribution of Variants

Improved signal detection by MI may be attributed to several causes. In observing the additional variance component in the multiple imputation model, s_B^2 (see Methods), we note that variability introduced by genotypic uncertainty should result in decreased rankings for variants regardless of trait being analyzed. Uncertainty in probabilities also differs with variant-wide imputation quality r^2, implying that different association tests may lead to different expected distributions of variants in a ranked association study across the quality spectrum, whether variants are trait-associated or not.

We sought to evaluate the null distribution of variant ranks across imputation quality. We calculated the percentile rank of each variant in the BMI GWAS and sorted the variants into bins across imputation quality. Results from this investigation are shown in Fig 4. All tested methods have a statistically significant correlation between imputation quality and average rank (all Pearson correlation test $p < 2 \cdot 10^{-16}$; comparable results for nonparametric tests). PLINK and SNPTEST have indistinguishable magnitudes of effect (shared effect size -0.017, indistinguishable with $p = 0.44$). Multiple Imputation shows a significantly stronger correlation than the other tests (effect size -0.351, greater than other tests with $p = 3.4 \cdot 10^{-7}$). MI produces test statistics that much more significantly incorporate uncertainty, through in particular the between-draw variance component.

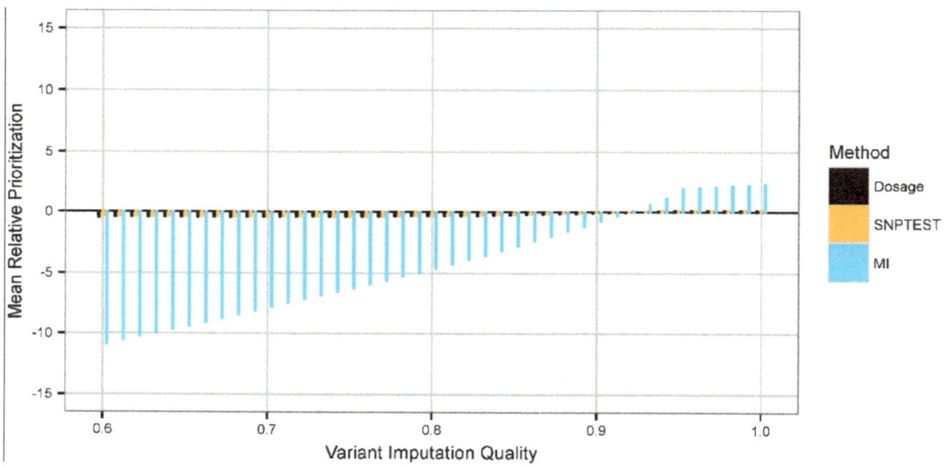

Figure 4. Evaluation of the null distribution of variants across an association study ranking.

x-axis: variant imputation quality bin; y-axis: absolute deviation from uniform random expected rank across all variants at given quality (that is, 50%). Data tracks correspond to PLINK dosage analysis, SNPTEST exact testing, and MI.

Published trait-associated variants tend to impute with higher quality than random variants from a dataset due to selection bias, leading to the possibility that this global incorporation of quality by MI is leading to better performance in a manner unrelated to the trait itself. To control for trait-unrelated differences between published variants and the global SNP distribution, we computed empirical matched null sets for every published variant by drawing 1000 SNPs matched to this variant with parameters $r^2 \pm 0.01$ and frequency ± 0.01 of the true variant. Here we are drawing variants from the association study itself; this null allows us to detect effects specifically affecting the significant tail of the distribution over the bulk of variants. For most traits, these variants will overwhelmingly be unassociated with the outcome, and thus this null will correspond to a true null of no genetic association; in the case that this condition is untrue, this null will lead to relatively conservative assumptions about the added performance of MI. We then regenerated ROC curves for each analysis, this time controlling for the null rank of SNPs matched to the published variant list based on these parameters. These results approximately correspond to trait-specific enrichment effects caused by the various analysis methods. We find that adjustment for trait-secular shifts in variant quality affects BMI and height differently. For BMI, MI continues to outperform PLINK and

SNPTEST (one-tailed DeLong $p < 1.177 \cdot 10^{-10}$). For height, null adjustment reverses the previously-observed trends, such that MI tends to underperform PLINK and SNPTEST (one-tailed DeLongp < 0.0025). We note that for this trait in particular, the null derived from drawing from the association study itself may be conservative given the broad genetic basis for human height [16].

Extensibility

To underscore the benefits of MI not simply on regression with existing uncertainty handling methoods, but additionally on more complex algorithms more difficult to directly adapt, we applied MI to EMMAX [4]. We ran EMMAX on both the Health ABC BMI GWAS and the NFBC66 height GWAS, with default parameter settings and the IBS-based kinship matrices. We compared EMMAX with thresholded genotype data and MI on imputed probabilities. The published version of EMMAX only accepts integral count genotypes, thus no other comparisons were included in this test.

We detect significant improvement in relative percentile increase for BMI-associated variants that is abrograted by null adjustment (one-sided DeLong test $p = 6.663 \cdot 10^{-12}$ and $p = 0.09933$ respectively). We find weak evidence for improved overall efficiency for known height variants (one-sided DeLong test $p = 0.01994$), which under null adjustment becomes a significant underperformance of MI relative to rounded genotype control (one-sided DeLong test $p = 2.242 \cdot 10^{-7}$); again, we note that this null may be overly conservative in this trait context [16]. Evaluation of the null distribution of variants for this experiment, analogous to the analysis inFig 4, shows that the MI-mediated rank shift is much smaller across both the frequency and variant quality spectrum. We propose that the error model used in EMMAX is partially compensating for the additional uncertainty variance component redundantly modeled by MI.

DISCUSSION

In this paper, we analyze the application of Multiple Imputation in the particular context of genotype imputation. We find that representative existing analysis methods tend to increase noise in association testing by incompletely modeling the uncertainty of genotype estimates across the entire set of imputed variants. This results not just in lower quality variants, for which information is limited, receiving inappropriately high ranking, but variants for which underpowered but significant trait association is present becoming lost in statistical noise introduced by imputation. We furthermore detect imputation program-specific inconsistencies in posterior genotype probabilities that differently affect the three genotype classes. Overall, we characterize the complexity of imputation probabilities and show that MI can improve association testing with uncertain data at the cost of increased post-imputation computational time.

This study particularly elaborates on the interpretation of a p-value from a probabilistic association study. Based on the results in Fig 4, we see that existing analysis tends to rank variants uniformly across r^2: the p-value weakly incorporates imputation quality, enough so that the tests are not correctly calibrated but insufficiently so to actually correct for differential uncertainty. This poor calibration is verifiable with a true null: observing the null distribution of variants in our study regressed against random standard normal traits, we observe a comparable correlation between variant imputation quality and SNP ranking for SNPTEST ($p = 0.001953$). Dosage analysis does not, in that context, recapitulate the correlation effect observed in our data, suggesting that the trend is specific to our trait-associated null. This poor calibration is potentially shared by many analysis methods in the field: following the simulation work of Acar and Sun [17], we have found low magnitude but significant miscalibration when operating on probabilistic genetic data and null traits for linear regression and a Kruskal-Wallis test on best-guess variants; dosage analysis; and their generalized Kruskal-Wallis test that directly handles uncertainty (all Wilcoxon rank sum $p < 2 \cdot 10^{-16}$). There is also a significant correlation between uncertainty for the Kruskal-Wallis based tests in this simulation context (ANOVA $p < 2 \cdot 10^{-16}$). Association p-values are intrinsically affected by genotype uncertainty, altering the expected null distribution from uniform random, but this is simply an uncharacterized bias introduced by incompletely handling uncertainty, not a formal characteristic with proven properties.

We suggest that this behavior is undesirable: if a SNP estimate is uncertain, then the behavior of an ideal inference should be to proportionally downweight the ranking of that SNP in that particular study in a predictable fashion. With Multiple Imputation, this uncertainty-induced variability is correctly apportioned to the between-draw variance component s_B^2, resulting in unmodified effect estimates that are still suitable for cross-cohort meta-analysis. In the case of our example BMI association study, the positive control variants used were all imputed with high confidence, yet MI still showed a trait-specific rank improvement in these SNPs, due to the selective downranking of low confidence variants with no or lesser phenotype association. In short, we see little reason to continue using dosage or score test methods for handling imputation probabilities, when a straightforward alternative with superior statistical properties exists.

The results in Figs 1 and 2 broadly characterize imputation performance across variant quality, frequency, and genotype class. Although parts of these results are hinted at in various imputation papers (in particular, [18], but also [2, 12, 19, 20]), we have not before encountered a presentation of the severity of quality degradation across the full spectrum of frequencies. We urge analysts in all contexts to avoid genotype thresholding, in particular using IMPUTE2 probabilities: with decreasing frequency and quality, the likelihood of rounding to an incorrect genotype grows extremely high. We also observe strong per-genotype class differences in performance, most severely affecting heterozygotes. This is not a surprising result, given the integral nature of computational prephasing in genotype imputation. In the modern genotype imputation protocol, prephasing is a one-time burdensome computation that is not repeated, whereas the imputation step itself is comparatively rapid and repeated many times as new reference panels become available. A useful future analysis would investigate the specific impact of differential phasing quality on imputation probability bias, and our results emphasize that prephasing should be reconducted as advancements in the field yield higher quality phasing solutions. We have observed in the literature a tendency to ignore uncertainty in genotype data when developing new algorithms. This elision is understandable in the sense that complete-case analysis is typically substantially more straightforward to implement, and as a first approximation, uncertain data may be converted seemingly straightforwardly to genotype "calls" via techniques such as rounding. Yet in the case study of simple regression, we see that this approximation bears with it a cost in loss of statistical power to detect trait-associated variants. One of the great benefits of MI is its simple application to complete-case methods, as each round of MI generates complete case data. In the case of standard regression, this is a straightforward benefit; in the case of a method such as EMMAX, one must balance the desirable avoidance of rounded probabilities with potential complications of the standard MI variance component model.

One of the strongest justifications for the widespread use of imputation is the facilitation of multisite multicohort meta-analysis, in which summary statistics from separate association studies are combined to increase statistical power. The benefits of integrating imputation quality into inference are magnified in this context. Under the current regime, either $\{\beta, s^2\}$ or $\{N, p\}$ pairs are the exclusive data provided to meta-analysis tools [21], leading to a downstream analysis that treats different estimates of variants with different imputation qualities as estimates identical to one another in expectation ascertained with perfect confidence. With nested model multiple imputation ([22], Methods), the improved model described in this paper may be extended to meta-analysis. A nested model MI meta-analysis will explicitly compensate for variable imputation quality across contributing studies with inflated variance components corresponding to noise in the mean effect estimate or inflated standard error from contributing studies (i.e., imprecision in effect estimate introduced either by variable imputation quality, fluctuations in allele frequency, or differential effect due to LD changes in different studies). The cost of this extended meta-analysis regime is limited. In addition to the standard $\{\beta, s^2\}$ pairs currently used to combine analysis, the within- and between-draw variance components must also be submitted. These data require additional disk space but are relatively trivial to provide. Crucially, the summary statistics from each individual draw are not required for this meta-analysis, such that the growth in memory requirements for meta-analysis does not scale with the number of draws conducted.

We note that by explicitly handling variable imputation quality in different studies, this meta-analysis regime introduces potential sources of heterogeneity in the final meta-analysis result. Studies with aberrantly high uncertainty may strongly influence the resulting meta-analyzed association statistic. Note that this source of heterogeneity already exists, but is not rigorously modeled and currently must be addressed by ad hoc filtering and quality control. We propose that heterogeneity from differential imputation quality may be quantified by a heterogeneity test analogous to the effect estimate heterogeneity I^2 metric in METAL. This test would quantify heterogeneity specifically in the between-test variance component s_B^2 from contributing studies, which captures the noise between individual MI draws introduced by meaningfully uncertain data. This test would enable standardized detection of cases in which low imputation quality may require custom secondary genotyping for validation.In the statistics literature, starting with [9] and moving forward, the recommended number of MI draws has varied widely. The original recommendation was that oftentimes 3–5 draws were sufficient to retain most of the accuracy while minimizing computational burden. More recent publications (i.e. [23]) have suggested that the original estimates of draws were insufficiently stringent. In this paper, we have used an a priori setting of 10 draws after testing various draw numbers' effects on quality of MI output, and balancing this impact with the added burden of multiple additional MI rounds. We find that this draw count surpasses the point at which MI effect estimates tend to converge (S6 Fig), but may in the case of particularly poorly imputed variants lead to suboptimal estimates of between-draw variance (S7 Fig). A useful target for future work would be the integration of dynamic computation of the number of draws for convergence for individual variants, which in this study is complicated by the manner in which our software interfaces externally, rather than reimplements internally, with existing analysis tools to maximize compatibility.

The existence of program-specific differences in the consistency of imputation probabilities is an intriguing result that raises meaningful questions for the field. Though each program has its own algorithmic features and drawbacks, the practical choice between imputation software often reduces to the banal: ease of use, runtime and memory requirements. These features are important for imputation study designs that may take weeks to months to complete. Yet here we show a more substantive trend of probability bias that follows a distribution specific to particular programs. The precise cause of these distortions is not clear. Further investigation may be warranted to determine a method of adjusting the native probabilities generated from imputation using empirical distributions based on masked comparison data.

We interpret the potential performance improvement of MI over other methods as a call to reevaluate the use of thresholded genotype calls in other contexts. In particular, as the field continues transitioning to sequence-derived variant data, the impact of thresholded certainty in sequencing data analysis cannot be overlooked. We note that standard methods for rare variant analysis, including burden testing, adapt to the high uncertainty in low frequency variant calls by using strict quality control and relying on bulk information to resist the noise introduced by false positives. Yet interpreting the probabilistic output of sequencing technology as a mechanism for completing data in a NMAR setting, Multiple Imputation straightforwardly provides a consistent solution for even complex statistical analyses.

In the case of statistical tests that analyze linked variants together, per-site marginal information is no longer sufficient, as each MI draw must be taken from the joint distribution of all tested sites. Yet with sequencing read data, this kind of analysis is not impossible: joint information can be directly estimated from shared reads, creating a computationally challenging and yet feasible method of rigorously handling genetic uncertainty without even linkage assumptions. The creation of a standard module for interfacing with sequencing read data and dynamically generating such joint probability information would be a significant contribution to the field.

Similarly, the independent draws conducted in multiple imputation implicitly assume independence of samples. In the case of pedigrees or cryptic relatedness of samples, the sampling problem becomes much more challenging. The imputation software analyzed in this study (IMPUTE2, minimac3) is designed to handle unrelated population-based samples. The marginal probabilities generated by the algorithms are not reflective of explicit joint distribution between related samples and thus are not directly compatible with correlated genotype draws without additional modeling. One could synthesize probabilities that scale with both the imputed probabilities and the Mendelian transmission rules, for example

$$P(\mathbf{child}|\mathbf{data},\mathbf{parents}) = \frac{P(\mathbf{child}|\mathbf{data})P(\mathbf{child}|\mathbf{parents})}{\sum_{i=0}^{2} P(\mathbf{child}=i|\mathbf{data})P(\mathbf{child}=i|\mathbf{parents})}$$

Unfortunately, such an approximation of the joint distribution would not be equivalent to actually modeling the combined structure of the data in the imputation software itself: for example, when the parents and children are modeled separately, certain genotypes will be given nonzero probabilities that would be rendered impossible by Mendelian transmission. In the case of BEAGLE [11], duos and trios are specially handled according to externally specified pedigrees. The resulting genotype probabilities then are reasonably considered to be conditional probabilities: for example P(**child|data, parents**). In this case, the appropriate probabilistic relationships should hold:

for example,

$$P(\mathbf{child}=aa) = \left[P(\mathbf{mother}=aa) + \frac{P(\mathbf{mother}=Aa)}{2}\right] \cdot \left[P(\mathbf{father}=aa) + \frac{P(\mathbf{father}=Aa)}{2}\right]$$

and thus consistent drawing could be conducted in a trio by first drawing the child, then drawing the parent probabilities conditional on the result of the child's draw. Ultimately, the suitability of MI to a given application is restricted to situations where the probability-generating method is itself appropriately suited.

Recent work ([24–26]) has produced algorithms (MIX, DISTMIX, ImpG-Summary) capable of imputing association statistics from summary data, without the need for individual-level genotype information. These methods offer substantial time savings relative to genotype imputation, at the cost of reduced overall quality of estimates relative to existing HMM methods. The imputed test statistic at a particular site is the mean of a multidimensional Gaussian distribution based on neighboring test statistics and linkage disequilibrium data: this intuitively corresponds to an MLE dosage estimate from genotype imputation probabilities. It is likely the method thus suffers from analogous disadvantages to those of incomplete uncertainty handling in genotype imputation. One could imagine replacing a single mean imputed test statistic with instead a set of random variates drawn from the underlying Gaussian; these draws would act as drawn genotypes in the analysis in this study. Although multiple test statistics per variant would prove less useful for analysts of individual studies, they would be more completely reflective of the uncertain nature of these estimates. Furthermore, using sample size weighting, one could generate an MI regime in multicohort meta-analysis in, for example, METAL, in which each set of drawn test statistics is used to generate a separate meta-analysis dataset, and the resulting sets are combined using MI. Such a regime would require further investigation, and most likely would require a substantial number of iterations if many contributing cohorts used uncertain input data.

The use of MI is not completely foreign to the field of statistical genetics. We note, however, that its use is very limited, and has not been extensively compared to other, prevalent methods of handling genotype probabilities. We evaluate MI in comparison to existing methods and show MI performance is typically comparable to existing methods, and in certain contexts significantly outperforms other existing algorithms. Furthermore, we emphasize the ease with which MI is extended to, conceptually, all existing and future genotype call analysis methods with little additional effort. We foresee MI as a simple and effective component of all probabilistic genotype analysis.

METHODS

Study Datasets

For this project, we applied for access to and downloaded two SNP array and phenotype datasets from the Database of Genotypes and Phenotypes (dbGaP) [27]. The Whole Genome Association Study of Visceral Adiposity in the Health Aging and Body Composition (Health ABC) Study, dbGaP accession phs000169.v1.p1, contains 2802 individuals genotyped on the Illumina Human1M-Duo SNP array. STAMPEED: Northern Finland Birth Cohort 1966 (NFBC1966), phs000276.v2.p1, contains 5415 individuals assayed on the Illumina HumanCNV370 array. Both datasets were requested and approved under project 7955; they are available from the dedicated General Research Use collection and do not require IRB approval.

The phenotype data released under this collection are quite limited. For this study we limited analysis to simple anthropometric traits. For Health ABC, we conducted a BMI association study with BMI (μ = 27.4, σ = 4.77) determined by age (μ = 73.6, σ = 2.87) and sex (51.2% female). For NFBC66, we conducted a height association study with height in centimeters stratified by sex (μ_W = 153.2, σ_W = 68.9; μ_M = 286.1, σ_M = 66.4; 52% female); age was not included for this single-year birth cohort.

Sample Quality Control

Datasets on dbGaP have already been subjected to a round of cleaning by their depositors. Nevertheless, for thoroughness we cleaned the SNP array data using a standard QC protocol. Briefly, variants with minor allele frequency less than 1%, Hardy-Weinberg Equilibrium p-value and either per-individual or per-SNP missingness greater than 5% were removed. Cryptic relatedness was estimated using genome-wide IBS estimation in PLINK [28]. A large cluster of approximate first-cousins was detected (IBS $\hat{\pi} \sim 0.125$). For the purposes of this analysis, whether this is indicative of unreported pedigree structure or technical artifacts in genotype collection is irrelevant, as we are not undertaking novel variant discovery, rather conducting comparisons relative to control data.

The remaining SNPs were pruned to an independent subset of SNPs using PLINK--indep with default parameters, and these variants along with the maximal independent subset of individuals were used for unrooted principal component analysis in EIGENSOFT [6]. Standard population stratification along geographical axes is observed, confounding novel variant discovery but not effecting within-sample comparisons. To prepare for genotype imputation, SNPs with complementary variant alleles were removed from the dataset, and positions and SNP rsIDs were updated to those of the 1000 Genomes reference panel we used. Complementary allele variants are challenging to reconcile with datasets of potentially different strand alignments. This is true when handling external datasets subject to unknown prior manipulation, but in particular in the case of modern Illumina arrays, which are only annotated with challenging "TOP/BOT" annotations instead of reference strand calls.

Prephasing and Genotype Imputation

Following modern genotype imputation guidelines [12], we first prephased our data using SHAPEITv2 [29] with the recommended parameters. Phased haplotype data were then probabilistically imputed to the Version 3 1000 Genomes Phase 1 Integrated global reference haplotypes [30] using IMPUTE2 [19]. For comparison purposes, to establish whether effects observed were specific to the software in use, in parallel we phased the genotype data using MACH [18] and imputed the resulting phased haplotypes to the same reference panel using minimac3 [20]. Using the global reference data, a large proportion of the approximately 40 million variants in the reference dataset are expected to not segregate in the study samples and impute very poorly; thus, before downstream analysis, variants with program-specific quality metric less than 0.4 were removed entirely. No per-genotype filtering was conducted, to avoid reintroducing NMAR bias.

Standard Analysis Methods

For standard association models under generalized linear models (in this case linear regression), various methods currently exist for analyzing probabilistic genotypes. We selected two widely-used methods of analysis for the purposes of this study. The genetics software PLINK, as of version 1.07, has an "allelic dosage" method of genotype imputation, in which the additive predictor **dosage** = 2P(aa) + P(Aa) is included in a generalized linear model (note that this value is not equivalent to a perfect confidence genotype, as it is permitted to be a decimal number between 0 and 2). This method projects the two parameter posterior probability into a single dimension, thus losing information in many cases: for example, this would consider the posterior probabilities {0, 1, 0} and $\{\frac{1}{3}, \frac{1}{3}, \frac{1}{3}\}$ to be equivalent.

The IMPUTE2 software used for imputation in this study has an accompanying analysis software package, called SNPTEST [2]. This software comes with a custom score test for explicitly handing genotype probabilities from imputation. The software has changed substantially since initial release; the best documentation available for the probability-handling methods is at https://mathgen.stats.ox.ac.uk/genetics_software/snptest/snptest.v2.pdf. For this investigation, we solely use SNPTEST's frequentist methods, which can explicitly handle uncertainty.

Statistical Missingness

Genotype imputation is a discipline-specific solution to a general statistical problem called "informative missingness" [9]. Consider a conceptual data matrix Y containing all phenotype and covariate data for a study. Classical statistical analysis assumes Y is complete, containing no null entries, and that all entries are known with perfect confidence. Study designs with null entries can be compelled into this format by removing all null datapoints before statistics are performed, resulting in a so-called "complete-case analysis."

The effect of deviations from these assumptions vary depending on the characteristics of the missingness itself. Now assume that Y is the conceptual matrix containing all true datapoints with perfect confidence. Missingness observed in realistic studies is encapsulated by a second matrix, M, where each entry M_{ij} is 1 if Y_{ij} is missing in the true study, and 0 otherwise.

Using this framework, missingness can be partitioned into three general classes. If the distribution of M is independent of Y, the missingness is called "missing completely at random" (MCAR). In this situation, corresponding to the classical model, all missingness can be safely ignored in downstream analysis, with a potential loss in statistical power but no introduction of bias.

If instead the distribution of M is dependent on the data matrix Y, missingness can be classified in two separate cases. If the dependency can be reduced to simply the observedsubset of Y_{obs}, where $Y = Y_{obs} \cup Y_{mis}$, then the missingness is, somewhat misleadingly, termed "missing at random" (MAR). Data that are MAR cannot be ignored while safely avoiding the introduction of bias. However, due to the restriction on Y_{obs}, the missing values can be probabilistically imputed from Y_{obs} and added into downstream statistical analysis.

In the worst case, the distribution of M is irreducibly dependent on Y; such missingness is called "not missing at random" (NMAR). NMAR data cannot be removed without potentially introducing bias, and furthermore cannot be predicted solely from the observed data Y_{obs}. The case of genetic data collection is invariably NMAR, as missingness created by collection technologies such as SNP arrays and sequencers exhibit different performance at different underlying genotypes, and the selection of variants for SNP arrays is itself biased by numerous factors including but not limited to predominant ancestry in early variation projects such as HapMap, variant location in the genome and neighboring sequence content, and allele class at the site of interest.

Genotype imputation is an attempt to project the NMAR missingness of genetic data collection into an MAR condition. Due to linkage disequilibrium (LD), the nonrandom segregation of neighboring variants over a limited number of generations, one can add externally collected, ancestrally related haplotypes to the data (the Y matrix). The resulting partition of this matrixY_{obs} now ideally contains sufficient information to probabilistically estimate missing genotype data in the original dataset at both typed and untyped variants.

Multiple Imputation

The framework for Multiple Imputation is established in [9]. Briefly, the method assumes that missing datapoints have been probabilistically estimated using some external method. From these probabilities, an arbitrary d complete datasets are drawn from the probability distributions. In the case of standard single-variant analysis, conducting these draws is straightforward as linkage disequilibrium can be ignored.

Each draw is independently subjected to the desired statistical test. This results in d sets of $\{\beta_i, s_i^2\}$ effect and standard at each variant. The Multiple Imputation consensus test statistic is computed from the following values:

$$\beta_{MI} = \frac{1}{d}\sum_{i=1}^{d}\beta_i$$

$$s_W^2 = \frac{1}{d}\sum_{i=1}^{d}s_i$$

$$s_B^2 = \frac{1}{d-1}\sum_{i=1}^{d}(\beta_i - \beta_{MI})^2$$

$$s_{MI}^2 = S_W^2 + \left(1+\frac{1}{d}\right)s_B^2$$

Here, β_{MI} is the consensus effect estimate; s_W^2 is the within-draw sample variance; s_B^2 is the between-draw sample variance; and s_{MI}^2 is the total sample variance. The test statistic $\frac{\beta_{MI}}{\sqrt{s_{MI}^2}}$ is the ratio of the test statistic and sample standard error, which is distributed as T with $(d-1)\left(1+\frac{ds_W^2}{(d+1)s_B^2}\right)^2$ degrees of freedom. The resulting probability may be interpreted as a posterior probability incorporating both the evidence for association in the study and the actual reliability of the genetic data.

Software implementing this Multiple Imputation regime (in beta) may be found athttps://github.com/cpalmer718/statgen-mi. This package features modularized, extensible interfacing with existing analysis software, and bsub/qsub integration. In total, this implementation of MI requires d times as long to run, and d times as much disk space, as a single analysis run, though running in tranches per chromosome on a cluster can reduce the maximum memory and effective time use by removal of intermediate files and quasiparallelization.

Meta-Analysis of Multiple Imputation

With Multiple Imputation, a simple regime for seamlessly correcting for different proportions of uncertainty in the contributing analyses is available. Extending the logic used when combiningd individual MI draws, the following meta-analysis regime applies [22], for M contributing cohorts to a multisite meta-analysis:

$$\hat{\beta} = \frac{1}{M}\sum_{i=1}^{M}\beta_{MI,i}$$

$$\hat{s}_W^2 = \frac{1}{M}\sum_{i=1}^{M}s_{MI,W}^2$$

$$\hat{s}_B^2 = \frac{1}{M}\sum_{i=1}^{M}s_{MI,B}^2$$

$$\hat{s}_{\mathbf{meta}}^2 = \frac{1}{M-1}\sum_{i=i}^{M}(\beta_{MI,i} - \hat{\beta})^2$$

The new variance component $\hat{s}_{\mathbf{meta}}^2$ is the between-site variance of estimated test statistics. Assuming a balanced study design in which each site runs the same number of MI rounds, the total variance of this nested model multiple imputation is $\hat{s}^2 = \hat{s}_W^2 + (1+\frac{1}{d})\hat{s}_B^2 + (1-\frac{1}{M})\hat{s}_{\mathbf{meta}}^2$.

The ratio of $\hat{\beta}$ to $\sqrt{\hat{s}^2}$ is distributed approximately T with degrees of freedom $\frac{1}{M(d-1)}\left(\frac{(1-\frac{1}{d})\hat{s}_W^2}{\hat{s}^2}\right)^2 + \frac{1}{M-1}\left(\frac{(1+\frac{1}{M})\hat{s}_{\mathbf{meta}}^2}{\hat{s}^2}\right)^2$. In the case of imbalances in the number of draws conducted in each contributing cohort, more complex expressions might be derived, or alternatively a conservative estimate of min(d_m) may be used for the weighting factor in the total variance and degrees of freedom.

Supporting Information

Data are estimated from 10% of the original chip masked from imputation. Discordance of predicted allelic dosage (y-axis) is the fraction difference between dosage computed from imputation probabilities and dosage based on masked genotype data: for example, if the true genotype is reference homozygote and the allelic dosage from imputation is 1.4, the discordance is . Left panel: imputation quality greater than 0.9; right panel: quality between 0.8 and 0.9. Clusters correspond to minor allele frequencies of 10%; individual bars represent quality stratified by masked genotype. Error bars represent 95% confidence intervals of mean discordance estimate.

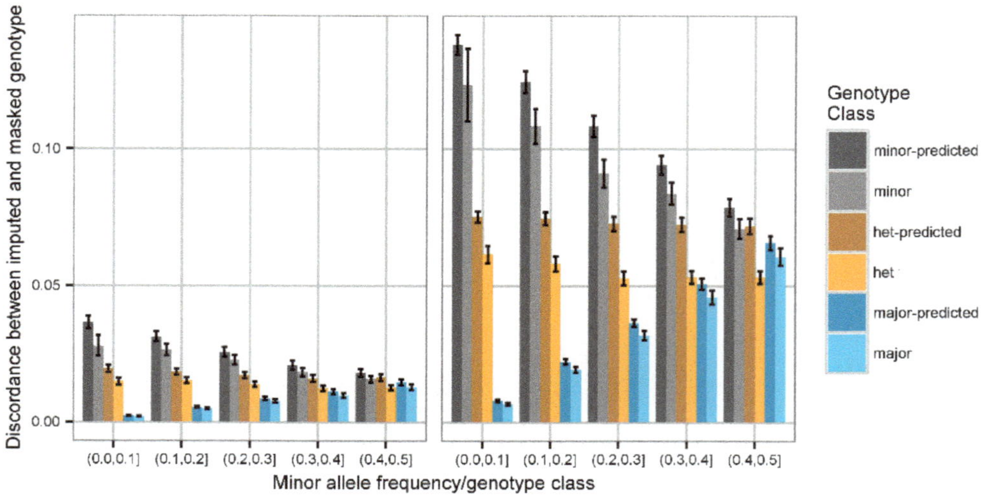

S1 Fig. Relationship between quality of estimated allelic dosage from minimac3 imputation and predictors of imputation quality.

Data are estimated from 10% of the original chip masked from imputation. Discordance of predicted allelic dosage (y-axis) is the fraction difference between dosage computed from imputation probabilities and dosage based on masked genotype data: for example, if the true genotype is reference homozygote and the allelic dosage from imputation is 1.4, the discordance is $\frac{|2-1.4|}{2} = 0.3$. Left panel: imputation quality greater than 0.9; right panel: quality between 0.8 and 0.9. Clusters correspond to minor allele frequencies of 10%; individual bars represent quality stratified by masked genotype. Error bars represent 95% confidence intervals of mean discordance estimate.

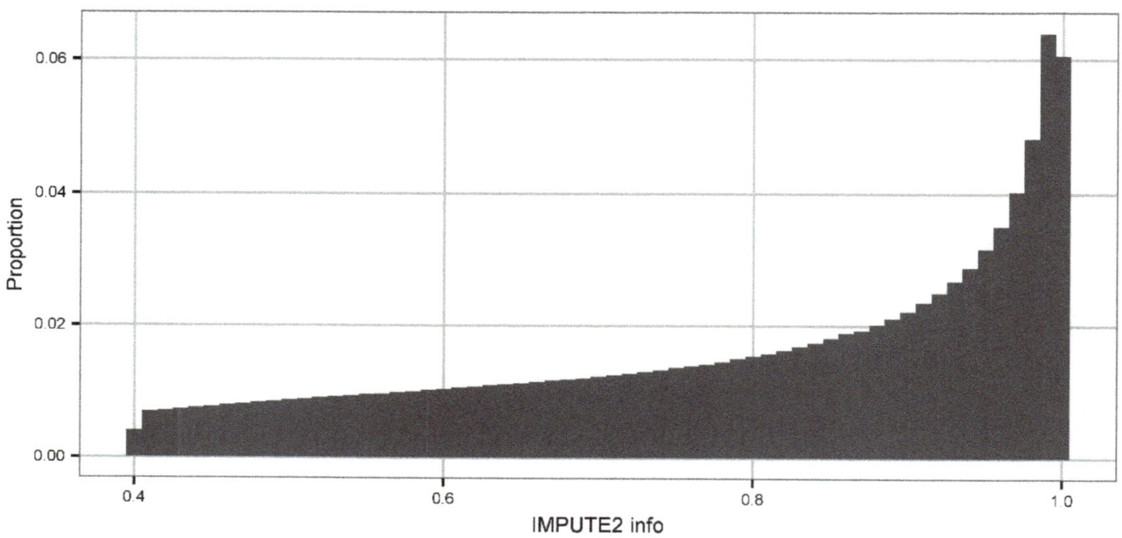

S2 Fig. Distribution of imputation quality from IMPUTE2 imputation.

x-axis: IMPUTE2 info (quality) metric; y-axis: proportion of full set of variants within this quality bin. Distribution is left-truncated at common quality threshold.

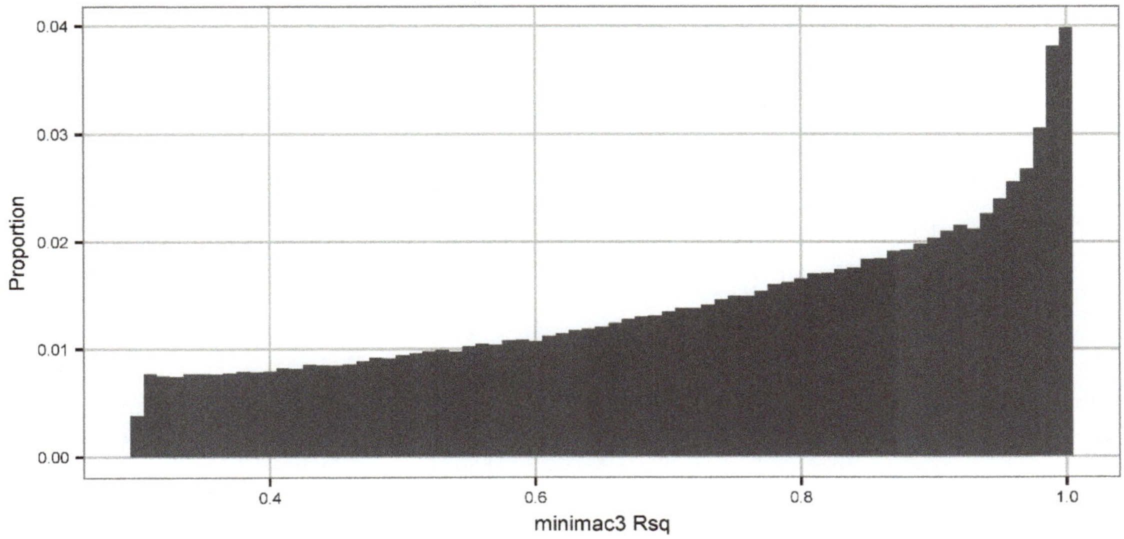

S3 Fig. Distribution of imputation quality from minimac3 imputation.

x-axis: minimac3 r^2 metric; y-axis: proportion of full set of variants within this quality bin. Distribution is left-truncated at common quality threshold. Final bin with quality greater than 1 indicates small percentage of variants where empirical variance exceeds that of the expected binomial distribution.

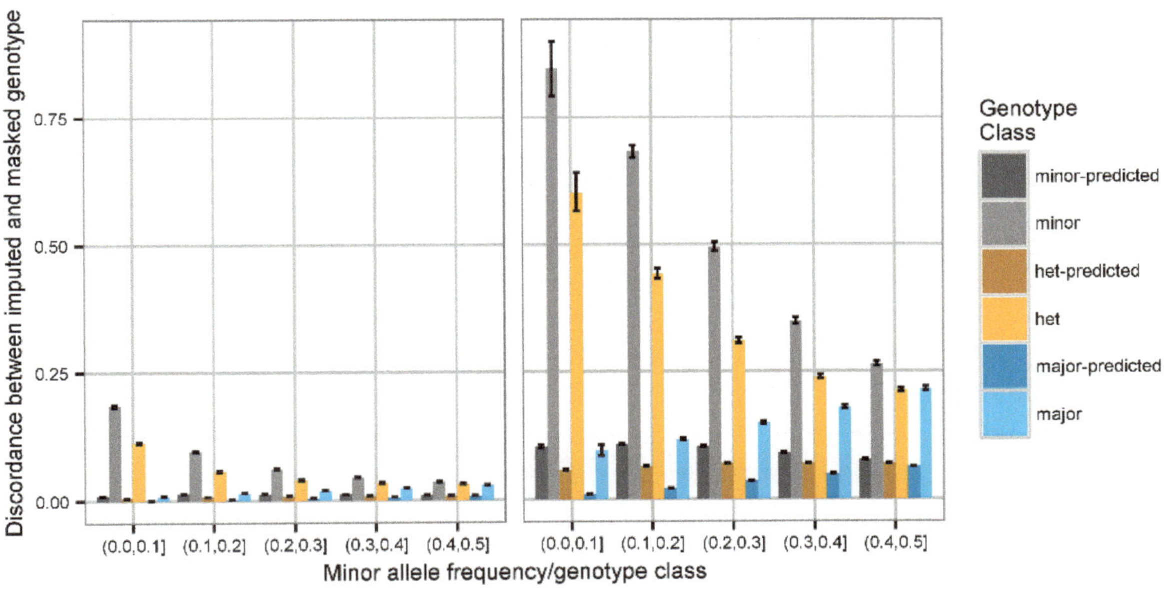

S4 Fig. Relationship between quality of best guess genotypes from IMPUTE2 imputation and predictors of imputation quality.

Data are estimated from 10% of the original chip masked from imputation. Discordance of predicted genotypes (y axis) is the fraction of best guess genotypes for a given bin that do not match the corresponding masked genotype. Left panel: imputation quality greater than 0.9; right panel: quality between 0.8 and 0.9. Clusters correspond to minor allele frequencies of 10%; individual bars represent quality stratified by masked genotype. Error bars represent 95% confidence intervals of mean discordance estimate.

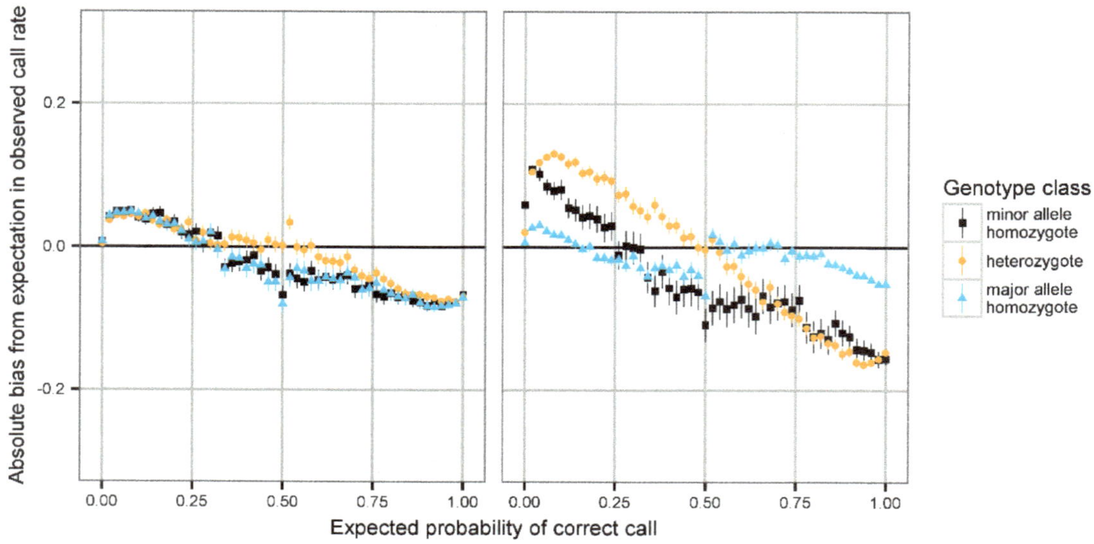

S5 Fig. Evaluation of the consistency of probability scores from IMPUTE2 imputation, stratified by allele frequency instead of imputation quality.

Data are estimated from 10% of the original chip (59808 SNPs) masked from imputation. x-axis: 0.02-width bins of imputation probabilities; y-axis: mean deviation between expected and observed accuracy. Data series correspond to results stratified by genotype class. Left panel: minor allele frequency greater than 0.4; right panel: minor allele frequency less than 0.1. Error bars represent 95% confidence intervals around mean consistency estimate.

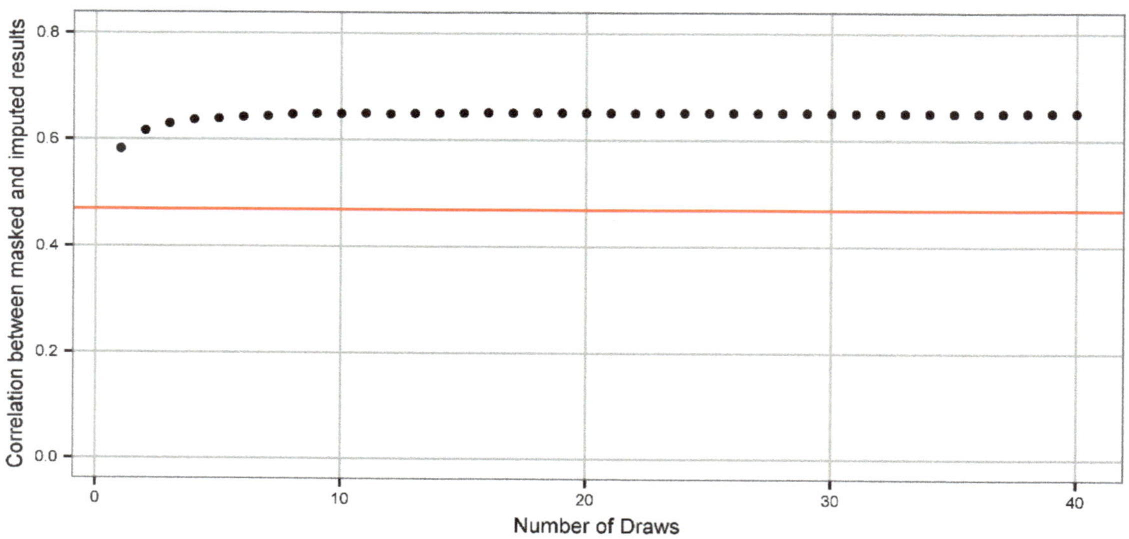

S6 Fig. Evaluation of the effect of Multiple Imputation draw count on estimated regression coefficients.

x-axis: number of MI draws; y-axis: observed Pearson correlation coefficient between regression coefficient estimates from masked data and estimates from MI on imputed estimates over masked sites. Horizontal line corresponds to correlation between masked data and "best guess" genotypes using imputation probabilities.

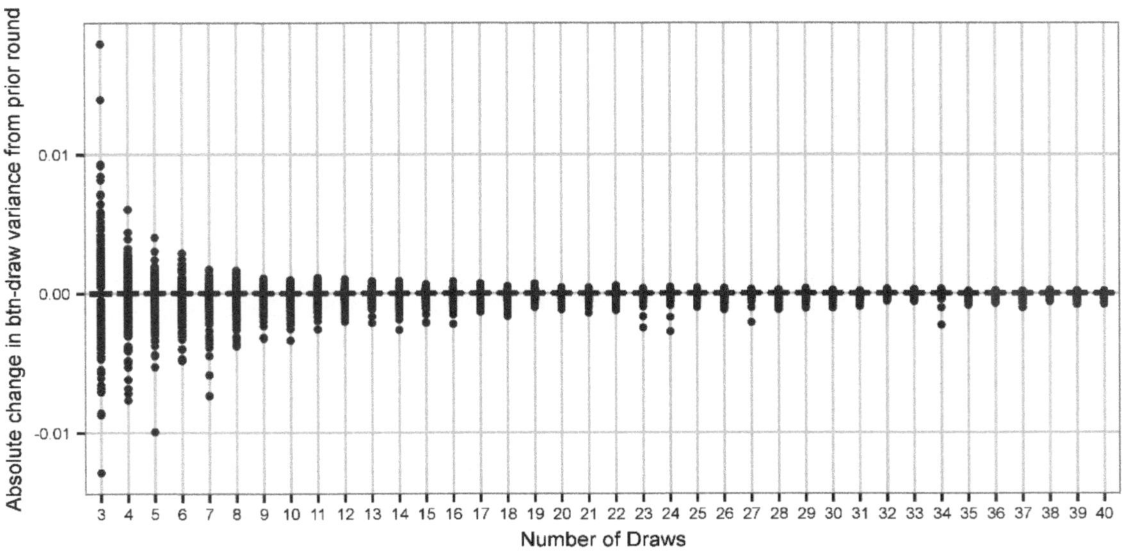

S7 Fig. Evaluation of the effect of Multiple Imputation draw count on estimated between-test variance component.

x-axis: number of MI draws; y-axis absolute change in between-draw variance component from one MI round to the next. Note this is a traditional boxplot but the boxes are tightly clustered around y = 0, leading to the boxes rendering as the small thick back lines for each x value at y = 0. The emphasis of these results is on the distribution of outliers, corresponding to low-quality imputed variants with trait-correlated uncertainty.

ACKNOWLEDGMENTS

We would like to thank the individuals from the contributing studies for the valuable contribution of their genetic and phenotypic data.

AUTHOR CONTRIBUTIONS

Conceived and designed the experiments: CP IP. Performed the experiments: CP. Analyzed the data: CP. Contributed reagents/materials/analysis tools: CP. Wrote the paper: CP IP.

REFERENCES

1. Browning SR. Missing data imputation and haplotype phase inference for genome-wide association studies. Hum Genet. 2008 Dec;124(5):439–450. doi: 10. 1007/s00439-008-0568-7. pmid:18850115
2. Marchini J, Howie B, Myers S, McVean G, Donnelly P. A new multipoint method for genome-wide association studies by imputation of genotypes. Nat Genet. 2007 Jul;39(7):906–913. doi: 10. 1038/ng2088. pmid:17572673
3. Price AL, Tandon A, Patterson N, Barnes KC, Rafaels N, Ruczinski I, et al. Sensitive detection of chromosomal segments of distinct ancestry in admixed populations. PLoS Genet. 2009 Jun;5(6):e1000519. doi: 10. 1371/journal. pgen. 1000519. pmid:19543370
4. Kang HM, Sul JH, Service SK, Zaitlen NA, Kong Sy, Freimer NB, et al. Variance component model to account for sample structure in genome-wide association studies. Nature Genetics. 2010 Apr;42(4):348–354. Available from:http://www. nature. com/doifinder/10. 1038/ng. 548. doi: 10. 1038/ng. 548. pmid:20208533
5. Prabhu S, Pe'er I. Ultrafast genome-wide scan for SNP-SNP interactions in common complex disease. Genome Res. 2012 Nov;22(11):2230–2240. doi: 10. 1101/gr. 137885. 112. pmid:22767386
6. Price AL, Patterson NJ, Plenge RM, Weinblatt ME, Shadick NA, Reich D. Principal components analysis corrects for stratification in genome-wide association studies. Nat Genet. 2006 Aug;38(8):904–909. Available from:http://www. nature. com/ng/journal/v38/n8/abs/ng1847. html. doi: 10. 1038/ng1847. pmid:16862161
7. Abecasis GR, Cherny SS, Cookson WO, Cardon LR. Merlin–rapid analysis of dense genetic maps using sparse gene flow trees. Nat Genet. 2002 Jan;30(1):97–101. doi: 10. 1038/ng786. pmid:11731797
8. Neale BM, Rivas MA, Voight BF, Altshuler D, Devlin B, Orho-Melander M, et al. Testing for an unusual distribution of rare variants. PLoS Genet. 2011 Mar;7(3):e1001322. doi: 10. 1371/journal. pgen. 1001322. pmid:21408211
9. Little RJA, Rubin DB. Statistical Analysis with Missing Data. 2nd ed. Hoboken, NJ: Wiley-Interscience; 2002.
10. Pei YF, Li J, Zhang L, Papasian CJ, Deng HW. Analyses and comparison of accuracy of different genotype imputation methods. PLoS ONE. 2008;3(10):e3551. doi: 10. 1371/journal. pone. 0003551. pmid:18958166
11. Browning BL, Browning SR. Genotype Imputation with Millions of Reference Samples. Am J Hum Genet. 2016 Jan;98(1):116–126. doi: 10. 1016/j. ajhg. 2015. 11. 020. pmid:26748515
12. Howie B, Fuchsberger C, Stephens M, Marchini J, Abecasis GR. Fast and accurate genotype imputation in genome-wide association studies through pre-phasing. Nat Genet. 2012 Aug;44(8):955–959. doi: 10. 1038/ng. 2354. pmid:22820512
13. Nothnagel M, Ellinghaus D, Schreiber S, Krawczak M, Franke A. A comprehensive evaluation of SNP genotype

imputation. Hum Genet. 2009 Mar;125(2):163–171. doi: 10. 1007/s00439-008-0606-5. pmid:19089453

14. Nho K, Shen L, Kim S, Swaminathan S, Risacher SL, Saykin AJ, et al. The effect of reference panels and software tools on genotype imputation. AMIA Annu Symp Proc. 2011;2011:1013–1018. pmid:22195161

15. Locke AE, Kahali B, Berndt SI, Justice AE, Pers TH, Day FR, et al. Genetic studies of body mass index yield new insights for obesity biology. Nature. 2015 Feb;518(7538):197–206. doi: 10. 1038/nature14177. pmid:25673413

16. Wood AR, Esko T, Yang J, Vedantam S, Pers TH, Gustafsson S, et al. Defining the role of common variation in the genomic and biological architecture of adult human height. Nat Genet. 2014 Nov;46(11):1173–1186. doi: 10. 1038/ng. 3097. pmid:25282103

17. Acar EF, Sun L. A generalized Kruskal-Wallis test incorporating group uncertainty with application to genetic association studies. Biometrics. 2013 Jun;69(2):427–435. doi: 10. 1111/biom. 12006. pmid:23441822

18. Li Y, Willer CJ, Ding J, Scheet P, Abecasis GR. MaCH: using sequence and genotype data to estimate haplotypes and unobserved genotypes. Genet Epidemiol. 2010 Dec;34(8):816–834. doi: 10. 1002/gepi. 20533. pmid:21058334

19. Howie BN, Donnelly P, Marchini J. A flexible and accurate genotype imputation method for the next generation of genome-wide association studies. PLoS Genet. 2009 Jun;5(6):e1000529. doi: 10. 1371/journal. pgen. 1000529. pmid:19543373

20. Fuchsberger C, Abecasis GR, Hinds DA. minimac2: faster genotype imputation. Bioinformatics. 2014 Oct;p. btu704. Available from:http://bioinformatics. oxfordjournals. org/content/early/2014/10/22/bioinformatics. btu704.

21. Willer CJ, Li Y, Abecasis GR. METAL: fast and efficient meta-analysis of genomewide association scans. Bioinformatics. 2010 Sep;26(17):2190–2191. doi: 10. 1093/bioinformatics/btq340. pmid:20616382

22. Harel O, Schafer JL. Multiple Imputation in Two Stages. Arlington, VA; 2003. Available from: http://fcsm. sites. usa. gov/files/2014/05/2003FCSM_Harel. pdf.

23. Graham JW, Olchowski AE, Gilreath TD. How many imputations are really needed? Some practical clarifications of multiple imputation theory. Prev Sci. 2007 Sep;8(3):206–213. doi: 10. 1007/s11121-007-0070-9. pmid:17549635

24. Lee D, Bigdeli TB, Riley BP, Fanous AH, Bacanu SA. DIST: direct imputation of summary statistics for unmeasured SNPs. Bioinformatics. 2013 Nov;29(22):2925–2927. doi: 10. 1093/bioinformatics/btt500. pmid:23990413

25. Pasaniuc B, Zaitlen N, Shi H, Bhatia G, Gusev A, Pickrell J, et al. Fast and accurate imputation of summary statistics enhances evidence of functional enrichment. Bioinformatics. 2014 Oct;30(20):2906–2914. doi: 10. 1093/bioinformatics/btu416. pmid:24990607

26. Lee D, Bigdeli TB, Williamson VS, Vladimirov VI, Riley BP, Fanous AH, et al. DISTMIX: direct imputation of summary statistics for unmeasured SNPs from mixed ethnicity cohorts. Bioinformatics. 2015 Oct;31(19):3099–3104. doi: 10. 1093/bioinformatics/btv348. pmid:26059716

27. Mailman MD, Feolo M, Jin Y, Kimura M, Tryka K, Bagoutdinov R, et al. The NCBI dbGaP database of genotypes and phenotypes. Nat Genet. 2007 Oct;39(10):1181–1186. doi: 10. 1038/ng1007-1181. pmid:17898773

28. Purcell S, Neale B, Todd-Brown K, Thomas L, Ferreira MAR, Bender D, et al. PLINK: a tool set for whole-genome association and population-based linkage analyses. Am J Hum Genet. 2007 Sep;81(3):559–575. doi: 10. 1086/519795. pmid:17701901

29. Delaneau O, Marchini J, Zagury JF. A linear complexity phasing method for thousands of genomes. Nature Methods. 2011 Dec;9(2):179–181. Available from:http://www. nature. com/doifinder/10. 1038/nmeth. 1785. doi: 10. 1038/nmeth. 1785. pmid:22138821

30. The 1000 Genomes Project Consortium. An integrated map of genetic variation from 1,092 human genomes. Nature. 2012 Nov;491(7422):56–65. Available from:http://www. nature. com/nature/journal/v491/n7422/full/nature11632. html. doi: 10. 1038/nature11632. pmid:23128226

CHAPTER 8 GENOME-WIDE SEARCH FOR MIRNA-TARGET INTERACTIONS IN ARABIDOPSIS THALIANA WITH AN INTEGRATED APPROACH

Jiandong Ding, Danqing Li, Uwe Ohler, Jihong Guan, Shuigeng Zhou

BACKGROUND

MicroRNAs (miRNAs) [1] are a class of 20-nt to 24-nt small non-coding RNA (sncRNA) that has emerged as a key regulator of gene activity. MiRNAs regulate virtually every aspect of biology, including developmental timing, differentiation, proliferation, antiviral defence and metabolism [2]. In plants, miRNAs are processed from larger precursor stem-loops (pre-miRNAs) in the nucleus, mainly by DICER-LIKE1 (DCL1) which excises a double-stranded RNA consisting of a miR and its near-complementary miR* sequence from the other arm of the stem-loop. The miRNA:miRNA* duplex is methylated and translocated to the cytoplasm where it can be loaded into an RNA-induced silencing complex (RISC) that includes a member of the ARGONAUTE (AGO) family as catalytic component. The RISC can then recognize mRNAs containing sequences complementary to the loaded miRNA [3]. In plants, cleavage of the target mRNA is the main mechanism for miRNA action, but there are also direct effects on protein accumulation [4, 5], as reported for many animal miRNAs [6, 7].

Unlike animals, plant miRNAs generally show a near-perfect complementary target mRNA which immensely facilitates computational predictions [8]. Taking advantage of this property, several methods were developed to search for antisense hits to known miRNAs on *Arabidopsis* mRNAs [9, 10]. While both animals and plants rely to a different extent on RNA complementarity to define their targets, some comparable features are employed in target prediction methods/tools for both animal and plant miRNAs. Notably, RNAhybrid [11] was first developed to identify miRNA-Target duplexes in *D. melanogaster, D. pseudoobscura*, and *A. gambiae*, and was more recently adapted to the specific requirements of plant miRNA target prediction, with outstanding results in *Arabidopsis thaliana* [12, 13].

Features reported for plant miRNA-target interactions in previous studies can be divided into three categories: (i) duplex pairing, with specific consideration of the seed region (2-8nt) in particular for animals, and the central region in plants (9-11nt), (ii) evolutionary conservation of MTI sites, and (iii) MTI site accessibility.

While experimental studies have already identified a certain amount of MTIs, this issue is far from resolved. On one hand, plant miRNA and miRNA-target related research increased yearly during the last decade (Figure 1). The list of known miRNAs is large and increasing rapidly [14, 15]. In the latest miRBase (Release 17.0), over 3,000 plant miRNAs are registered. On the other hand, only a few miRNA-target interactions are experimentally validated; thus, predicting and validating miRNA targets is one of the key topics in understanding miRNA biology. Although many target prediction methods/tools have been developed, several new discoveries are still worth considering.

First, the effect of different seed site matches has been evaluated by different means. In animals, this led to the definition of several canonical seed types that differ in abundance and downstream effect [7]. Recent studies suggested that the majority of functional target sites are formed by less specific seeds of only 6 nt indicating a crucial role of this type, and they also suggest that the majority of functional sites remain uncovered by common prediction methods [16]. Second, not all animal targets are defined by 5' seed matches,

Citation: Jiandong Ding, Danqing Li, Uwe Ohler, Jihong Guan and Shuigeng Zhou, Genome-wide search for miRNA-target interactions in Arabidopsis thaliana with an integrated approach, DOI: 10.1186/1471-2164-13-S3-S3.

but other types of complementarity, including a small number of near-perfect target sites inducing cleavage [17]. This feature was considered in a target prediction method for human/mouse miRNAs [18]. Third, increasing numbers of reports emphasize the importance of multiplicity of target sites in *Arabidopsis*. As example, some primary and secondary trans-acting siRNAs are generated from regions of *Arabidopsis*genes with two or more known miRNA/siRNA complementary sites [19, 20]. Fourth, miRNA-target interaction is determined by multiple factors. Considering the extent of influence of each of these factors in recognition mechanisms is still unclear to date, and current predictive approaches are often based on only some factors [21]. As result, our study clearly shows that current methods can give different predictions on identical miRNA/mRNA sets (see Results).

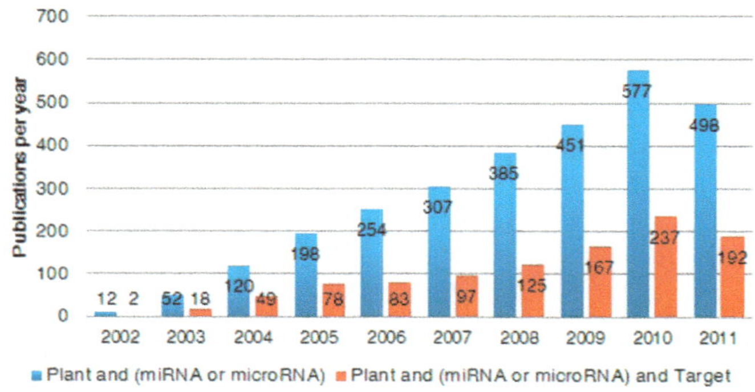

Figure 1. Growth of plant 'miRNA' and 'miRNA Target' in PubMed. In last decade, miRNA changed to be a hot research topic. It's impossible to establish the exact number of how many labs are studying this small molecule and how much funding is spent. However, the number of relevant papers can broadly reflect this trend. We then collect plant miRNA related articles indexed by PubMed (collected on Jun.13th, 2011). Statistical results show that these articles grow in an exponential way.

All the problems mentioned above exist in predicting miRNA-target interactions of both animal and plant miRNAs. One successful attempt to address these is by integrating diverse approaches and datasets in a comprehensive manner that may substantially improve animal MTIs prediction. To date, miRNAmap 2.0 [22], miRecords [23], miRGator 2.0 [24], miRGene 2.0 [25], miRror [26] provide miRNA targets by integrating extensively adopted target prediction methods. Moreover, Tarbase [27], miRDB [28], miR2Disease [29] and miRTarBase [30] are established to provide experimentally validated MTIs.

Here, we present the first integrated MTI identification toolkit--imiRTP (i ntegrated miR NA T arget P rediction) for *Arabidopsis thaliana*, the most studied plant model species. It integrates 4 powerful predictors based on different factors, and is evaluated on 142 experimentally validated MTIs and 25,688 MTIs predicted by CleaveLand [31] on several Degradome data sets. Besides integrating different prediction methods and data sources, imiRTP also offers 4 effective filters to select high quality MTIs and supports diverse outputs to facilitate further analysis.

METHODS

Over the last decades, studying the biogenesis and function of miRNA has been an important task. Here, we integrate several plant miRNA target prediction methods and collect data from various sources, aiming to effectively identify *Arabidopsis thaliana* MTIs on the genome-wide scale. Details of the imiRTP pipeline are shown in Figure 2.

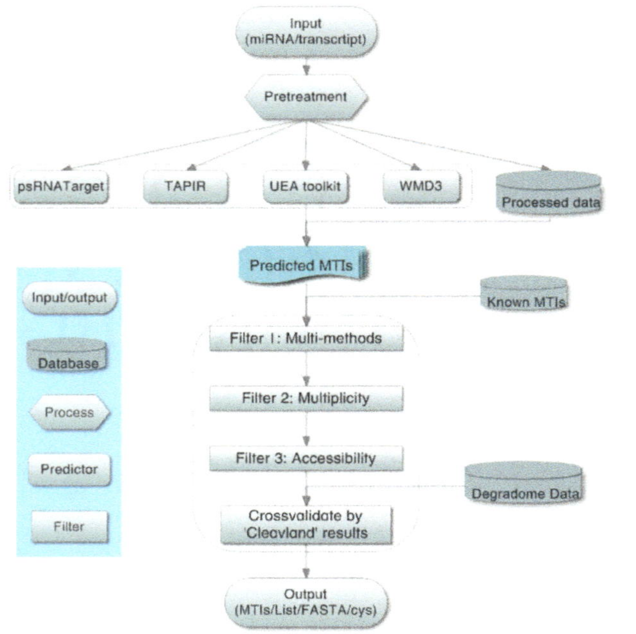

Figure 2. The pipeline of imiRTP. Here we present the first integrated miRNA Target Prediction toolkit (imiRTP) to search MTIs for *Arabidopsis*. In this toolkit, four online plant miRNA target prediction tools are considered. We then employ four local filters to select high quality candidates. Finally, it could output predicted results in several different formats. As for data, we collect 142 experimentally validated *Arabidopsis* MTIs and also 25,688 Degradome-seq support *Arabidopsis* MTIs.

Considering target prediction is extremely computation time consuming, imiRTP submits input miRNA and/or transcript sequences to corresponding online predictors and then collects results for local analysis to save time. Moreover, data will be processed before submission with the aim to further save time. First, all input miRNAs are searched against a pre-processed miRNA dataset, consisting of all *Arabidopsis* miRNAs in miRBase (Release 17). Matched miRNA will not be submitted to online predictors; instead, their MTIs will be searched from already computed prepared genome-wide results. Second, MIR genes contained in transcript sequences will be removed. Then, all online collected and locally searched MTIs are combined together. In post-processing, imiRTP provides four filters to narrow results, thus substantially improving the predictions.

Dataset

We downloaded all 255 *Arabidopsis thaliana* miRNAs arising from 231 pre-miRNAs in the miRNA database miRBase [32] (http://www.mirbase.org/). Transcript sequences (CDS, 5›UTR and 3›UTR) were downloaded from the central database TAIR [33] (http://www.arabidopsis.org/, Release 9).

A previous study [13] has collected 102 experimentally validated *Arabidopsis* MTIs from several publications [34, 35, 36], and these MTIs have been used as benchmark in comparison [13, 37]. As the most complete online experimentally validated MTI database, miRTarBase has accumulated nearly 4,000 MTIs by manually surveying over 1,100 pertinent publications after systematic text mining to filter research articles related to functional studies of miRNAs [30]. Sixty two experimentally validated *Arabidopsis thaliana* MTIs were downloaded from miRTarBase (http://mirtarbase.mbc.nctu.edu.tw/, Release 2.4). After removing duplicates, a total of 142 experimentally validated MTIs were collected. Recently, high-throughput CLIP-Seq (HITS-CLIP [38], PAR-CLIP [39]) and Degradome-seq [34, 36] methods have been applied to identify the sites of Argonaute interaction and miRNA cleavage, respectively. 25,688 degradome sequencing supported *Arabidopsis thaliana* MTIs were downloaded from starBase [40] (http://starbase.sysu.edu.cn/, Release 2.0). These MTIs are predicted by CleaveLand (version 2.0) [31] with a cutoff of 7.

Online Predictors

A number of algorithms and tools have been developed to predict complementarity between miRNAs and their targets (Table 1). But the types of methods applied, the input miRNA and transcript sequences used and the performance evaluation vary widely between tools. In this work, we prudentially chose four existing predictors to construct the core component of imiRTP's first stage. All of them rely on different combinations of seed pairing, central pairing, and hybridization energy of target site.

Table 1. Summary of target prediction tools for plant miRNA

Method	Link	AUTS[1]	Limit[2]	Spe[3]	Ref
miRU	N/A	N	1 miR	N	[57]
psRNATarget	http://plantgrn.noble.org/psRNATarget/?function=3	Y	20 M/200 M	EH	[45]
TAPIR	http://bioinformatics.psb.ugent.be/webtools/tapir/	Y	50 kb/40 M	H	[13]
UEA_sRNA	http://srna-tools.cmp.uea.ac.uk/plant/cgi-bin/srna-tools.cgi?rm=input_form&tool=target	N	50 miRs	S	[42]
WMD3	http://wmd3.weigelworld.org/cgi-bin/webapp.cgi?page=TargetSearch;project=stdwmd	N	1 miR	H	[41]
TargetAlign	http://www.leonxie.com/targetAlign.php#	Y	locale	ES	[37]
Targetfinder	http://jcclab.science.oregonstate.edu/node/view/56334	Y	locale	N	[58]

[1] AUTS - Accepts User-supplied Transcript Sequences.

[2] Input limitations. Limitations for miRNA and transcript input are on the left and right sides of the slash.

[3] Running speed at the time of testing. E-Extremely, H-High ($\leq$ 5 min), N-Normal (5-30 min), S-Slow ($\geq$ 30 min).

WMD3 [41] is based on principles of artificial miRNAs, which support the notion that extensive base pairing with targets is required for plant miRNA function. It predicts targets using previously determined parameters of target selection for natural miRNAs. The number of mismatches (cutoff 5) and hybridization energy ratio ($\geq$ 70%) are two critical parameters when searching targets. In this method, a GU wobble pair is counted as 1 mismatch.

UEA_sRNA is included in the UEA toolkit [42] which identifies plant sRNA (miRNA/siRNA) targets. The rules used for target prediction are based on factors suggested in previous studies [35, 43]. Both seed region and central region are considered. Mismatches in the central region (9-11nt) are not allowed. The hybridization energy ratio is computed as the MFE (minimum free energy) of miRNA:miRNA* instead of the traditional optimal energy that is calculated by the miRNA and its perfect reverse complement. Considering the similar rules used in UEA_sRNA and Targetfinder [44], the latter is not integrated in imiRTP.

TAPIR offers potential plant miRNA targets using a fast (FASTA) search engine and a precise (RNAhybrid) engine. A miRNA target score is modified from a previous study [35]. Mismatch, gap and wobble pairs inside and outside the core region (2-12nt) are counted differently. Again, the hybridization energy ratio is considered ($\geq$ 70%). Considering a previous assessment [13], we chose to integrate the fast FASTA algorithm. Another Smith-Waterman-like alignment, Target-align, has been shown to perform better than TAPIR [37]. However it is not practical for prediction of MTIs on genome-wide scale since too many parameters are considered.

psRNATarget [45] is designed for plant sRNA target prediction with an efficient distributed computing back-end pipeline that runs on a Linux cluster. This tool can rapidly search for potential MTIs and it is the first to provide multiplicity information and functional type (cleavage or translation) determined by the occurrence of a mismatch in central region (9-11nt). Unfortunately, the multiplicity is only reported but not considered in prediction.

In Table 1, we list the input limitations of existing online predictors. Here, the third mission of the pre-processing procedure is rearranging user-submitted files, in order to guarantee flexibility when working with imiRTP.

Local filters

The secondary stage of imiRTP includes several effective filters. The user can remove predicted MTIs with one filter or various ensembles. When comparing performance among predictors, there are usually two levels: mRNA level and target-site level. Here, we use the latter. Putative target sites that overlap at least 90% will be grouped into one common MTI.

Multi-method

MTI predicted by single method is usually not as credible as those identified by multiple methods. Keep this in mind, we introduce the multi-method filter to help user to select multiple predicted MTIs.

Multiplicity

Strong miRNA targets tend to have multiple target sites instead of one single site [46]. Considering the number of putative miRNA site per mRNA can therefore significantly enhance MTI prediction. In reported plant miRNA target prediction tools, the importance of the target site multiplicity was generally underestimated. Default cutoff of multiplicity is 2.

Accessibility

The frequently considered free energy of interaction of a miRNA and its target is generally not a very good predictor [21]. An effective MTI needs an open structure on the target site to begin the hybridization reaction, an issue which has been extensively explored in animals [47, 48, 49]. The RNAup program in Vienna package is used to calculate secondary structure in target site regions [50]. The RNAup takes into account the hybridization energy and the free energy needed to open the target site, which turns out to be the real accessibility. The default threshold of accessibility is set to the highest value that observed for all 125 validated MTIs recovered by imiRTP.

Degradome-seq Support

Degradome-seq (also known as PARE and GMUCT) directly sequences degradome tags derived from the 5' ends of uncapped mRNAs and delivers an empirical overview of cleaved sRNA targets without computational predictions or overexpression. In this work, 25,688 Degradome-seq results were collected from [40], which were then used to filter computationally predicted MTIs at the mRNA level. The default cutoff 4.5 is suggested by [31].

Input and Output

The imiRTP toolkit accepts user-submitted miRNA and/or transcript sequences for analysis, i.e. (i) searching user-submitted miRNAs against included TAIR transcripts; and (ii) searching user-submitted miRNAs and user-submitted transcripts. After all files are successfully submitted, imiRTP will search targets based on selected predictors and combine all results into one group.

Once the submitted analysis is completed, imiRTP outputs details of predicted MTIs to one file and outputs statistics of every unique miRNA-target (mRNA level) predicted by which predictor to another file. A sort tool is implemented to easily browse through the results. In addition, imiRTP allows users to extract several essential columns from results related to single miRNAs or mRNAs, which greatly facilitate further analysis, i.e. motif discovery, SNP detection and regulatory network analysis.

Implementation

imiRTP was implemented in C++. Online interaction programs were implemented in C# and java. Both are tested on Windows platform. Computation of the accessibility profiles in the post-processing steps is performed with the help of RNAup program. When calculating the accessibility, imiRTP extracts a maximum of 100nt flanking sequences on both upstream and downstream of a target site instead of using the whole sequence, thus greatly reduces the calculating time.

RESULTS

To test the toolkit, we evaluated imiRTP on a reference set with 142 experimentally validated mRNA level MTIs [13, 40] (Additional file 1). All comparisons are executed at the target-site level, except Degradome-seq support. The numbers of validated MTIs listed in Table 2 are therefore always larger than 142. To facilitate the comparison, we defined and considered several criteria:

Table 2. Performance of four predictors*

Method	PM†	VM†	CM†	AP#(%)	TP#(%)
psRNATarget	541	366	100	32.35	70.42
TAPIR_FASTA	622	411	116	33.92	**81.69**
UEA_sRNA	362	269	110	**25.69**	77.46
WMD3	615	411	98	33.17	69.01
Average	535	364	106	31.28	76.41

† PM - predicted MTI; VM - experimentally validated MTI; CM - collapsed MTI.

AP - additional prediction; TP - true positive.

* Results achieved with default parameters.

- Additional prediction Percentage of predicted target-site level MTIs that do not belong to the reference set. Smaller is better.
- True positive Percentage of MTIs that each predictor or predictor ensembles can recover from the reference set. Since all validated MTIs are on mRNA level, predicted target-site level MTIs are first collapsed to mRNA level. Larger is better.
- Filter power Geometric mean of filter ratio and additional prediction. Filter ratio is defined as the

fraction of predicted MTIs that are filtered by a given filter compared to the number of total predictions. Smaller is better.

Performance of Online Predictors

First, we tested the four selected predictors with the reference set and compiled the results in Table 2. At default settings TAPIR_FASTA identifies the most validated MTIs (116/142), while WMD3 identifies the least (90/142). This demonstrates the specific importance of the core region (2-12nt), which covers both the seed region and central region. UEA_sRNA gets the lowest additional prediction with only 362 predicted MTIs, which is considerably smaller than other three methods. For one reason, UEA_sRNA uses stringent parameters. The other reason might be the special hybridize energy ratio computed by this method.

Moreover, on the reference set, different methods lead to different results at the target-site level and mRNA level. The percentage of common MTIs that predicted by any two predictors lies between 42.14% and 83.25% (Additional file 2, Table S1). We first selected three methods (psRNATarget, TAPIR_FASTA and WMD3) and show their results in Figure 3A, since these three methods give the most similar predictions. However, the fraction of highest credible MTIs, those that are predicted by all three methods, is still lower than 50% both at the target-site level (Figure 3B) and mRNA level (Figure 3C) on the genome-wide scale. Indeed, the results change very little at different levels, except WMD3, for which 2,240 duplicate MTIs are removed at the mRNA level. A certain number of targets are identified by only one method, as a result of the various factors considered by different methods (Figure 3B-D). A similar fraction of common MTIs are identified by TAPIR/psRNATarget and TAPIR/UEA_sRNA on the genome-wide scale, while psRNATarget and UEA_sRNA share fewer common predictions. One likely reason might be the opposite decision made on mismatches in the central region (9-11nt). Another reason might be that psRNATarget does not pay specific attention to the seed region as UEA_sRNA does. WMD3 leads to the highest number of predictions, as it does not consider any specific regions (like seed or central region). Yet, it identifies only 98 validated MTIs. All these observations show that it is necessary to develop a more general and accurate method to search qualified targets of plant miRNA through combining various sources.

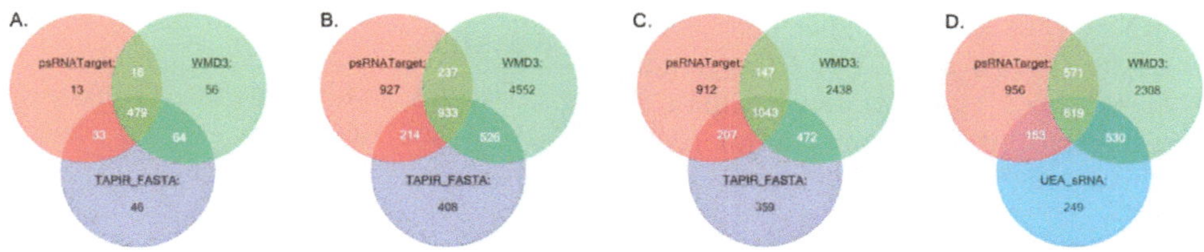

Figure 3. The degree of overlap between the four MTI prediction tools at target-site level and mRNA level. In order to directly compare different online predictors, we run them on a conducted reference set and the whole *Arabidopsis Thaliana* cDNA sequences. Results turn to be that different predictors could give different results. (A.) Target site level predictions on reference set. (B.) Target site level predictions on whole cDNA sequences. (C.) mRNA level predictions on whole cDNA sequences. (D.) mRNA level predictions on whole cDNA sequences.

Performance of Local Filters

Direct combination of different predictors can lead to fewer additional predictions, but also can greatly decrease the number of true positives (Additional file 2, Table S2). imiRTP therefore accepts user-defined cutoff to meet different needs; e.g. when 3 predictors are chosen, the user can use a loose cutoff, like 2, to select more predicted results. Results show that with more predictors and looser cutoff, additional predictions increase slowly, while true positives increase and the filter power decreases rapidly (Figure 4). Specifically, with a combination of 4 predictors and the multi-method cutoff 2, imiRTP identifies only one experimentally validated MTI less than TAIR_FASTA but 9 more high quality predicted MTIs.

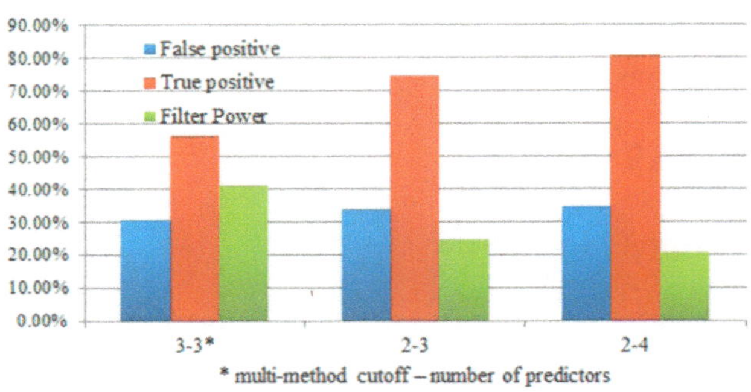

Figure 4. Performance of imiRTP by integrating multiple predictors.

It's clear that directly combine results of single online predictors, we can't expect imiRTP achieves higher true positive than the best single method. At the other side, we will get the lowest additional prediction, which contains fewest true negatives. Here, with the multi-method cutoff, imiRTP can achieve the best balance between true positive and additional prediction.

We next compared the effect of other filters. To achieve reliable results, we constructed a benchmark set by selecting several best combinations of predictors and/or multi-method cutoff from the different groups mentioned above (highlighted in Table 2, and in Additional file 2, Tables S1 & S2).

Based on this benchmark, we tested the other three filters: multiplicity, accessibility and Degradome-seq support (Figure 5). We first find that multiplicity (cutoff 2) and Degradome-seq support (cutoff 4.5) get similar performances. However, more validated MTIs are removed by multiplicity, which indicates that in *Arabidopsis*, maybe one fifth of target genes contain only one unique functional miRNA site (Additional file 2, Tables S3 & S4).

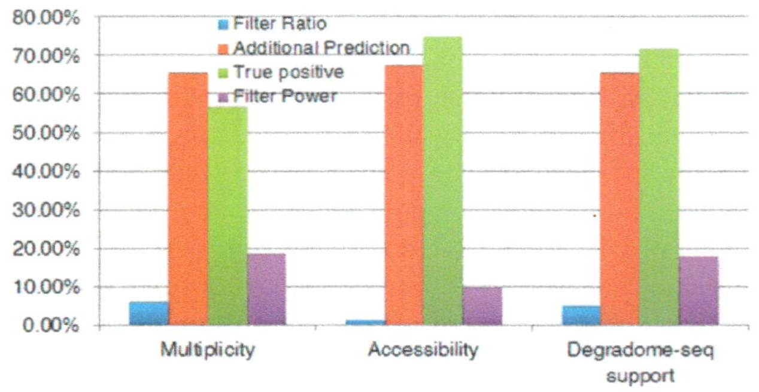

Figure 5. Performances of three locale filters. Based on the benchmark, we also compare other three locale filters. Results shown here are achieved by best cutoffs (multiplicity: 2, accessibility: -15.87 kal/mol, Degradome-seq support: 4.5).

As for accessibility, the default cutoff for RNAup program is -15.87 kcal/mol, which is the maximum value of 119 out of all 125 validated MTIs that could be recovered by imiRTP. Thermodynamic related features are considered by all four online predictors but with different calculation methods. For example, the RNAup program has been employed by psRNATarget, while RNAcofold was set as default in WMD3, and the flanking regions around the target site are different. Here, we employ RNAup to compute the accessibility uniformly. Because of the specific cutoff (-15.87 kcal/mol), only 6 validated MTIs, whose accessibilities couldn't be calculated by RNAup, are removed. Correspondingly, it results in the highest true positives. On the other hand, the filter ratio is extremely low (Additional file 2, Table S5), which then gives rise to contain a little bit more additional predictions. When validating the effectiveness of the three local filters, results also show that the combinations of multiple methods always achieve similar or better predictions than any single method.

Performance on Whole Transcripts

Plant miRNA binding sites occur typically in the coding region of target genes [51], whereas in animals, they are most often found within the 3'UTR [52]. However, new findings indicate that both animal and plant miRNAs can target 5'UTR, 3'UTR and coding regions [53, 54]. We therefore run the programs specifically on *Arabidopsis thaliana* CDS, 5'UTR and 3'UTR sequences downloaded from TAIR (version 9).

Because only psRNATarget and TAPIR accept user-submitted transcript files, only these two predictors are considered here. Consistent with previous studies, 74.63% (897/1202) miRNA target sites identified by imiRTP falls within the coding region. 15.46% miRNAs (32/207) that come from 5 families are predicted to target mRNAs in the 3›UTR. Only 4 miRNAs belonging to 2 families (MIR399 and MIR827_3) can bind to the 5›UTR region. Results are shown in Table 3. The statistics of MTIs that predicted by different methods and filters are compiled in Additional file 2, Table S6-S12. Considering that secondary structure plays less of an importance in coding region than in the UTRs, accessibility here is less effective as in animal target prediction (Figure 5).

Table 3. Genome-wide results*

	5' UTR	Coding region	3' UTR
Predicted MTI[1]	52	897	253
Validated MTI[2]	5	254	81
Collapsed MTI[3]	2	80	10

[1] Common MTIs predicted by psRNATarget and TAPIR.

[2] Number of validated MTIs on target site level.

[3] Number of validated MTIs on mRNA level.

* All MIR genes are removed.

DISCUSSION

In order to verify the effectiveness of the imiRTP toolkit, we collected 142 experimentally validated MTIs from previous studies within a reference set. We find that four online predictors integrated within imiRTP give highly different target-site level results (Additional file 2, Table S1), especially on the genome-wide scale (Additional file 2, Table S9).

Degradome-seq is a novel technology that is independent of computational methods. However, if we directly compare the results of imiRTP and CleaveLand at the target-site level, the fraction of common MTIs decreases dramatically from ~50% to ~2% (data not shown). Moreover, even the combination of all four predictors could only identify 88.03% (125/142) validated MTIs.

Besides psRNATarget, all existing target prediction methods and Degradome-seq for plant miRNA are looking for features specific to target cleavage. As a consequence, a portion of additional predictions might in fact be true positive, although many of them are indeed false positives.

All these results indicate the importance of integrating multiple methods and the introduction of translational repression related factors. Additionally, our results have indicated that proper filters can efficiently identify potential MTIs from large candidate sets.

Future work mainly includes the following parts. (i) Integrate additional existing and novel target prediction methods, (ii) support more plant species, (iii) improve and consider other efficient filters, like computing the accessibility with Raccess [55] and RNAplex [56] and selection of predicted MTIs by evolutionary conservation, (iv) maintain imiRTP with future experimentally and Degradome-seq validated MTIs.

CONCLUSIONS

In this work, we propose the first integrated miRNA target prediction toolkit for *Arabidopsis thaliana*. The imiRTP toolkit brings new features compared to existing methods. The ability to use different predictors and filters to search qualified MTIs, the rich output results, and the use pre-computed results should make imiRTP a useful and efficient resource for the plant research community.

DECLARATIONS

Acknowledgements

This article has been published as part of *BMC Genomics* Volume 13 Supplement 3, 2012: Selected articles from the IEEE International Conference on Bioinformatics and Biomedicine 2011: Genomics. The full contents of the supplement are available online at http://www.biomedcentral.com/bmcgenomics/supplements/13/S3.

We are grateful to Molly Megraw (Duke University) for providing comments and code. JD, DL and SG were supported by Major State Basic Research and Development Program of China (973 Program) under grant no.2010CB126604. JG was also supported by the Shuguang Program of Shanghai Education Foundation.

REFERENCES

1. Lee RC, Feinbaum RL, Ambros V: The C. elegans heterochronic gene lin-4 encodes small RNAs with antisense complementarity to lin-14. Cell. 1993, 75 (5): 843-854. 10.1016/0092-8674(93)90529-Y.
2. Schickel R, Boyerinas B, Park SM, Peter ME: MicroRNAs: key players in the immune system, differentiation, tumorigenesis and cell death. Oncogene. 2008, 27 (45): 5959-5974. 10.1038/onc.2008.274.
3. Voinnet O: Origin, biogenesis, and activity of plant microRNAs. Cell. 2009, 136 (4): 669-687. 10.1016/j.cell.2009.01.046.
4. Lanet E, Delannoy E, Sormani R, Floris M, Brodersen P, Crete P, Voinnet O, Robaglia C: Biochemical evidence for translational repression by Arabidopsis microRNAs. Plant Cell. 2009, 21 (6): 1762-1768. 10.1105/tpc.108.063412.
5. Brodersen P, Voinnet O: Revisiting the principles of microRNA target recognition and mode of action. Nat Rev Mol Cell Biol. 2009, 10 (2): 141-148.
6. Selbach M, Schwanhausser B, Thierfelder N, Fang Z, Khanin R, Rajewsky N: Widespread changes in protein synthesis induced by microRNAs. Nature. 2008, 455 (7209): 58-63. 10.1038/nature07228.
7. Bartel DP: MicroRNAs: target recognition and regulatory functions. Cell. 2009, 136: 215-233. 10.1016/j.cell.2009.01.002.
8. Mendes ND, Freitas AT, Sagot M-F: Current tools for the identification of miRNA genes and their targets. Nucleic Acids Res. 2009, 37 (8): 2419-2433. 10.1093/nar/gkp145.
9. Rhoades MW, Reinhart BJ, Lim LP, Burge CB, Bartel B, Bartel DP: Prediction of plant microRNA targets. Cell. 2002, 110 (4): 513-520. 10.1016/S0092-8674(02)00863-2.
10. Wang X-J, Reyes Je L, Chua N-H, Gaasterland T: Prediction and identification of Arabidopsis thaliana microRNAs and their mRNA targets. Genome Biol. 2004, 5 (9): R65-10.1186/gb-2004-5-9-r65.
11. Rehmsmeier M, Steffen P, Hochsmann M, Giegerich R: Fast and effective prediction of microRNA/target duplexes. RNA. 2004, 10 (10): 1507-1517. 10.1261/rna.5248604.
12. Alves L, Niemeier S, Hauenschild A, Rehmsmeier M, Merkle T: Comprehensive prediction of novel microRNA targets in Arabidopsis thaliana. Nucleic Acids Res. 2009, 37 (12): 4010-4021. 10.1093/nar/gkp272.
13. Bonnet E, He Y, Billiau K, Van de Peer Y: TAPIR, a web server for the prediction of plant microRNA targets, including target mimics. Bioinformatics. 2010, 26 (12): 1566-1568. 10.1093/bioinformatics/btq233.
14. Ding J, Zhou S, Guan J: miRFam: an effective automatic miRNA classification method based on n-grams and a multiclass SVM. BMC Bioinformatics. 2011, 12 (1): 216-10.1186/1471-2105-12-216.
15. Ding J, Zhou S, Guan J: MiRenSVM: towards better prediction of microRNA precursors using an ensemble SVM classifier with multi-loop features. BMC Bioinformatics. 2010, 11 (Suppl 11): S11-10.1186/1471-2105-11-S11-S11.
16. Ellwanger DC, Buttner FA, Mewes HW, Stumpflen V: The sufficient minimal set of miRNA seed types. Bioinformatics. 2011, 27 (10): 1346-1350. 10.1093/bioinformatics/btr149.
17. Shin C, Nam JW, Farh KK, Chiang HR, Shkumatava A, Bartel DP: Expanding the microRNA targeting code: functional sites with centered pairing. Mol Cell. 2010, 38 (6): 789-802. 10.1016/j.molcel.2010.06.005.
18. Elefant N, Berger A, Shein H, Hofree M, Margalit H, Altuvia Y: RepTar: a database of predicted cellular targets of host and viral miRNAs. Nucleic Acids Res. 2011, 39: D188-D194. 10.1093/nar/gkq1233.
19. Axtell MJ, Jan C, Rajagopalan R, Bartel DP: A two-hit trigger for siRNA biogenesis in plants. Cell. 2006, 127 (3): 565-577. 10.1016/j.cell.2006.09.032.
20. Montgomery TA, Howell MD, Cuperus JT, Li D, Hansen JE, Alexander AL, Chapman EJ, Fahlgren N, Allen E, Carrington JC: Specificity of ARGONAUTE7-miR390 interaction and dual functionality in TAS3 trans-acting siRNA formation. Cell. 2008, 133 (1): 128-141. 10.1016/j.cell.2008.02.033.
21. Dai X, Zhuang Z, Zhao PX: Computational analysis of miRNA targets in plants: current status and challenges. Brief Bioinform. 2011, 12 (2): 115-121. 10.1093/bib/bbq065.
22. Hsu SD, Chu CH, Tsou AP, Chen SJ, Chen HC, Hsu PW, Wong YH, Chen YH, Chen GH, Huang HD: miRNAMap 2.0: genomic maps of microRNAs in metazoan genomes. Nucleic Acids Res. 2008, D165-D169. 36 Database
23. Xiao F, Zuo Z, Cai G, Kang S, Gao X, Li T: miRecords: an integrated resource for microRNA-target interactions. Nucleic Acids Res. 2009, 37: D105-D110. 10.1093/nar/gkn851.
24. Cho S, Jun Y, Lee S, Choi HS, Jung S, Jang Y, Park C, Kim S, Kim W: miRGator v2.0: an integrated system for functional investigation of microRNAs. Nucleic Acids Res. 2011, 39: D158-D162. 10.1093/nar/gkq1094.
25. Alexiou P, Vergoulis T, Gleditzsch M, Prekas G, Dalamagas T, Megraw M, Grosse I, Sellis T, Hatzigeorgiou AG: miRGen 2.0: a database of microRNA genomic information and regulation. Nucleic Acids Res. 2010, 38: D137-D141. 10.1093/nar/gkp888.
26. Friedman Y, Naamati G, Linial M: MiRror: A combinatorial analysis web tool for ensembles of microRNAs and their targets. Bioinformatics. 2010, 26 (15): 1920-1921. 10.1093/bioinformatics/btq298.

27. Papadopoulos GL, Reczko M, Simossis VA, Sethupathy P, Hatzigeorgiou AG: The database of experimentally supported targets: a functional update of TarBase. Nucleic Acids Res. 2009, 37: D155-D158. 10.1093/nar/gkn809.

28. Wang X, El Naqa IM: Prediction of both conserved and nonconserved microRNA targets in animals. Bioinformatics. 2008, 24 (3): 325-332. 10.1093/bioinformatics/btm595.

29. Jiang Q, Wang Y, Hao Y, Juan L, Teng M, Zhang X, Li M, Wang G, Liu Y: miR2Disease: a manually curated database for microRNA deregulation in human disease. Nucleic Acids Res. 2009, 37: D98-D104. 10.1093/nar/gkn714.

30. Hsu SD, Lin FM, Wu WY, Liang C, Huang WC, Chan WL, Tsai WT, Chen GZ, Lee CJ, Chiu CM, et al: miRTarBase: a database curates experimentally validated microRNA-target interactions. Nucleic Acids Res. 2011, 39: D163-D169. 10.1093/nar/gkq1107.

31. Addo-Quaye C, Miller W, Axtell MJ: CleaveLand: a pipeline for using degradome data to find cleaved small RNA targets. Bioinformatics. 2009, 25 (1): 130-131. 10.1093/bioinformatics/btn604.

32. Kozomara A, Griffiths-Jones S: miRBase: integrating microRNA annotation and deep-sequencing data. Nucleic Acids Res. 2011, 39: D152-D157. 10.1093/nar/gkq1027.

33. Poole RL: The TAIR database. Methods Mol Biol. 2007, 406: 179-212.

34. Addo-Quaye C, Eshoo TW, Bartel DP, Axtell MJ: Endogenous siRNA and miRNA targets identified by sequencing of the Arabidopsis degradome. Curr Biol. 2008, 18 (10): 758-762. 10.1016/j.cub.2008.04.042.

35. Allen E, Xie Z, Gustafson AM, Carrington JC: microRNA-directed phasing during trans-acting siRNA biogenesis in plants. Cell. 2005, 121 (2): 207-221. 10.1016/j.cell.2005.04.004.

36. German MA, Pillay M, Jeong DH, Hetawal A, Luo S, Janardhanan P, Kannan V, Rymarquis LA, Nobuta K, German R, et al: Global identification of microRNA-target RNA pairs by parallel analysis of RNA ends. Nat Biotechnol. 2008, 26 (8): 941-946. 10.1038/nbt1417.

37. Xie F, Zhang B: Target-align: a tool for plant microRNA target identification. Bioinformatics. 2010, 26 (23): 3002-3003. 10.1093/bioinformatics/btq568.

38. Kishore S, Jaskiewicz L, Burger L, Hausser J, Khorshid M, Zavolan M: A quantitative analysis of CLIP methods for identifying binding sites of RNA-binding proteins. Nat Methods. 2011, 8 (7): 559-564. 10.1038/nmeth.1608.

39. Hafner M, Landthaler M, Burger L, Khorshid M, Hausser J, Berninger P, Rothballer A, Ascano M, Jungkamp AC, Munschauer M, et al: Transcriptome-wide identification of RNA-binding protein and microRNA target sites by PAR-CLIP. Cell. 2010, 141 (1): 129-141. 10.1016/j.cell.2010.03.009.

40. Yang JH, Li JH, Shao P, Zhou H, Chen YQ, Qu LH: starBase: a database for exploring microRNA-mRNA interaction maps from Argonaute CLIP-Seq and Degradome-Seq data. Nucleic Acids Res. 2011, 39: D202-D209. 10.1093/nar/gkq1056.

41. Schwab R, Ossowski S, Riester M, Warthmann N, Weigel D: Highly specific gene silencing by artificial microRNAs in Arabidopsis. Plant Cell. 2006, 18 (5): 1121-1133. 10.1105/tpc.105.039834.

42. Moxon S, Schwach F, Dalmay T, Maclean D, Studholme DJ, Moulton V: A toolkit for analysing large-scale plant small RNA datasets. Bioinformatics. 2008, 24 (19): 2252-2253. 10.1093/bioinformatics/btn428.

43. Schwab R, Palatnik JF, Riester M, Schommer C, Schmid M, Weigel D: Specific effects of microRNAs on the plant transcriptome. Dev Cell. 2005, 8 (4): 517-527. 10.1016/j.devcel.2005.01.018.

44. Fahlgren N, Carrington JC: miRNA target prediction in plants. Methods Mol Biol. 2010, 592: 51-57. 10.1007/978-1-60327-005-2_4.

45. Dai X, Zhao PX: psRNATarget: a plant small RNA target analysis server. Nucleic Acids Res. 2011, 39: W155-W159. 10.1093/nar/gkr319.

46. John B, Enright AJ, Aravin A, Tuschl T, Sander C, Marks DS: Human microRNA targets. PLoS Biol. 2004, 2 (11): e363-10.1371/journal.pbio.0020363.

47. Kertesz M, Iovino N, Unnerstall U, Gaul U, Segal E: The role of site accessibility in microRNA target recognition. Nat Genet. 2007, 39 (10): 1278-1284. 10.1038/ng2135.

48. Long D, Lee R, Williams P, Chan CY, Ambros V, Ding Y: Potent effect of target structure on microRNA function. Nat Struct Mol Biol. 2007, 14 (4): 287-294. 10.1038/nsmb1226.

49. Lekprasert P, Mayhew M, Ohler U: Assessing the utility of thermodynamic features for microRNA target prediction under relaxed seed and no conservation requirements. PloS One. 2011, 6 (6): e20622-10.1371/journal.pone.0020622.

50. Hofacker IL: Vienna RNA secondary structure server. Nucleic Acids Res. 2003, 31 (13): 3429-3431. 10.1093/nar/gkg599.

51. Axtell MJ, Bowman JL: Evolution of plant microRNAs and their targets. Trends Plant Sci. 2008, 13 (7): 343-349. 10.1016/j.tplants.2008.03.009.

52. Stark A, Brennecke J, Bushati N, Russell RB, Cohen SM: Animal microRNAs confer robustness to gene expression and have a significant impact on 3'UTR evolution. Cell. 2005, 123 (6): 1133-1146. 10.1016/j.cell.2005.11.023.

53. Meng Y, Chen D, Jin Y, Mao C, Wu P, Chen M: RNA editing of nuclear transcripts in Arabidopsis thaliana. BMC Genomics. 2010, 11 (Suppl 4): S12-10.1186/1471-2164-11-S4-S12.

54. Lytle JR, Yario TA, Steitz JA: Target mRNAs are repressed as efficiently by microRNA-binding sites in the 5' UTR as in the 3' UTR. Proc Natl Acad Sci USA. 2007, 104 (23): 9667-9672. 10.1073/pnas.0703820104.

55. Kiryu H, Terai G, Imamura O, Yoneyama H, Suzuki K, Asai K: A detailed investigation of accessibilities around target sites of siRNAs and miRNAs. Bioinformatics. 2011, 27 (13): 1788-1797. 10.1093/bioinformatics/

btr276.

56. Tafer H, Amman F, Eggenhofer F, Stadler PF, Hofacker IL: Fast accessibility-based prediction of RNA-RNA interactions. Bioinformatics. 2011, 27 (14): 1934-1940. 10.1093/bioinformatics/btr281.

57. Zhang Y: miRU: an automated plant miRNA target prediction server. Nucleic Acids Res. 2005, 33: W701-W704. 10.1093/nar/gki383.

58. Fahlgren N, Howell MD, Kasschau KD, Chapman EJ, Sullivan CM, Cumbie JS, Givan SA, Law TF, Grant SR, Dangl JL, et al: High-throughput sequencing of Arabidopsis microRNAs: evidence for frequent birth and death of miRNA genes. PloS One. 2007, 2 (2): e219-10.1371/journal.pone.0000219.

CHAPTER 9

IDENTIFICATION OF DIFFERENTIALLY EXPRESSED GENES FROM MICROARRAY DATA

Jianjun Hu and Jia Xu

INTRODUCTION

Statistical methods for identifying differentially expressed genes are now routinely used by biologists. There are two main categories of algorithms. The first category includes single gene testing approaches such as fold change [1], rank product [2], t-test and its variants [3]. These methods are characterized by a single statistics score used to rank genes from significantly differentially expressed genes to no- change ones. The second category includes gene set testing approaches such as gene set enrichment analysis [4, 5]. These methods are featured by exploiting externally determined gene sets to rank a group of genes. The shortcoming of these methods is that in many cases such gene set information is not available, especially for under-studied species. Despite increasing usage of gene set analysis methods [4], single-gene based identification algorithms for differentially expressed genes (DEGs) still dominate the practice of biological differential gene expression analysis [6, 7, 8, 9] from microarray data. This is partially due to their simplicity as well as little requirement on gene annotation. Thus improving single-gene DEG identification algorithms still has great implication for DEG microarray analysis practice in biology. Currently, a major purpose of DEG algorithm design is to reduce their false positive and false negative errors since experimental biologists usually only afford to test only a very limited number of predicted DEGs. Biologically interesting DEGs are those genes that have significant phenotypic changes along with their change of gene expression levels. Most current single-gene DEG identification algorithms, however, take it as a statistical significance test problem without referring to the real characteristics of differentially expressed genes [10]. Unfortunately, limited number of samples of microarray datasets in most biological studies makes such statistical test methods ineffective [11, 12]. This issue has been addressed recently using multiple strategies. A popular strategy is to gather information across similar genes to improve DEG identification. This includes the Bayes t-test approach [13], the local pooled error algorithm [14], the famous SAM algorithm [15], and et cetera. Another strategy is to use external information to improve variance estimation. Wille et. al. [16] proposed an external variance estimation algorithm called EVE, which exploits the relationships between variances of gene expression and gene function. Kim and Park [17] proposed a normalization method to make multiple microarray datasets with different chips comparable, which then facilitates the estimation of gene variance with those external datasets. Their method showed big improvement over the basic regularized t-test algorithm on experiments with 1x1, 2x2 and 3x3 samples. Hack- stadt and Hess [18] investigated three filtering methods for pruning genes before statistical tests: MAS detection call, variance, and average signal. They showed that gene filtering by MAS detection call and mean signal lead to increased performance of DEG identification. They also suggested that filtering 50% of probe sets is reasonable due to majority genes are expected to be equally expressed.

Here we propose a pattern recognition strategy for improving DEG identification algorithms. This pruning algorithm shares some similarity to all-gene-analysis DEG identification algorithms as discussed in [19]. The first step of our algorithm is to apply pattern recognition algorithms to prune non-DEGs from the whole gene list based on the

Citation: Jianjun Hu and Jia Xu, Identification of differentially expressed genes from microarray data, DOI: 10.1186/1471-2164-11-S2-S3.

characteristics of experimentally verified differentially expressed genes. In this paper, a density based pruning (DB Pruning) is developed based on two features of DEGs: the average difference of gene expression level between two classes and the average gene expression level. It is motivated by the observation that a majority of true DEGs experimentally verified by RT-PCR tend to have high expression levels in 38 real-world datasets [20]. The tendency for high expression genes to be over-represented in the list of DEGs is also suggested in [18]. And we found that the true DEGs tend to be sparsely located in the boundary regions in the average-difference—expression level space (peripheral areas of the gene distribution map) as shown in Fig. 1. In the second step, common statistics-based DEG identification algorithms such as t-test are applied to rank genes. The non-DEG pruning will be able to enrich true DEGs in the remaining gene lists. This is especially desirable for small-size microarray datasets. It can also be used to greatly reduce the computational cost of DEG algorithms that search gene combinations [21], in which all gene-pairs need to be ranked. Based on systematic evaluation on 17 real-world microarray datasets with a total of 184 true DEGs applied to four existing DEG algorithms, we showed that DB pruning can significantly improve the performance of these traditional algorithms for both large and small datasets in terms of false positive rates. For example, DB Pruning can prune 83% (19156) genes out of 22283 while keeping 89% (164) true DEGs out of 184 for 17 datasets we tested. The enrichment of true DEGs in the pruned gene list is almost six times of the original gene list. DB pruning is also shown to increase the AUC score of rank product by up to 21% and helps it to find 33% more true DEGs when the cutoff top K=550. For fold change and t-test, it can find 11% and 15.8% more true DEGs. When the sample size is 4x4, DB pruning improves t-test by 26.8% in terms of the number of identified true DEGs. When the sample size is 2x2, t-test is improved by 50%.

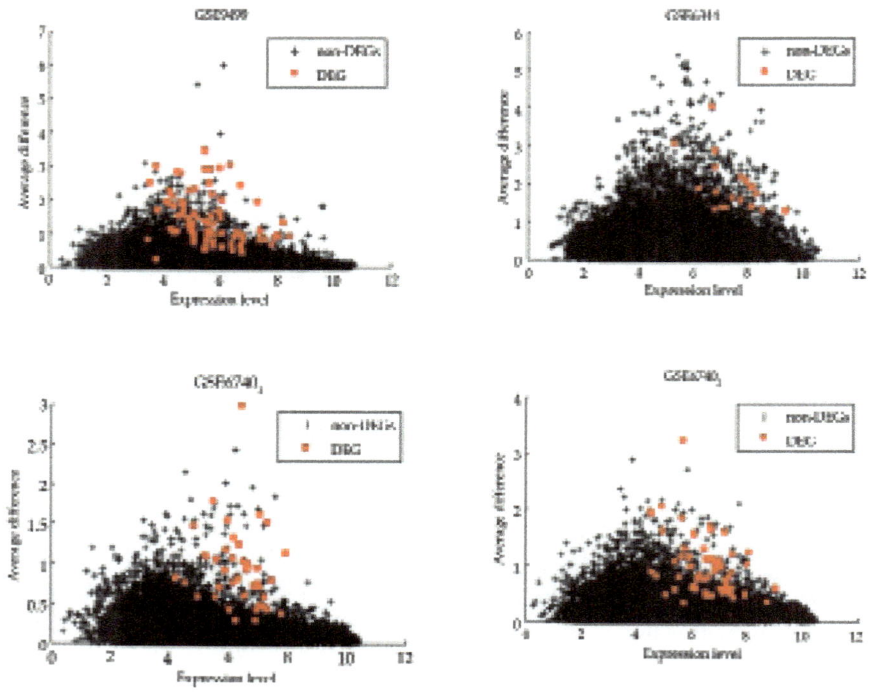

Figure 1. istribution of true DEGs in the boundary regions of the AG-AD feature space for four datasets. Most DEGs are located in the boundary regions in the figure. Screening out boundary genes has the potential to improve the power of gene ranking methods such as t-test for DEG identification.

METHODS

Differentially expressed genes are those genes with significant difference in expression levels among two or more classes/ conditions. Such expression changes should not be caused by random variation in gene expression. DEGs resulting from a specific perturbation to corresponding pathways tend to share some functional or physiological characteristics. It is thus justified that DEG identification can be improved by considering the characteristics of true DEGs. One characteristic is that true DEGs experimentally identified to date tend to have high average expression values across all conditions [20]. The resulting WAD algorithm is very competitive compared to other DEG algorithms based on evaluation over 38 GEO microarray datasets. In WAD, the product of the gene expression ratio and relative gene expression level are used to rank genes. The limitation of this ranking scheme is that it biases to genes with balanced expression ratios and expression levels.

The main idea of the proposed DB pruning is that differentially expressed genes between two conditions are usually located in the boundary region in the 2-D feature space of average gene expression (AG) versus average difference of gene expression (AD). Fig.1. shows the distribution of true DEGs in the 2D space for four datasets: GSE9499, GSE6342, GSE6740_1, and GSE6740_2 from GEO database [22]. Based on the fact that boundary region is characterized with scarcity of genes, a density based pruning algorithm is proposed here for pre-filtering non-DEG genes located outside the boundary region so that the false positive rate of current DEG algorithms can be improved.

Density-based Pruning Algorithm for DEG Identification

The main idea of density based pruning is to remove non-DEGs that usually appear within the dense part of the AG-AD space. Assume M is a microarray matrix with N genes (rows) and P profiles (columns). There are total P1 profiles in P corresponding to condition A and P2=P-P1 profiles corresponding to condition B. The average expression level (AG) of a gene X_i is defined as $(X_i^A + X_i^B)/2$, where X_i^A and X_i^B are the average expression level (log-scaled) of gene X_i under condition A and B. The average difference of gene expression of a gene X_i is defined as $|X_i^A - X_i^B|$ Since the expression values used in calculating $|X_i^A - X_i^B|$ are log-transformed, the average differences of expression calculated here are actually equivalent to expression ratios as in fold change method.

The density based pruning algorithm works as follows: each gene X_i is mapped into the (AG, AD) feature space. Pairwise Euclidian difference between two genes X_i and X_j is calculated, where $i \neq j$. If the distance is smaller than a user-defined radius threshold R_0, these two genes will be declared as neighbors. Then the number of neighbors (n_i) will be calculated for each gene. If $n_i \geq N_0$ then gene X_i will be pruned from the gene list, where N_0 is a user-specified density parameter. The final output gene list is composed of genes that are mostly outliers located in the boundary region of the AG-AD feature space.

For different datasets, an important step of our algorithm is to determine appropriate parameters R_0 and N_0 such that all or most DEGs are kept in the final list and that a maximum number of non-DEGs are pruned. Through our experiments, we found that $N_n = 4$ is an appropriate parameter for most of 17 datasets used in our experiments. The value of threshold radius R_0 has a large effect on the number of pruned genes. The minimum value of R_0 is 0 and maximum value is the max AD value. A binary search procedure is used to identify R_0 value that can generate the desired number (K) of candidate DEGs.

DEG Identification Algorithms

We tested four popular DEG identification algorithms on the 17 GEO datasets with or without DB pruning.

- Fold Change (FC) is one of early DEG identification algorithms that are still widely used by biologists. It was recently recommended to be used with a non-stringent P cutoff to generate more reproducible DEG lists [11, 23]. FC ranks genes based on the ratio of average gene expression under two conditions. Usually a 2-fold change is regarded as significant in many biological studies. A major criticism of FC is that it doesn't consider the case that genes with low expression level in both conditions but with small variances can be ranked high.
- Rank Product (RP) [2, 24] ranks genes based on product of rank ratios for multiple A-B conditions. The results and simplicity of RP is similar to FC but overcomes its most significant limitations. It also provides a statistically rigorous estimation of significance. It was reported to have good performance for small or noisy datasets.
- T-statistics (tTest) is one of the earliest and popular methods used in DEG identification. The major advantage is that it considers the variation of genes in its ranking. The limitation is that the estimation of gene expression variances is not reliable for small datasets, which can lead to poor performance.
- Weighted Average Difference (WAD) [20] is a DEG algorithm based on the observation that experimentally verified true DEGs tend to have high expression level across the conditions. Genes are ranked by the product of fold change times normalized expression level. It was shown to have significantly better and robust performance than most other standard algorithms including FC, RP and tTest.

For each of these methods, we compare their DEG prediction performance with or without DB pruning. Comprehensive evaluation is conducted on 17 real-world microarray datasets from GEO database with experimentally verified DEGs.

RESULTS

Data set preparation

Most DEG identification algorithms are tested using unverified "statistically" significant genes plus a few (if any) experimental verifications [2, 3, 16, 25, 26]. These unverified DEGs may be quite different from biologically meaningful DEGs and have bias toward statistical algorithms. In this paper, we used real-world microarray datasets with experimentally verified DEGs as collected by Kadota et. al. [20]. They collected 38 microarray datasets with experimentally determined true DEGS by real-time polymerase chain reaction (RT-PCR). Thirty six of the datasets are downloaded from GEO database [22]. Without losing generality, we experimented with 17 disease or dose response datasets of Homo sapiens out of the 36 GEO datasets (Table 1). The 17 datasets are reported just for convenience so that we can use a single set of DB pruning parameters. Other datasets have also been tested with different DB pruning parameters and similar results are obtained. All 17 datasets are normalized and transformed into log scale. Table 1 shows the statistics of the datasets with the sample sizes of normal and disease conditions and also the number of true DEGs. Out of the 17 datasets, only 7 have more than 10 samples for both conditions. Four datasets have less than 5 samples per condition. These datasets show that real-world GEO datasets, especially historical ones, tend to have small sample size.

Table 1. 17 Datasets with 284 DEGs in total. Each dataset has 22833 genes.

Dataset	Conditions		True DEG
A	B		
GSE1462	4	4	4
GSE1615_1	4	5	8
GSE1650	18	12	8
GSE2666_2	5	5	6
GSE3524	16	4	4
GSE3860	9	9	8

GSE4917	3	3	5
GSE5667_1	5	6	3
GSE6236	14	14	7
GSE6344	10	10	19
GSE6740_1	10	10	40
GSE6740_2	10	10	62
GSE7146	6	6	6
GSE7765	3	3	13
GSE8441	11	11	9
GSE9499	15	7	77
GSE9574	15	14	5

The 17 Datasets used here cover a variety of biological or medical studies: GSE1462 (mitochondrial DNA mutations), GSE1615_1 (Valproic acid treatment), GSE1650 (chronic obstructive pulmonary disease), GSE2666_2(bone marrow Rho level effect), GSE3524 (tumor of epithelial tissue), GSE3860 (Hutchinson-Gilford progeria syndrome), GSE4917 (breast cancer), GSE5667_1 (atopic dermatitis), GSE6236 (Adult vs. fetal reticulocyte transcriptome comparison), GSE6344 (renal cell carcinoma disease), GSE6740_1 (HIV-infection), GSE6740_2 (HIV-infection, disease state), GSE7146 (hyperinsulinaemic, does response), GSE7765 (dose response, DMSO or 100 nM Dioxin), GSE8441 (dietary intake response), GSE9574 (breast cancer), and GSE9499 (hypomorphic germline mutations). The diversity of these datasets ensures that the observed performance of the proposed pruning algorithm is not due to some specific characteristics of the data.

Bias of DEG Identification Algorithms

DEG identification algorithms such as t-test and fold change all have different bias in their ranking schemes. Three factors have been commonly used in their gene ranking criteria: $r(y) = (d, e, v)$ where d is the difference of expression levels between two conditions; v is the overall gene expression level of the gene; and v is the variance of the gene's gene expression. T-statistics based algorithms may make false positive prediction for genes with low $d$because of small v. Fold change algorithm instead suffers from the fact that a gene with large variances tend to have larger fold changes. Both methods may make mistakes by neglecting the overall gene expression levels, which has been explicitly addressed by the WAD algorithm which rank genes by $d \times e$. Indeed, it is shown that when the expression level was considered, the WAD algorithm achieves significantly better prediction performance than all previous methods based on extensive tests on 38 datasets with known true DEGs. This shows that expression levels of true DEGs are usually high. It is thus interesting to visualize the bias of different DEG algorithms in the (d, e) feature space. For simplicity, the variance$v$ feature is neglected as it is not correlated to true DEGs as strongly as (d, e) features.

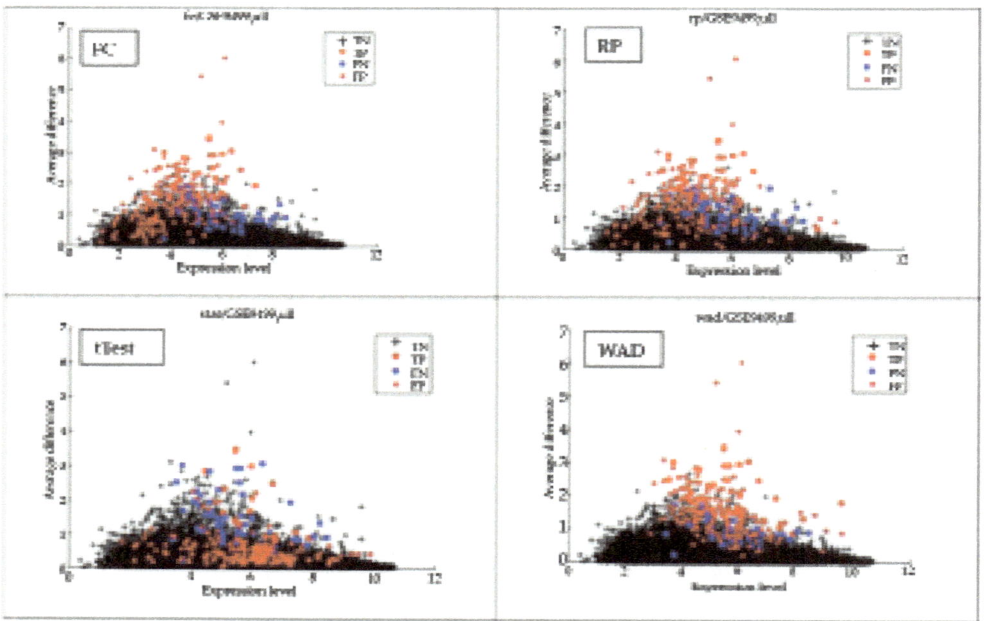

Figure 2. Visualization of bias of popular DEG identification algorithms. FC has many false positive predictions for genes with low average expressions or small expression differences. RP's false positives are sparsely located in low expression and small average difference region. tTest's false positives are dominated by genes with low average difference. WAD has less false positives than other algorithms.

In Fig. 1, it is shown that most true DEGs are outliers located in the sparse boundary region in the (d, e) space. A smaller portion of true DEGs are mixed with other non-DEGs in the dense regions and cannot be differentiated by the algorithms such as WAD and FC. To illustrate the bias of popular DEG identification algorithms, Fig. 2 shows true positive (TP), true negative (TN), false positive (FP), and false negative (FN) DEGs for dataset GSE9499 which has 77 true DEGs. Fig.2. (a) shows that fold change (FC) misses most true DEGs (FN genes), which are located in the region below the threshold average difference and with high expression levels.

This is because FC uses a fixed ratio as cutoff value. It also made many false positive predictions mostly in the region with low expression levels (see FP genes). Rank product (Fig.2b) misses similar true DEGs as fold change algorithm does but the false positive genes have different distributions. Fig. 2 (c) shows the predicted DEGs of t-test. This method misses many true DEGs that have high average difference between two conditions. Most of its false positives are located across the expression level with low average difference, reflecting the fact that it can be misled by genes with small variances. Fig.2 (d) shows the distribution of predicted DEGs of WAD algorithm. WAD has a better performance in terms of capturing true DEGs located in the boundary region. The main false positives are mixed together with the true DEGs, which are difficult to distinguish without extra information.

Improving DEG Identification Algorithms using Density Based Pruning Effect of density based pruning of non-DEGs

One way to test the performance of DB pruning is to calculate the enrichment score of true DEGs after pruning. It is defined as the ratio of true DEGs and the number of all genes. We applied DB pruning algorithm to 17 microarray datasets each having 22283 genes. For simplicity, we use the same set of parameters ($N_0 = 4$ and $R_0 = 0.0017$) to prune all the datasets. The idea is that by pruning those non-DEGs, true DEGs are more enriched in the remaining gene list and should be easier to be identified by current DEG algorithms. The reduced search range of candidate DEGs can also greatly reduce computational cost for detecting combinatorial gene sets. Table 2 shows the effect of applying DB pruning. It shows that this procedure can prune more than ≥86% (19156) genes out of 22283 while keeping ≥89% (164) out of 184 true DEGs. The enrichment of true DEGs in the pruned gene sets is 6 times of original gene list. Note that a binary search procedure is available to determine the DB pruning parameters for obtaining a user-specified number of candidate DEGs.

Table 2. Comparison of No. of missing true DEGs after DB pruning. ($N_0 = 4$, $R_0 = 0.0017$)

Total Gene: 22283	After DP-pruning	True DEG	DP missed
GSE1462	2054	4	0
GSE1615_1	2449	8	3
GSE1650	1317	8	2
GSE2666_2	1618	6	2
GSE3524	814	4	0
GSE3860	2073	8	0
GSE4917	785	5	1
GSE5667_1	1316	3	0
GSE6236	2231	7	0
GSE6344	3127	19	0
GSE6740_1	1183	40	1
GSE6740_2	1801	62	5
GSE7146	1274	6	1
GSE7765	1607	13	1
GSE8441	978	9	1
GSE9499	1805	77	3
GSE9574	1448	5	0

Improvement of ranks of true DEGs in the rank list by DB Pruning

Here we check how DB pruning can improve existing DEG identification algorithms. We compare the ranks of true DEGs in the original gene list and in the pruned gene list ranked by different algorithms including t-test, fold change, rank product and Wad. Table 3 shows that after DB pruning, ranks of most true DEGs by t-test and fold change statistics are improved, usually with significant improvements. For example, ranks of true DEG were improved from 1404 to 808, 3800 to 1713, 1321 to 768 and etc by the t-test after DB pruning. We also observe considerate improvements of DEG ranks for fold change and rank product algorithms via DB pruning. The improved enrichment of true DEGs toward top of gene rank lists implies that it can help current DEG algorithms to achieve better performance as shown in next subsections. DB pruning has moderate effect on Wad algorithm since Wad also used the feature of true DEGs, namely, the tendency of true DEG to have high expression levels and high expression difference.

Table 3. Ranks of true DEGs in original gene list and pruned gene list. Genes are sorted by four DEG identification algorithms on the GSE1577 dataset. Increase of ranks of true DEGs means that DB pruning have correctly filtered out many non-DEGs.

t-test/ tTest	1404/808	7/6	1321/768	3800/1713	4741/1975	3633/1659	4145/1828	606/388	210/155
FC/FC'	167/153	154/142	39/33	18/13	1/1	22/17	6/5	1601/1249	80/72
Rp/Rp'	111/85	91/70	18/12	9/8	1/1	16/15	6/6	4520/980	97/68
Wad/Wad'	31/31	25/25	32/25	7/7	3/3	15/15	6/6	515/515	10/10

Improving Standard DEG Algorithms using DB Pruning

To evaluate the improvement of prediction performance of DEG identification algorithms with DB pruning, we used the receiver operating characteristic (ROC), or simply ROC curve. It is a graphical plot of the fraction of true positives (TPR = true positive rate) vs. the fraction of false positives (FPR = false positive rate) as the K (the number of genes predicted to be DEGs) varies. We use the area under curve (AUC) value of the ROC curve as the criterion for comparison, which has been used in previous work [20]. To make the comparison relevant to real-world practice, we only plot and compare the AUC value with K varies from 1 to 1000 rather than to the total number of genes (22832) as done previously. The reason is that biologists rarely have the resources to check all 22832 genes and usually only care about top K predicted DEGs for experimental verification.

We calculate AUC values with K up to 1000 for four DEG algorithms with or without DB pruning. The experiments are conducted on all 17 datasets with a total of 284 true DEGs. DB priming is run with the following parameters: neighborhood radius $R_0 = 0.03$, no. of neighbors, $N_0 = 4$. Table 4 shows that DB pruning significantly increased the AUC values for all four popular DEG algorithms especially for rank product algorithm with 21% increase of AUC score. The smallest improvement is for WAD algorithm, which is reasonable considering that WAD uses the same information as DB pruning, though in different way. To obtain more intuitive understanding of how DB pruning improves current DEG algorithms, we showed in Table 5 the total numbers of true DEGs out of top K predictions identified by different algorithms from the 17 datasets with or without DB pruning. First, the results showed that rank product and fold change have worse performance than tTest and WAD algorithms in the number of identified true DEGs. For example, tTest and WAD can detect 132 and 156 true DEGs from the 17 datasets when K=150 predictions are allowed for each dataset. Instead, RP and FC can only detect 74 and 97 true DEGs respectively. When the no. of predictions K increases, all algorithms retrieve more true DEGs with the highest coverage by WAD algorithm which retrieves 240 out of 284 true DEGs when 550 genes are allowed to predict for each dataset. A major observation of Table 4 is that all 4 algorithms can benefit from DB pruning with the maximum improvement for tTest and the minimum improvement for WAD. When DB pruning is used, the 38 true DEG discrepancy between tTest and WAD is reduced to 6 when K=550. In other words, DB pruning can significantly improve the performance of t-statistics based DEG identification algorithms up to level of the most competitive DEG algorithm-WAD. In the case of RP, DB pruning helps RP to find 35 (nearly 33%) more true DEGs for K=550. For FC and tTest, 11% and 15.8% more true DEGs are identified with the help of DB pruning. The DB pruning shows only moderate to zero improvement for WAD algorithm because they use the same information, the gene expression levels and average difference of gene expressions.

Table 4. Increase of AUC values for DEG algorithms after DB pruning: Rp, Wad, Fc, and tTest.

	Partial AUC (up to K=1000)	Percentage of Improvement
Rp/Rp'	0.0162/0.0196	21%
Fc/Fc'	0.0245/0.0263	7.3%
tTest/tTest'	0.0284/0.0310	9.2%
Wad/Wad'	0.032/0.033	3.1%

Table 5. Increase of No. of identified true DEGs out of top K predictions with or without DB pruning. Rp', Wad', tTest', FC' are algorithms with DB pruning. The total number of true DEGs of the 17 datasets is 284.

	K=150	K=250	K=350	K=450	K=550
Rp/Rp'	74/78	81/91	92/104	98/122	106/141
Fc/Fc'	97/98	120/137	146/159	164/184	178/198
tTest/tTest'	132/150	163/181	179/206	191/218	202/234
Wad/Wad'	156/156	195/198	221/221	227/227	240/240

To further investigate the improvement of DB pruning over classic DEG algorithms, Fig. 3. shows the ROC curves of the algorithms with and without pruning with K=1 to 1000. It is shown that WAD algorithm has the best performance and there exists dominance relationship of WAD>t-test>FC>RP. It also shows that after DB pruning, the performance of t-test was significantly improved up to that of WAD algorithm. Both RP and FC were also greatly improved. Indeed, Fig.3 clearly demonstrates that DB pruning is able to significantly improve the AUC values with improvements across all K values ranging from 1 to 1000. Compared to the improvements of ROC curves as shown by the variance estimation algorithms [22], our improvement is much more significant.

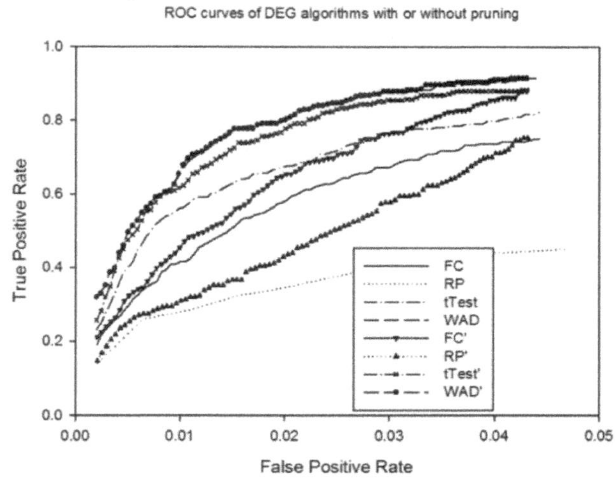

Figure 3. Comparison of ROC curves of DEG algorithms with/out DB pruning. It shows that WAD and t-Test have higher AUC values than FC and RP. Using DB pruning, tTest's AUC value can be improved to be close to that of WAD. Actually, DB pruning significantly improves all DEG algorithms.

DB Pruning's Performance on Microarray Datasets with a Small Number of Samples

A major issue of current DEG algorithms is that they have difficulty to deal with small-size microarray datasets. Unfortunately, many biological studies only generate limited profiling samples due to cost or labor constraints. Here we show DB pruning can help improve the performances of popular DEG algorithms for such small datasets. Four algorithms were applied to 17 datasets with a total of 284 true DEG. These full datasets are sub-sampled to generate small datasets with 2, 3, and 4 samples for each condition. Each algorithm was also run with different K, the number of predicted DEGs by DEG algorithms. Table 6 shows how the number of samples of the data set affects the number of true DEGs predicted by current algorithms with or without DB pruning.

Firstly, the table shows that with the increase of K, more true DEGs will be predicted. For each specific K, decreasing the number of samples reduces the number of true DEG identified. For example, when the number of samples of each condition decreases from 4 to 2, the number of predicted true DEGs will drop from 119 to 92 for WAD, from 60 to 45 for RP, from 62 to 43 for FC, and from 67 to 16 for tTest, which has the largest reduction of performance. DB pruning is shown to be able to significantly improve the prediction performance, especially for tTest, RP and FC. With 4x4 samples, DB pruning helps tTest to identify 18 more true DEGs, a 26.8% improvement. When the sample size is reduced to 2x2, the improvement is 16, or a 50% improvement. Improvement upon RP and FC is less significant, but still achieves 20% improvement when K=550 for FC with 2x2 samples and 14% for RP with K=450 and 3x3 samples. All these prove that the DB pruning is a useful procedure for DEG identification.

Table 6. The no. of predicted true DEGs using partial samples from condition A and B with or without using DB Pruning. Rp', Wad', tTest', FC' are algorithms with DB pruning. The total number of true DEGs of the 17 datasets is 284.

		K=150	K=250	K=350	K=450	K=550
2x2 samples	Rp/Rp'	45/46	61/61	68/71	78/79	86/92
	Fc/Fc'	43/44	58/62	62/71	69/82	74/89
	tTest/tTest'	16/32	24/47	31/60	37/77	45/88
	Wad/Wad'	92/92	116/116	127/128	140/141	149/149
3x3 samples	Rp/Rp'	52/53	60/64	71/75	76/81	81/90
	Fc/Fc'	54/54	61/63	71/77	79/87	90/100
	tTest/tTest'	32/52	48/76	62/98	72/115	82/132
	Wad/Wad'	91/91	128/129	150/150	166/166	171/175
4x4 samples	Rp/Rp'	60/63	70/74	78/86	85/97	97/105
	Fc/Fc'	62/63	74/81	86/92	94/108	115/128
	tTest/tTest'	67/85	83/111	100/141	108/157	119/174
	Wad/Wad'	119/119	155/155	173/174	189/190	193/196

DISCUSSION

We have proposed a density based pruning algorithm for removing non-differentially expressed genes with high confidence from the total gene list. This pruning procedure can significantly improve the prediction accuracy of popular DEG identification algorithms such as fold change, t-test, and rank product. The key idea of DB pruning is based on the observation that DEGs tend to have high average expression values across conditions.

In this paper, the golden standard true differentially expressed genes are those verified by the RT-PCR method, which may comprise of only a portion of true DEGs. The fact that most true DEGs used here show high average expression levels may be due to the technical limitation of RT-PCR and/or microarray: only highly expressed genes can be identified. In this case our method should be qualified to be able to improve DEG identification algorithms for these types of true DEGs.

DB pruning has two parameters to set to pre-filter non-DEGs. Even though there is no theoretical guideline for setting their perfect parameter values, these two values can be easily set to achieve significant improvements. Both parameters can be set such that an expected number of predicted DEGs are obtained. In our experiments, a single set of R0 (=0.0017) and N0 (=4) have been able to reduce the DEG prediction accuracy for all 17 datasets. This demonstrates the stability of the algorithm in terms of the parameters for different datasets. In addition, an improved pruning algorithm based on Pareto set concept is being developed which can completely remove the parameters in DB pruning.

There are several further improvements following this pattern recognition based DEG identification. One common problem of DEG identification is lack of sufficient data points for reliable estimation of gene expression levels and their differences. This usually hurt the performance of most DEG algorithms including our pruning algorithm. One potential is to use additional external datasets to help estimate gene expression levels and their differences for the dataset of the study. Our preliminary experiments showed that estimating gene expression levels using external datasets is straightforward and feasible but estimating difference of gene expression needs more study. Another improvement is to introduce additional features of DEGs, e.g. the variance of gene expressions across multiple datasets. For example, the variance estimation method using multiple datasets [16] can be combined with DB pruning algorithm. Functional annotation information from gene ontology or pathways can also be integrated to aid gene pruning. Current DB pruning focuses on identifying DEGs between two groups. The extension to multiple groups is straightforward since calculation of average expression level remains the same. And the average difference of expression can be defined as sum of average difference among pairwise comparisons.

Our DB pruning is implemented using C++ and Perl and can be downloaded from http://mleg.cse.sc.edu/degprune.

DECLARATIONS

Acknowledgements

This work is supported by National Science Foundation CAREER AWARD BIO-DBI-0845381

This article has been published as part of BMC Genomics Volume 11 Supplement 2, 2010: Proceedings of the 2009 International Conference on Bioinformatics & Computational Biology (BioComp 2009). The full contents of the supplement are available online at http://www.biomedcentral.com/1471-2164/11?issue=S2

REFERENCES

1. Derisi JL, Iyer VR, Brown PO: Exploring the metabolic and genetic control of gene expression on a genomic scale. Science. 1997, 278: 680-686. 10.1126/science.278.5338.680.
2. Breitling R, Armengaud P, Amtmann A, Herzyk P: Rank products: a simple, yet powerful, new method to detect differentially regulated genes in replicated microarray experiments. FEBS Lett. 2004, 573: 83-92. 10.1016/j.febslet.2004.07.055.
3. Jeffery IB, Higgins DG, Culhane AC: Comparison and evaluation of methods for generating differentially expressed gene lists from microarray data. Bmc Bioinformatics. 2006, 7:
4. Nam D, Kim SY: Gene-set approach for expression pattern analysis. Briefings in Bioinformatics. 2008, 9: 189-197. 10.1093/bib/bbn001.
5. Shi J, Walker MG: Gene set enrichment analysis (GSEA) for interpreting gene expression profiles. Current Bioinformatics. 2007, 2: 133-137. 10.2174/157489307780618231.
6. Chen R, Morgan AA, Dudley J, Deshpande T, Li L, Kodama K, Chiang AP, Butte AJ: FitSNPs: highly differentially expressed genes are more likely to have variants associated with disease. Genome Biol. 2008, 9: R170-10.1186/gb-2008-9-12-r170.
7. Nevarez L, Vasseur V, Le DG, Tanguy A, Guisle-Marsollier I, Houlgatte R, Barbier G: Isolation and analysis of differentially expressed genes in Penicillium glabrum subjected to thermal stress. Microbiology. 2008, 154: 3752-3765. 10.1099/mic.0.2008/021386-0.
8. Estler M, Boskovic G, Denvir J, Miles S, Primerano DA, Niles RM: Global analysis of gene expression changes during retinoic acid-induced growth arrest and differentiation of melanoma: comparison to differentially expressed genes in melanocytes vs melanoma. Bmc Genomics. 2008, 9: 478-10.1186/1471-2164-9-478.
9. Satish L, Laframboise WA, O'Gorman DB, Johnson S, Janto B, Gan BS, Baratz ME, Hu FZ, Post JC, Ehrlich GD: Identification of differentially expressed genes in fibroblasts derived from patients with Dupuytren's Contracture. BMC Med. Genomics,. 2008, 1: 10-10.1186/1755-8794-1-10.
10. Datta S, Satten GA, Xia JZ, Heslin MJ, Datta S: An empirical bayes adjustment to increase the sensitivity of detecting differentially expressed genes in microarray experiments. Bioinformatics. 2004, 20: 235-242. 10.1093/bioinformatics/btg396.
11. Shi L, Jones WD, Jensen RV, Harris SC, Perkins RG, Goodsaid FM, Guo L, Croner LJ, Boysen C, Fang H: The balance of reproducibility, sensitivity, and specificity of lists of differentially expressed genes in microarray studies. BMC Bioinformatics. 2008, 9 (Suppl 9): S10-10.1186/1471-2105-9-S9-S10.
12. Yang K, Li J, Gao H: The impact of sample imbalance on identifying differentially expressed genes. Bmc Bioinformatics,. 2006, 7 (Suppl 4): S8-10.1186/1471-2105-7-S4-S8.
13. Baldi P, Long AD: A Bayesian framework for the analysis of microarray expression data: regularized t -test and statistical inferences of gene changes. Bioinformatics. 2001, 17: 509-519. 10.1093/bioinformatics/17.6.509.
14. Jain N, Thatte J, Braciale T, Ley K, O'Connell M, Lee JK: Local-pooled-error test for identifying differentially expressed genes with a small number of replicated

microarrays. Bioinformatics. 2003, 19,: 1945-1951. 10.1093/bioinformatics/btg264.

15. Tusher VG, Tibshirani R, Chu G: Significance analysis of microarrays applied to the ionizing radiation response. Proc. Natl. Acad. Sci. U. S A. 2001, 98: 5116-5121. 10.1073/pnas.091062498.

16. Wille A, Gruissem W, Buhlmann P, Hennig L: EVE (external variance estimation) increases statistical power for detecting differentially expressed genes. Plant Journal. 2007, 52: 561-569. 10.1111/j.1365-313X.2007.03227.x.

17. Kim RD, Park PJ: Improving identification of differentially expressed genes in microarray studies using information from public databases. Genome Biology. 2004, 5:

18. Hackstadt AJ, Hess AM: Filtering for increased power for microarray data analysis. Bmc Bioinformatics. 2009, 10:

19. Zhou Y, Cras-Meneur C, Ohsugi M, Stormo GD, Permutt MA: A global approach to identify differentially expressed genes in cDNA (two-color) microarray experiments. Bioinformatics. 2007, 23: 2073-2079. 10.1093/bioinformatics/btm292.

20. Kadota K, Nakai Y, Shimizu K: A weighted average difference method for detecting differentially expressed genes from microarray data. Algorithms for Molecular Biology. 2008, 3:

21. Dettling M, Gabrielson E, Parmigiani G: Searching for differentially expressed gene combinations. Genome Biol. 2005, 6: R88-10.1186/gb-2005-6-10-r88.

22. Barrett T, Troup DB, Wilhite SE, Ledoux P, Rudnev D, Evangelista C, Kim IF, Soboleva A, Tomashevsky M, Edgar R: NCBI GEO: mining tens of millions of expression profiles - database and tools update. Nucleic Acids Research. 2007, 35: D760-D765. 10.1093/nar/gkl887.

23. Kadota K, Nakai Y, Shimizu K: Ranking differentially expressed genes from Affymetrix gene expression data: methods with reproducibility, sensitivity, and specificity. Algorithms for Molecular Biology. 2009, 4:

24. Hong FX, Breitling R, McEntee CW, Wittner BS, Nemhauser JL, Chory J: RankProd: a bioconductor package for detecting differentially expressed genes in meta-analysis. Bioinformatics. 2006, 22: 2825-2827. 10.1093/bioinformatics/btl476.

25. Xiaodong Cai, Giannakis GB: Identifying differentially expressed genes in microarray experiments with model-based variance estimation. IEEE Transaction on Signal Processing. 2008, 54: 2418-2426.

26. Shaik JS, Yeasin M: A unified framework for finding differentially expressed genes from microarray experiments. Bmc Bioinformatics. 2007, 8:

CHAPTER 10 GENETIC EPIDEMIOLOGICAL STUDIES OF INFECTIOUS DISEASES

Catherine M. Stein, Noémi B. Hall, LaShaunda L. Malone2 and Ezekiel Mupere

Keywords: extended pedigrees, genetic association, whole genome studies, cohort study, case-contact

INTRODUCTION

The advantages of family studies for genetic epidemiology have long been established (Stein and Elston, 2009). Early methods in genetic epidemiology utilized twins, sibling pairs, and other relative pairs to establish the relative recurrence risk of a disease. Segregation analysis and traditional linkage analysis can only be conducted using pedigree data. Concerns of population stratification are easily accounted for. In addition to these analytical issues, family studies have the advantage of investment of relatives; if someone in the family has a particular disease, family members are more likely to participate in research in order to somehow help their relative and others affected with the disease. Today, with the advent of whole exome and whole genome sequencing technologies, there are additional advantages of family studies, which we shall review below.

These advantages of family studies are further amplified for genetic epidemiological studies of infectious diseases. It was once believed that tuberculosis (TB) was a familial disease because it occurred within families. Once the disease was determined to be caused by a mycobacteria, the ideas surrounding the familial component recessed to the background. Now decades after the causal pathogen, Mycobacterium tuberculosis (Mtb), has been identified, many studies have shown that human genetic factors influence risk for development of TB infection and disease (Moller and Hoal, 2010; Stein, 2011). Development of TB infection and disease is essentially a phenotype resulting from a gene by environment interaction, so a well-constructed genetic epidemiological study must account for host genetics, shared environment, and gene x environment interaction. In this paper, we provide an overview of our household contact (HHC) study of TB and its advantages for genetic epidemiological studies, particularly in light of study designs best suited to identify rare genetic variants.

OVERVIEW OF THE HOUSEHOLD CONTACT STUDY DESIGN

In its natural history, TB is a two-stage process of infection followed by disease (Comstock, 1982). The household provides a natural setting to study TB because the genetic epidemiology of the two stages of infection and disease can be characterized. In our previous studies (Guwatudde et al., 2003), we defined a household as a group of people living within one residence and share meals together with a head of family who makes decisions for the household. Extensive epidemiological data are collected on individual risk factors, such as proximity and frequency of contact with the index case as well as other factors that may increase susceptibility, characteristics of the home that may increase the risk of transmission, as well as clinical data. Blood samples are obtained at baseline and longitudinally for genetic and immunologic studies.

In our HHC study, the first TB patient is identified in the household and referred to as the index case. Thereafter individuals who reside in the same household with the index case for a certain period prior to the diagnosis of the index case are identified and screened for TB as HHCs. Each HHC is also evaluated clinically for latent Mtb infection with the tuberculin skin test (or interferon-γ response assay in the future). Individuals who are tuberculin skin test negative have repeated skin tests several times over the 2-year study follow-up. Thus, the HHC evaluation is efficient in identification of individuals with different phenotypes or stages of TB infection in a household including: (1) exposed and uninfected, (2)

Citation: Catherine M. Stein, Noémi B. Hall, LaShaunda L. Malone and Ezekiel Mupere, genetic epidemiological studies of infectious diseases, http://dx.doi.org/10.3389/fgene.2013.00061.

exposed and infected without disease, (3) recent infection, and (4) active TB. These different household phenotypes or categories can provide the basis to compare genetic factors associated with TB infection and disease. As all of these stages of infection and disease are diagnosed, both the index case and his/her contacts receive appropriate clinical care and treatment, which is an immediate benefit to all study participants.

The design of the HHC study is ideal for evaluating genetic susceptibility to TB (Stein et al., 2003,2005, 2007, 2008). The family structure and the ability to identify sibling pairs can form the basis for linkage analysis studies. Evaluation for new candidate genes for TB can be done through conduct of association studies such as case–control, family based, and/or case–parent studies. Heritability to TB can be determined using standard quantitative genetic approaches which can be based on host immune responses as intermediate phenotypes (Stein et al., 2005; Tao et al., 2013). Studies of HHCs have demonstrated that young children are at greater risk for developing TB and the clustering of cases within families does give hint at a familial susceptibility (Brailey, 1940;Puffer et al., 1952).

In sum, the essence of an HHC design is the recruitment of an entire household through an index case/proband, and collection of extensive clinical and epidemiological data. All age ranges and relative pair types are enrolled, and the entire spectrum of disease is captured. There is flexibility for collection of biological samples and a longitudinal component to observe changes in phenotypes and biomarkers.

ADVANTAGES OF THE HHC DESIGN FOR CURRENT GENETIC EPIDEMIOLOGICAL STUDIES

Recruitment and Phenotype Collection

As summarized above, the household is ascertained through an index case with TB (aka proband). Thus, as long as each individual in the household provides informed consent (or assent in the case of children), an entire family is enrolled in the study. Sometimes, there is another individual with TB in the household at the time of enrollment (co-prevalent case). In some households, another individual develops TB later on during the course of study follow-up (incident case). In this respect, no additional recruitment efforts are needed to identify additional affected individuals. The longitudinal component of the HHC design is valuable, especially for TB, where individuals have a 5–10% lifetime risk of developing active disease after exposure. In our studies, we have observed incident cases develop 2 years after initial enrollment of the household. If related individuals are desired for analytical and study design reasons (see "Analytical Considerations" below), the HHC design allows for easier enrollment of relatives, particularly in settings where literacy is low and roads are impassable (Bennett et al., 2002). Since both HIV co-infected and uninfected individuals may live within the same household, both will be enrolled in the study; this enables the examination of gene by HIV interaction effects (Stein et al., 2007). Finally, the ideal setting for a case-contact study is where the balance of household vs. community spread of disease is in favor of the household (Hill and Ota, 2010).

Both pediatric and adult TB cases may be diagnosed because the HHC design does not restrict enrollment by age. Studies suggest that the genetic influences on pediatric vs. adult TB differ (Malik et al., 2005; Alcais et al., 2010) and the HHC study design is an efficient method for ascertaining both types of cases. By contrast, studies that focus solely on recruitment of pediatric TB cases are challenging – school-based studies are limited because children living in poverty may not have access to education, and hospital- and clinic-based studies may also miss out on enrolling children because many babies are born at home in developing countries and families in poverty who are most at risk for developing TB may not have access to medical care. Door-to-door case finding strategies would require a great number of resources in order to identify a sufficient number of pediatric cases.

The HHC design also enables the enrollment of appropriate "controls." For a proper case–control study, controls must be similar in every way to the cases except that they do not have the disease of interest. For infectious diseases like TB, this is especially true, and in order for an individual to have the opportunity to become a case, he/she must have been exposed to an infectious TB case. This is particularly important for TB, because clinical status of the controls determines whether observed genetic associations are with susceptibility to latent infection or progression to active disease (Stein, 2011). By virtue of the HHC design, all the household members have been exposed to the index case. The selection of appropriate controls in community-based studies of TB is problematic (Hill and Ota, 2010).

Finally, studies of large pedigrees often include extensive and highly detailed phenotype information (Wijsman, 2012). This is extraordinarily useful for infectious diseases such as TB for a number of reasons. As the natural history of Mtb infection and disease follows a two-stage process, the longitudinal HHC design captures all of these stages, and progression from one stage to another. Furthermore, the HHC design can also include collection of extensive immunological data. The HHC design therefore is flexible enough to analyze immunological correlates of the natural history of TB (Whalen et al., 2006; Mahan et al., 2012), and also genetic influences on the immune response to Mtb (Stein et al., 2007, 2008). Omics technologies, such as gene expression and proteomic arrays, can also be incorporated into a study that has an established blood draw protocol and rigorous clinical classification. Finally, as we describe later, data are also collected on important epidemiological factors, which can be incorporated as covariates as well as in gene by environment interaction models.

Analytical Considerations

One unique aspect of HHC studies is that households may contain all sorts of relationship types – nuclear families, extended relatives, and unrelated individuals. Half-siblings are common in African settings where polygamy is practiced (Bennett et al., 2002). Similarly, adoption by extended relatives is common when children are orphaned, which may be particularly relevant in areas with a heavy AIDS burden.

A few studies have developed strategies for jointly analyzing family based and case–control/population-based data (Chen and Lin, 2008; Gray-McGuire et al., 2009; Lasky-Su et al., 2010; Zheng et al., 2010; Mirea et al., 2012). Though they differ in how they combine data from these two different study designs – some analyze them all together, and some combine p-values or test statistics – there are some common themes. First, joint analysis of data from these two different study designs results in increased power due to increased sample size, enabling the detection of smaller effect sizes. Second, family based data have the advantage of controlling for population substructure, which alleviates this common concern of population-based studies.

There have been many recent reports detailing the usefulness of extended pedigrees for the analysis of sequence data and detection of rare variants. Cirulli and Goldstein (2010) explain how the analysis of distantly related, co-affected individuals is an economical design, because there will be fewer genetic variants in common, thereby reducing the search space for rare variants. Stringent filtering could use identity-by-descent sharing to capitalize on this biological phenomenon (Akula et al., 2011). Large pedigrees also have increased power to detect linkage, even in the presence of linkage heterogeneity among families, and are enriched for variants of interest (Wijsman, 2012). Linkage analysis with pedigree data can be used as a filtering strategy of chromosomal regions, and can guide the selection of subjects to sequence (Wijsman, 2012). In addition, linkage analysis may be conducted to examine co-segregation between the trait and variant(s) of interest (Clerget-Darpoux and Elston, 2007; Ziegler and Sun, 2012). Consanguineous marriages are common in West Africa, which increases the power to detect rare recessive alleles (Bennett et al., 2002). To summarize, all of the relationship types that are useful for the identification of rare variants are easily obtainable in the HHC design.

Impact of Environment

A well-designed HHC study includes vast epidemiologic data about environmental risk factors for transmission of disease within homes. For TB, these include factors related to ventilation and crowding within the home, poverty, clinical characteristics of the index case that make him/her more infectious, and proximity to the index case that increase degree of contact (Stein et al., 2005;Mandalakas et al., 2012). Risk of infection by Mtb is determined by a number of epidemiological risk factors (Guwattude et al., 2003; Lienhardt et al., 2003; Mandalakas et al., 2012), and many variables associated with high risk of TB transmission are automatically present in the HHC design. Analysis of foster relationships as seen in adoptions may be useful for the estimation of effects due to shared environment (Bennett et al., 2002), and many such relationships occur in HHC studies in the developing world.

Genetic substrains of Mtb may differ in their transmissibility. All of these factors relate to the risk of an individual to acquire infection, and develop disease, and thus are important in epidemiological characterization of affected individuals. Furthermore, recent studies have also suggested that substrains of Mtb have synergistic effects with host genes, thus resulting in gene x environment interaction effects related to TB risk (Caws et al., 2008). Case-only designs can be nested within HHC studies to examine these gene x environment effects (Bennett et al., 2002). Because exposure to the index case is generally highest, and in turn exposure to that individual's strain of Mtb, the HHC design provides a natural setting to test both transmissibility, gene x environment interaction, and role of shared environment.

Nutrition and nutritional status are also important factors in TB-related outcomes (Jaganath and Mupere, 2012; Mupere et al., 2012a). We have shown that nutritional status of a patient may be an indicator on how the food basket is shared in the household and the subsequent macro- and micronutrient intake (Mupere et al., 2012b). Because of the shared environmental and genetic components of diet and obesity (or in the case of TB, malnutrition), the HHC design provides a robust setting to test the role of nutritional status on infectious disease outcomes.

Examples from Our Studies

Our genetic association studies have taken the approach by Gray-McGuire et al. (2009). We identified the first reported association between TNFR1 gene and TB and also a gene by HIV interaction for this same gene (Stein et al., 2007). Our genome-wide linkage scan (Stein et al., 2008) and subsequent fine mapping studies (Baker et al., 2011) replicated previously a novel set of genes on chromosome 20, CTSZ, and MC3R. We have also identified novel chromosomal regions linked to a unique resistance phenotype (Stein et al., 2008); we are uniquely able to clinically and epidemiologically characterize this phenotype because of our solid study design. Our future plans will incorporate structural equation modeling (SEM to multivariately analyze the influences of host genetics, immunology, and environment on clinical outcome; this shall be done using a SEM approach that jointly models familial relationship and covariance among variables (Morris et al., 2011).

CONCLUSION

Certainly HHC designs may be expensive to implement, because they include repeated clinical visits, longitudinal data collection, and travel to the homes. However, the wealth of data collected through HHC studies is invaluable for genetic epidemiological studies, as described here. HHC study designs offer unique advantages for genetic epidemiological studies, including the presence of related and unrelated individuals, and the ability to quantify environmental factors that are important for both shared environmental influences on the phenotype as well as gene x environment interaction. Though our focus has been primarily on studies of TB, this study design has advantages for the study of infectious diseases in general (Hill and Ota, 2010).

Conflict of Interest Statement

The authors declare that the research was conducted in the absence of any commercial or financial relationships that could be construed as a potential conflict of interest.

ACKNOWLEDGMENTS

We would like to thank Drs. Christopher Whalen and W. Henry Boom for their key roles in the design and implementation of the Household Contact Studies in Kampala, Uganda.

Funding for this work was provided by the Tuberculosis Research Unit (grant N01-AI95383 and HHSN266200700022C/ N01-AI70022 from the NIAID), and

National Heart Lung and Blood Institutes (NHLBI) grants R01HL096811, R01HL-10566113, and T32HL007567.

REFERENCES

1. Akula, N., Detera-Wadleigh, S., Shugart, Y., Nalls, M., Steele, J., and McMahon, F. J. (2011). Identity-by-descent filtering as a tool for the identification of disease alleles in exome sequence data from distant relatives. BMC Proc. 5(Suppl. 9):S76. doi: 10.1186/1753-6561-5-S9-S76
2. Alcais, A., Quintana-Murci, L., Thaler, D. S., Schurr, E., Abel, L., and Casanova, J. L. (2010). Life-threatening infectious iseases of childhood: single-gene inborn errors of immunity? Ann. N. Y. Acad. Sci. 1214, 18–33.
3. Baker, A. R., Zalwango, S., Malone, L. L., Igo, R. P. Jr, Qiu, F., Nsereko, M., et al. (2011). Genetic Susceptibility to Tuberculosis Associated with CTSZ Haplotype in Ugandan Household Contact Study. Hum. Immunol. 72, 426–430.
4. Bennett, S., Lienhardt, C., Bah-Sow, O., Gustafson, P., Manneh, K., Del Prete, G., et al. (2002). Investigation of environmental and host-related risk factors for tuberculosis in Africa. II. Investigation of host genetic factors. Am. J. Epidemiol. 155, 11, 1074–1079.
5. Brailey, M. (1940). Mortality in the children of tuberculous households. Am. J. Public Health Nations Health 30, 816–823.
6. Caws, M., Thwaites, G., Dunstan, S., Hawn, T. R., Lan, N. T., Thuong, N. T., et al. (2008). The influence of host and bacterial genotype on the development of disseminated disease with Mycobacterium tuberculosis. PLoS Pathog. 4:e1000034. doi: 10.1371/journal.ppat.1000034
7. Chen, Y. H., and Lin, H. W. (2008). Simple association analysis combining data from trios/sibships and unrelated controls.Genet. Epidemiol. 32, 520–527.
8. Cirulli, E. T., and Goldstein, D. B. (2010). Uncovering the roles of rare variants in common disease through whole-genome sequencing. Nat. Rev. Genet. 11, 415–425.
9. Clerget-Darpoux, F., and Elston, R. C. (2007). Are linkage analysis and the collection of family data dead? Prospects for family studies in the age of genome-wide association. Hum. Hered. 64, 91–96.
10. Comstock, G. (1982). Epidemiology of tuberculosis. Am. Rev. Respir. Dis. 125, 8–15.
11. Gray-McGuire, C., Bochud, M., Goodloe, R., and Elston, R. C. (2009). Genetic association tests: a method for the joint analysis of family and case–control data. Hum. Genomics 4, 2–20.
12. Guwattude, D., Nakakeeto, M., Jones-Lopez, E. C., Maganda, A., Chiunda, A., Mugerwa, R. D., et al. (2003). Tuberculosis in household contacts of infectious cases in Kampala, Uganda. Am. J. Epidemiol. 158, 887–898.
13. Guwatudde, D., Zalwango, S., Kamya, M. R., Debanne, S. M., Diaz, M. I., Okwera, A., et al. (2003). Burden of tuberculosis in Kampala, Uganda. Bull. World Health Organ. 81, 799–805.
14. Hill, P. C., and Ota, M. O. (2010). Tuberculosis case-contact research in endemic tropical settings: design, conduct, and relevance to other infectious diseases. Lancet Infect. Dis. 10, 723–732.
15. Jaganath, D., and Mupere, E. (2012). Childhood tuberculosis and malnutrition. J. Infect. Dis. 206, 1809–1815.
16. Lasky-Su, J., Won, S., Mick, E., Anney, R. J., Franke, B., Neale, B., et al. (2010). On genome-wide association studies for family-based designs: an integrative analysis approach combining ascertained family samples with unselected controls. Am. J. Hum. Genet. 86, 573–580.
17. Lienhardt, C., Fielding, K., Sillah, J., Tunkara, A., Donkor, S., Manneh, K., et al. (2003). Risk factors for tuberculosis infection in sub-Saharan Africa: a contact study in The Gambia. Am. J. Respir. Crit. Care Med. 168, 448–455.
18. Mahan, C. S., Zalwango, S., Thiel, B. A., Malone, L. L., Chervenak, K. A., Baseke, J., et al. (2012). Innate and adaptive immune responses during acute M. tuberculosis infection in adult household contacts in Kampala, Uganda. Am. J. Trop. Med. Hyg. 86, 690–697.
19. Malik, S., Abel, L., Tooker, H., Poon, A., Simkin, L., Girard, M., et al. (2005). Alleles of the NRAMP1 gene are risk factors for pediatric tuberculosis disease. Proc. Natl. Acad. Sci. U.S.A. 102, 12183–12188.
20. Mandalakas, A. M., Kirchner, H. L., Lombard, C., Walzl, G., Grewal, H. M., Gie, R. P., et al. (2012). Well-quantified tuberculosis exposure is a reliable surrogate measure of tuberculosis infection. Int. J. Tuberc. Lung Dis. 16, 1033–1039.
21. Mirea, L., Infante-Rivard, C., Sun, L., and Bull, S. B. (2012). Strategies for genetic association analyses combining unrelated case–control individuals and family trios. Am. J. Epidemiol. 176, 70–79.
22. Moller, M., and Hoal, E. G. (2010). Current findings, challenges and novel approaches in human genetic susceptibility to tuberculosis. Tuberculosis (Edinb.) 90, 71–83.
23. Morris, N. J., Elston, R. C., and Stein, C. M. (2011). A framework for structural equation models in general pedigrees. Hum. Hered. 70, 278–286.
24. Mupere, E., Malone, L., Zalwango, S., Chiunda, A., Okwera, A., Parraga, I., et al. (2012a). Lean tissue mass wasting is associated with increased risk of mortality among women with pulmonary tuberculosis in urban Uganda. Ann. Epidemiol. 22, 466–473.
25. Mupere, E., Parraga, I. M., Tisch, D. J., Mayanja, H. K., and Whalen, C. C. (2012b). Low nutrient intake among adult women and patients with severe tuberculosis disease in Uganda: a cross-sectional study. BMC Public Health 12:1050. doi: 10.1186/1471-2458-12-1050.:1050-12
26. Puffer, R. R., Zeidberg, L. D., Dillon, A., Gass, R. S., and Hutcheson, R. H. (1952). Tuberculosis attack and death rates of household associates; the influence of age, sex, race, and relationship. Am. Rev. Tuberc. 65, 111–127.
27. Stein, C. M. (2011). Genetic epidemiology of

tuberculosis susceptibility: impact of study design. PLoS Pathog. 7:e1001189. doi: 10.1371/journal.ppat.1001189

28. Stein, C. M., and Elston, R. C. (2009). Finding genes underlying human disease. Clin. Genet. 75, 101–106.

29. Stein, C. M., Nshuti, L., Chiunda, A. B., Boom, W. H., Elston, R. C., Mugerwa, R. D., et al. (2005). Evidence for a major gene influence on tumor necrosis factor-alpha expression in tuberculosis: path and segregation analysis. Hum. Hered. 60, 109–118.

30. Stein, C. M., Zalwango, S., Chiunda, A. B., Millard, C., Leontiev, D. V., Horvath, A. L., et al. (2007). Linkage and association analysis of candidate genes for TB and TNFalpha cytokine expression: evidence for association with IFNGR1, IL-10, and TNF receptor 1 genes. Hum. Genet. 121, 663–673.

31. Stein, C. M., Zalwango, S., Malone, L. L., Won, S., Mayanja-Kizza, H., Mugerwa, R. D., et al. (2008). Genome scan of M. tuberculosis infection and disease in Ugandans. PLoS ONE 3:e4094. doi: 10.1371/journal.pone.0004094

32. Stein, C., Guwatudde, D., Nakakeeto, M., Peters, P., Elston, R. C., Tiwari, H. K., et al. (2003). Heritability analysis of cytokines as intermediate phenotypes of tuberculosis. J. Infect. Dis. 187, 1679–1685.

33. Tao, L., et al. (2013). Genetic and shared environmental influences on interferon-gamma production in response toMycobacterium tuberculosis antigens in a Ugandan population. Am. J. Trop. Med. Hyg. (in press).

34. Whalen, C. C., Chiunda, A., Zalwango, S., Nshuti, L., Jones-Lopez, E., Okwera, A., et al. (2006). Immune correlates of acuteMycobacterium tuberculosis infection in household contacts in Kampala, Uganda. Am. J. Trop. Med. Hyg. 75, 55–61.

35. Wijsman, E. M. (2012). The role of large pedigrees in an era of high-throughput sequencing. Hum. Genet. 131, 1555–1563.

36. Zheng, Y., Heagerty, P. J., Hsu, L., and Newcomb, P. A. (2010). On combining family-based and population-based case–control data in association studies. Biometrics 66, 1024–1033.

37. Ziegler, A., and Sun, Y. V. (2012). Study designs and methods post genome-wide association studies. Hum. Genet. 131, 1525–1531.

CHAPTER 11

SOFTWARES AND METHODS FOR ESTIMATING GENETIC ANCESTRY IN HUMAN POPULATIONS

Yushi Liu, Toru Nyunoya, Shuguang Leng, Steven A Belinsky, Yohannes Tesfaigzi and Shannon Bruse

Keywords: Ancestry, Genetic, Polymorphism, Structure

INTRODUCTION

The analysis of population structure based on genetic ancestry is an increasingly important component of many genetic studies. Genetic ancestry estimation is a broad term which is concerned with a number of different population genetics problems, including: (1) detection of population structure (2) defining the number of subpopulations in a sample (3) assigning individuals to subpopulations (4) defining the number of ancestral populations in admixed populations (5) assigning ancestral population proportions to admixed individuals and (6) identifying the genetic ancestry of distinct chromosomal segments within an individual [1]. No single method or software can optimally solve all of these problems. This review will present a number of softwares for defining these various facets of genetic ancestry, with an emphasis on their use in medical genetic studies.

Genetic ancestry arose from the biogeographical distribution of human populations, and is a concept distinct from ethnicity, which is a social construct with no clear genetic definition [2]. The establishment of inexpensive single nucleotide polymorphism (SNP) genotyping platforms in the previous decade has allowed for relatively facile collection of markers to assess genetic ancestry in human populations. With prior knowledge of population-specific allele frequencies, panels of SNPs referred to as ancestry informative markers (AIMs) can be used to estimate genetic ancestry [3, 4, 5, 6]. AIMs are markers whose frequencies are significantly different, and thus able to distinguish, between two or more populations [7]. Panels of AIMs vary in size, depending on the intended purpose. Relatively small panels numbering in the dozens to hundreds of SNPs can be used when the purpose is to define continental genetic ancestry, whereas hundreds or thousands of SNPs are required for more refined sub continental estimation or for traditional mapping by admixture linkage disequilibrium (MALD) [8, 9, 10]. Alternatively, the advent of genome-wide association studies (GWAS) has made it increasingly common to use the large amount of SNP data already present on genome-wide arrays to estimate genetic ancestry [11]. Some of the methods presented in this review do not require the use of specific AIM panels, but work more effectively with dense genotyping data, though different softwares are more or less adept at handling different sized marker sets. Subsets of AIMs can also be selected from GWAS data using traditional approaches based on SNP informativeness [12] or more recent principal components analysis (PCA) approaches [13].

In medical genetics, perhaps the most common use of estimated genetic ancestry is as a control against cryptic population stratification in genetic association studies [8, 14]. Confounding by population stratification can occur when (a) the allele frequencies of a disease causing SNP are substantially different between populations (b) population proportions are not matched in cases and controls (c) population structure isn't accounted for in the statistical modeling of genetic association. Self-identified ethnicity can be used to control for this potential confounding, often by simply including individual ethnicity as a covariate in the regression models or by performing population stratified analyses. However, using self-identified ethnicity can result in misclassification [15], and also cannot account for varying degrees of admixture within self-identified ethnic groups. Direct estimates of genetic ancestry based on genotype data are therefore preferred as a control for population substructure, given the advantage in precision and informativeness over self-identified ethnicity [16]. In addition to serving as a control for population stratification, estimation of genetic ancestry has become particularly important in

Citation: Yushi Liu, Toru Nyunoya, Shuguang Leng, Steven A Belinsky, Yohannes Tesfaigzi and Shannon Bruse, Softwares and methods for estimating genetic ancestry in human populations, DOI: 10.1186/1479-7364-7-1.

studies of recently admixed populations, such as African-Americans and Latinos [3,17]. Admixed populations which show protection or susceptibility to common diseases provide an unprecedented opportunity for disease gene mapping [18, 19].

Genetic ancestry can be divided into "local" and "global" estimates [20]. Local estimates are concerned with identifying the ancestral origin of distinct chromosomal segments within an individual genome, and these methods are a more recent development in the field. Global estimates seek to establish ancestral proportions averaged across the genome of an individual, so that proportions of each ancestry (summing to 1) can be assigned to each individual. In general, the softwares for estimating genetic ancestry can also be divided into methods that rely on multivariate statistical methods (like PCA and cluster analysis) versus methods that make use of explicit genetic models, although this distinction does not imply that there aren't important similarities between algorithmic and model-based methods. The purpose of this survey is to describe some of the better known algorithmic and model-based programs for estimating both local and global genetic ancestry. Table 1contains a list of the softwares under discussion, usefulness in estimating global or local ancestry, the computing environment, and a link to software website. All softwares presented in this review are free to academic users.

Table 1. Softwares for estimating genetic ancestry

Software	Global/local estimation	Operating Environments	**Link**
STRUCTURE	Global	Windows/DOS/Linux/ Solaris/Mac	http://pritch.bsd.uchicago.edu/structure.html
frappe	Global	Windows/Linux/Mac	http://med.stanford.edu/tanglab/software/ frappe.html
ADMIXTURE	Global	Linux/Mac	http://www.genetics.ucla.edu/software/ admixture/index.html
EIGENSTRAT/ smartpca	Global	Linux	http://www.hsph.harvard.edu/faculty/alkes-price/software/
ipPCA/EigenDev	Global	Windows/Linux (MatLab)	http://www4a.biotec.or.th/GI/tools/ippca
GEMTools	Global	Windows/Linux	http://www.wpic.pitt.edu/wpiccompgen/ GemTools/GemTools.htm
PLINK	Global	Windows/Linux/Mac/C/ C++	http://pngu.mgh.harvard.edu/~purcell/plink/
LAMP	Local and Global	Windows/Linux	http://lamp.icsi.berkeley.edu/lamp/
SABER	Local and Global	Linux	http://med.stanford.edu/tanglab/software/ saber.html
HAPMIX	Local and Global	Unix/Linux/Windows	http://www.stats.ox.ac.uk/~myers/software. html
ANCESTRYMAP	Local and Global	Unix/Linux	http://genepath.med.harvard.edu/~reich/ Software.htm

ESTIMATING GLOBAL ANCESTRY

Structure

STRUCTURE, perhaps the most widely used program for estimating global genetic ancestry, was developed by Pritchard et. al. in 2000 [1]. STRUCTURE is a model-based clustering approach which utilizes genotype data to infer the presence of distinct populations, assign individuals to populations, identify admixture proportions at the individual level, and to estimate ancestral population allele frequencies in admixed populations. There are four main models within STRUCTURE: (1) No admixture model, which assumes individuals come from distinct populations (2) admixture model (3) linkage model [21], which accounts for admixture linkage disequilibrium (i.e. the phenomenon whereby recently admixed populations have larger regions of LD between loci), and (4) prior population information models, which can use location or self-identified ethnicity (if they are informative) to enhance the detection of population structure [22]. The model which utilizes prior population information is particularly useful when working with a small number of markers or when population structure is weak.

Prior to running STRUCTURE, parameters must be set, with perhaps the most critical being K, the number of populations. The authors took an ad hoc approach for K, estimating the conditional mean and variance of Bayesian deviance based on the data [1]. It is also useful to consider known information on the populations under study when choosing an appropriate K. As with any method used to estimate global ancestry proportions, a highly informative marker set and better representation of ancestral populations allows for more exquisite resolution of population structure, and thus will influence the selection of K. In order to run STRUCTURE, individual genotypes are required as input. For the linkage model, phase and genetic map data can also be used.

Briefly, STRUCTURE models the probability of observed genotypes given the individual ancestry proportions and ancestral population allele frequencies. The program assigns individuals to ancestral populations (or proportions of individuals in the case of the admixture model) based on genotype data, while simultaneously estimating the allele frequencies of those populations. Given prior information about the probability of the populations of origin for individuals and the probability of allele frequencies for all populations, traditional Bayesian methods using Markov chain Monte Carlo (MCMC) and Gibbs Sampling are used to obtain the corresponding posterior distribution [1]. A burn-in period is required to reach a stationary posterior distribution, and this burn-in period (and the number of MCMC iterations) is set by the user. MCMC methods are useful in obtaining samples from a posterior distribution when direct sampling is not possible. The method utilizes the Metropolis-Hastings algorithm to obtain a sequence of random samplings which can approximate the distribution.

Admixture

Similar to STRUCTURE, the ADMIXTURE program models the probability of observed genotypes using ancestry proportions and population allele frequencies, simultaneously estimating population allele frequencies along with ancestry proportions. An input file of genotypes from unrelated individuals is required, as is an estimate of K. The ADMIXTURE program uses a cross-validation approach to help estimate K, unlike STRUCTURE which computes the model evidence for each value of K. The ADMIXTURE cross validation procedure helps identify which value of K has the best predictive value, by masking or holding out a subset of genotype data and then predicting those masked genotypes.

Unlike STRUCTURE, ADMIXTURE focuses on maximum likelihood estimation (MLE) rather than sampling the posterior distribution using MCMC, and calculates the estimates via a block relaxation approach which results in improvements in speed [20, 23]. This computational efficiency provides an advantage over STRUCTURE when using very large numbers of markers, for example when using dense GWAS data instead of smaller AIM panels. Briefly, ADMIXTURE updates the allele frequency parameter and ancestry fraction parameter alternatively by maximizing the second-order Taylor's expansion of the likelihood function. It does this iteratively, based on allele frequencies and ancestry proportions associated with the current parameter values. This is typically known as sequential quadratic programming and coincides with Newton's method in the absence of constraints [24]. Newton's method can be used to find the optimal point to solve x-M(x) =0. However, obtaining the differential of M(x) is challenging; therefore a quasi-Newton method is used. This accelerates the convergence, and has been shown to provide an advantage in speed over convergence methods like the Expectation Maximization (EM) algorithm, as employed in the MLE-based program frappe(discussed below). Alexander and coworkers showed that on real world datasets, ADMIXTURE is much faster than STRUCTURE but with comparable estimation, and has been shown to be faster and more accurate thanfrappe[20].

Frappe

Frappe uses a full maximum likelihood approach to estimate individual admixture [25]. frappe requires a genotype and parameter file, containing individual genotypes and a specification of K. Unlike STRUCTURE and ADMIXTURE, frappe does not provide measures to choose an optimal K value. frappe is far more computationally efficient than STRUCTURE [25], but as stated above, less computationally efficient than ADMIXTURE. In simulations using few SNPs (n=60), few individuals from ancestral populations (n=20 and n=60), and low information content of the SNPs (average delta=0.33), frappe produced significantly less biased estimates than STRUCTURE [25]. Thus, frappe appears to perform well when population structure is weak. However, STRUCTURE can use population information to inform the prior probabilities, and this model is also effective in the case of weak population structure [22].

Eigenstrat and ipPCA

PCA can be used for dimensionality reduction to group those with similar genetic ancestry together [26]. PCA is a computationally efficient method which can handle large numbers of markers, and is useful for visualizing population structure [27, 28]. The first few principal components are often used to correct for population stratification in genetic association studies. The EIGENSOFT software package contains EIGENSTRAT (and its helper routine smartpca), and is the most cited PCA method for population structure applications [29].

Briefly, the PCA methods focus on the spectral decomposition of a variance covariance matrix for dimensionality reduction. Both the eigenvalues and eigenvectors are important for underlying population structure identification. The eigenvectors present the linear combination of the covariates which in turn serve as the new dimensions. All the dimensions are orthogonal to each other. These linear combinations are known as the principal components. If there is underlying structure among populations, PCA tends to separate them based on the principal components. A question, however, is when to stop dividing individuals into subpopulations. Patterson and colleagues provided an answer which allows determination of the probability of structure based on the Tracy-Widom distribution [29]. The Tracy-Widom theory considers that when the dimension for a matrix M is suitably large, the distribution of the largest eigenvalue follows approximately the Tracy Widom distribution as identified by Johnstone [30]. This allows assessment of the probability that the largest eigenvalue is random, and thus, whether or not structure exists [29].

In large, highly structured samples, particularly when subpopulations are closely related or when there is a genetically distant subpopulation, traditional PCA methods have difficulty assigning individuals to the correct subpopulation [31]. However, ipPCA (and an extension termed EigenDev-ipPCA) is a refinement of the PCA method which efficiently assigns individuals to populations and provides accurate estimates of K, even in highly structured populations [31, 32]. Although there is no general agreement on what constitutes a subpopulation, on simulated and real datasets, ipPCA was more accurate (ie. fit better with population assignments based on prior knowledge of population structure) than STRUCTURE in determining K, particularly as the number of subpopulations increased [31].

Plink and GEMTools

Other algorithmic approaches statistically related to the PCA exist as well. PLINK implements multidimensional scaling (MDS) to assess population structure. Given that PLINK is commonly used for genetic association testing, it is convenient that the output file from MDS analysis in PLINK can be directly used as a covariate file in PLINK-based association testing. In the current version of PLINK, genome-wide coverage of SNPs is required to perform the MDS analysis. MDS is a class of statistical analysis that provides a view of the proximities for objects. Therefore, the similarities of people based on genetic ancestry can be viewed using MDS. Theoretically, the MDS method tries to find a matrix from the dissimilarity matrix that preserves the distances, allowing the data to be projected into low dimensional space [33]. PLINK utilizes a distance measure based on genome-wide pairwise IBS (identity-by-state) to construct an MDS plot. In a comparative study, PCA structure analysis as implemented in EIGENSOFT performed slightly better than PLINK-based MDS analysis in correcting for population stratification in a GWAS dataset [34].

Another algorithmic approach is a recently introduced package called GEMTools which uses spectral graph theory for dimensionality reduction and clustering by genetic ancestry [35]. This approach may be more flexible than PCA [36], and the package contains a convenient function for matching cases and controls based on genetic similarity.

ESTIMATING LOCAL ANCESTRY

Lamp

LAMP (Local Ancestry in adMixed Populations) is a program used to infer locus-specific ancestry in admixed populations using sliding windows of contiguous SNPs [37, 38]. A significant advantage of LAMP relative to other methods for local ancestry is that it does not require genotypes from unadmixed ancestral populations as input. This is advantageous when working with an uncharacterized populations or when ancestral genotypes aren't available. When available, ancestral genotype information can be utilized by the LAMP program using LAMP-ANC. The LAMP-ANC program then infers local ancestry based on the ancestral populations, rather than the de novo inference used by LAMP.

Similar to other local ancestry programs, LAMP does require input parameters, including the recombination rate, global ancestry proportion, and an upper limit on time since admixture. Global recombination rates have previously been calculated [39], and global ancestral proportion can be calculated using a program such as STRUCTURE. Simulations indicate that LAMP is more robust to inaccuracies in time since admixture and less so to inaccuracies in global ancestral proportions, and performs somewhat less well as this proportion nears 0.5 [37]. On simulated admixed populations representing African-Americans, LAMP and LAMP-ANC were on average more accurate and considerably faster than SABER (discussed below) [37]. However on simulations of admixed populations with very closely related ancestral populations (Chinese and Japanese), SABER was more accurate than LAMP but less accurate than LAMP-ANC. However, all methods perform rather poorly when the ancestral populations are very closely related. All of the local ancestry methods can be used to estimate global ancestry by chromosomal or genome-wide averaging of the local ancestry estimates. On simulated data, relative to STRUCTURE, LAMP was more accurate in estimating global genetic ancestry [37]. Again on simulated data, LAMP is capable of accurately estimating admixture proportions in cases of three-way, and presumably greater, admixture. In contrast to SABER and HAPMIX (reviewed in following sections), LAMP does not model LD and assumes uncorrelated SNPs, though the program is somewhat robust to this assumption [37].

Briefly, the idea of LAMP is to select a suitable window length, and then a clustering algorithm known as Iterated Conditional Modes (ICM) is used to estimate the likelihood that an individual chromosome has a particular ancestry within this window. The ancestry of individual SNPs is determined by majority vote using all such overlapping windows containing that SNP [37]. For this procedure, the most important step is the Iterated Conditional Modes. This algorithm differs from the traditional Expectation Maximization (EM) algorithm in the E step [37]. In the EM algorithm, the expected classification based on the minor allele frequencies of the SNPs within the given window will be obtained; in contrast, in the ICM algorithm, the maximized posterior estimate for the classification based on the minor allele frequencies and genotype will be obtained instead, assuming the initial classification is reasonable [37]. Therefore, ICM can have a greatly accelerated convergence compared to the EM algorithm. Since this algorithm involves the accurate estimation of the minor allele frequency as the starting point, the authors of this software considered two scenarios: (1) in the case of two ancestral populations with unknown allele frequencies in the ancestral population, the MAXVAR algorithm will be used, in which the individuals will be grouped according to the measurement of similarity (2) in the case when there are two or more ancestral populations and the minor allele frequency is known, the question is simpler and the given ancestral allele frequencies will be used [37].

Hapmix

HAPMIX is an extension of a Hidden Markov Model (HMM) [40] used to model linkage disequilibrium in population genetic data [41]. HAPMIX requires as input phased data from ancestral populations, unphased data from the admixed population, and a recombination rate file which give the physical and genetic position (in cM) of each SNP. Like LAMP and SABER, HAPMIX is used to determine genetic ancestry for each chromosomal position or segment in the genome. Unlike those other programs, HAPMIX makes use of haplotype information. This requires the use of phased genotype data from unadmixed ancestral populations, and the current version of HAPMIX can only handle two-way admixture.

In admixed populations, linkage disequilibrium exists at a coarse scale and fine scale [41]. Course scale admixture linkage disequilibrium is due to relatively recent recombination events which result in individual genomes being comprised of distinct chromosomal segments inherited from particular ancestral populations. Fine scale linkage disequilibrium is based on historical recombination events in the ancestral populations. Modeling of both, using a program such as HAPMIX, may increase the power of genetic association testing [41], as demonstrated in a recent study of breast cancer in African-American women [11]. Full modeling of the ancestral LD may also lead to more accurate estimates of local genetic ancestry, as demonstrated using simulated and real world data of African-Americans, where HAPMIX outperformed both ANCESTRYMAP and LAMP-ANC [41]. Further simulations demonstrated that the HAPMIX performance advantage increased with increasing time since admixture, indicating its utility across a range of admixed populations [41].

Briefly, in HAPMIX the haplotype of an individual is viewed as a mosaic of the haplotypes from the ancestral populations. At each position in the genome the likelihood that the haplotype arises from a particular ancestral population is estimated, and a Hidden Markov Model combines these likelihoods with information from neighboring loci to give probabilistic evidence that particular segments come from one ancestral population versus another [41]. Importantly, HAPMIX treats the ancestral population as unambiguously phased, but uses a built in phasing algorithm on the admixed population and doesn't assume that any one haplotype phasing is correct. This flexible approach can help avoid inappropriate inferences of ancestry transitions [41]. Additional advantages of HAPMIX are very accurate inferences of date of admixture and the ability to accurately estimate 0, 1, or 2 ancestral alleles at each locus [41].

Saber

SABER is a program suitable for genome-scale data which uses a "Markov-hidden Markov model" to estimate local ancestry [42]. This local ancestry is referred to as "ancestral blocks". Like HAPMIX, it models the ancestral LD; however it does not model haplotype structure. Input files are typical and include genotype data from ancestral and admixed individuals, global ancestry estimates of admixed individuals, and physical map location of the SNPs. In addition to providing localized ancestry (with graphical output), SABER can be used to estimate time since admixture.

Ancestrymap, admixmap, and maldsoft

A number of other methods can infer local (and global) ancestry, but are not computationally efficient when working with genome-scale data. These include ANCESTRYMAP [43], ADMIXMAP [44], and MALDSOFT [45]. These are all well-established methods which use Hidden Markov Models to combine data across loci to infer ancestry at each locus, and these programs require that there be no LD between markers. The primary focus of these programs is for traditional admixture mapping on AIM panels, and not the evaluation of local genetic ancestry using dense panels of markers [25].

CONCLUSION

The programs presented here offer tools to deal with a number of population genetics problems related to genetic ancestry. No single program is sufficient for dealing with the variety of research questions being asked, and using combinations of these programs may be most helpful for the next generation of medical genetics studies. For example, while global ancestry has historically been used to control for population stratification in association studies, it may be more appropriate to control for both local and global ancestry [46], which may be optimally resolved using separate programs. New uses for these programs are also arising. Several recent studies have assessed the correlation of individual ancestry proportions with disease risk or treatment response [47, 48, 49, 50]. For example, it was reported that the percent Native American genetic ancestry in a cohort of children was associated with risk for relapse after chemotherapeutic treatment of acute lymphoblastic leukemia [49]. Understanding why ancestry proportions in admixed populations correlate with phenotypes will require precise identification of the ancestry specific loci that are responsible. Recent reports have demonstrated that statistical tests combining admixture and ancestral linkage disequilibrium signals is a more powerful method of testing for genetic association than MALD or traditional LD mapping individually [11,41]. Genetic ancestry softwares which give refined and accurate estimates of local ancestry are critically important to this next generation of genetic studies in admixed populations.

DECLARATIONS

Competing interests

We declare that we have no competing interests.

Authors' contribution

YL and SB made substantial contributions to conception and design of the manuscript, and interpretation of statistical methods. YL, TN, SL, SAB, YT, and SB made substantial contributions to drafting the article or revising it critically for important intellectual content. All authors read and approved the final manuscript.

REFERENCES

1. Pritchard JK, Stephens M, Donnelly P: Inference of population structure using multilocus genotype data. Genetics. 2000, 155 (2): 945-959.
2. Tishkoff SA, Kidd KK: Implications of biogeography of human populations for "race" and medicine. Nat Genet. 2004, 36 (11 Suppl): S21-S27.
3. Mao X, Bigham AW, Mei R, et al: A genomewide admixture mapping panel for Hispanic/Latino populations. Am J Hum Genet. 2007, 80 (6): 1171-1178. 10.1086/518564.
4. Tian C, Hinds DA, Shigeta R, et al: A genomewide single-nucleotide-polymorphism panel for Mexican American admixture mapping. Am J Hum Genet. 2007, 80 (6): 1014-1023. 10.1086/513522.
5. Tian C, Hinds DA, Shigeta R, et al: A genomewide single-nucleotide-polymorphism panel with high ancestry information for African American admixture mapping. Am J Hum Genet. 2006, 79 (4): 640-649. 10.1086/507954.
6. Hou L, Phillips C, Azaro M, Brzustowicz LM, Bartlett CW: Validation of a cost-efficient multi-purpose SNP

panel for disease based research. PLoS One. 2011, 6 (5): e19699-10.1371/journal.pone.0019699.

7. Rosenberg NA, Li LM, Ward R, Pritchard JK: Informativeness of genetic markers for inference of ancestry. Am J Hum Genet. 2003, 73 (6): 1402-1422. 10.1086/380416.

8. Chakraborty R, Weiss KM: Admixture as a tool for finding linked genes and detecting that difference from allelic association between loci. Proc Natl Acad Sci U S A. 1988, 85 (23): 9119-9123. 10.1073/pnas.85.23.9119.

9. Briscoe D, Stephens JC, O'Brien SJ: Linkage disequilibrium in admixed populations: applications in gene mapping. J Hered. 1994, 85 (1): 59-63.

10. Stephens JC, Briscoe D, O'Brien SJ: Mapping by admixture linkage disequilibrium in human populations: limits and guidelines. Am J Hum Genet. 1994, 55 (4): 809-824.

11. Pasaniuc B, Zaitlen N, Lettre G, et al: Enhanced statistical tests for GWAS in admixed populations: assessment using African Americans from CARe and a breast cancer consortium. PLoS Genet. 2011, 7 (4): e1001371-10.1371/journal.pgen.1001371.

12. Tandon A, Patterson N, Reich D: Ancestry informative marker panels for African Americans based on subsets of commercially available SNP arrays. Genet Epidemiol. 2011, 35 (1): 80-83. 10.1002/gepi.20550.

13. Paschou P, Ziv E, Burchard EG, et al: PCA-correlated SNPs for structure identification in worldwide human populations. PLoS Genet. 2007, 3 (9): 1672-1686.

14. Lander ES, Schork NJ: Genetic dissection of complex traits. Science. 1994, 265 (5181): 2037-2048. 10.1126/science.8091226.

15. Burnett MS, Strain KJ, Lesnick TG, et al: Reliability of self-reported ancestry among siblings: implications for genetic association studies. Am J Epidemiol. 2006, 163 (5): 486-492. 10.1093/aje/kwj057.

16. Rosenberg NA, Pritchard JK, Weber JL, et al: Genetic structure of human populations. Science. 2002, 298 (5602): 2381-2385. 10.1126/science.1078311.

17. Smith MW, Patterson N, Lautenberger JA, et al: A high-density admixture map for disease gene discovery in African Americans. Am J Hum Genet. 2004, 74 (5): 1001-1013. 10.1086/420856.

18. Brehm JM, Celedón JC: Chronic obstructive pulmonary disease in Hispanics. Am J Respir Crit Care Med. 2008, 177 (5): 473-478.

19. González Burchard E, Borrell LN, Choudhry S, et al: Latino populations: a unique opportunity for the study of race, genetics, and social environment in epidemiological research. Am J Public Health. 2005, 95 (12): 2161-2168. 10.2105/AJPH.2005.068668.

20. Alexander DH, Novembre J, Lange K: Fast model-based estimation of ancestry in unrelated individuals. Genome Res. 2009, 19 (9): 1655-1664. 10.1101/gr.094052.109.

21. Falush D, Stephens M, Pritchard JK: Inference of population structure using multilocus genotype data: linked loci and correlated allele frequencies. Genetics. 2003, 164 (4): 1567-1587.

22. Hubisz MJ, Falush D, Stephens M, Pritchard JK: Inferring weak population structure with the assistance of sample group information. Mol Ecol Resour. 2009, 9 (5): 1322-1332. 10.1111/j.1755-0998.2009.02591.x.

23. Alexander DH, Lange K: Enhancements to the ADMIXTURE algorithm for individual ancestry estimation. BMC Bioinforma. 2011, 12: 246-10.1186/1471-2105-12-246.

24. Nocedal J, Wright SJ: Numerical optimization. 2006, Springer, New York, Available at: http://site.ebrary.com/id/10228772. Accessed January 22, 2012

25. Tang H, Peng J, Wang P, Risch NJ: Estimation of individual admixture: analytical and study design considerations. Genet Epidemiol. 2005, 28 (4): 289-301. 10.1002/gepi.20064.

26. Menozzi P, Piazza A, Cavalli-Sforza L: Synthetic maps of human gene frequencies in Europeans. Science. 1978, 201 (4358): 786-792. 10.1126/science.356262.

27. Bryc K, Auton A, Nelson MR, et al: Genome-wide patterns of population structure and admixture in west Africans and African Americans. Proc Natl Acad Sci U S A. 2010, 107 (2): 786-791. 10.1073/pnas.0909559107.

28. Bryc K, Velez C, Karafet T, et al: Colloquium paper: genome-wide patterns of population structure and admixture among Hispanic/Latino populations. Proc Natl Acad Sci U S A. 2010, 107 (Suppl 2): 8954-8961.

29. Patterson N, Price AL, Reich D: Population structure and eigenanalysis. PLoS Genet. 2006, 2 (12): e190-10.1371/journal.pgen.0020190.

30. Johnstone I: On the distribution of the largest eigenvalue in principal components analsysis. Ann Statist. 2001, 29 (2): 295-327. 10.1214/aos/1009210544.

31. Intarapanich A, Shaw PJ, Assawamakin A, et al: Iterative pruning PCA improves resolution of highly structured populations. BMC Bioinforma. 2009, 10: 382-10.1186/1471-2105-10-382.

32. Limpiti T, Intarapanich A, Assawamakin A, et al: Study of large and highly stratified population datasets by combining iterative pruning principal component analysis and structure. BMC Bioinforma. 2011, 12: 255-10.1186/1471-2105-12-255.

33. Cox TF, Cox MAA: Multidimensional scaling. 2001, Chapman & Hall/CRC, Boca Raton

34. Wang D, Sun Y, Stang P, et al: Comparison of methods for correcting population stratification in a genome-wide association study of rheumatoid arthritis: principal-component analysis versus multidimensional scaling. BMC Proc. 2009, 3 (Suppl 7): S109-10.1186/1753-6561-3-s7-s109.

35. Lee AB, Luca D, Klei L, Devlin B, Roeder K: Discovering genetic ancestry using spectral graph theory. Genet Epidemiol. 2010, 34 (1): 51-59.

36. Anon. 1104, Available at: http://arxiv.org/PS_cache/arxiv/pdf/1104/1104.1162v1.pdf. Accessed January 9, 2012, .1162v1.pdf

37. Sankararaman S, Sridhar S, Kimmel G, Halperin E: Estimating local ancestry in admixed populations. Am J Hum Genet. 2008, 82 (2): 290-303. 10.1016/j.

ajhg.2007.09.022.

38. Pasaniuc B, Sankararaman S, Kimmel G, Halperin E: Inference of locus-specific ancestry in closely related populations. Bioinformatics. 2009, 25 (12): i213-i221. 10.1093/bioinformatics/btp197.

39. Myers S, Bottolo L, Freeman C, McVean G, Donnelly P: A fine-scale map of recombination rates and hotspots across the human genome. Science. 2005, 310 (5746): 321-324. 10.1126/science.1117196.View

40. Li N, Stephens M: Modeling linkage disequilibrium and identifying recombination hotspots using single-nucleotide polymorphism data. Genetics. 2003, 165 (4): 2213-2233.

41. Price AL, Tandon A, Patterson N, et al: Sensitive detection of chromosomal segments of distinct ancestry in admixed populations. PLoS Genet. 2009, 5 (6): e1000519-10.1371/journal.pgen.1000519.

42. Tang H, Coram M, Wang P, Zhu X, Risch N: Reconstructing genetic ancestry blocks in admixed individuals. Am J Hum Genet. 2006, 79 (1): 1-12. 10.1086/504302.

43. Patterson N, Hattangadi N, Lane B, et al: Methods for high-density admixture mapping of disease genes. Am J Hum Genet. 2004, 74 (5): 979-1000. 10.1086/420871.

44. Hoggart CJ, Shriver MD, Kittles RA, Clayton DG, McKeigue PM: Design and analysis of admixture mapping studies. Am J Hum Genet. 2004, 74 (5): 965-978. 10.1086/420855.

45. Montana G, Pritchard JK: Statistical tests for admixture mapping with case–control and cases-only data. Am J Hum Genet. 2004, 75 (5): 771-789. 10.1086/425281.

46. Shriner D, Adeyemo A, Rotimi CN: Joint ancestry and association testing in admixed individuals. PLoS Comput Biol. 2011, 7 (12): e1002325-10.1371/journal.pcbi.1002325.

47. Bruse S, Sood A, Petersen H, et al: New Mexican Hispanic smokers have lower odds of chronic obstructive pulmonary disease and less decline in lung function than non-Hispanic whites. Am J Respir Crit Care Med. 2011, 184 (11): 1254-1260. 10.1164/rccm.201103-0568OC.

48. Kumar R, Seibold MA, Aldrich MC, et al: Genetic ancestry in lung-function predictions. N Engl J Med. 2010, 363 (4): 321-330. 10.1056/NEJMoa0907897.

49. Yang JJ, Cheng C, Devidas M, et al: Ancestry and pharmacogenomics of relapse in acute lymphoblastic leukemia. Nat Genet. 2011, 43 (3): 237-241. 10.1038/ng.763.

50. Choudhry S, Burchard EG, Borrell LN, et al: Ancestry-environment interactions and asthma risk among Puerto Ricans. Am J Respir Crit Care Med. 2006, 174 (10): 1088-1093. 10.1164/rccm.200605-596OC.

CHAPTER 12

HERITABILITY FROM GENOME-WIDE IDENTITY-BY-DESCENT SHARING BETWEEN FULL SIBLINGS

Peter M Visscher, Sarah E Medland, Manuel A. R Ferreira, Katherine I Morley, Gu Zhu, Belinda K Cornes, Grant W Montgomery, Nicholas G Martin

INTRODUCTION

The theoretical basis for the resemblance between relatives due to genetic factors was developed by R.A. Fisher in a now famous and classic paper that reconciled Mendelian and biometrical genetics [1]. Following that theoretical basis, quantitative genetic parameters are estimated from the resemblance between different types of relatives by equating the observed phenotypic covariance to the degree of genetic relationship, which is estimated from pedigree data. The degree of relationship is usually expressed as the coefficient of kinship [2] or the additive coefficient of relationship [2,3]. In a non-inbred population, the coefficient of relationship is the expected proportion of alleles identical-by-descent (IBD) between relatives and determines the additive genetic covariance between a pair of relatives. Maximum likelihood (ML) methods and software have been developed to estimate genetic (co)variances in simple [4] and large complex pedigrees [5–7], for univariate and multivariate models. What all these methods have in common is that they estimate genetic parameters from observed variation between and within families, assuming an underlying model for causative components of variance [3]. For example, in twin studies it is commonly assumed that the variance between families is due to common environmental and additive genetic effects, and that the variance within families reflects individual environmental effects (for monozygotic [MZ] pairs) or both individual environmental and additive genetic effects (for dizygotic [DZ] pairs).

Citation: Peter M Visscher , Sarah E Medland, Manuel A. R Ferreira, Katherine I Morley, Gu Zhu, Belinda K Cornes, Grant W Montgomery, Nicholas G Martin, Heritability from Genome-Wide Identity-by-Descent Sharing between Full Siblings, http://dx.doi.org/10.1371/journal.pgen.0020041.

In human populations, the interplay of genetic, environmental, and cultural factors that cause family resemblance is complex; and crucially, the ultimate separation of nature and nurture effects can generally not be tested empirically through controlled experiments. If the true (unknown) effects causing between-family variance deviate from the assumed model of family resemblance, then the resulting estimates of genetic parameters, and their estimated standard errors (SE), will be biased. This bias could be severe if strong assumptions are necessary to estimate genetic parameters. In the classical twin design, only three underlying parameters are estimated, and strong assumptions regarding the causes of familial resemblance are necessary. For example, the assumption that twin resemblance due to common environmental effects is the same for MZ and DZ pairs is often made. Although some of these assumptions can and have been tested empirically [8,9], the use of twin data to estimate heritability, in particular for traits such as cognitive function, has been controversial [10].

Until now, it has been impossible to exclude a possible confounding between genetic and non-genetic causes of family resemblance. We propose an alternative approach to estimate genetic variance that is based upon the observed proportion of the genome that is shared by relatives and does not make any assumptions about the variation between families.

The actual genome-wide relationship, defined as the proportion of the genome that two relatives share IBD, varies around its expectation because of Mendelian segregation [11–14], except for MZ twins and parent-offspring pairs. We use the term "actual" throughout, but other possibilities are "realized relationships" or "the proportion of the genome-shared IBD." It is possible to estimate this relationship with the use of genetic markers. If these estimates are accurate, then it is, in principle, feasible to estimate genetic parameters within families, obviating the need for contentious assumptions about the sources of between-family variation. In this study, we estimated heritability for height in humans without making any assumptions regarding the causes of resemblance between relatives. We present the relevant theory and estimate the heritability of height from collections of 3,375 full-sib pairs, using genome-wide estimates of actual additive genetic relationships. Bias and accuracy of our estimation approach was explored analytically and by computer simulation. Ours is the first example of an estimate of heritability in humans for which a possible confounding between nature and nurture can be excluded.

RESULTS

Simulated Data

We first assessed bias and accuracy of the estimates of variance components from our method using simulation studies and analytical predictions (see Materials and Methods). Table 1 shows the empirical mean and SE of the ML estimate of the heritability from actual relationships between sibling pairs and statistical power, and their theoretical predictions, for a range of population parameters. As predicted by theory (see Materials and Methods), the SE of the estimates are large, unless the number of pairs is large (10,000), the heritability is large (>0.6), or there is no residual family effect. For 2,500 sib pairs, the SE of the heritability is approximately 0.2 when the true value is 0.8. For 10,000 sib pairs, the range of SE is from 0.08–0.19. The theoretical predictions are accurate, in particular for the special case when the proportion of variance due to non-genetic family effects (f^2) is zero. When the proportion of variance due to non-genetic family effects is zero, the estimate of the heritability is biased downwards, in particular when the sample size is small (Table 1). This is because we constrain variance components to be non-negative in our ML estimation procedure. An analytical prediction of the bias is given in Materials and Methods. When the heritability is large (0.8), its estimate is biased downwards, even when the proportion of variance due to non-genetic family effects was larger than zero. Again this is the result of ML estimation, because the sum of the proportion of variance due to genetic and non-genetic factors cannot be larger than unity.

Table 1. Predicted and Empirical Power and Standard Errors of Heritability Estimation from Genome-Wide IBD Sharing between Sib Pairs

n	h^{2a}	f^{2b}	Simulations Mean $(h^2)^c$	Simulations SE(h^2)	Simulations Power	Theory Mean (h^2)	Theory SE(h^2)	Theory Power[d]
2,500	0.4	0.0	0.27	0.17	0.13	0.21	0.28	0.22
		0.2	0.41	0.28	0.28	0.40	0.39	0.27
	0.6	0.0	0.43	0.22	0.36	0.43	0.26	0.40
		0.2	0.60	0.29	0.58	0.60	0.34	0.56
	0.8	0.0	0.65	0.21	0.66	0.64	0.23	0.66
		0.2	0.70	0.16	0.92	0.80	0.27	0.90
10,000	0.4	0.0	0.31	0.13	0.52	0.31	0.14	0.52
		0.2	0.39	0.19	0.64	0.40	0.20	0.65
	0.6	0.0	0.52	0.12	0.87	0.51	0.13	0.87
		0.2	0.60	0.17	0.97	0.60	0.17	0.97
	0.8	0.0	0.73	0.11	1.00	0.72	0.11	0.99
		0.2	0.75	0.08	1.00	0.80	0.14	1.00

[a]Proportion of phenotypic variance due to additive genetic effects.
[b]Proportion of phenotypic variance due to non-genetic family effects.
[c]The mean and SE of the estimated heritability were calculated using equations given in the Materials and Methods.
[d]Power was calculated at 0.05 significance, using Purcell et al. [43].

Data Application

There were a total of 4,401 quasi-independent sibling pairs with estimates of genome-wide IBD sharing statistics. The average proportion of the genome-shared IBD between the sib pairs (the coefficient of additive genetic variance) was 0.498 (SE 0.0005, standard deviation [SD] 0.036), with a range of 0.374–0.617. The distribution of the genome-wide additive coefficients is shown in Figure 1. The mean and range of the proportion of the genome for which a sibling pair shared two alleles IBD (the coefficient of dominance variance, also termed IBD2) was 0.248 (SE 0.0006, SD 0.040) and 0.116–0.401, respectively. Hence, both mean sharing statistics were slightly lower than the expected values of 0.50 and 0.25, respectively. When comparing the mean sharing statistics to their SE, there was evidence for a small but significant departure from expectation ($p = 0.002$ and 0.0002, for genome-wide additive and dominance coefficients, respectively, assuming a normal distribution of the test statistic). However, the SE is under-estimated because not all pair-wise sib comparisons are independent, so that the departure from expectation is less significant than it appears from the reported p-values. The SD of the mean (additive) IBD and mean IBD2 (dominance) sharing proportions were 0.036 and 0.040, respectively. One quality control measure of our IBD calculations is to test for independence of chromosome-specific additive and dominance relationships. For the combined dataset, 8/231 and 2/231 Spearman rank correlations of the mean IBD sharing between chromosomes were significant at the 0.05 and 0.01 level, respectively, when 12 and 2 were expected under the assumption of independent segregation. For IBD2 sharing the corresponding numbers were 9/231 and 1/231. The observed numbers are not significantly different from expectation under the null hypothesis of independent segregation of chromosomes (the SD of the number of significant correlations at the 0.05 and 0.01 level under the null hypothesis is 3.3 and 1.5, respectively).

Figure 2 shows the empirical variance of genome-wide mean IBD and IBD2 sharing, relative to the expected value from theoretical considerations (see Materials and Methods). There is a remarkably good agreement between theory and data, with a correlation between the theoretical and empirical SDs across chromosomes of 0.98 for both mean IBD sharing and mean IBD2 sharing. The correlation between mean IBD and mean IBD2 sharing for 4,401 pairs was 0.91, close to the theoretical value of 0.89 (Figure 3). This large correlation implies a strong sampling correlation between the estimates of additive and dominance variance.

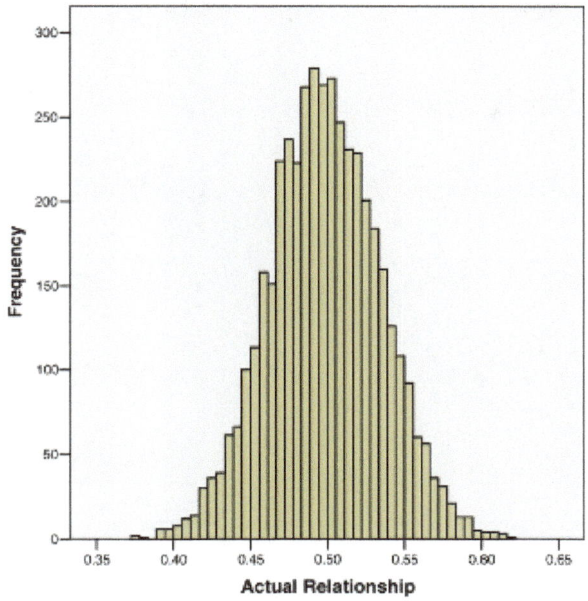

Figure 1. Empirical Distribution of Actual Additive Genetic Relationships of 4,401 Quasi-Independent Pairs of Full Sibs, Histogram of the genome-wide additive genetic relationships of full-sib pairs estimated from genetic markers.

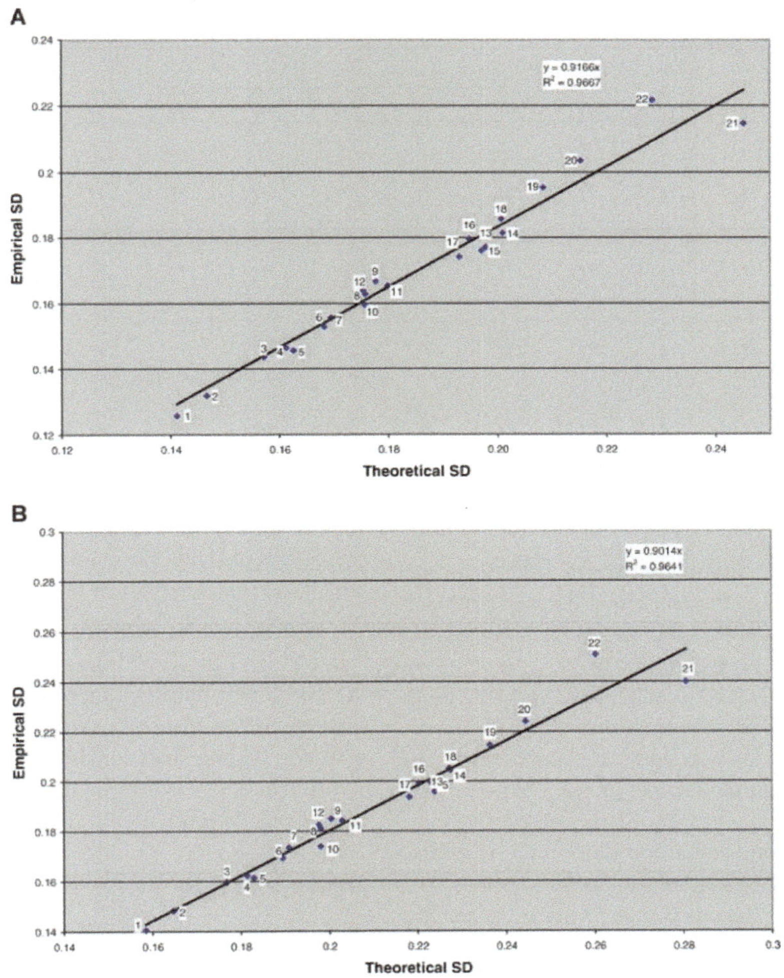

Figure 2. Comparison of the Empirical and Theoretical Standard Deviations in Genome-Wide Sharing in 4,401 Quasi-Independent Pairs of Full Sibs,IBD sharing (A) and genome-wide IBD2 sharing (B) from marker data on 22 autosomes. The x- and y- axes are the theoretical and empirical SD, respectively. Numbers around the regression line indicate chromosomes.

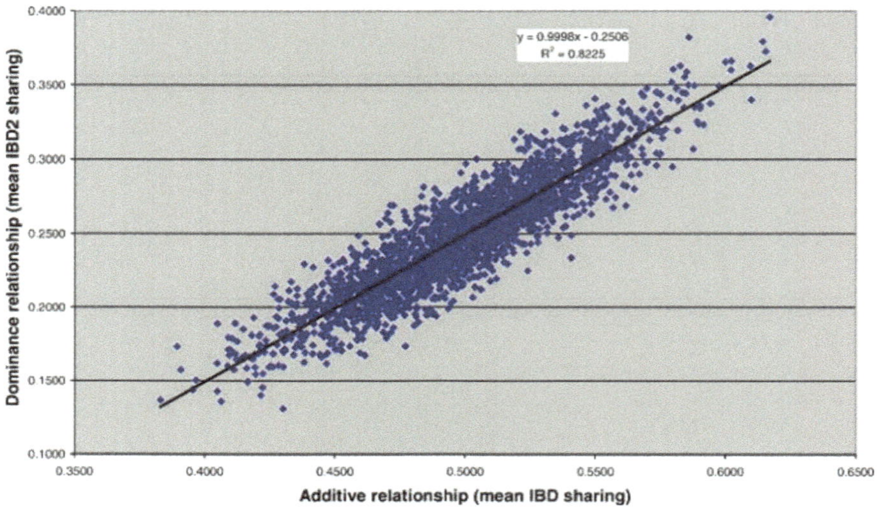

Figure 3. Correlation between Genome-Wide Mean IBD and Mean IBD2 Sharing

Table 2. ML Estimates of Heritability of Height from Genome-Wide IBD Sharing between Sib Pairs

Table 2. ML Estimates of Heritability of Height from Genome-Wide IBD Sharing between Sib Pairs

Data	Model	Estimates (95% CI)		LRT[a]	*p*-Value[b]
		f^2	h^2		
Adolescents (n = 931)	FAE	0.00 (0.00–0.43)	0.80 (0.00–0.90)		
	FE	0.40 (0.34–0.45)		1.850	0.0869
Adults (n = 2,444)	FAE	0.00 (0.00–0.18)	0.80 (0.43–0.86)		
	FE	0.39 (0.36–0.43)		9.817	0.0009
Combined (n = 3,375)	FAE	0.00 (0.00–0.17)	0.80 (0.46–0.85)		
	FE	0.39 (0.36–0.42)		11.553	0.0003

[a]Likelihood ratio test statistic for the null hypothesis that $h^2 = 0$, calculated from the difference in log-likelihood between models FAE and FE.
[b]*p*-Value calculated assuming that the LRT is distributed as zero with a probability of ½ and $\chi_{(1)}^2$ with a probability of ½.
LRT, likelihood ratio test.

The x- and y- axes are the genome-wide additive and dominance relationships, respectively. Each point represents the genome-wide additive and dominance relationship for a sibling pair, estimated from genetic markers (n = 4,401 pairs).

ML estimators of heritability are shown in Table 2 for the two datasets separately and for the combined dataset. For each dataset, two models were fitted: a full model (FAE), containing a non-genetic family effect (F), a genome-wide additive effect (A), a residual error effect (E); and a reduced model containing F and E effects only (FE). In all analyses, the estimate of the residual family component was zero, and the estimate of heritability 0.8. For the combined dataset (n = 3,375 pairs), the 95% confidence interval (CI) was from 0.46 to 0.85 (a SE of approximately 0.1) with strong statistical support (p = 0.0003) for a variance associated with genome-wide IBD. The SE of the estimated proportion of variance due to additive genetic variance (h^2) is large relative to the estimate. However, because the sampling correlation of the estimates of the non-genetic and genetic variance is large and negative, the estimate of the total proportion of variance explained by genetic and non-genetic effects (i.e., the predicted MZ correlation) is more accurate. For the combined dataset, the ML estimate of this proportion is 0.80, with a 95% CI of 0.62–0.85. Hence, we have estimated the equivalent of an MZ correlation without having such pairs in our data. The estimates from the FE model reflect the sibling correlation of 0.40 and 0.39 for the adolescent and adult datasets. Estimates of the proportion of variance due to additive genetic effects from the AE model (not shown in Table 2) were very close to twice the estimates of the proportion of variance due to the family effect in the FE model.

When genome-wide dominance was fitted in addition to F and A, the log-likelihood did not increase significantly for the combined dataset (unpublished data). However, there is unlikely to be sufficient power to distinguish these components with our sample size, consistent with our observed correlation coefficient of 0.89 between the additive genetic and dominance coefficients (Figure 3).

DISCUSSION

We have shown that it is feasible to estimate genetic parameters solely from segregation within families, without making any assumptions regarding an underlying model for between-family effects. In fact, our only assumption in the analysis is that the additive genetic covariance between relatives is proportional to the actual proportion of the genome that is shared IBD. The resulting estimates of the heritability for height (0.80, 95% CI, 0.46–0.85) and residual family effects (0.00, 95% CI, 0.00–0.17) are very close to estimates from twin studies [15], where the information comes from the difference in correlation between MZ and DZ twin pairs. Essentially, we have estimated the same parameters from DZ and full-sib pairs only.

Previously, methods have been proposed to estimate kinship and genetic parameters from marker data when pedigree data are not available, for example, in natural populations [16–18]. Relationship estimation and reconstruction in these methods are based upon identity-by-state sharing of marker alleles. These methods have the same principle as our approach, i.e., first estimating kinship from marker data and subsequently estimating genetic variance from the association between phenotype similarity and estimated kinship. However, there are some important differences between the methods. Firstly, our method is based upon IBD sharing, i.e., we know the pedigree and estimated actual relationships from marker data conditional on the pedigree. The resulting estimates of actual kinship are unbiased and have lower error variance, provided that the pedigree is correct. Secondly, we estimate genetic variance free from possible confounding with environmental factors. In natural populations, even if the kinship were to be estimated without error, there can still be a confounding between genetic and environmental similarities and this could lead to bias.

We do not suggest that all estimation of genetic (co) variance from classical designs that utilize between-family comparisons should be abandoned. On the contrary, such designs, for example, those employing twin families, are in principle powerful enough to separate genetic and non-genetic causes of family resemblance if the statistical models are correct or at least a good approximation of the true underlying causes of variation. With sufficient data, our approach allows the testing of hitherto untestable underlying assumptions in other models and, for large samples, allows the estimation of non-additive genetic variation for disease susceptibility and quantitative traits. Therefore, the two methods should be seen as complementary.

There is a continuum in the estimation of genetic parameters from genome-wide IBD sharing to quantitative trait loci (QTL) mapping. In QTL mapping, variation in IBD sharing is maximal but many estimations/tests are performed. For sib pairs, the variance of IBD sharing at a single location is $^1/_8$ [14,19–21], whereas it is only 0.039^2 genome-wide. Hence, relative to the mean there is about 82 times more variation in IBD sharing between sib pairs at a particular locus than in the genome-wide average [22]. The disadvantage of QTL mapping is that a genome-wide search is performed at many correlated locations, whereas the estimation of genetic variance from genome-wide IBD sharing is a single estimate. An intermediate between the two is to estimate the proportion of additive genetic variance associated with a chromosome [23–25]. The variance in proportion of a chromosome-shared IBD is intermediate between the sharing proportion at a single location and genome-wide, as shown in Table 3. We note that the emphasis in this study is on the estimation of genetic parameters rather than its detection. Hence, in contrast to QTL mapping where hypothesis testing and p-values are important, we have concentrated on the sampling variance of the estimated parameters, because for most traits it is usually known that there is genetic variance, and the scientific question is what proportion of observed variation is genetic.

Table 3. Theoretical Standard Deviation of IBD Sharing between Sibs per Chromosome

Chromosome	Length (Mb)[a]	Length (Morgan)[a]	SD(π)	Equivalent Number of Segments[b]
1	245.13	2.865	0.1411	6.28
2	243.16	2.633	0.1466	5.82
3	198.96	2.251	0.1571	5.06
4	191.51	2.122	0.1612	4.81
5	180.32	2.082	0.1625	4.73
6	169.96	1.922	0.1682	4.42
7	158.06	1.89	0.1694	4.36
8	145.7	1.733	0.1757	4.05
9	135.81	1.687	0.1777	3.96
10	134.6	1.735	0.1756	4.05
11	134.08	1.638	0.1798	3.87
12	131.43	1.742	0.1753	4.07
13	94.45	1.289	0.1978	3.19
14	85.13	1.238	0.2009	3.10
15	79.69	1.302	0.1971	3.22
16	89.51	1.342	0.1948	3.29
17	81.18	1.375	0.1929	3.36
18	75.33	1.242	0.2007	3.10
19	62.78	1.122	0.2084	2.88
20	61.38	1.025	0.2153	2.70
21	33.22	0.685	0.2451	2.08
22	33.11	0.861	0.2284	2.40
Total	2,764.5	35.781		84.79

[a]From [41].
[b]The number of independent loci for which the mean variance in IBD sharing would be equivalent to the observed variance for the whole chromosome (= $1/[8\text{var}(\pi)]$).

Although our estimates of the variation in mean IBD and IBD2 sharing per chromosome are very similar to the theoretical values (Figure 2) and consistent with recently reported genome-wide sharing statistics from a sample of 498 sib pairs [22], a few caveats are required. Firstly, the theoretical value may be too low for the true variance in IBD sharing on a chromosome because in reality there may be more crossovers than modeled [13,14]. Secondly, the empirical variance of IBD sharing is likely to be an underestimate because the marker information was not perfect. If we assume that our genome-wide average multipoint marker information content was approximately 80%, then we would expect to find a regression slope of the empirical on theoretical SD in IBD sharing of $\sqrt{0.80} = 0.89$, close to the observed value of 0.92 (Figure 2A). Nevertheless, the correlations of 0.98 between empirical and theoretical values are extremely high.

We detected a small genome-wide deviation of the observed IBD sharing statistics from expectation. Genome-wide transmission distortion, which results in excess allele sharing between relatives, has been reported previously [26]. Our results were driven by a deficit of the probability of sharing two alleles IBD, hence we do not replicate the findings of [26] with our large sample of 4,401 pairs.

Our simulation studies confirmed that a large number of pairs is needed for accurate estimation, and showed that the estimates of heritability were biased downwards when there was no underlying source of non-genetic family resemblance. This bias is the result of ML estimation because of the usual constraints that estimated variance components have to be non-negative and that the sum of the partitioned variance ratios is bounded by zero and one. The observed bias is not particular to our method because it applies to any variance partitioning approach by ML, in particular when sampling variances are large [27,28].

We have estimated a single additive genetic variance from genome-wide segregation of marker loci within families, after adjusting phenotypes for the fixed effects of sex and age at measurement. However, genetic variances for males and females and younger and older siblings may be different, and the genetic correlation across these groups may be smaller than unity. Although we have ignored these potential sources of heterogeneity of genetic variance in this study because of sample size considerations, models that include, for example, sex-limitation effects are, in principle, straightforward to implement.

We have ignored the contribution of the sex chromosomes to genome-wide IBD. In humans, the X chromosome accounts for 4% of genes and 5% of physical length [29]. If all chromosomes account for genetic variation in proportion to the number of genes or physical length, then our estimate of heritability will be biased downwards by about 4% to 5%.

Although our sample size of 3,375 was sufficient to estimate the heritability of height with reasonable accuracy, for phenotypes with smaller heritability (and to distinguish additive from dominance variance), larger sample sizes are necessary. Such large datasets are in the process of being generated, either from large national studies or by combining samples across countries. For example, the GenomEUtwin study will accrue over 10,000 sib pairs for linkage studies [30]. Therefore, in the near future we will be able to estimate unbiased genetic parameters for traits that have been controversial in the past due to the assumptions regarding the (non-genetic) resemblance between relatives. If a large population resource of relatives with measured phenotypes were to be available, then a selective genotyping strategy in which only concordant and discordant pairs are genotyped may be efficient in estimating quantitative genetic parameters accurately, for the same reason that such a design can be powerful in gene mapping studies [31,32].

Our application was on a single quantitative trait and using a simple pedigree structure. However, the method is entirely general and can be applied to disease phenotypes, multiple traits, and large arbitrary pedigrees. All that is required is genome-wide estimates of IBD sharing between relatives, observations on relevant phenotypes, large samples, and software to estimate components of (co)variance.

There are limitations of the applied method, the main one being that large sample sizes are required with dense marker coverage of genotyped individuals. This may be unachievable for most single labs now, but future large population-based studies that have a family component, or pooling of sample resources across studies, will have the desired effect of increasing sample size. A second limitation is that sufficient markers need to be genotyped to obtain an accurate estimate of genome-wide sharing statistics. This is less of a problem because many samples that are suitable for our suggested analyses are genotyped for linkage studies, and marker density is likely to increase in the near future because of the availability of relatively cheap single nucleotide polymorphism genotyping. With the advent of high density single nucleotide polymorphism genotyping platforms, the error in estimation of genome-wide IBD sharing between relatives is likely to be small, and we have assumed, in the present study, that it is negligible. If the estimation of genome-wide IBD sharing is less than 100% accurate, then the variation in IBD sharing between pairs is less than the true variation, resulting in less powerful analysis but still unbiased estimates [33]. With less complete marker coverage, the estimate of the proportion of alleles shared IBD is unbiased $(E(\pi|\hat{\pi}) = \hat{\pi})$ but has larger prediction error variance. For a single location in the genome, we derived the prediction error variance as: $\mathrm{var}(\pi|\hat{\pi}) = \frac{1}{4}P_1(1-P_1) + P_2(1-P_2) - P_1P_2$, with P_i, with P_i the probability of having i alleles IBD; note that this variance could be used as a weight in gene mapping studies. To a first order approximation, the sampling variance of the estimate of the heritability, relative to the situation of perfect marker information, is increased by the reciprocal of the average genome-wide information content [34]. A third limitation is that it is difficult to disentangle additive from non-additive effects. However, with sufficient data the large correlation between additive and dominance coefficients is not an issue, and one could even consider estimating additional non-additive effects, for example additive-by-additive or additive-by-dominance effects.

In conclusion, we have shown that it is feasible to estimate genetic variance entirely within families, by correlating phenotypes and genome-wide similarity. Our assumption-free method facilitates a complete separation of genetic and environmental causes of family resemblance and will allow the estimation and testing of non-additive sources of variation.

MATERIALS AND METHODS

Variance of genome-wide IBD sharing.

The variance of the proportion of chromosome segments that are IBD between relatives has been derived by a number of authors for pairs of full sibs [13,14,23,33,35], complex pedigrees [12,36,37], for inbred individuals [38], and for experimental backcross populations [39,40]. In the case of full sibs we give a derivation for both the additive and dominance component of covariance, and their correlation, following the approach of Hill [39].

Additive effects.

For a given sib pair, the genome-wide mean IBD sharing (π) is the sum of the proportion shared from the paternal (p) and maternal (m) contribution,

$$\pi = \tfrac{1}{2}\pi^{\mathrm{p}} + \tfrac{1}{2}\pi^{\mathrm{m}}, \text{ and } \mathrm{var}(\pi) = \tfrac{1}{4}\mathrm{var}(\pi^{\mathrm{p}}) + \tfrac{1}{4}\mathrm{var}(\pi^{\mathrm{m}}) \quad (1)$$

Hence, to calculate the variance it is sufficient to consider the contribution from a single parent only. For parent k, the sharing of alleles by progeny depends on the proportion of alleles shared due to the parent's paternal or maternal gamete. Let δ_i be an indicator variable for locus i, which is one if both sibs have inherited the paternal allele or both sibs have inherited the maternal allele, and zero otherwise. Then,

$$E(\delta_i) = \tfrac{1}{2} \text{ and } \mathrm{var}(\delta_i) = \tfrac{1}{4} \quad (2)$$

The covariance of the indicator variables at two loci (i and j) is:

$$\begin{aligned}\mathrm{cov}(\delta_i,\delta_j) &= \mathrm{E}(\delta_i\delta_j) - \mathrm{E}(\delta_i)\mathrm{E}(\delta_j) = \tfrac{1}{4}[1 + (1-2r)^2] - (\tfrac{1}{2})^2 \\ &= \tfrac{1}{4}(1-2r)^2.\end{aligned} \quad (3)$$

Assuming the Haldane mapping function, the covariance can

be written as:

$$\mathrm{cov}(\delta_i, \delta_j) = \tfrac{1}{4}\exp(-4d_{ij}) \tag{4}$$

with d_{ij} the distance (in Morgan) between the loci. For n loci, the variance of chromosome-wide sharing between two sibs is:

$$\mathrm{var}(\pi^k) = (1/n^2)(\tfrac{1}{4})\Sigma\Sigma\exp(-4d_{ij}) \tag{5}$$

(following [39]). If n becomes very large this equation can be expressed as an integral [12,39], $\mathrm{var}(\pi^k) = \frac{1}{4}\int_0^l \int_0^l e^{-4|x_1-x_2|}dx_1dx_2 = \frac{1}{8l^2}(l - r_{2l}/2)$ with l the length of the chromosome (in Morgan) and r_{2l} the recombination fraction for a segment of length 2l. Hence, the total variance in IBD sharing between two siblings for chromosome i of length l is:

$$\mathrm{var}(\pi_i) = 2(\tfrac{1}{4})\mathrm{var}(\pi^k) = (16l^2)^{-1}(l - \tfrac{1}{2}r_{2l}) \tag{6}$$

Finally, genome-wide π is, $\pi_g = (1/L)\,\Sigma(l_i\,\pi_i)$, with $L = \Sigma(l_i)$, and:

$$\begin{aligned}\mathrm{var}(\pi_g) &= (1/L^2)\Sigma l_i^2(16l_i)^{-1}(1 - \tfrac{1}{2}r_{2l_i}/l_i)\\ &= [1/(16L^2)][L - \tfrac{1}{2}\Sigma r_{2l_i}]\\ &\approx 1/(16L) - 1/(3L^2),\end{aligned} \tag{7}$$

because there are 22 autosomes and $r_{2li} \approx \tfrac{1}{2}$. These results are the same as those of Guo [11], whose derivations were based upon Markov chains. They imply, that to a first order approximation, the variance in genome-wide IBD sharing is a function of the total genome length only [12,36,38,39]. For L = 35 Morgan, the SD of genome-wide IBD sharing is approximately 0.039. Table 3 shows a breakdown in the variance of IBD sharing per chromosome and the equivalent number of independent loci. It was constructed using the above equations, with physical and genetic lengths from [41], and using the sex-averaged recombination map. For comparison, the SD of the proportion of alleles shared at a given locus is 0.354.

Dominance.

Dominance variance is a function of the probability that two siblings share both alleles IBD (= IBD2). In a non-inbred population, this probability is also called the coefficient of fraternity [2]. The prior probability that full sibs share two alleles IBD is ¼, and the mean and variance of an indicator variable that is one if both alleles are shared IBD and zero otherwise is ¼ and $^3/_{16}$, respectively. Note that the variance of IBD2 sharing at a single locus is 1.5 times the variance of mean IBD sharing. The probability that the sibs share two alleles IBD at a linked locus, given that they are IBD2, is $(1 - r)^4 + 2[(1 - r)r]^2 + r^4 = [(1 - r)^2 + r^2]^2$. Hence the covariance of the indicator variable (δ) at loci i and j is:

$$\mathrm{cov}(\delta_i, \delta_j) = E(\delta_i\delta_j) - E(\delta_i)E(\delta_j) = \tfrac{1}{4}[(1 - r)^2 + r^2]^2 - 1/16 \tag{8}$$

After some algebra it can be shown that the variance of the mean IBD2 sharing (π_{di}) on a chromosome of length l is:

$$\mathrm{var}(\pi_{di}) = [1/(16l^2)][(5/4)l - \tfrac{1}{2}r_{2l} - (1/16)r_{4l}] \tag{9}$$

The genome-wide variance in mean IBD2 sharing is:

$$\begin{aligned}\mathrm{var}(\pi_d) &= [1/(16L^2)][(5/4)L - \tfrac{1}{2}\Sigma r_{2l_i} - (1/16)\Sigma r_{4l_i}]\\ &\approx 5/(64L) - 99/(256L^2) \approx 5/(64L) - 1/(3L^2).\end{aligned} \tag{10}$$

Hence, the variance of the genome-wide IBD2 sharing is larger (by about 30% if L = 35) than the variance of the genome-wide mean IBD sharing. The correlation between mean genome-wide allele sharing and mean genome-wide IBD2 sharing is the ratio of the SD,

$$r(\pi_a, \pi_d) = \sigma(\pi_a)/\sigma(\pi_d) \approx [1/(16L)/\{5/(64L)\}]^{0.5} = 0.89 \tag{11}$$

The actual relationship between full sibs can be estimated with genetic markers. For fully informative markers and close relatives, only a few markers are needed per chromosome to capture the proportion of alleles shared IBD [23,24]. This is because the number of recombination events per chromosome is small.

Sampling variance of estimators of genetic variance.

For n sib pairs, the simplest estimation procedure is to apply the Haseman-Elston regression analysis [33] of the squared difference between the phenotypes (Y_{i1} and Y_{i2}) of the ith pair of siblings on the estimate of their genome-wide IBD proportion (π_i),

$$(Y_{i1} - Y_{i2})^2 = \alpha + \beta\pi_I. \tag{12}$$

The parameter β is proportional to the within-family additive genetic variance, adjusted for inbreeding in the parents,

$$\beta = -2\sigma_A^2[1 - \tfrac{1}{2}F_{mum} - \tfrac{1}{2}F_{dad}] \tag{13}$$

[2,3,33]. We will assume that parents are not inbred, so that the regression slope equals minus twice the additive genetic variance. Then, an estimate of the narrow sense heritability is simply,

$$\hat{h}^2 = -\hat{\beta}/(2\hat{\sigma}_p^2) \tag{14}$$

with $\hat{\sigma}_p^2$ an estimate of the total phenotypic variance. If we ignore the sampling correlation between the estimate of the regression coefficient and the total phenotypic variance, then the sampling variance of the heritability is, using a Taylor series expansion [2]:

$$\begin{aligned}\mathrm{var}(\hat{h}^2) &\approx (\tfrac{1}{4})[\beta/\sigma_p^2]^2[\mathrm{var}(\hat{\beta})/\beta^2 + \mathrm{var}(\hat{\sigma}_p^2)/\sigma_p^4]\\ &= h^4[\mathrm{var}(\hat{\beta})/(4\sigma_p^4h^4) + 1/n].\end{aligned} \tag{15}$$

The variance of the regression coefficient is approximately,

$$\mathrm{var}(\hat{\beta}) \approx \left[8(1 - t)^2/(n\mathrm{var}(\pi) - 4h^4/n)\right]\sigma_p^4 \tag{16}$$

with t the sib intra-class correlation [20,21]. Hence, the sampling variance of the estimate of the narrow sense heritability is, approximately,

$$\text{var}(\hat{h}^2) \approx 2(1-t)^2/[n\text{var}(\pi)] \quad (17)$$

This is fully analogous to the estimation of the proportion of variance explained by a single QTL, the only difference being the variance in genome-wide IBD sharing. The non-centrality-parameter (NCP) for a test of significance of genome-wide additive genetic variance is,

$$\text{NCP} = nh^4\text{var}(\pi)/[2(1-t)^2] \quad (18)$$

which reduces to the form given by Sham and Purcell [20] and Visscher and Hopper [21] for a single QTL when var(π) = 1/8. Following the derivations in Sham and Purcell [20] and Visscher and Hopper [21], the SE of the estimate of the heritability and NCP when using both the squared difference and squared sum of the sib pairs are, approximately,

$$\text{var}(\hat{h}^2) \approx (1-t^2)^2/[(1+t^2)\{n\text{var}(\pi)\}] \quad (19)$$

and

$$\text{NCP} = nh^4\text{var}(\pi)(1+t^2)/(1-t^2)^2 \quad (20)$$

Hence, power calculations for QTL mapping can be used to assess the sample size required to "detect" genome-wide additive genetic variance. For example, to detect a heritability of a given size is equivalent to detecting a QTL at a fully informative locus explaining q^2 of the phenotypic variance when h^4 var(π) = $(^1/_8)q^4$, i.e., a QTL explaining about $0.11h^2$ of the phenotypic variance.

ML estimation uses more information than the difference between the sib pairs, and the resulting estimate of the heritability is more accurate. For a single QTL asymptotically (large sample size and a QTL that explains a small amount of variance), the sampling variance of the ML estimator is that of the least squares estimator, when both the squared differences and sums are used in the regression analysis [20,21]. For genome-wide estimation, the proportion of variance explained by π is small (~ $0.11h^2$), so it seems reasonable to use the predictions for the regression analysis. However, the predictions differ dramatically if there is no other source of family resemblance than sharing of genetic effects. The following approximate results were derived assuming the simple equation:

$$\hat{t}_0 = \hat{f}^2 + 0.5\hat{h}^2 \quad (21)$$

with $\hat{t}_0$ the estimate of the intra-class correlation under the null hypothesis of no genome-wide additive genetic effect, $\hat{f}^2$ the estimate of the proportion of the variance due to residual familial effects under the alternative hypothesis, and $\hat{h}^2$ the estimate of the heritability under the full model. Equation 21 is a good approximation because the intra-class correlation, which is estimated relatively precisely under the reduced model, is essentially partitioned into a genetic and non-genetic component in the full model. The sampling correlation between the estimates of f^2 and h^2 is approximately −1. If there are no constraints imposed on the estimates, then, using results from [42],

$$\text{var}(\hat{t}_0) \approx (1-t^2)^2/n \quad (22)$$

$$\text{var}(\hat{h}^2) \approx (1-t^2)^2/[n\,\text{var}(\pi)(1+t^2)] \quad (23)$$

(from [20,21]). By difference,

$$\text{var}(\hat{f}^2) \approx \text{var}(\hat{t}_0) + \frac{1}{4}\text{var}(\hat{h}^2) \approx \frac{1}{4}\text{var}(\hat{h}^2) \quad (24)$$

Hence, the SE of the estimate of the non-genetic familial resemblance is approximately half of the SE of the estimate of the genome-wide heritability. The above SE of the estimates can be used to calculate the probability that the ML estimate is zero, using standard normal distribution truncation theory [3] with truncation values of $-f^2/\sigma(\hat{f}^2)$ and $-h^2/\sigma(\hat{h}^2)$, respectively. This was validated using simulations (unpublished data).

Conditional on $f^2 = 0$.

When the true residual familial component is zero, the ML estimate is zero with a probability of ½, and > 0 with a probability of ½ [27,28]. When the estimate of $f^2 = 0$ then the estimate of the heritability is approximately twice the intra-class correlation of the sibs. Hence, asymptotically,

$$\hat{h}^2 | \hat{f}^2 = 0 \sim N(h^2, 4(1-t^2)^2/n) \quad (25)$$

When the estimate of $f^2 > 0$, the mean estimate of the familial component is, approximately,

$$E(\hat{f}^2 | \hat{f}^2 > 0) = i\sigma(\hat{f}^2) \quad (26)$$

with i the mean value of a truncated standard normal distribution. For a truncation value of 0, as is the case here, i = 0.798 [3]. The variance of the truncated distribution is:

$$\text{var}(\hat{f}^2 | \hat{f}^2 > 0) = (1-i^2)\text{var}(\hat{f}^2) \quad (27)$$

Taking the whole of the distribution of the estimate of f^2 gives the mean and variances as:

$$E(\hat{f}^2 | f^2 = 0) = 0.5i\sigma(\hat{f}^2) = 0.4\sigma(\hat{f}^2) \quad (28)$$

and

$$\text{var}(\hat{f}^2 | f^2 = 0) = 0.5(1-0.5i^2)\text{var}(\hat{f}^2) = 0.34\text{var}(\hat{f}^2) \quad (29)$$

Similarly for the estimate of the heritability,

$$E(\hat{h}^2 | f^2 = 0) \approx h^2 - i\sigma(\hat{f}^2) \quad (30)$$

and

$$\mathrm{var}(\hat{h}^2 | f^2 = 0) \approx 0.5(1 - 0.5i^2)\mathrm{var}(\hat{h}^2) = 0.34\mathrm{var}(\hat{h}^2) \quad (31)$$

Equations 23, 30, and 31 were used to predict the mean and SE of the estimate of the heritability and were found to be close to simulation results for large samples (Table 1). For small samples the distribution of the estimates of the two variance ratios could be approximated by a truncated bivariate distribution. This situation is more complex because the probability that either estimate is zero as well as the probability that the estimates are constrained at unity needs to be considered jointly. If there is no residual non-genetic family resemblance then the SE of the estimate of the heritability is nearly halved relative to the case where such effects are present. The case of no residual family resemblance is very unlikely for QTL mapping (where the effects of genes elsewhere in the genome and common environmental effects cause resemblance) but realistic for genome-wide analysis of highly heritable phenotypes. The reduction in SE is at the expense of a downward bias in the estimate of the heritability.

Models.

The basic additive genetic model, fitted in both the simulation study and data application, is $Y_{ij} = \mu + F_i + A_{ij} + E_{ij}$, with μ the fixed effects of the mean and F, A, and E the random effects of non-genetic family, additive genetic, and residual factors, respectively. The covariance between the phenotypes of two siblings is modeled as $\mathrm{cov}(Y_{i1},Y_{i2}) = \mathrm{var}(F_i) + \mathrm{cov}(A_{i1},A_{i2}) = \sigma_F^2 + \pi_{a(i)}\sigma_A^2$, and $\mathrm{cov}(Y_{ij},Y_{kl}) = 0$ if $i \neq j$. Extensions to non-additive models are straightforward, in principle. For example, the covariance for a model containing dominance (D) and additive-by-additive (AA) effects is: $\mathrm{cov}(Y_{i1},Y_{i2}) = \sigma_F^2 + \pi_{a(i)} \sigma_A^2 + \pi_{d(i)}\sigma_D^2 + \pi_{a(i)}\pi_{a(i)}\sigma_{AA}^2$.

Simulation.

Simulations were performed to validate the predictions of the sampling variance of the heritability and statistical power. Genome-wide IBD sharing between pairs of sibs and their phenotypes were simulated from a simple model,

$$\pi_i \sim N(0.5, 0.04^2), Y_{ij} = \mu + F_i + A_{ij} + E_{ij} \quad (32)$$

with μ, F, A, and E defined as before, with distributions

$$F_i \sim N(0, f^2), A_{i1} \sim N(0, h^2), A_{i2}|A_{i1} \sim N(\pi_{a(i)}A_{i1}, (1 - \pi^2_{a(i)})h^2) \text{ and } E_{ij} \sim N(0, 1 - f^2 - h^2). \quad (33)$$

Regression and ML analyses were performed (for details, see [21]). The number of pairs (n) in the simulation was either 2,500 or 10,000; heritability values were 0.4, 0.6, and 0.8; and the proportion of variance due to non-genetic family effects was either 0.0 or 0.2. For each set of population parameters, 1,000 replicates were run. Power was calculated using Web-based software for power of QTL analysis [43] at a type-I error rate of 0.05, which is appropriate because we performed a single hypothesis test.

Application to data.

We estimated the mean and variance of genome-wide IBD sharing from 4,401 quasi-independent full-sib pairs, and applied the ML estimation method to 3,375 quasi-independent full-sib pairs with both marker data and phenotypic measurements on height. These data were collected from two cohorts of Australian twins and their siblings. Phenotypes for the adolescent cohort were collected in the context of continuing longitudinal studies examining risk factors for melanoma [44] and cognitive functioning [45]. For this cohort, height was measured during a clinical examination using a stadiometer at ages 12, 14, and 16; the most recent measurement being used in the current analyses. In the first instance phenotypes for the adult cohort (consisting of twins registered with the Australian Twin Registry born prior to 1971) were collected from self-report questionnaires. Through their subsequent participation in a variety of studies, 58% of the twins included here attended a clinical examination in which height was measured using a stadiometer [15,46]; self-reported height was analyzed if no clinical measurement existed. Correlation between clinically measured and self-reported height was 0.92 in individuals measured both ways [15]. Age at time of measurement was used as a covariate in both cohorts.

Genotypic information was available for a subset of the adolescent and adult participants. For the adolescent cohort, genotypic information was available for 1,201 individuals from 500 families, yielding 950 quasi-independent full-sib pairs. Genotypic information was available for up to 791 autosomal markers. The number of markers per participant in the current study ranged from 211 to 791, with a mean and SD of 588 and 194, respectively, giving an average marker spacing of 6 cM per genotyped individual. The genotyping, error checking, and cleaning of these data have been described in detail elsewhere [47]. For the adult cohort, genotypic information was available for 3,804 individuals from 1,512 families, yielding 3,451 quasi-independent full-sib pairs. Genotypic information was available for up to 1,717 autosomal markers. The number of markers per participant in the current study ranging from 201 to 1,717, with mean and SD of 628 and 264, respectively, and the average marker spacing was 5.6 cM per individual. Details of the genotyping, error checking, and cleaning strategies of these data are given elsewhere [48].

Phenotypes for height were missing on 481 individuals, eight in the adolescent cohort and 473 in the adult cohort. The number of sib pairs for which both individuals had a measured phenotype for the adolescent cohort, the adult cohort, and the combined cohort was 931, 2,444, and 3,375, respectively.

IBD probabilities at 1 cM intervals were calculated using Merlin [49], and the estimate of chromosome and genome-wide IBD sharing was enumerated by averaging the IBD probabilities over the length of a chromosome and the whole genome, respectively.

Each dataset was first adjusted for fixed effects, using a general linear model in which sex was fitted as a fixed factor and age at measurement as a linear covariate. Residuals from this analysis were standardized by the residual variance for each dataset because there was some evidence of heterogeneity of variance: the residual SD for the adolescent and adult dataset was 7.71 cm and 6.89 cm, respectively.

ML analysis was performed using Mx [4]. The full model, termed FAE, contained F and A and E. The covariance between the phenotypes of sibs one and two of pair i was modeled as $cov(Y_{i1},Y_{i2}) = \sigma_F^2 + \pi_{a(i)}\sigma_A^2$, with $\pi_{a(i)}$ the estimate of the genome-wide actual additive relationship of the sibling pair. Reduced models FE and AE were subsequently fitted. A likelihood-ratio-test was performed to test the null hypothesis that A was zero, by comparing the MLs of models FAE and FE. A p-value was calculated assuming that the test statistic has an asymptotic distribution that is 0 with a probability of ½ and a one degree of freedom χ^2 with a probability of ½ [27,28]. CIs of the variance ratios were calculated by Mx and verified by a profile likelihood approach, in which one variance component at a time was changed from its ML value, while maximizing the likelihood for the remaining parameters, until a drop in twice the log-likelihood of 3.84 was reached. In addition to estimating the ML estimate of the variance components for F, A, and E, the ML estimate of (F + A) and its 95% CI were estimated. This was performed because the estimates of F and A have a large negative sampling correlation, so that the estimate of their sum is more precise than the estimate of the individual components.

ACKNOWLEDGMENTS

The authors thank Pam Saunders, Ann Eldridge, and Marlene Grace for phenotype collection; Dixie Statham and Alison MacKenzie for project coordination; Anjali Henders and Megan Campbell for managing sample processing and preparation; David Smyth and Scott Gordon for data management; David Evans for his role in integration of the genome scans; David Duffy for collation of the genetic map; and the twins for their generous participation. For genome scans of the adult twins, we acknowledge and thank the Mammalian Genotyping Service, Marshfield, Wisconsin, United States (Director, Dr. James Weber) for genotyping under a grant to Dr. Daniel T. O'Connor, Dr. Eline Slagboom, Dr. Bas Heijmans, and Dr. Dorret Boomsma for the Leiden genome scan; Dr. Peter Reed for the Gemini genome scan; and Dr. Jeff Hall for the Sequana genome scan. We thank Dr. Kelly Ewen White and Mary Jewell, respectively, for their supervision of these scans. We thank Bill Hill for helpful comments.

Author Contributions

NGM initiated and led the studies from which the data were collected. PMV and NGM conceived the main idea for this study. SEM, MARF, KIM, GZ, and BKC error-checked, cleaned, and stored genotypic and phenotypic data, estimated IBD probabilities, and performed preliminary statistical analyses. GWM supervised the storage and quality control of DNA samples and genotypes. PMV performed theoretical calculations, statistical analyses and simulation studies, and wrote the manuscript.

REFERENCES

1. Fisher RA (1918) The correlation between relatives on the supposition of Mendelian inheritance. Trans Roy Soc Edin 52: 399–433.
2. Lynch M, Walsh B (1998) Genetics and analysis of quantitative traits. Sunderland (Massachusetts): Sinauer Associates. 980 p.
3. Falconer DS, Mackay TFC (1996) Introduction to quantitative genetics. London: Longman Press. 180 p.
4. Neale MC, Boker SM, Xie G, Maes HH (2003) Mx: Statistical modeling. Richmond (Virginia): Virginia Institute for Psychiatric and Behavioral Genetics.
5. Patterson HD, Thompson R (1971) Recovery of interblock information when block sizes are unequal. Biometrika 58: 545–555.
6. Lange K, Westlake J, Spence MA (1976) Extensions to pedigree analysis. III. Variance components by the scoring method. Ann Hum Genet 39: 485–491.
7. Gilmour AR, Thompson R, Cullis BR (1995) Average information REML: An efficient algorithm for variance parameter estimation in linear mixed models. Biometrics 51: 1440–1450.
8. Hettema JM, Neale MC, Kendler KS (1995) Physical similarity and the equal-environment assumption in twin studies of psychiatric disorders. Behav Genet 25: 327–335.
9. Kendler KS, Neale MC, Kessler RC, Heath AC, Eaves LJ (1993) A test of the equal-environment assumption in twin studies of psychiatric illness. Behav Genet 23: 21–27.
10. Devlin B, Daniels M, Roeder K (1997) The heritability of IQ. Nature 388: 468–471.
11. Guo SW (1996) Variation in genetic identity among relatives. Hum Hered 46: 61–70.
12. Stam P (1980) The distribution of the fraction of the genome identical-by-descent in finite random mating populations. Genet Res 35: 131–155.
13. Risch N, Lange K (1979) Application of a recombination model in calculating the variance of sib pair genetic identity. Ann Hum Genet 43: 177–186.
14. Suarez BK, Reich T, Fishman PM (1979) Variability in sib pair genetic identity. Hum Hered 29: 37–41.
15. Silventoinen K, Sammalisto S, Perola M, Boomsma DI, Cornes BK, et al. (2003) Heritability of adult body height: A comparative study of twin cohorts in eight countries. Twin Res 6: 399–408.
16. Thomas SC (2005) The estimation of genetic relationships using molecular markers and their efficiency in estimating heritability in natural populations. Philos Trans R Soc Lond B Biol Sci 360: 1457–1467.
17. Ritland K (2000) Marker-inferred relatedness as a tool for detecting heritability in nature. Mol Ecol 9: 1195–1204.
18. Lynch M, Ritland K (1999) Estimation of pair-wise relatedness with molecular markers. Genetics 152: 1753–1766.
19. Rijsdijk FV, Hewitt JK, Sham PC (2001) Analytic power calculation for QTL linkage analysis of small pedigrees. Eur J Hum Genet 9: 335–340.
20. Sham PC, Purcell S (2001) Equivalence between Haseman-Elston and variance-components linkage analyses for sib pairs. Am J Hum Genet 68: 1527–1532.
21. Visscher PM, Hopper JL (2001) Power of regression and maximum likelihood methods to map QTL from sib-pair and DZ twin data. Ann Hum Genet 65: 583–601.
22. Gagnon A, Beise J, Vaupel JW (2005) Genome-wide

identity-by-descent sharing among CEPH siblings. Genet Epidemiol 29: 215–224.

23. Goldgar DE (1990) Multipoint analysis of human quantitative genetic variation. Am J Hum Genet 47: 957–967.
24. Visscher PM (1996) Proportion of the variation in genetic composition in backcrossing programs explained by genetic markers. J Hered 87: 136–138.
25. Schork NJ (2001) Genome partitioning and whole-genome analysis. Adv Genet 42: 299–322.
26. Zollner S, Wen X, Hanchard NA, Herbert MA, Ober C, et al. (2004) Evidence for extensive transmission distortion in the human genome. Am J Hum Genet 74: 62–72.
27. Self SG, Liang KY (1987) Asymptotic properties of maximum likelihood estimators and likelihood ratio tests under nonstandard conditions. J Am Stat Assoc 82: 605–610.
28. Stram DO, Lee JW (1994) Variance components testing in the longitudinal mixed effects model. Biometrics 50: 1171–1177.
29. Ross MT, Grafham DV, Coffey AJ, Scherer S, McLay K, et al. (2005) The DNA sequence of the human X chromosome. Nature 434: 325–337.
30. Peltonen L (2003) GenomEUtwin: A strategy to identify genetic influences on health and disease. Twin Res 6: 354–360.
31. Risch N, Zhang H (1995) Extreme discordant sib pairs for mapping quantitative trait loci in humans. Science 268: 1584–1589.
32. Risch NJ, Zhang H (1996) Mapping quantitative trait loci with extreme discordant sib pairs: Sampling considerations. Am J Hum Genet 58: 836–843.
33. Haseman JK, Elston RC (1972) The investigation of linkage between a quantitative trait and a marker locus. Behav Genet 2: 3–19.
34. Sham PC, Cherny SS, Purcell S, Hewitt JK (2000) Power of linkage versus association analysis of quantitative traits, by use of variance-components models, for sibship data. Am J Hum Genet 66: 1616–1630.
35. Guo SW (1994) Computation of identity-by-descent proportions shared by two siblings. Am J Hum Genet 54: 1104–1109.
36. Guo SW (1995) Proportion of genome shared identical by descent by relatives: Concept, computation, and applications. Am J Hum Genet 56: 1468–1476.
37. Guo SW (1996) Gametogenesis processes and multilocus gene identity by descent. Am J Hum Genet 58: 408–419.
38. Franklin IR (1977) The distribution of the proportion of the genome which is homozygous by descent in inbred individuals. Theor Popul Biol 11: 60–80.
39. Hill WG (1993) Variation in genetic composition in backcrossing programs. J Hered 84: 212–213.
40. Stam P, Zeven AC (1981) The theoretical proportion of the donor genome in near-isogenic lines of self-fertilizers bred by backcrossing. Euphytica 30: 227–238.
41. Kong X, Murphy K, Raj T, He C, White PS, et al. (2004) A combined linkage-physical map of the human genome. Am J Hum Genet 75: 1143–1148.
42. Fisher RA (1921) On the "probable error" of a coefficient of correlation deduced from a small sample. Metron 1: 3–32.
43. Purcell S, Cherny SS, Sham PC (2003) Genetic power calculator: Design of linkage and association genetic mapping studies of complex traits. Bioinformatics 19: 149–150.
44. Zhu G, Duffy DL, Eldridge A, Grace M, Mayne C, et al. (1999) A major quantitative-trait locus for mole density is linked to the familial melanoma gene CDKN2A: A maximum-likelihood combined linkage and association analysis in twins and their sibs. Am J Hum Genet 65: 483–492.
45. Wright M, De Geus E, Ando J, Luciano M, Posthuma D, et al. (2001) Genetics of cognition: Outline of a collaborative twin study. Twin Res 4: 48–56.
46. Healey SC, Kirk KM, Hyland VJ, Munns CF, Henders AK, et al. (2001) Height discordance in monozygotic females is not attributable to discordant inactivation of X-linked stature determining genes. Twin Res 4: 19–24.
47. Zhu G, Evans DM, Duffy DL, Montgomery GW, Medland SE, et al. (2004) A genome scan for eye color in 502 twin families: Most variation is due to a QTL on Chromosome 15q. Twin Res 7: 197–210.
48. Cornes BK, Medland SE, Morley KI, Ferreira MAR, Gordon S, et al. (2005) Sex-limited genome-wide linkage scan for body mass index in an unselected sample of 933 Australian Twin Families. Twin Res Hum Genet 8: 616–632.
49. Abecasis GR, Cherny SS, Cookson WO, Cardon LR (2002) Merlin—rapid analysis of dense genetic maps using sparse gene flow trees. Nat Genet 30: 97–101.

CHAPTER 13

LOCATING DISEASE GENES USING BAYESIAN VARIABLE SELECTION WITH THE HASEMAN-ELSTON METHOD

Cheongeun Oh, Kenny Q Ye, Qimei He and Nancy R Mendell

BACKGROUND

In this work, we analyzed the slope of the cholesterol increase with age in the simulated data (Problem 2). Our objective was to identify the markers that are linked to the disease genes related to a high rate of increase in cholesterol. Genetic Analysis Workshop 13 provided information that the disease genes are located on chromosomes 7(s7), 15(s8), and 21(s9), respectively, and that the gene on chromosome 21(s9) only affects cholesterol rate in the females, i.e., it interacts with gender. The Haseman-Elston [1] method allowed one to apply linear regression methods for linkage analysis. For each sibling pair, it used the number of alleles identical by descent (IBD) at each marker as the explanatory variables and a statistic measuring similarity of values of the quantitative traits in the sibling pair as the response variable. The original Haseman-Elston method [1] used the squared difference between the traits of the siblings. In a recent publication, Elston et al. [1] proposed the cross-product of the two trait values in a sib pair as the response, which was used in this paper. Suh et al. [2] applied Stochastic Search Variable Selection (SSVS), a Bayesian variable selection method proposed by George and McCulloch [3] for the linear regression model, to the Haseman-Elston method. Although the scope of Suh et al was very preliminary, with only the IBD values at the linked markers plus 10 unlinked markers used as candidate explanatory variables in the variable selection, it showed the Bayesian variable selection approach to be very promising. The study presented here extended these methods in two respects. First, we took advantage of SSVS by including all 399 markers as candidate explanatory variables. It is computationally impossible to consider all subsets of 399 markers using a traditional frequentist approach. Secondly, a hierarchical prior probability structure as discussed by Chipman [4] was imposed on the model space to study the interaction effects (epistasis). The results were reported and compared with those obtained with the more traditional forward and backward step-wise regression.

Citation: Cheongeun Oh, Kenny Q YeEmail author, Qimei He and Nancy R Mendell, Locating disease genes using Bayesian variable selection with the Haseman-Elston method, DOI: 10.1186/1471-2156-4-S1-S69.

METHODS

Haseman-Elston method

We chose to analyze the rate of change in cholesterol over time in the simulated data. First, for each individual, we obtained the least square (LS) estimate for the slope of cholesterol over the time. For the i^{th}sibling pair, using the LS estimate of slope as the trait (Y_{1i}, Y_{2i}), we computed their cross-product CP_i = (Y_{1i}-m)(Y_{2i}- m) as our response values, where m is the mean of the slopes over all siblings in the same family. Elston et al. [1] introduced the cross-product CP, as the replacement of the squared difference $D_i^2 = (Y_{1i} - Y_{2i})^2$. In our regression analysis, we adopted CP as the response, and also used squared-difference for comparison. For simplicity, we assumed the errors to be independent but a correlation structure could be implemented into our method in a straightforward way.

There are about 1500 full sib pairs and a few half sib pairs in each replicate. In the replicate we considered there are 1522 full sib pairs. The number of alleles shared in each pair was obtained for each sib pair at each marker using the SIBPAL program of the SAGE software [5]. There were a total of 399 markers. We had

$$\text{Response} = \beta_0 + \sum_{j=1}^{p} \beta_j X_j + \varepsilon,$$

where the $\varepsilon \sim N(0, \sigma^2)$ were assumed to be independent and X values were IBD scores.

To study the effect of gender, we also included the genders of the siblings as an explanatory variable. It was in fact coded as two dummy explanatory variables as follows: (male, male) = (0, 0), (male, female) = (0,1), and (female, female) = (1,1).

SSVS

George and McCulloch [3] proposed a Bayesian model selection method for variable selection based on the Gibbs sampler. The criterion of interest was taken to be the posterior probability of a model conditional on the data that could be obtained using the stochastic search variable-selection. For the simplest case of linear regression with normal errors:

$$Y = X'\beta + \varepsilon,\ \varepsilon \sim N(0, \sigma^2 I),$$

where β may contain main effects or interactions effects. They set the prior distribution of β as mixtures of two normal distributions by introducing the latent variable γ:

$$\beta_k|\gamma_k \sim (1 - \gamma_k)\,N(0, \tau^2) + \gamma_k N(0, c^2\tau^2),$$

where much larger variance ($c > 1$) allowed for $\gamma_k = 1$ to have a large influence. A recommended choice for these parameter values is given by George and McCulloch [3]. The value of c was set equal to 10 in our analysis. A model was represented by a vector $\gamma = (\gamma_1, \gamma_2, ..., \gamma_p)$, where $\gamma_k = 0$ or 1. If $\gamma_k = 0$, then the marker X_j was considered to be excluded from the model and if $\gamma_k = 1$, it was considered to be included in the model. Note that β_0 was taken to be always included, thus we could set β_0 $N((0, c^2\tau^2)$. With appropriate prior on $\gamma = (\gamma_1, \gamma_2, ..., \gamma_p)$ and σ^2, we obtained a posterior distribution of γ using Gibbs sampling. Therefore, by examining the posterior probability of γ, we identified the optimal model with the largest posterior probability and rank the markers using the marginal distribution of each γ_k. A prior for γ corresponds to a prior on the model. The commonly used independence prior implies that the importance of any variable is independent of any other variable. In other words, under this prior, each X_i enters the model independently of the other coefficients, with probability $p(\gamma_i = 1) = 1 - p(\gamma_i = 0) = p_i$. A smaller p_i can be used to downweight X_i values that are costly or of less interest. For our case, a useful reduction was to set $p_i = p$, in which p is the a priori expected proportion of X_i values in the model. When only main effects but no interaction were considered, the importance of any variable was independent of the importance of any other variable. Thus the independence prior implied that the prior of γ was simply set as $\text{prob}(\gamma) = p^n$, where n is the number of ones in γ. Increased weight on parsimonious models could instead be obtained by setting p small. So in our case, p was set to be small, 0.02 first, and next to see how our method is robust to this choice of p, we chose a new value of p = 0.002 for comparison. The details on the MCMC algorithms can be found in George and McCulloch [3].

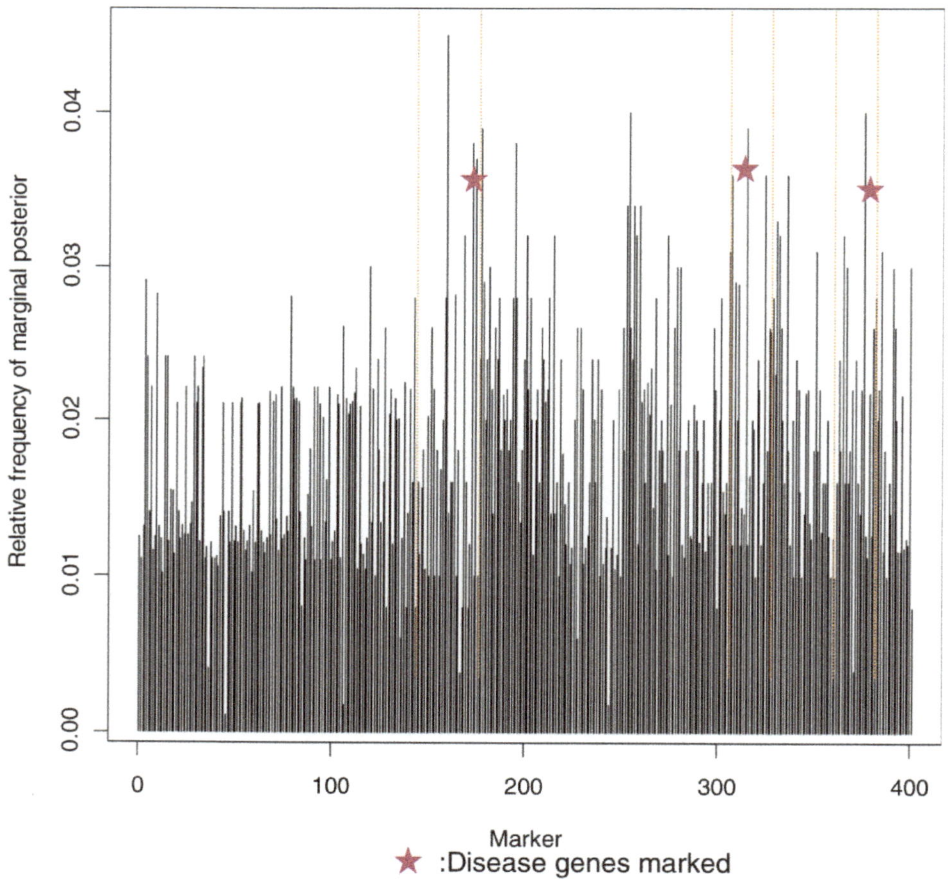

Figure 1 Top ranked markers based upon SSVS The markers are ranked according to their marginal posterior obtained using 10,000 cycles of Gibbs algorithm. Disease loci are located on chromosomes 7, 15, and 21, and gender effect is ranked at the 15th (Replicate 1 of the simulated data).

We applied SSVS to select markers linked to cholesterol rate from all 399 markers under consideration. Since it is impractical to track the complete posterior of γ, only the marginal posterior of each marker is obtained. Although both posterior probability of the models and marginal probabilities of each marker are sensitive to the prior settings, especially c and p, we showed that the ranking of the marginal posterior of the markers are not.

Figure 2 illustrates the robustness through plots of the ranking of the markers obtained using two different priors p = 0.02 and 0.002. Other prior settings showed similar high correlations in the rankings of the markers.

We followed the Markov chain Monte Carlo (MCMC) algorithms described in Chipman [4] and implemented it using the JAVA programming language. The programs were run on a Linux cluster using Intel processors. The length of the MCMC chain was set to 10,000. The running time was approximately 30 minutes on a single 1.0 GHz CPU under the above specified environment. The first 1000 samples were used as the burn-in period and not included in estimating the posterior.

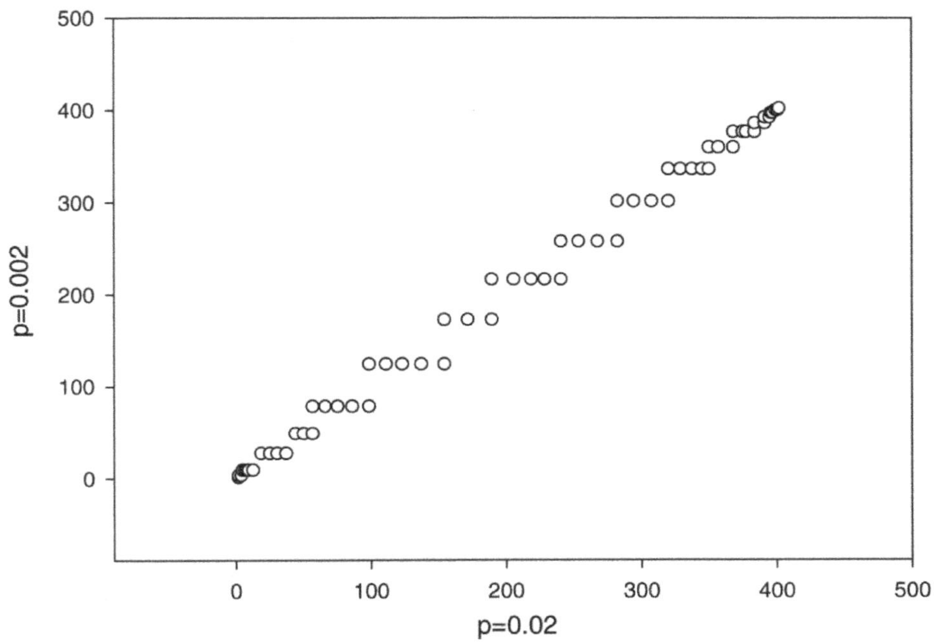

Figure 2 Rankings of markers with p = 0.02 and p = 0.002 Ranking of the markers for two different prior settings (p = 0.02 and p = 0.002) is plotted, which shows its robustness to the choice of p.

Hierarchical prior structure

When interaction effects (epistasis) are considered in the model selection, the model space becomes enormous and the common independence prior for γ is not appropriate anymore. With interactions, the prior for gamma can capture the dependence relation between the importance of a higher order term and those lower order terms from which it was formed. Chipman [4] proposed a hierarchical prior structure for this model space. The importance of the interactions such as X_iX_j will depend only on whether the main effects X_i and X_j are included in the model. This belief can be expressed by a prior for $\gamma = (\gamma_{X_i}, \gamma_{X_j}, \gamma_{X_iX_j})$ of the form

$$p(\gamma) = p(\gamma_{X_i})p(\gamma_{X_j})p(\gamma_{X_iX_j} | \gamma_{X_i}, \gamma_{X_j}).$$

The probability that the term $X_i X_j$ is active $\Pr(\gamma_{X_iX_j} = 1 | \gamma_{X_i}, \gamma_{X_i})$ may take on four different values, depending on the values of the pair $(\gamma_{X_i}, \gamma_{X_j})$.

$$\Pr(\gamma_{X_iX_j} = 1 | \gamma_{X_i}, \gamma_{X_i}) = \begin{cases} p_{00} & \text{if } (\gamma_{X_i}, \gamma_{X_j}) = (0,0) \\ p_{01} & \text{if } (\gamma_{X_i}, \gamma_{X_j}) = (0,1) \\ p_{10} & \text{if } (\gamma_{X_i}, \gamma_{X_j}) = (1,0) \\ p_{11} & \text{if } (\gamma_{X_i}, \gamma_{X_j}) = (1,1) \end{cases}.$$

In our analysis, we set $(p_{00}, p_{01}, p_{10}, p_{11}) = (0, 0, 0, p)$. This corresponded to the prior belief that if the interaction effect between two factors exists in a model, the main effects of the two factors must be included in the same model.

Our study was conducted in two stages. At the first stage, all 399 candidate markers and gender were the candidate variables in SSVS, but interactions were not considered. At the second stage, SSVS was applied to the same sib-pair responses with the top 30 candidate variables selected from the first stage and their interactions as the candidate variables. Among the third were the gender and 29 markers. This brought the total number of candidate variables in SSVS to 465. We chose only the top 30 variables from the first stage for two reasons. First, it is reasonable to assume that only a few linked loci exist and they should be contained in the top 30. Second, this is the maximum size that the current SSVS algorithm handles comfortably in the second stage.

Step-wise regression

In order to compare the traditional method to our method, we used a step-wise method based on Akaike information criterion (AIC) [6] to select a formula-based model, which was implemented under R, the "GNU S". The details of this method can be found in the R manual [7].

Results

Only the first of the 100 simulated data sets was used. Figure 1 displays the marginal posterior of each marker obtained from SSVS with all 399 markers but no interactions. The marginal posterior was computed from the relative frequency of each markers in the MCMC sample of γ. It clearly showed that the high posterior values are concentrated on chromosomes 7, 15, and 21. Table 1 shows the top 30 markers, a marker from chromosome 7 is rated as most significant, and there are seven, four, and two markers from chromosomes 7, 15, and 21, respectively. The variable gender was ranked as 15th. Table 2 shows the most significant 20 markers obtained from the univariate LS regression and from the step-wise regression. These markers were very much evenly distributed in all chromosomes.

When we considered the results from the univariate regression, a marker from chromosome 13 was most significant. One each from chromosome 7 and chromosome 15 were only marginally significant; none from chromosome 21 (where a linked marker was located) are in the top 20 most significant markers. Similar results were obtained when backward and forward step-wise regression methods were used. Among the top 20, only two markers were from chromosome 15, and one each from chromosomes 7 and 21. Also, these two traditional methods failed to locate the gender effect as significant.

Table 1 Top rank markers based on their marginal posterior probability.

Posterior Ranking	Markers
1	**M160 (chr7)** ^{A}
2	M254
3	**M315(chr15)**
4	**M173(chr7)**
tied at 5	M336, M325, **M387(chr21)**
tied at 8	M260, M257, M201, **M169(chr7)**
tied at 12	M385, M351, **M306(chr15)**
tied at 15	**400(gender)**, M367, M281, M279, M182
tied at 19	**M175(chr7)**, M120
tied at 22	**M391(chr21), M178(chr7)**
tied at 24	**M309(chr15), M179(chr7)**
tied at 26	**M311(chr15)**
tied at 27	**M164(chr7)**

^{A}Disease loci are located all on chromosomes 7, 15, and 21. Markers on these three chromosomes are shown in bold face. p = 0.02 is used in SSVS.

Table 2 Top 20 markers selected in step-wise regression and univariate regression.

Chromosome	Step-wise	Univariate
1	M13^{A}	M3
2	M57^{A}	M43
3		M64^{A}, M69^{A}, M70^{A}, M81^{A}
4		
5	M114^{A}	M114^{A}, M128^{A}
6	M142^{A}	M142, M158^{A}
7	M162^{A}	M169^{A}
8	M182^{A}, M193^{A}	M182^{A}
9	M211^{A}, M216^{B}	M211^{A}, M216^{B}
10	M227^{A}	
11	M244^{A}, M253^{A}	M257^{A}
12		

13	M278[C]	M278[B]
14		
15	M313[A], M318[A]	M318[A]
16		M341
17	M347[A]	M347[B]
18	M359[A]	M355[A]
19	M372[C]	
20		
21	M389[B]	
22	M397[A]	

[A]$p < 0.05$, [B]$p < 0.01$, [C]$p < 0.001$

The result from the second stage SSVS is shown in Figure 3. The marginal posterior probabilities of the interaction effects are displayed. The existence of the gender-gene interaction on chromosome 21 is clear.

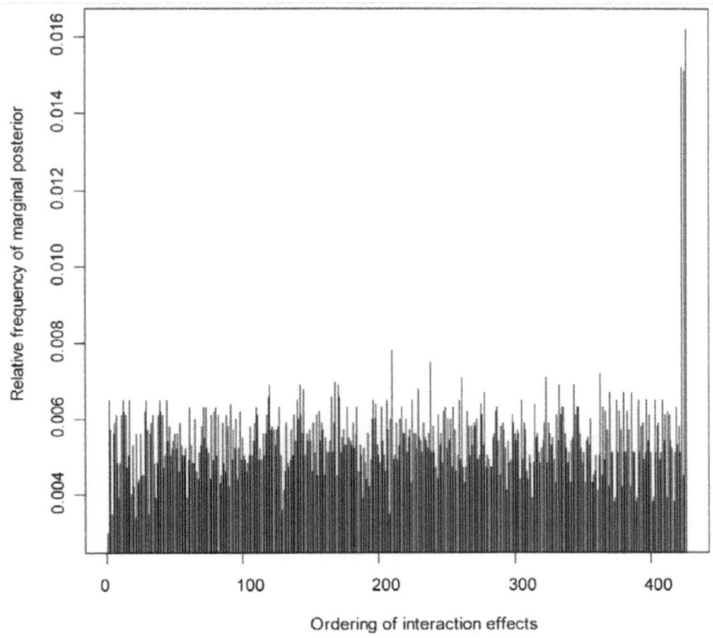

Figure 3 Gene × gene and gene × gender interaction effects The top ranked 30 markers selected from the first stage and their interactions are considered in the second stage. The interaction between chromosome 21 and gender are observed.

The same analysis was also carried out on the third simulated data set and similar results were obtained.

CONCLUSION

We showed that SSVS is a powerful method in identifying linked markers using the Haseman-Elston method, even for weak effects. SSVS is very effective because it does a smart search over the entire model space, while the frequentist best subset model selection procedures are constrained by computing power required to examine all candidate models. The former can work on problems with many more candidate variables, which is essential when interaction effects are studied. By using the prior structures that reflect the relation among the candidate variables, SSVS can accommodate a good number of candidate markers as well as their interactions. The two-stage strategy used in this study worked well. It identified the chromosomes of the linked markers in the first stage and the interaction effects were located in the second stage. Both univariate regression and the step-wise regression failed to identify the chromosomes of the linked markers.

DISCUSSION

One thing found to be interesting was that when we also use the squared-difference as response for comparison, its false positives did not overlap with those of cross-product. As we can see in Figure 4, the red strip covers those unlinked markers with high posterior probability when squared-difference is used, the posterior of these markers when cross-product are used are just average. So the information obtained from these two responses is complementary. This result is not a surprise because many recent works [8] have proposed the use of both the squared-sum and squared-difference as responses and combined the results of two regressions together in drawing the inference. As a special case, the cross-product response weights these two equally. For a comprehensive review on these "new" Haseman-Elston methods, see Feingold [8]. A natural extension of the methods proposed in this paper is to combine the posterior probability from regressions on both squared-sum and squared-difference. We will investigate this in our future research.

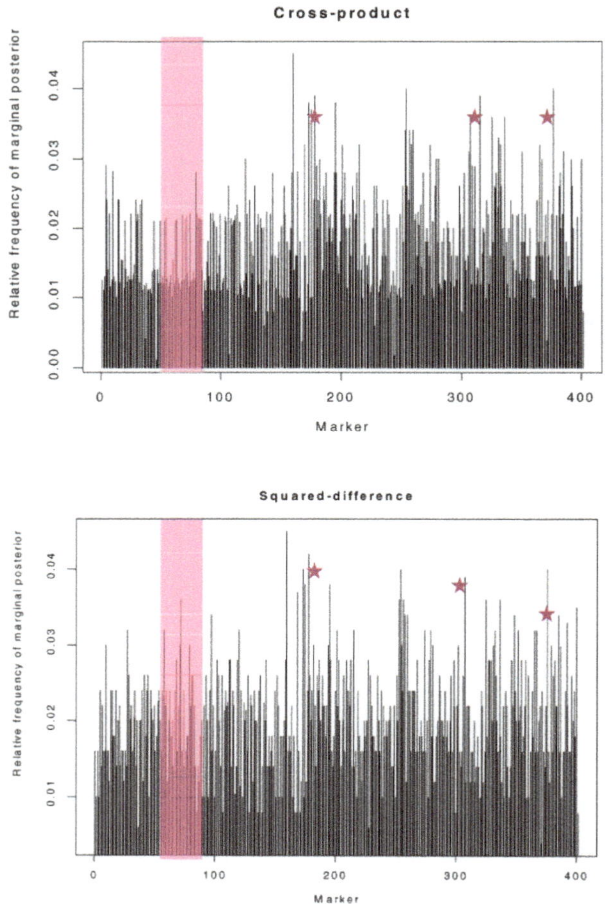

Figure 4 Type I error of Haseman-Elston methods with D^2 and CP as responses False positives when squared-difference is used do not overlap with ones of cross-product. This suggests that complementary information are contained in each responses.

REFERENCES

1. Elston RC, Buxbaum S, Jacobs KB, Olson JM: Haseman and Elston revisited. Genet Epidemiol. 2000, 19: 1-17. 10.1002/1098-2272(200007)19:1<1::AID-GEPI1>3.0.CO;2-E.
2. Suh YJ, Finch SJ, Mendell NR: Application of a Bayesian method for optimal subset regression to linkage analysis of Q1 and Q2. Genet Epidemiol. 2001, 21 (suppl 1): S706-S711.
3. George EI, McCulloch RE: Variable selection via Gibbs sampling. J Am Stat Assoc. 1993, 88: 881-889. 10.2307/2290777.
4. Chipman H: Bayesian variable selection with related predictors. Can J Stat. 1996, 24: 17-36.
5. Case Western University: SAGE, Statistical Analysis of Genetic Epidemiology release 3.1. Cleveland, Ohio, Department of Genetic Epidemiology and Biostatistics, Rammelkamp Center for Education and Research, Case Western Reserve University. 1997
6. Sakamoto Y, Ishiguro M, Kitagawa G: Akaike Information Criterion Statistics. Dordrecht: Reidel Publishing Company. 1986
7. R Development Core Team: The R Referene Index. [http://cran.r-project.org/doc/manuals/refman.pdf]
8. Feingold EL: Regression-based quantitative-trait-locus mapping in the 21st century. Am J Hum Genet. 2002, 71: 217-22. 10.1086/341964.

CHAPTER 14

NETWORK ANALYSIS OF GENOME-WIDE SELECTIVE CONSTRAINT REVEALS A GENE NETWORK ACTIVE IN EARLY FETAL BRAIN INTOLERANT OF MUTATION

Jinmyung Choi, Parisa Shooshtari, Kaitlin E. Samocha, Mark J. Daly, Chris Cotsapas

INTRODUCTION

Genetic variation is introduced into the human genome by spontaneously arising de novomutations in the germline. The majority of these mutations have, at most, modest effects on phenotype; they are thus subject to nearly neutral drift and can be transmitted through the population, with some increasing in frequency to become common variants. Conversely, de novo mutations with large effects on phenotype may be subject to many different selective forces, both positive and negative, with the latter resulting in either the variant being completely lost from the population or maintained at very low frequencies [1].

Large-scale DNA sequencing can now be used to comprehensively assess de novo mutations, with many current applications focusing on the protein-coding portion of the genome (the exome). This approach has been used to identify causal genes and variants in rare Mendelian diseases: for example, exome sequencing of ten affected individuals with Kabuki syndrome identified the methyl transferase KMT2D (formerly MLL2) as causal, after substantial post hocdata filtering [2]. In complex traits, this approach has successfully identified pathogenic genes harboring de novo mutations in autism spectrum disorders [3], intellectual disability [4] and two epileptic encephalopathies [5]; notably, all these studies sequenced the exomes of parent-affected offspring trios and quantified the background rate of de novo mutations in each gene using formal analytical approaches. They were thus able to identify genes harboring a statistically significant number of mutations, which are likely to be causal for disease [5,6].

These large-scale exome sequencing studies have demonstrated that the rate of non-synonymous de novo mutations is markedly depleted in some genes, and that these genes are more likely to harbor disease-causing mutations [6]. As synonymous de novo mutations occur at expected frequencies, this depletion is not driven by variation in the local overall mutation rate; instead, these genes appear to be intolerant of changes to amino acid sequence and are thus under selective constraint, with non-synonymous mutations removed by purifying selection. These genes represent a limited number of fundamental biological roles, which suggests that entire processes, rather than single genes, are under selective constraint. This is consistent with the extreme polygenicity of most human traits, where hundreds of genes play a causal role in determining organismal phenotype [7,8]. These genes must participate in the same cellular processes, but uncovering the relevant connections and the cell populations and developmental stages in which they occur remains a challenge. We and others have described statistical frameworks to test connectivity within a nominated set of genes [9–11] by considering how genes interact either in annotated pathways or in networks derived from protein interactions or gene co-expression across tissues, and these approaches have been successfully applied to detecting networks of genes underlying neurodevelopmental disease [12]. These studies have demonstrated that genes underlying complex diseases tend to aggregate in networks; we hypothesize that the same is true of constrained genes. However, unlike disease traits where the relevant organ system is known and hypotheses about pathogenesis can by formulated, the phenotypic targets of selective forces are usually unknown. Thus, systematic

Citation: Choi J, Shooshtari P, Samocha KE, Daly MJ, Cotsapas C (2016) Network Analysis of Genome-Wide Selective Constraint Reveals a Gene Network Active in Early Fetal Brain Intolerant of Mutation. PLoS Genet 12(6): e1006121. doi:10.1371/ journal.pgen.1006121.

genome-wide approaches to assessing connectivity between a set of genes of interest and to identify relevant tissues are required to investigate how selective constraint acts on groups of genes and uncover the relevant physiology.

To address these issues we have developed a robust, unbiased framework and applied it to genome-wide selective constraint data derived from exome sequences of 6,503 individuals [6]. We identified a single, statistically significant subnetwork of 72 interacting genes highly intolerant of non-synonymous variation, with no other interacting groups of genes showing evidence of such coordinate constraint. To establish biological context for this subnetwork, we developed a robust approach to test for preferential expression of the module as a whole, rather than the individual constituent genes. Using gene expression data from the cosmopolitan atlas of tissues in the Roadmap Epigenome Project [13,14], we found that this subnetwork is preferentially expressed in several early-stage tissues, with the strongest enrichment in fetal brain. To more carefully dissect the role of this subnetwork in the central nervous system, we analyzed expression data from BrainSpan [15], an atlas of the developing human brain, and found that the constrained gene subnetwork is preferentially expressed in the early development of the hippocampus. Consistent with this observation, this module is enriched for genes mutated in neurological, but not other, Mendelian disorders. We thus show that selective constraint acts on a set of interacting genes active in early brain development, and that these genes are in fact intolerant of mutation. Our **P**rotein **I**nteraction **N**etwork **T**issue**S**earch (PINTS) framework is publicly available at https://github.com/cotsapaslab/PINTSv1.

RESULTS

Calculating selective constraint scores

We have previously described a framework to assess selective constraint across coding sequences in the genome [6]. Briefly, we calibrated an expectation for all possible conversions of one base to another by mutation from non-coding sequence. For each transition, we modeled the effect of the surrounding sequence and its conservation across species to correct for context effects. We then counted the number of synonymous and non-synonymous variants in the coding sequence of each gene in the genome and derived a statistic of constraint on each class of variation compared to this global expectation. We found that a number of genes show decreased rates of non-synonymous substitution but expected rates of synonymous substitution, consistent with purifying selection removing the non-synonymous alleles from the population.

Analysis framework description

If constrained genes lie in biologically meaningful networks, we expect them to (i) interact and (ii) be expressed in the same tissues. We developed a robust, modular workflow (**PINTS**–**P**rotein **I**nteraction **N**etwork **T**issue **S**earch; Fig 1) to test both of these hypotheses at a genome-wide level. To detect interactions between constrained genes we used a high-confidence protein-protein interaction network (InWeb [16]), and employed a clustering algorithm previously validated on such networks [17]. We assessed significance empirically by randomly reassigning constraint scores to genes (see Materials and Methods and).

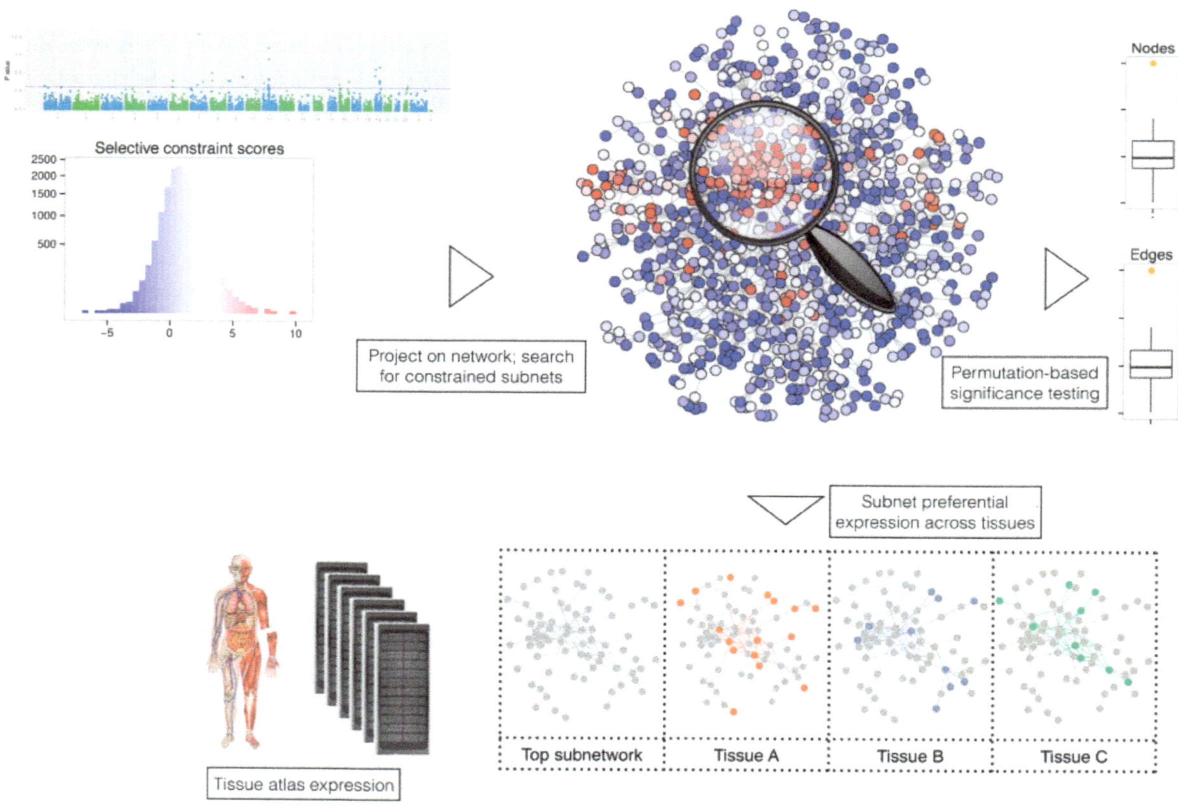

Figure 1. The Protein Interaction Network Tissue Search (PINTS) workflow.

We then tested any significant subnetworks for preferential expression in the diverse tissue atlas provided by the Roadmap Epigenome Project (REP), which assays gene expression in 27 human primary samples across the developmental spectrum [14]. Our final dataset is comprised of 9729 genes both present in InWeb and detected in at least one REP tissue.

We project gene-wise selective constraint scores [6] onto the InWeb protein-protein interaction dataset [16] and use a heuristic version of the prize-collecting Steiner Tree algorithm [17,29] to detect clusters of interacting constrained genes. We assess significance empirically, by randomly assigning the scores to genes 1000 times and calibrating detected subnetwork parameters. We then test any significant subnetwork for usual patterns of preferential expression [32] across the Roadmap Epigenome Project expression data [14], a cosmopolitan tissue atlas, using a Markov random field approach. The approach is flexible and modular, so gene interaction and tissue expression reference datasets can be altered according to the application.

Our workflow is both modular and flexible: clustering algorithms, gene-gene relationships and tissue atlases can be replaced as required, so that analyses can be tailored to suit specific biological problems. A flexible implementation, including all data described here, is freely available as an R package at https://github.com/cotsapaslab/PINTSv1.

Highly constrained genes form a protein interaction module expressed in fetal tissues and the immune system

We define highly constrained genes as those with evidence of constraint on non-synonymousde novo substitutions ($p < 5 \times 10^{-6}$, Bonferroni correction for the number of genes in our InWeb dataset) but null synonymous constraint scores, indicating intolerance to functionally relevant mutation rather than fluctuations in the local mutation rate [6]. Of these, 107/9729 genes pass this stringent threshold (binomial $p < 2.2 \times 10^{-16}$;), and form the core of the analysis presented here. We found that 67/107 form a connected subnetwork (Fig 2A; Table 1). Five additional genes are included as our cluster detection algorithm by design looks for a backbone of null nodes connected to many signal nodes. To assess the significance of this observation, we randomly distribute constraint scores to InWeb nodes 1000 times and find that the constrained subnetwork is larger (number of nodes: $p < 0.001$) and more densely connected (number of edges: $p < 0.001$; clustering coefficient: $p = 0.008$) than expected by chance (Fig 2B). As such, it also explains more total constraint in the genome than expected (sum of constraint scores: $p < 0.001$). After accounting for the genes forming this subnetwork, we found no evidence that the remaining 35 genes form statistically significant subnetworks by our criteria.

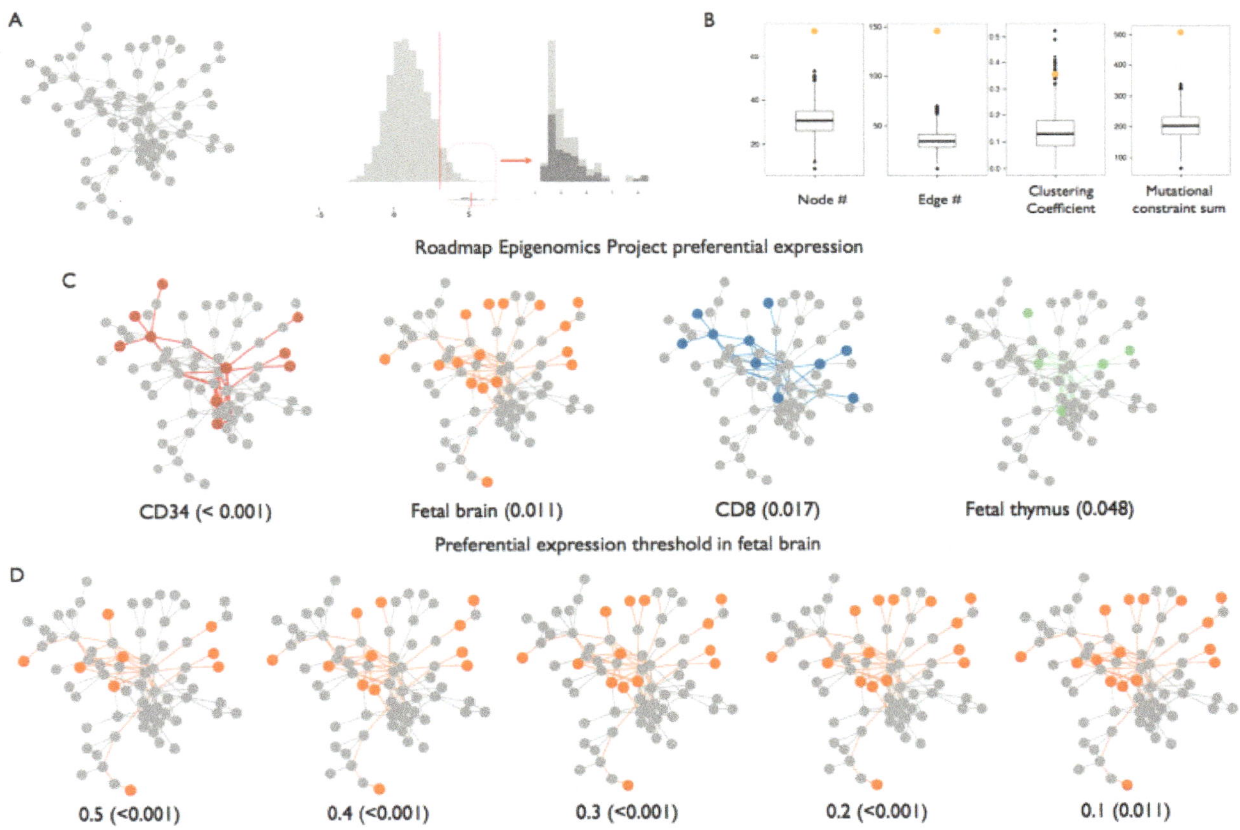

Figure 2. selectively constrained genes form a 72-member network, preferentially expressed in fetal brain, heart and immune cell populations.

A: constrained genes form a connected subnetwork of genes in the extreme of the constraint score distribution. B: the constrained subnetwork contains more genes (nodep < 0.001), has more connections (edge p < 0.001), is more densely connected (clustering coefficient p = 0.008) and explains more total constraint (sum p < 0.001) than expected by chance (orange dots) compared to networks discovered in 1000 permutations of the constraint data (boxplots and black dots). C: the constrained subnetwork is preferentially expressed in a subset of Roadmap Epigenome Project tissues, including fetal brain. Preferentially expressed nodes and the shortest paths connecting them are in color; grey nodes are not preferentially expressed in each displayed tissue. D: The most consistent preferential expression signal is seen in fetal brain, which is robust to stringency of preferential expression threshold.

Table 1. A 72-member constrained gene subnetwork.

Gene	Constraint score	Chr	Start	End	Gene	Constraint score	Chr	Start	End
DYNC1H1	9.977	14	101964528	102050792	*UBR4*	4.940	1	19074506	19210276
PRPF8	8.302	17	1650629	1684882	*CHD3*	4.905	17	7884806	7912760
HUWE1	7.973	X	53532096	53686729	*USP7*	4.866	16	8892094	8964514
SMARCA4	6.604	19	10961001	11065395	*PRPF6*	4.826	20	63981135	64033100
POLR2A	6.578	17	7484366	7514618	*GNAS*	4.806	20	58839718	58911192
RYR2	6.436	1	237042205	237833988	*THOC2*	4.791	X	123600561	123733056
MED12	6.388	X	71118556	71142454	*FRY*	4.772	13	32031300	32299122
SNRNP200	6.166	2	96274336	96305515	*OGT*	4.753	X	71533083	71575897
CHD4	6.162	12	6570083	6607476	*POLR2B*	4.729	4	56977722	57031168
MTOR	5.974	1	11106535	11262507	*KCNMA1*	4.687	10	76869601	77638595
GRIN1	5.971	9	137138390	137168762	*TAOK1*	4.685	17	29390464	29551904
PPFIA3	5.794	19	49119389	49151026	*BRWD3*	4.683	X	80670854	80809688
MLL	5.747	11	118436490	118526832	*SPTAN1*	4.671	9	128552558	128633665
UBR5	5.720	8	102253012	102412841	*PHIP*	4.670	6	78935867	79078236
ITPR1	5.589	3	4493348	4847840	*DDB1*	4.670	11	61299451	61342596
CLTC	5.547	17	59619689	59696956	*HSPA2*	4.665	14	64535905	64546173
FLNA	5.541	X	154348524	154374638	*SPEG*	4.644	2	219434846	219498287
UPF1	5.514	19	18831938	18868236	*SMC3*	4.639	10	110567691	110604636
HCFC1	5.450	X	153947553	153971807	*MYH10*	4.629	17	8474205	8630761
DHX30	5.428	3	47802909	47850195	*XPO1*	4.621	2	61477849	61538626
SPTBN1	5.423	2	54456285	54671445	*CUL3*	4.610	2	224470150	224585397
SF3B1	5.418	2	197389784	197435091	*IRS2*	4.592	13	109752698	109786568
SMARCA2	5.387	9	2015219	2193624	*ADCY1*	4.587	7	45574140	45723116
CACNA1I	5.363	22	39570753	39689737	*APC2*	4.564	19	1446302	1473244
SMC1A	5.360	X	53374149	53422728	*ZBTB17*	4.547	1	15941869	15976132
GRIN2B	5.334	12	13537337	13980119	*TLN1*	4.517	9	35696948	35732395
GRIN2D	5.211	19	48394875	48444931	*MYH9*	4.496	22	36281281	36388018
TAF1	5.178	X	71366239	71532374	*EEF2*	4.478	19	3976056	3985469
VCP	5.162	9	35056064	35073249	*PDS5A*	4.451	4	39822863	39977956
CNOT1	5.146	16	58519951	58629886	*PRKD2*	4.438	19	46674275	46717127
TRIO	5.109	5	14143702	14532128	*BRD4*	4.436	19	15235519	15332545
CYFIP2	5.100	5	157266079	157395598	*HSPA8*	4.364	11	123057489	123063230
SUPT5H	5.065	19	39436156	39476670	*CTNNB1*	4.198	3	41194837	41260096
FZD8	5.028	10	35638249	35642278	*UBC*	3.997	12	124911604	124917368
TNPO2	4.993	19	12699194	12724011	*PIK3CD*	3.858	1	9651732	9729114
GTF2I	4.945	7	74657667	74760692	*PIK3R1*	2.170	5	68215720	68301821

We find that 67/107 significantly constrained genes form a single protein-protein interaction subnetwork. Five additional genes are also included (gray shading), as our cluster detection algorithm by design looks for a backbone of null nodes connected to many signal nodes. As shown in Fig 2, the subnetwork is significantly larger and more densely connected than expected by chance, and is preferentially expressed in a subset of early-stage neural and immune tissues.

The genes in the constrained subnetwork appear to represent several fundamental cell processes, most notably mitosis and cell proliferation (SMC1A, SMC3, CTNNB1) and transcriptional regulation (CHD3, CHD4, SMARCA4). We performed a formal pathway analysis to further test this and found enrichment of several annotated pathways reflecting these fundamental processes (Table 2). Encouraged that our detected subnetwork represents one or more biological processes under constraint, we sought to add cellular context to our observations. In particular, we wanted to determine if this group of genes is preferentially expressed in particular tissues, indicating a likely site of action. We thus developed an approach to estimate the joint probability of preferential expression of the genes in the subnetwork in each tissue of an atlas of expression data, while accounting for how frequently each gene is detected across the entire atlas. We applied our approach, which uses Markov random fields, to the expression data on 27 primary tissues and cell lines available from the Roadmap Epigenome Project. Using two conservative permutation-based significance tests, we find the constrained subnetwork is preferentially expressed in a number of fetal and immune tissues (Fig 2C and Table 3), including fetal brain (permuted $p < 0.001$), the immune cell subpopulations marked by CD34 (permuted $p < 0.001$) and CD8 (permuted $p = 0.017$) and fetal thymus (permuted $p = 0.048$). We note that, whilst only a subset of genes are expressed in any one tissue, the combinations of genes expressed in these tissues is highly statistically significant: each gene is only expressed in a small subset of the tissues interrogated, so the cumulative probability of seeing these genes coordinately expressed in any one tissue is small.

Table 2. The 72-member constrained gene subnetwork is enriched for canonical pathways reflecting neuronal and immune functionality and basic aspects of cell cycle control.

Name	All	Mapped	Subnetwork	KS	HG
Developmental biology (Reactome)	397	344	10	2.53E-19	1.83E-05
Immune system (Reactome)	934	702	9	4.98E-08	1.96E-02
Adaptive immune system (Reactome)	540	421	8	3.13E-10	2.08E-03
Axon guidance (Reactome)	252	220	8	4.62E-16	1.65E-05
mRNA Processing (Reactome)	162	120	8	9.06E-12	1.05E-07
Calcium signaling pathway (KEGG)	179	163	7	6.00E-08	1.36E-05
Spliceosome (KEGG)	129	85	7	5.32E-21	9.60E-08
mRNA splicing (Reactome)	112	74	7	6.26E-20	3.19E-08
Processing of capped intron containing pre-mRNA (Reactome)	141	102	7	3.21E-13	3.99E-07
Pathways in cancer (KEGG)	329	301	6	4.05E-12	4.21E-03
Regulation of actin cytoskeleton (KEGG)	217	188	6	8.08E-13	2.74E-04
Cell cycle (Reactome)	422	332	6	7.95E-03	7.12E-03
mRNA splicing minor pathway (Reactome)	46	20	6	2.90E-05	3.56E-11
Signalling by NGF (Reactome)	218	191	6	3.04E-21	3.02E-04
Focal adhesion (KEGG)	202	188	5	9.72E-07	1.70E-03
Long term potentiation (KEGG)	71	60	5	9.64E-15	2.97E-06
MAPK signaling pathway (KEGG)	268	233	5	3.02E-15	4.92E-03
HIV infection (Reactome)	208	163	5	1.32E-06	8.12E-04
HIV life cycle (Reactome)	126	95	5	1.03E-02	4.27E-05
Late phase of HIV life cycle (Reactome)	105	85	5	1.36E-02	2.27E-05
Neuronal system (Reactome)	280	219	5	3.80E-28	3.64E-03
NGF signalling via TRKa from the plasma membrane (Reactome)	138	120	5	1.09E-14	1.57E-04
Signaling by GPCR (Reactome)	921	415	5	1.63E-11	6.21E-02

We tested pathways from two sources (the Reactome database and KEGG, the Kyoto Encyclopedia of Genes and Genomes), assessing how many genes are in each pathway (All), how many map onto the 9729 inteconnected genes in our analysis (Mapped), and how many are present in the constrained subnetwork (Subnetwork). We assess significance using both the GSEA approach of a Kolmogorov-Smirnov (KS) test and a simple hypergeometric (HG) test of expected overlaps.

Table 3. The 72-member constrained gene subnetwork is preferentially expressed in a range of tissues and brain structures.

Source	Tissue	Developmental stage	Permutation p-value	Resampled p-value	Tissue-specific genes
REP	$CD34^+$	Perinatal (cord blood)	0.00100	0.00100	10
REP	Fetal brain	Fetal	0.01100	0.00100	16
REP	$CD8^+$	Adult (>20 years)	0.01700	0.00100	10
REP	Fetal thymus	Fetal	0.04800	0.00100	5
BrainSpan	Caudal ganglionic eminence	2A (8–9 pcw)	0.00125	0.00125	20
BrainSpan	Dorsolateral prefrontal cortex	2A (8–9 pcw)	0.00125	0.00125	16
BrainSpan	Hippocampal anlage	2A (8–9 pcw)	0.00125	0.00125	17
BrainSpan	Lateral ganglionic eminence	2A (8–9 pcw)	0.00125	0.00125	19
BrainSpan	Primary motor-sensory cortex	2A (8–9 pcw)	0.00125	0.00125	20
BrainSpan	Medial frontal cortex	2A (8–9 pcw)	0.00125	0.00125	19
BrainSpan	Orbital frontal cortex	2A (8–9 pcw)	0.00250	0.00125	14
BrainSpan	Parietal neocortex	2A (8–9 pcw)	0.00250	0.00125	18
BrainSpan	Medial ganglionic eminence	2A (8–9 pcw)	0.00375	0.00125	18
BrainSpan	Occipital neocortex	2A (8–9 pcw)	0.00500	0.00125	18
BrainSpan	Hippocampus	2B (10–12 pcw)	0.00625	0.00125	18
BrainSpan	Hippocampus	3A (13–15 pcw)	0.00625	0.00125	19
BrainSpan	Primary somatosensory cortex	3A (13–15 pcw)	0.01250	0.00125	20
BrainSpan	Primary visual cortex	4 (19–24 pcw)	0.01750	0.00125	22
BrainSpan	Posterior superior temporal cortex	3B (16–18 pcw)	0.01875	0.00125	22
BrainSpan	Posteroventral parietal cortex	3A (13–15 pcw)	0.02250	0.00125	19
BrainSpan	Cerebellar cortex	4 (19–24 pcw)	0.02500	0.00125	19
BrainSpan	Primary motor cortex	3A (13–15 pcw)	0.02750	0.00125	19
BrainSpan	Striatum	3A (13–15 pcw)	0.04125	0.00125	17
BrainSpan	Dorsolateral prefrontal cortex	4A (19–24 pcw)	0.04625	0.00250	21

We find strong enrichment in a variety of tissues, predominantly neural and immune-derived samples sourced from the Roadmap Epigenome Project (REP) and the BrainSpan Atlas. We report only tissues passing significance with two conservative independent empirical approaches: random permutation of preferential expression values for the subnetwork across tissues (permutation); and comparison to the largest subnetworks detected when we permute constraint scores for all 9729 InWeb genes. As several tissues are enriched for subnetwork expression, we sought to understand whether we were capturing the same signature across multiple tissues reflecting a shared process. We assessed whether the same genes are preferentially expressed in each tissue, and found a distinct signature in the fetal brain and heart samples and the immune cell subpopulations ($CD34^+$, $CD8^+$, $CD3^+$, thymus; pairwise $p < 0.05$ hypergeometric test;). To ensure our tissue expression results are not an artifact of the threshold we set for preferential expression, we repeated the entire analysis with a range of threshold values and found consistent results across tissues; this is most notable in fetal brain (Fig 2D), which remains significant irrespective of threshold used.

Genes under selective constraint are more likely to harbor pathogenic mutations causing Mendelian diseases, consistent with intolerance of functional mutations [6]. Accordingly, we found that our subnetwork of 72 genes is significantly enriched for OMIM annotations (Fisher's exact $p = 0.0013$). To further elucidate this observation, we mapped all OMIM entries to Medical Subject Headings (MeSH) disease categories and assessed enrichment per organ system category. We found that our subnetwork is significantly enriched for genes mutated in Mendelian diseases affecting the central nervous system (Fisher's exact $p = 0.0017$), validating our observation of enrichment in fetal brain. We note that this enrichment is not in the inflammatory/immune neurological disease sub-category, suggesting no overlap with the discrete immune signature we found. Samocha et al [6] have previously reported that constrained genes are also enriched for de novo mutations associated with autism spectrum disorders, further strengthening our conclusion that this constrained subnetwork represents a brain-related biological process.

The constrained module is preferentially expressed in early brain development

To further elucidate the relevance of our constrained module to brain physiology, we interrogated expression data for multiple brain structures across developmental stages from the BrainSpan project [15]. We found a strong signature of preferential expression in very early stages of development, which declines rapidly and is absent by mid-gestation and remains inactive after birth into adulthood (Fig 3A and Table 3). Several transitional structures in the early brain exhibit significant preferential expression levels, including the ganglionic eminences that eventually form the ventral forebrain and the early structures of the hippocampus. The latter structure shows the most consistent signature across developmental time, with the module's pattern of expression gradually weakening and becoming non-significant by mid gestation (post-conception weeks 16–18; Fig 3B). These results, taken with the likely involvement of constrained genes in fundamental processes of mitosis and transcriptional regulation, suggest this gene module is relevant to developmental patterning at crucial time points in early brain development.

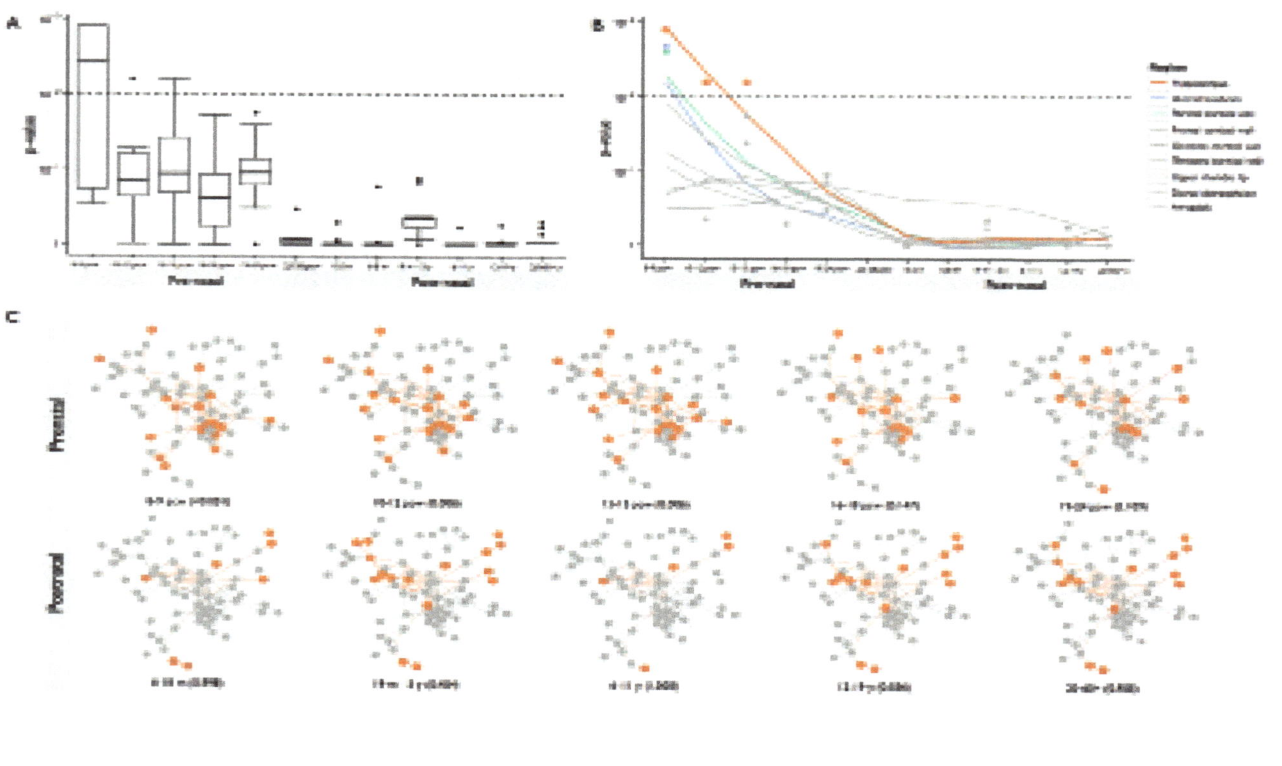

Figure 3. The 72-member selectively constrained gene subnetwork is active in early brain development, particularly in the hippocampus.

A: the constrained subnetwork shows elevated signatures of preferential expression in early stages of brain development. B: the signature is most robust in the hippocampus and its ancestral structures (orange), with some enrichment in ventral forebrain and parietal cortical wall structures very early in development (8–9 post-conception weeks). C: The constrained subnetwork shows significant preferential expression in early developmental stages, with patterns of expression losing this enrichment signature by mid-gestation. Preferentially expressed nodes and the shortest paths connecting them are colored orange; grey nodes are not preferentially expressed in each displayed tissue. Overall, these data suggest the constrained subnetwork is specifically active in very early stages of hippocampal formation.

DISCUSSION

We have shown that selective constraint influences sets of interacting genes involved in core cellular control processes, and that these have elevated expression levels in early stages of central nervous system development. We found the strongest enrichment in the early hippocampal stages at post-conception weeks eight and nine, with additional signals in ventral forebrain structures and the parietal cortical wall. This stage of development involves neuronal proliferation through carefully orchestrated sequences of cell differentiation during developmental patterning across the brain. As the constrained subnetwork we have detected is enriched for genes involved in the control of mitosis and transcription, we speculate that it plays a fundamental role in these processes. Our finding that neurological Mendelian disease genes are over-represented, combined with previous reports of de novo mutations affecting autism spectrum disorders [6,18], intellectual disability [6] and epileptic encephalopathy [5], further support this notion, indicating that most perturbation leads to severe phenotype. This strong limitation in tolerance may also explain our observation of enrichment in immune cell populations, as precise control of developmental decisions is crucial to the correct differentiation of the lymphoid and myeloid lineages throughout life. As the selective constraint scores are by design corrected for both coding sequence length and GC bias [6], constraint is more likely to be due to intolerance of changes to protein function rather than structural characteristics of the encoded proteins.

Network analyses have been used to identify interacting groups of genes conserved across species [19], and to identify groups of co-expressed genes in both healthy individuals [20] and groups of genes whose expression is coordinately altered in neurological disease [21]. In particular, network analyses of expression data across species suggest that co-regulated genes form stable interaction networks that evolve in a coordinate fashion [19]. These diverse analyses all suggest that functionally linked genes form stable networks and are targets of natural selection due to their group contribution to specific biological processes [22]. Our own results support this notion, demonstrating that interacting protein networks are under remarkable constraint within the human species, presumably because they underlie carefully orchestrated biological processes.

More broadly, our results present a glimpse into how natural selection may affect entire groups of genes involved in central homeostatic functions. Most studies of selection aim to identify specific alleles inconsistent with the nearly neutral model of drift, with particular success in studies of recent positive selection [23,24]. We suggest that the majority of these effects represent near-Mendelian effects on relevant phenotypes, which are the actual targets of selective forces: for example, variability in lactase persistence is almost entirely explained by any one of handful of necessary and sufficient alleles [25]. However, the majority of human traits are polygenic, and selection would likely exert far weaker effects on risk alleles, most of which have been revealed by GWAS to only explain a fraction of phenotypic variance. Although such polygenic adaptation [26] has proven difficult to detect thus far, our data provide confirmation that selective forces can act on groups of genes involved in the same process, supporting the notion that purifying selection can act coordinately on multiple genes. We describe how selective constraint acts on groups of genes, suggesting such coordination, though we note that the constraint statistics contain no information about whether multiple genes are targets of the same pressure. We further note that the substantial preferential expression we see does not apply to the entire constrained subnetwork—this may be due either to imprecise specification of the network itself or limitations in detecting preferential expression in a limited tissue atlas. However, our results clearly support a coherent physiological role for this network in early fetal development.

We have presented a robust approach to identifying sets of interacting genes under selective constraint and placing these into biological context, using the wealth of genome-scale data produced by large-scale public projects. Our approach builds on robust statistical frameworks to interrogate single variants or genes and thus provides previously lacking biological context from which further hypotheses can be drawn. The approach is flexible and not restricted to studies of constraint: per-gene measures derived from studies of other forms of natural selection, non-human hominid introgression, common and rare variant disease association can be analyzed in our framework. Further, as PINTS is modular, appropriate tissue atlases can be used to meaningfully interpret results. We believe our work represents a new class of approaches that can leverage multiple genome-scale datasets to gain new insight into biological activities responsible for health and disease.

MATERIALS AND METHODS

Selective constraint data

We have used selective constraint scores as previously described [6]. Briefly, we used a mutation rate table—containing the probability of every trinucleotide XY_1Z mutating to every other possible trinucleotide XY_2Z—based on intergenic SNPs from the 1000 Genomes project and the sequence of a gene to determine that gene's probability of mutation. These sequence context-based probabilities of mutation were additionally corrected for regional divergence between humans and macaques as well as the depth of coverage for each base in an exome sequencing study. Given the high correlation (Pearson's $r = 0.94$) between the probability of a synonymous mutation in a gene with the number of rare (MAF < 0.01%) synonymous variants in that gene seen in the NHLBI's Exome Sequencing Project, we used a linear model to predict the number of rare missense variants expected per gene in the same dataset. The difference between observation and expectation was quantified as a signed Z score of the chi-squared deviation. The missense Z score was used as the basis for determining selective constraint. In this study, we took a conservative approach to assessing selective constraint, using the Bonferroni correction for number of InWeb genes to derive a significance threshold of $p_c < 5 \times 10^{-6}$.

Detecting selectively constrained subnetworks in protein-protein interaction data

We used InWeb, a previously described comprehensive map of protein-protein interactions, containing 169,736 high-confidence interactions between 12,687 gene products, compiled from a variety of sources [16]. By mapping ENSEMBL IDs, we were able to identify 9729 genes with constraint scores from Samocha et al [6] also present in the REP expression data (below), to which we restricted our analysis.

To detect clusters of interacting constrained genes, we used a heuristic form of the prize-collecting Steiner tree (PCST) algorithm [27,28], which has been previously applied to protein-protein interaction data[17]. The canonical form of the PCST algorithm takes a connected, undirected graph G(V,E,w,u) with V vertices and E edges, with vertex weights w and edge weights u; it then finds the connected subgraph T(V',E') with maximal profit(T), which is some function of (w'-u'). By definition, T is a minimal spanning tree. The algorithm thus identifies the set of nodes with the strongest signal given the cost of their connecting edges. The classical PCST algorithm is, however, NP-hard, which makes it computationally intractable on the scale of InWeb [27]. Several heuristic simplifications have been proposed, including one previously validated as suitable for protein-protein interaction networks which we use here [17]. This approach partitions the set V into null (with weights $w < 0$) and signal (with weights $w > 0$) vertices (genes) and equal edge weights e before searching for T. Beisser et al have implemented this approach in the BioNet package for the R statistical language [29]. Here, we define signal genes as those with constraint scores passing the Bonferroni threshold of $p_c < 5 \times 10^{-6}$, and calculate the weights as $w = -\log(p_c) + \log(5 \times 10^{-6})$. The PCST algorithm returns a single, maximal T solution; to discover further independent subnetworks, we apply the method iteratively after we assign gene nodes in the previously discovered solution to be null.

The algorithm always returns a solution for T, so we sought to assess the significance of our observations empirically. To understand if the observed solution is unlikely by chance, we permuted the constraint scores of genes 1000 times and for each iteration ran the heuristic PCST to generate 1000 random resampled subnetworks (these are also used in the tissue-specificity analyses described below). We then quantified the following key parameters and assessed how many random subnetworks had values exceeding those of the true discovered subnetwork: size (number of gene nodes); density (number of connections); clustering coefficient and total amount of constraint explained (sum of constraint scores). To address the possible contribution of degree bias to these results, we also performed biased permutations to select signal nodes with the same degree distribution as we had previously done for DAPPLE [9]. We found weak correlation between degree and significance and opted for random permutations where the number of combinations of random genes selected as signal nodes is much larger.

Gene expression data processing and preferential expression analysis

We obtained gene expression data for a cosmopolitan set of tissues from the Roadmap Epigenome Project (REP) [14]. The REP data consists of 88 samples across 27 tissue types from diverse human organs, profiled on the Affymetrix HuEx-1_0-st-v2 exon array, which we downloaded on 9/25/2013 from http://www.genboree.org/EdaccData/Current-Release/experiment-sample/Expression_Array/. We processed these data using standard methods available from the BioConductor project [30,31]. Briefly, we removed cross-hybridizing probesets, applied RMA background correction and quantile normalization and then summarized probesets to transcript-level intensities. We then mapped transcripts to genes using the current Gencode annotations for human genes (version 12). Transcripts with no match in Gencode were removed and the remaining transcripts we again quantile normalized. We then assigned transcript expression levels to their matching genes. Where multiple transcripts mapped to the same gene we used the transcript with maximum expression over all cell types.

The Brainspan atlas [15] data are available as processed, gene-level expression levels fromhttp://www.brainspan.org/static/download.html. We mapped these genes to the InWeb gene set using ENSEMBL IDs, and quantile normalized data for the overlapping genes. We then grouped replicate data by developmental stage and brain structure and calculated preferential expression as described above.

We used a previously described approach to detect tissue-specific expression across each tissue atlas [32]. Briefly, we group together replicates from the same cell type and compute pairwise differential expression between all pairwise combinations of tissues, using an empirical Bayes approach to account for variance shrinkage [33]. Thus, for each gene there are 26 linear model coefficients and associated p values for each tissue, quantifying the comparison to all other tissues. For each gene in each tissue, we then capture the overall difference in expression from all other tissues as the sum of these coefficients. To reduce noise, only coefficients with $p < 0.0019$ ($p < 0.05$ with Bonferroni correction for 26 tissues) are considered. Rescaling all coefficient sums across all genes values to the range $[-1,1]$ gives us a final preferential expression score. Intuitively, a gene highly expressed in only one tissue would get a high positive enrichment score in that tissue, as it is differentially expressed compared to all other tissues. The score is directional, strong negative values indicate very low expression in one tissue compared to all others. We partition the overall distribution into deciles and define preferential expression in a tissue if a gene has a score > 0.1.

Scoring subnetwork tissue specificity

To score the tissue specific expression of a subnetwork, we detect which genes in the subnetwork are preferentially expressed in each tissue of our expression atlas and assess the joint probability of this observation. Rather than ask if some nodes of the subnetwork are preferentially expressed in a given tissue, we developed an approach to account for the connections between genes; we thus assess whether the pattern of preferential expression across the whole subnetwork is unusual for a given tissue, suggesting the subnetwork is operational. Formally, we consider the subnetwork as a Markov random field with a particular configuration of preferentially expressed nodes in each atlas tissue. We compute a score for each configuration using a standard scoring function [34]:

$$P(x_1, \ldots, x_n) = \frac{1}{Z} \prod_{(i,j) \in Edges} \Phi(x_i, x_j)$$

The partition function Z is defined as: $Z = \sum_{x_1, \ldots, x_n} \prod_{(i,j) \in Edges} \Phi(x_i, x_j)$ where $x_i (i = 1, \ldots, n)$ represents a binary tissue specificity of the genes in the subnetwork for a given tissue with values either 1 (expressed) or 0 (not expressed). The $\Phi(x_i, x_j)$ factor lists the co-occurrence of two connected nodes across tissues. This is calculated from the thresholded preferential expression data, and each pair of connected nodes is assigned exactly oneconfiguration in each tissue, so that $\Phi(x_i = 0, x_j = 0) + \Phi(x_i = 1, x_j = 0) + \Phi(x_i = 0, x_j = 1) + \Phi(x_i = 1, x_j = 1) = number\ of\ tissues$

We assess the significance of these scores using two conservative permutation approaches. First we assess how likely we are to see each observed configuration (i.e. each pattern of detected/not detected nodes) in each tissue of the atlas. We do this by permuting the preferential expression scores across tissues for each gene independently and rescoring the configuration found in each tissue. This alters the co-expression structure across genes and empirically assesses how likely we are to see a particular configuration of a specific subnetwork by chance. Second, we estimate the probability of observing the extent of tissue specificity in each tissue. We construct the null expectation by scoring the resampled subnetworks generated by permutation above in each tissue and compute the empirical significance from this distribution of scores.

To ensure our results are not artifacts of a specific preferential expression threshold, we repeat this analysis across a spectrum of preferential expression thresholds.

Pathway analysis

To test if any biological pathways are over represented in a subnetwork, we use the Gene Set Enrichment Analysis (GSEA) approach [35]. We obtained the full list of curated canonical pathways from the GSEA website (http://www.broadinstitute.org/gsea/msigdb/collections.jsp) and mapped the 9729 genes to each pathway using HUGO IDs. We then test for enrichment of subnetwork members over background using the hypergeometric test.

Online Mendelian Inheritance in Man (OMIM) analysis

To test if genes in the subnetwork are more likely to harbor pathogenic mutations causing Mendelian diseases than expected by chance, we retrieved OMIM records for all 9729 genes using the biomaRt package in BioConductor [31]. We then tested whether the proportion of 107 subnetwork genes with OMIM entries was higher than the background proportion of the full set of 9729 in our analysis using Fisher's exact test. We then mapped all OMIM entries to Medical Subject Headings (MeSH) disease categories using the Comparative Toxicogenomics Database (CTD) MEDIC disease vocabulary [36] and assessed enrichment in any disease category, again using Fisher's exact test.

SUPPORTING INFORMATION

Acknowledgments

We acknowledge our use of the gene set enrichment analysis, GSEA software, and Molecular Signature Database (MSigDB), available at http://www.broad.mit.edu/gsea/.

Author Contributions

Conceived and designed the experiments: JC PS CC. Performed the experiments: JC PS. Analyzed the data: JC PS CC. Contributed reagents/materials/analysis tools: KES MJD. Wrote the paper: JC PS CC.

REFERENCES

1. Nielsen R, Hellmann I, Hubisz M, Bustamante C, Clark AG. Recent and ongoing selection in the human genome. Nature Reviews Genetics. 2007;8: 857–868. doi: 10. 1038/nrg2187. pmid:17943193
2. Exome sequencing identifies MLL2 mutations as a cause of Kabuki syndrome. Nature Genetics. Nature Publishing Group; 2010;42: 790–793. doi: 10. 1038/ng. 646.
3. Sanders SJ, He X, Willsey AJ, Ercan-Sencicek AG, Samocha KE, Cicek AE, et al. Insights into Autism Spectrum Disorder Genomic Architecture and Biology from 71 Risk Loci. Neuron. Elsevier; 2015;87: 1215–1233. doi: 10. 1016/j. neuron. 2015. 09. 016.
4. Robinson EB, St Pourcain B, Anttila V, Kosmicki JA, Bulik-Sullivan B, Grove J, et al. Genetic risk for autism spectrum disorders and neuropsychiatric variation in the general population. Nature Genetics. 2016;48: 552–555. doi: 10. 1038/ng. 3529. pmid:26998691
5. Epi4K Consortium, Epilepsy Phenome/Genome Project, Allen AS, Cossette P, Delanty N, Eichler EE, et al. De novo mutations in epileptic encephalopathies. Nature. 2013;501: 217–221. doi: 10. 1038/nature12439. pmid:23934111
6. Samocha KE, Robinson EB, Sanders SJ, Stevens C, Sabo A, McGrath LM, et al. A framework for the interpretation of de novo mutation in human disease. Nature Genetics. 2014;46: 944–950. doi: 10. 1038/ng. 3050. pmid:25086666
7. Yang J, Manolio TA, Pasquale LR, Boerwinkle E, Caporaso N, Cunningham JM, et al. Genome partitioning of genetic variation for complex traits using common SNPs. Nature Genetics. 2011;43: 519–525. doi: 10. 1038/ng. 823. pmid:21552263
8. Yang J, Benyamin B, McEvoy BP, Gordon S, Henders AK, Nyholt DR, et al. Common SNPs explain a large proportion of the heritability for human height. Nature Genetics. 2010;42: 565–569. doi: 10. 1038/ng. 608. pmid:20562875
9. Rossin EJ, Lage K, Raychaudhuri S, Xavier RJ, Tatar D, Benita Y, et al. Proteins encoded in genomic regions associated with immune-mediated disease physically interact and suggest underlying biology. PLoS Genetics. 2011;7: e1001273. doi: 10. 1371/journal. pgen. 1001273. pmid:21249183

10. Hormozdiari F, Kichaev G, Yang W-Y, Pasaniuc B, Eskin E. Identification of causal genes for complex traits. Bioinformatics. Oxford University Press; 2015;31: i206–i213. doi: 10. 1093/bioinformatics/btv240.

11. Lee Y, Li H, Li J, Rebman E, Achour I, Regan KE, et al. Network models of genome-wide association studies uncover the topological centrality of protein interactions in complex diseases. Journal of the American Medical Informatics Association. 2013. doi: 10. 1136/ amiajnl-2012-001519.

12. Hormozdiari F, Penn O, Borenstein E, Eichler EE. The discovery of integrated gene networks for autism and related disorders. Genome Research. Cold Spring Harbor Lab; 2015;25: 142–154. doi: 10. 1101/gr. 178855. 114.

13. Maurano MT, Humbert R, Rynes E, Thurman RE, Haugen E, Wang H, et al. Systematic Localization of Common Disease-Associated Variation in Regulatory DNA. Science. 2012;337: 1190–1195. doi: 10. 1126/ science. 1222794. pmid:22955828

14. Bernstein BE, Stamatoyannopoulos JA, Costello JF, Ren B, Milosavljevic A, Meissner A, et al. The NIH Roadmap Epigenomics Mapping Consortium. Nat Biotechnol. Nature Publishing Group; 2010;28: 1045–1048. doi: 10. 1038/nbt1010-1045.

15. Kang HJ, Kawasawa YI, Cheng F, Zhu Y, Xu X, Li M, et al. Spatio-temporal transcriptome of the human brain. Nature. Nature Publishing Group; 2011;478: 483–489. doi: 10. 1038/nature10523.

16. Lage K, Karlberg EO, Størling ZM, Ólason PÍ, Pedersen AG, Rigina O, et al. A human phenome-interactome network of protein complexes implicated in genetic disorders. Nat Biotechnol. 2007;25: 309–316. doi: 10. 1038/nbt1295. pmid:17344885

17. Dittrich MT, Klau GW, Rosenwald A, Dandekar T, Muller T. Identifying functional modules in protein-protein interaction networks: an integrated exact approach. Bioinformatics. 2008;24: i223–i231. doi: 10. 1093/bioinformatics/btn161. pmid:18586718

18. Neale BM, Kou Y, Liu L, Ma'ayan A, Samocha KE, Sabo A, et al. Patterns and rates of exonic de novo mutations in autism spectrum disorders. Nature. 2012;485: 242–245. doi: 10. 1038/nature11011. pmid:22495311

19. Oldham MC, Horvath S, Geschwind DH. Conservation and evolution of gene coexpression networks in human and chimpanzee brains. Proceedings of the National Academy of Sciences. National Acad Sciences; 2006;103: 17973–17978. doi: 10. 1073/pnas. 0605938103.

20. Kircher M, He Z, Guo S, Fairbrother GL. Evaluating intra-and inter-individual variation in the human placental transcriptome. Genome …. 2015. doi: 10. 1186/s13059-015-0627-z

21. Voineagu I, Wang X, Johnston P, Lowe JK, Tian Y, Horvath S, et al. Transcriptomic analysis of autistic brain reveals convergent molecular pathology. Nature. Nature Publishing Group; 2011;: 1–7. doi: 10. 1038/ nature10110.

22. Wagner GP, Zhang J. The pleiotropic structure of the genotype–phenotype map: the evolvability of complex organisms. Nature Reviews Genetics. Nature Publishing Group; 2011;12: 204–213. doi: 10. 1038/nrg2949.

23. Grossman SR, Shlyakhter I, Shylakhter I, Karlsson EK, Byrne EH, Morales S, et al. A composite of multiple signals distinguishes causal variants in regions of positive selection. Science. American Association for the Advancement of Science; 2010;327: 883–886. doi: 10. 1126/science. 1183863.

24. Sabeti PC, Fry B, Lohmueller J, Hostetter E, Cotsapas C, Xie X, et al. Genome-wide detection and characterization of positive selection in human populations. Nature. 2007;449: 913–918. doi: 10. 1038/nature06250. pmid:17943131

25. Scheinfeldt LB, Tishkoff SA. Recent human adaptation: genomic approaches, interpretation and insights. Nature Reviews Genetics. 2013;14: 692–702. doi: 10. 1038/ nrg3604. pmid:24052086

26. Pritchard JK, Di Rienzo A. Adaptation—not by sweeps alone. Nature Reviews Genetics. Nature Publishing Group; 2010;11: 665–667. doi: 10. 1038/nrg2880.

27. Ljubić I, Weiskircher R, Pferschy U, Klau GW, Mutzel P, Fischetti M. An Algorithmic Framework for the Exact Solution of the Prize-Collecting Steiner Tree Problem. Math Program. Springer-Verlag; 2006;105: 427–449. doi: 10. 1007/s10107-005-0660-x.

28. Ljubic I, Weiskircher R, Pferschy U, Klau GW. Solving the prize-collecting Steiner tree problem to optimality. ALENEX/ANALCO. 2005.

29. Beisser D, Klau GW, Dandekar T, Müller T, Dittrich MT. BioNet: an R-Package for the functional analysis of biological networks. Bioinformatics. Oxford University Press; 2010;26: 1129–1130. doi: 10. 1093/ bioinformatics/btq089.

30. Gautier L, Cope L, Bolstad BM, Irizarry RA. affy—analysis of Affymetrix GeneChip data at the probe level. Bioinformatics. Oxford University Press; 2004;20: 307–315. doi: 10. 1093/bioinformatics/btg405.

31. Gentleman RC, Carey VJ, Bates DM, Ben Bolstad, Dettling M, Dudoit S, et al. Bioconductor: open software development for computational biology and bioinformatics. Genome Biol. BioMed Central Ltd; 2004;5: R80. doi: 10. 1186/gb-2004-5-10-r80.

32. Benita Y, Cao Z, Giallourakis C, Li C, Gardet A, Xavier RJ. Gene enrichment profiles reveal T-cell development, differentiation, and lineage-specific transcription factors including ZBTB25 as a novel NF-AT repressor. Blood. 2010;115: 5376–5384. doi: 10. 1182/blood-2010-01-263855. pmid:20410506

33. Smyth GK. limma: Linear Models for Microarray Data. Bioinformatics and Computational Biology Solutions Using R and Bioconductor. New York: Springer New York; 2005. pp. 397–420. doi: 10. 1007/0-387-29362-0_23.

34. Schmidt M. UGM: Matlab code for undirected graphical models [Internet]. Vancouver, Canada; [cited 28 Mar 2015]. Available:http://www. cs. ubc. ca/~schmidtm/ Software/UGM. html

35. Subramanian A, Tamayo P, Mootha VK, Mukherjee

S, Ebert BL, Gillette MA, et al. Gene set enrichment analysis: a knowledge-based approach for interpreting genome-wide expression profiles. Proc Natl Acad Sci USA. National Acad Sciences; 2005;102: 15545–15550. doi: 10. 1073/pnas. 0506580102.

36. Davis AP, Grondin CJ, Lennon-Hopkins K, Saraceni-Richards C, Sciaky D, King BL, et al. The Comparative Toxicogenomics Database's 10th year anniversary: update 2015. Nucleic Acids Research. Oxford University Press; 2015;43: D914–20. doi: 10. 1093/nar/gku935.

CHAPTER 15

A NOVEL METHOD TO DISCOVER FLUOROQUINOLONE ANTIBIOTIC RESISTANCE (QNR) GENES IN FRAGMENTED NUCLEOTIDE SEQUENCES

Fredrik Boulund, Anna Johnning, Mariana Buongermino Pereira, DG Joakim Larsson and Erik Kristiansson

Keywords: Metagenomics Antibiotic resistance, Fluoroquinolones, PMQR, Qnr, Hidden markov models

BACKGROUND

Antibiotics are one of our most powerful tools for treating and preventing bacterial infections and have since their introduction vastly improved human health and drastically reduced mortality rates. The high use of antibiotics in human and veterinary medicine has however resulted in an accelerated development of multiresistant bacteria [1, 2]. Bacteria can adapt to an antibiotic selection pressure by altering their genome, either by mutations in pre-existing DNA or through the acquisition of resistance genes [3]. Since resistance genes can be horizontally transferred between bacterial cells, antibiotic resistance can rapidly spread within and between bacterial communities [4, 5, 6]. Many types of antibiotics are derived from compounds that are naturally found in the environment and bacteria have developed resistance genes as a protection mechanism. Environmental bacterial communities have therefore been hypothesized to contain a large and unexplored collection of antibiotic resistance genes [7, 8, 9, 10]. Antibiotic resistance genes were present in environmental bacterial communities long before they emerged in human pathogens [11]. As a consequence, many of the antibiotic resistance genes found in clinical settings have been horizontally transferred from environmental bacteria [12, 13].

Citation: Fredrik Boulund, Anna Johnning, Mariana Buongermino Pereira, DG Joakim Larsson and Erik Kristiansson, A novel method to discover fluoroquinolone antibiotic resistance (qnr) genes in fragmented nucleotide sequences, DOI: 10.1186/1471-2164-13-695.

The broad-spectrum fluoroquinolone antibiotics were introduced in the early 1960's and are today extensively used in human and veterinary medicine. Fluoroquinolones interacts with the essential bacterial type II topoisomerases (topoisomerase IV and DNA gyrase) and thereby inhibits DNA replication. The most effective fluoroquinolone resistance mechanism is chromosomal mutations in the antibiotic target proteins which confers high levels of resistance in several bacterial species [14, 15]. Recently, a family of mobile fluoroquinolone antibiotic resistance genes called *qnr* was discovered [16, 17]. These mobile plasmid-mediated quinolone resistance genes (sometimes labeled PMQR) have been grouped into five recognized classes; *qnrA*, *qnrB*, *qnrC*, *qnrD*, and *qnrS* and it is currently unknown whether more classes exist. The *qnr*genes encode proteins that prevent fluoroquinolones from interacting with DNA/type-II-topoisomerase complexes formed during DNA replication, thus preventing fluoroquinolone inhibition. The levels of resistance conferred by *qnr* genes are generally lower than chromosomal mutations but can reach up to 1 mg/L (minimum inhibitory concentration) depending on the organism and specific antibiotic compound [18].

The *qnr* genes belong to the larger family of pentapeptide repeat proteins (PRP), which are ubiquitously present with more than 500 variants described in all forms of life [19]. All PRPs are characterized by a sequence feature consisting of repeating subunits of five amino acid residues following the form A(D/N)LXX. This repetitive pattern makes PRPs fold into a β-helix that performs a wide range of cellular functions and they are found both membrane bound and in the cytoplasm [20]. For *qnr* genes the β-helix resembles the structure of the DNA spiral and interacts with type II topoisomerases and thereby prevent fluoroquinolone antibiotics to inhibit the function of the complex [21, 22]. Despite the strong similarity in the repeating amino acid pattern between *qnr* sequences and other PRPs it is unclear exactly why *qnr* genes provide resistance to fluoroquinolones.

Further characterization of *qnr* genes is necessary to fully understand their function and estimate their diversity. Assuming the presence of antibiotic resistance genes in clinical settings is the result of transfer of mobile genetic elements from the environment, it is natural to search environmental microbial communities to find previously unidentified *qnr* genes. Recent culture-independent methods such as metagenomics enables unprecedented exploratory analysis of the genetic basis in microbial communities [23, 24]. This is especially true considering that more than 99% of environmental bacterial communities do not submit easily to cultivation and would consequently be missed with sampling and analysis of individual strains [25, 26]. In combination with next-generation DNA sequencing technologies metagenomics provide means for culture-independent studies of bacterial communities at a very high resolution. However, high-throughput sequencing equipment can currently only produce short DNA fragments (typically 75-400 nucleotides long) which substantially limits the sensitivity and specificity of identifying genes such as *qnr*[27].

In-silico approaches have previously been used to identify novel variants of *qnr* genes. For example, Fonseca*et al.* identified *qnr* VC1 and *qnr* VC2 in *Vibrio cholerae* using sequence comparison to existing plasmid-mediated *qnr* genes [28]. A similar approach was used by Sanches *et al.* to identify several chromosomal *qnr*variants, including multiple members of the class *Smqnr* from *Stenotrophomonas maltophilia*[29], and by Velasco *et al.* to discover *Smaqnr* in *Serratia marcescens*[30]. However, all of these studies used sequence alignment tools such as BLAST which do not explicitly make use of the repetitive structure of the *qnr* genes. Furthermore, none of the previous suggested methods were adapted to short sequence lengths and high volumes of data which makes them inapplicable to sequences from shotgun metagenomics.

In this paper, we describe a novel method to identify fluoroquinolone antibiotic resistance genes in DNA sequence data. By using hidden Markov models combined with a length-dependent classification rule, the method is able to discriminate between *qnr* and other pentapeptide repeat proteins not associated with a resistance phenotype. Cross-validation estimated that the method had a high statistical power of detecting fragments of *qnr* genes in metagenomic data, even at fragment lengths as short as 100 nucleotides. The method was applied to sequence data from various databases and both known and novel putative *qnr* genes were identified. An implementation of the method is freely available athttp://bioinformatics.math.chalmers.se/qnr/.

RESULTS

A hidden Markov model (HMM) was constructed from a multiple sequence alignment of all currently known and experimentally verified plasmid-mediated *qnr* resistance gene amino acid sequences [31]. Using the database search software HMMER3, we analyzed the empirical bit score distributions produced by applying the HMM to two sources of protein sequence data; a*)* true *qnr* fragments, created from randomly fragmented*qnr* sequences and *b)* non-*qnr* fragments, created from pentapeptide repeat protein (PRP) sequences not associated with a fluoroquinolone resistance phenotype (see Methods). To visualize the bit score distributions of fragmented sequences, random fragments of *qnr* and non-*qnr* sequences were created for each fragment length between 10 and 210 amino acid residues (i.e. full length *qnr* sequences) and their scores against the HMM were plotted as a function of fragment length. As indicated by Figure 1 true *qnr* fragments had bit scores that were approximately linear in relation to their fragment length while the bit score distribution of the non-*qnr* fragments was centered around 33. A two-part linear classification function was therefore introduced to discriminate between true *qnr* and non-*qnr* fragments. For fragments up to a length threshold (D), the classification function was linear with an intercept M and slope K. For fragments longer than D, the function used a fixed cutoff $C = K \times D + M$ (Figure 1A).

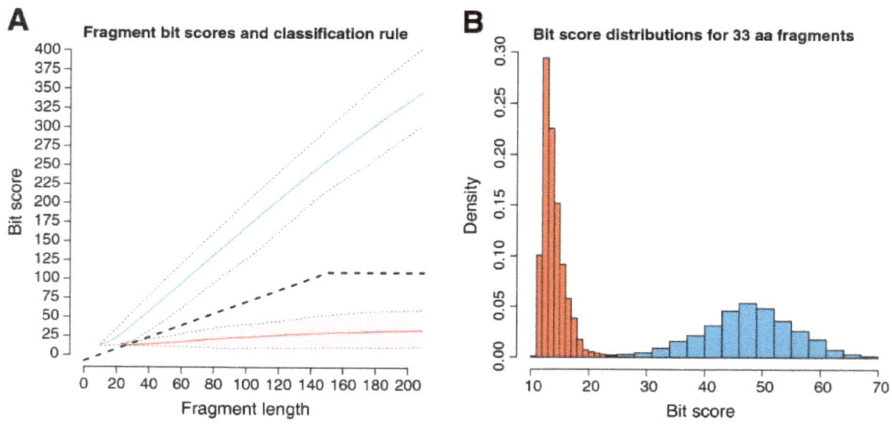

Figure 1 Fragment bit scores and classification rule. **A**) The figure shows the distribution of the fragment bit scores at different fragment lengths. The separation between the *qnr* fragments (light blue) and non-*qnr* fragments (light red) increase for longer fragment lengths. The solid blue and red lines show the average bit scores for *qnr* and non-*qnr*fragments, with their 99th and 1st percentiles in grey dashed lines above and below, respectively. The thick dashed line in black shows the classification function with the optimized parameters K=0.778, M=-7.89, D=150.64 . **B**) The bit scores when compared to the hidden Markov model for 33 amino acid long fragments, corresponding to the approximately 100 nucleotides long sequence reads common in next-generation sequencing

technologies. At this fragment length, the *qnr*fragments (blue) are clearly separated from the non-*qnr* (red) with only a small overlap.

Cross-validation was used to optimize the parameters M, K and D of the classification function for identification of novel classes of *qnr* genes. The optimization was performed for five different models where each model was created by excluding one class of plasmid-mediated *qnr* proteins (i.e. QnrA, QnrB, QnrC, QnrD and QnrS). The cross-validation was then performed using disjoint set of fragments, one for parameter estimation (training) and one for evaluation of the corresponding performance (validation). The training and validation data sets were created from fragments of both *qnr* genes and non-*qnr* PRP genes without any associated resistance phenotype. For each of the five models, the excluded *qnr* class was also removed from the training dataset. The corresponding performance was, on the other hand, evaluated only using the excluded *qnr* class and a set of non-*qnr* genes. Thus, the ability to classify novel *qnr* genes was evaluated on fragments of gene classes not included in the model. The cross-validation was performed with random fragments ranging from 10 to 209 amino acid residues, each length repeated 2500 times. The parameters of the classification function were estimated to M = -7.89 (1.37), K = 0.778 (0.084), D = 150.64 (27.05) (average over all five models, standard deviation in brackets). The corresponding fixed cutoff C was calculated to C = 109.64 (16.40).

The optimized classification function parameters were then used to validate the statistical power to detect novel putative fragments. At a fragment length as short as 33 amino acids the average power for correctly classifying fragments from novel putative *qnr* gene classes was 94% (Figure 2A). The results differed between the five models (Figure 2B): for a 33 amino acid long sequence, the power to identify a QnrD fragment (given a model built from QnrA, B, C and S) was highest (99.04%) while the power of identifying a QnrB fragment (given QnrA, C, D and S) was the lowest (88.02%). The specificity was estimated to be above 99.27% for all models and all fragment lengths. See Methods for full details.

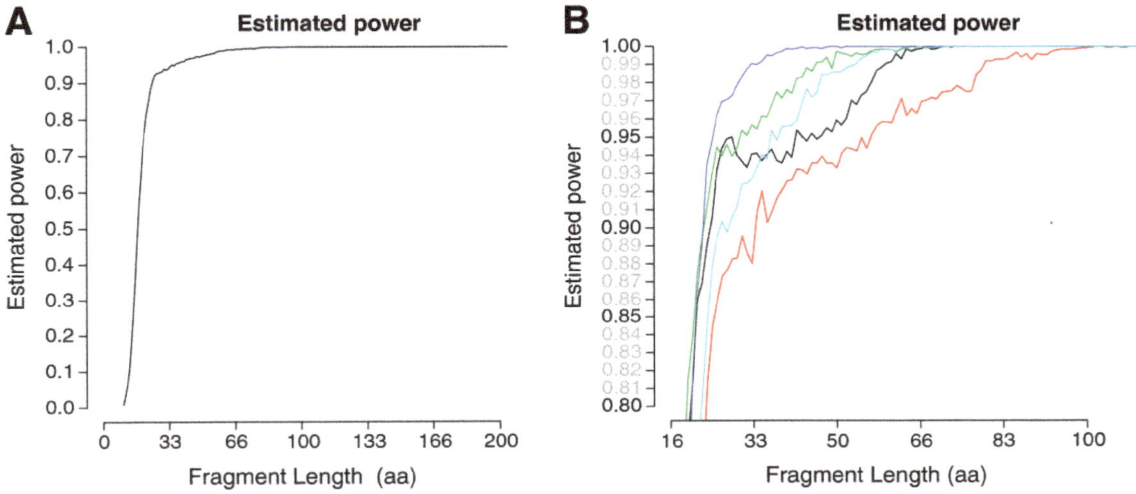

Figure 2 Estimated power. **A)** The figure shows the estimated power of detecting fragments from novel classes of *qnr* as a function of fragment length in nucleotides (averaged over the five different models used in the cross-validation). At a fragment length of 33 amino acids (approximately 100 nucleotides), the power to detect fragments from novel classes of *qnr* genes was estimated to 94% which increased to 100% for 100 amino acid long fragments. **B)** A magnification of the upper left region showing the power of detecting each class of *qnr* genes: QnrA (black), QnrB (red), QnrC (green), QnrD (dark blue) and QnrS (cyan). Corresponding plots for the specificity are available as.

To search for novel putative *qnr* gene variants a model based on all five classes of plasmid-mediated *qnr*genes together with the classifier with the optimized parameter values was applied to protein sequences from various databases and metagenomic sequencing projects; GenBank [32], CAMERA [33], MG-RAST [34], contigs from Meta-HIT [35], and several data sets from SRA [36] (see Table 1 and Methods). A smaller metagenomic dataset from a recent study where a high abundance of *qnr* genes was detected was also included [37]. The total number of fragments available in all datasets was 478,025,600 comprising 214,168,682,742 nucleotides. In total, 1733 (3.6×10^{-4}%) sequence fragments classified as *qnr* by the method. For the metagenomes the proportion of *qnr* fragments was estimated to 2.8×10^{-4}% (1275 out of 463,364,852 metagenomic fragments), reflecting the low abundance of *qnr* genes in the environment. All fragments that classified as *qnr* were stringently clustered into 475 groups (where 165 contained more than one fragments) and annotated against GenBank and the list of known *qnr* genes [31]. Among these clusters, all five classes of plasmid-mediated *qnr* were represented as well as 28 previously described chromosomally located variants [28, 29, 38, 39, 40, 41]. In addition, one contig in group #1, which consisted entirely of metagenomic fragments, represented a full length sequence of a novel putative *qnr* gene with 93% identity (97% similarity) to QnrB1. During the course of this project this sequence was accepted as a novel QnrB variant, QnrB35, and submitted to GenBank [GenBank:AEL00456] [39]. The method was hence capable of reconstructing complete*qnr* sequences directly from fragmented metagenomic data. This was particularly evident since the complete sequence of QnrB35 was not available in any of the datasets at the time of their retrieval in this project.

Table 1 Data sources searched for *qnr* gene fragments

Data source	Number of sequences	Number of nucleotides*(approximate)*	Identified putative *qnr*fragments
CAMERA [33]	161,016,287	57,118,358,119	217
GenBank (nt) [32]	14,627,404	35,003,500,149	392
GenBank (env_nt) [32]	18,438,927	7,602,413,875	54
GenBank (refseq) [32]	33,074	7,192,954,783	66
Meta-HIT [35]	6,589,348	10,322,657,198	2
MG-RAST [42]	74,767,763	29,132,992,517	226
SRA [36]	202,090,286	67,627,717,961	516
India Patancheru [37]	462,241	168,088,140	260
Total:	*478,025,600*	*214,168,682,742*	*1733*

Table 2 Examples of identified novel putative *qnr* sequences

Example #	Group	Source(s)	Contig length (aa)	Model bit score	Most similar plasmid-mediated*qnr*
1	1	Metagenome:	214	356.9	QnrB37 (79% identity)
		SRA: SRX032366			
2	12	Metagenome:	218	131.2	QnrC (33% identity)
		MG-RAST: 4441580			
3	78	Chromosome:	213	326.4	QnrB28 (68% identity)
		Dickeya dadantii 3937, NC_014500.1			
4	81	Chromosome:	211	294.6	Qnr19 (66% identity)
		Xenorhabdus bovienii SS-2004, NC_013892.1			
5	199	Chromosome:	218	350.0	QnrC (72% identity)
		Vibrio furnissii, CP002378.1			

The method discovered 732 fragments of metagenomic origin that clustered in 440 groups which did not contain any of the previously described plasmid-mediated or chromosomal *qnr* genes. An additional 11 sequences of novel putative *qnr* genes in the genomes of 9 sequenced bacteria were also discovered. Table 2 shows five examples of groups containing sequences classified as novel putative *qnr* genes by the method. Sequence #1 was constructed from fragments originating from baby stool metagenomes [43] [SRA accession SRX032366] and shared 79% sequence identity with QnrB37. Sequence #2 was discovered in an environmental samples from coastal sea water outside the North American coast [MG-RAST accession 4441580] as a part of the Gene Ocean Sampling Expedition [44]. This sequence is a 218 amino acid long fragment that shares 33% sequence identity with QnrC. The next three sequences were discovered in bacterial genomes in GenBank. Sequence #3 was discovered in the chromosome of *Dickey dadantii* 3937 [GenBank:NC_014500.1] and was a 213 amino acid long sequence with 68% identity to QnrB28. Sequence #4 was found in the chromosome of *Xenorhabdus bovienii* [GenBank:NC_013892.1] and was a 211 amino acid long sequence with 66% identity to QnrB19. Sequence #5 came from the chromosome of *Vibrio furnissii*[GenBank:CP002378.1] and was a 218 amino acid long sequence sharing 72% identity with QnrC. Full results, including all 475 groups and their annotation, are available in.

DISCUSSION

Qnr genes provide resistance to broad-spectrum fluoroquinolone antibiotics and can move between bacteria using horizontal gene transfer. However, the total number of *qnr* classes and their diversity in environmental bacterial communities is not clear. We therefore developed a novel method to identify new classes of *qnr*genes in fragmented metagenomic data. The method uses a hidden Markov model (HMM) to identify candidate *qnr* fragments which are then further classified based on their model score and sequence length. Cross-validation confirmed that the method had a high sensitivity and specificity to detect fragments from novel classes of known *qnr* genes, even at fragments as short as 33 amino acid residues. This makes the method applicable to many forms of nucleotide data, including sequences generated by next-generation DNA sequencers. From public sequence repositories the method classified 1733 sequence fragments (3.6×10^{-4}%) as *qnr*, which were further clustered into 475 groups. The method also identified 39 chromosomal *qnr*variants in 33 bacterial species.

Several of the novel putative *qnr* genes identified in this study have to the authors' best knowledge previously not been described in literature. Experimental verification, including phenotypic profiling in multiple bacterial hosts, is therefore necessary to fully evaluate the resistance potential of our predictions. However, the cross-validation demonstrated that the proposed method had a high sensitivity and could discriminate between fragments from classes of known *qnr* and pentapeptide repeat proteins without a resistance phenotype (Figure 2A). The method was also able to identify all previously reported classes of *qnr* genes, including the variant *qnr* B35 which was at the time for this analysis not submitted to the database and thus not included in the hidden Markov model. This shows that the method has a high predictive power and it is therefore possible that several of the predictions indeed represent previously unidentified novel classes or variants of *qnr* genes.

Many of the identified putative *qnr* gene fragments were discovered in metagenomes sampled from different types of environments, e.g. human gut [43], seawater [44] and river sediment [37]. This indicates that there is an unexplored diversity of *qnr* genes within environmental bacterial communities and that these can be identified by metagenomic sequencing. However, the amount of nucleotide data currently represented in the sequence repositories merely reflects a tiny fraction of the total microbial diversity on earth [45, 46, 47]. In addition, the estimated relative abundance of unknown fragments from putative *qnr* genes was 2.8 × 10-4% (1275 out of 463,364,852 metagenomic fragments) underlining the vast amounts of sequence data needed to identify and assemble *qnr* genes from environmental data. It is therefore possible, and even likely, that there are additional variants of *qnr* genes present in the environmental bacterial communities currently not represented in the sequence repositories due to the heavy undersampling. The data that is currently being generated by large-scale reference metagenome projects, such as the Earth Microbiome Project [48] and the Gene Ocean Sampling [44], will offer a substantially higher sequencing depth and may therefore reveal additional classes and variants of *qnr* genes.

Our results show that hidden Markov models are highly suitable for identifying sequence fragments from *qnr*genes. The model used in this study was derived from a multiple alignment of *qnr* genes and can thereby infer information on the degree of variability at different amino acid positions in the sequence [49]. This is especially useful for pentapeptide repeat proteins which generally have a low sequence similarity except in the conserved residues of the distinctive repetitive A(D/N)LXX motif. In contrast, traditional sequence alignment tools such as BLAST cannot distinguish between important variation in the repeating pattern and variation in the intermediate regions. Previous methods to identify novel *qnr* genes from DNA sequence data have used BLAST and may therefore have limited sensitivity and specificity [49]. The proposed method has, on the other hand, demonstrated a high power of detecting new classes of *qnr* genes (Figure 2) and is hence a more suitable approach for identification and annotation of *qnr* genes.

Controlling the number of false predictions is vital for large-scale data analysis. A low specificity can generate a massive amount of false positives and thereby decrease the quality of analysis and the biological interpretation of the downstream results (in this case the sequence groups). Based on the distribution of bit scores for the sequence fragments (Figure 1A) it is clear that a traditional cut-off would not be sufficient to discriminate between *qnr* and non-*qnr* PRPs with both a high sensitivity and specificity. Indeed, a single bit score cut-off would have to be set to 75 to minimize false positives across all fragment lengths, effectively removing the ability to classify fragments shorter than 100 amino acid residues (300 nucleotides). Instead, a linear classification function dependent on fragment length for short fragments enabled correct identification while maintaining a high specificity. This makes the method suitable for analysis of large datasets consisting of short sequence fragments and the method is therefore directly applicable to data from next-generation sequencing technologies such as Illumina's sequencing by synthesis, Life Technologies' sequencing by ligation (SOLiD) or Roche's 454 pyrosequencing [50].

The hidden Markov model used by the method was created from all known plasmid-mediated *qnr* genes with experimentally validated resistance phenotype. However, several recent studies have described chromosomally located *qnr* genes in wide range of species (e.g. *Vibrio spp. alginolyticus*, *Vibrio harveyi* and*Aeromonas hydrophilia*) [28, 29, 38, 40, 41]. These chromosomal *qnr* genes show a relatively high sequence similarity to their plasmid-mediated relatives and some have been shown to confer resistance towards fluoroquinolones when expressed in *E. coli* (e.g. SmaQnr and SmQnr) [29, 41]. Their potential to transfer horizontally between bacteria is however not clear. Even though the hidden Markov model was based on plasmid-mediated gene variants, the method demonstrated a high sensitivity to detect *qnr* genes in bacterial chromosomes. In fact, the method identified 28 previously reported chromosomally located *qnr* genes in 24 species. In addition, 11 potentially novel chromosomal *qnr* genes in 9 different species were also identified. Interestingly, four previously suggested chromosomal *qnr* genes were not classified as such by the method. These genes, which are located in *Alkaliphilus metalliredigens, Bacteroides thetaiotaomicron, Bacillus weihenstephanensis* and *Anabaena variabilis* have previously been identified as putative *qnr* genes using BLAST [38]. However, all these genes share low sequence similarity to other *qnr*genes and their resistance phenotype has so far not been validated. The four genes received very low scores by our model, which may indicate that these are false predictions and hence not *qnr* genes. All other previously described *qnr* genes received high scores by the model and were thus classified as *qnr*.

The method described in this study has been implemented as a freely available application in Python. The application searches any specified sequence dataset, classifies the matching sequences as *qnr* or non-*qnr* and clusters the results into groups of putative *qnr* genes. The implementation is straightforward to use, has been optimized to handle data sizes of the order of terabytes, and is suitable for use on standard desktop computers. The package is documented with internal functions thoroughly commented in the distributed source code, making it possible to interface them directly from related applications. The application can be installed and run on any modern GNU/Linux system and it is available from http://bioinformatics.math.chalmers.se/qnr/.

CONCLUSIONS

In this study we proposed a new method to detect and annotate novel classes of *qnr* antibiotic resistance genes in nucleotide sequence data. The method uses a hidden Markov model with a fragment length-dependent classification rule and has a high sensitivity and specificity, even for sequences as short at 100 nucleotides. This makes the method directly applicable to the immense amount of data generated by the next-generation DNA sequencing techniques. Based on sequence data currently available in the repositories, the method was able to identify all previously reported plasmid-mediated *qnr* genes as well as the vast majority of the previously reported chromosomal variants. In addition, the method predicted several novel putative *qnr*genes and some of these were discovered in shotgun metagenomes, which may indicate a large and unknown diversity of *qnr* genes in uncultured environmental bacteria.

METHODS

A hidden Markov model was based on a multiple sequence alignment of sequences from the reference list of acknowledged and experimentally verified plasmid-mediated *qnr* genes [31]. Peptide *qnr* sequences were aligned using MAFFT [51] with default settings. The alignment quality was manually assessed and then used as input for the construction of the hidden Markov model using HMMER3 [49] with default settings.

Investigation of the empirical bit score distribution of the HMM was performed by drawing random fragments of both *qnr* and non-*qnr* genes (Figure 1). This led to the creation of a classifier consisting of a two-part linear discrimination function using information of fragment length (L_f) and fragment bit score (S_f) from the hidden Markov model from HMMER. The classifier was defined by three parameters; linear intercept (M), linear slope (K), and long fragment definition (D). A fragment with length, L_f, and domain bit score, S_f, was classified as *qnr*if $L_f < D$ and $S_f \geq K \times L_f + M$, or if $L_f \geq D$ and $S_f \geq K \times D + M$.

Cross-validation was used to estimate the parameters and to evaluate the performance of the model. Five different models were created and for each model one class of plasmid-mediated *qnr* genes was excluded. Two different kinds of sequences were used in the cross-validation: true *qnr* genes and non-*qnr* pentapeptide repeat protein sequences. The source of true *qnr* sequences was the reference list of *qnr* sequences [31] and the source of non-*qnr* sequences was sequences from GenBank annotated as pentapeptide repeat proteins (PRP) with the COG1357 annotation, but without a known resistance phenotype.

Two sets of data were created for each model in the cross-validation; a training and a validation set. The training sets consisted of a combination of true *qnr* sequences excluding the class which was left out from the model in question and a set of 90 random non-*qnr* genes. The validation sets contained all known variants of the previously excluded *qnr* class plus a different set of 421 non-*qnr* genes. For example, the first model was based on all known plasmid-mediated *qnr* sequences excluding the sequences from the class *qnrA*. This model was then applied to training data consisting of true *qnr* sequences excluding *qnrA* and a set of non-*qnr*genes. The classification function was then applied to validation data consisting exclusively of *qnrA* and a different set of non-*qnr* sequences where the performance of the model to identify unknown (i.e. novel) classes of plasmid-mediated *qnr* was estimated. The fragments used in the cross-validation were randomly generated from the training and validation data sets for each model by randomly drawing a *qnr*/non-*qnr*fragments with equal probability. For each dataset, 2500 random fragments were created for each fragment length between 10-210 amino acids. A relatively high mutation rate on amino acid sequence was added by randomly substituting each residue for another with the probability of 5% to introduce a substantial amount of noise.

Parameter values for the classification function were optimized using particle swarm optimization where the parameter spaces for the three parameters were explored (ranges in brackets): M [-20, 30], K [0, 2], and D [30, 210]. Optimization was performed six times using a swarm size of 30 particles with 50 iterations in each run with randomized starting points in parameter space. The objective was to achieve a high true positive rate (TPR) without letting the false positive rate (FPR) becoming too high. The objective function was therefore set to TPR-FPR. The statistical power of the model for identifying novel plasmid-mediated *qnr* gene variants was computed by using the average parameter values from the six optimization runs when applying the model to the validation data sets (Figure 2).

The nucleotide datasets used in this project (Table 1) were public sequence data sets downloaded in April 2011 (GenBank version 183). Data from the NCBI Sequence Read Archive (SRA) was selected using the search string "metagenom* AND (454 AND (flx OR titanium)) NOT 16S NOT V6 NOT V9" which generated 1756 hits at the time data was sourced for this project. The sequence data was first translated into all six reading frames using bacterial translation table 11 in EMBOSS *transeq*[52]. The translated sequences were fed into HMMER3 program *hmmsearch* to find hits against the model. The only non-default settings used were --notextw and --cpu 8, with no change from default settings for inclusion or reporting thresholds. All hits discovered by HMMER3 were instead subjected to the classification function and hits that classified as *qnr* were clustered using Blastclust [53]. Clustering parameters used were fragment similarity threshold 90% and minimum length coverage 25%. Cluster groups (containing hits/sequence fragments) were aligned using MAFFT to produce overlapping multiple alignments. The aligned groups were then manually adjusted to identify overlapping fragments that formed longer contigs and complete *qnr* gene contigs. Finally, such contig sequences were annotated using a combination of the reference *qnr* compilation [31] and the GenBank data displayed in Table1.

DECLARATIONS

Acknowledgements

Thanks to Dr Carl-Fredrik Flach for valuable discussions on the topic of mobile fluoroquinolone resistance. This research was supported by the Life Science Area of Advance at Chalmers University of Technology, Sweden, the Swedish Research Council (VR), the Swedish Research Council for Environment, Agricultural Sciences and Spatial Planning (FORMAS) and the Swedish Society for Medical Research (SSMF). Support from the Gothenburg Bioinformatics Network (GOTBIN) is gratefully acknowledged.

Authors' original submitted files for images

Below are the links to the authors' original submitted files for images.

Competing interests

The authors declare no competing interests.

Authors' contributions

FB, EK and AJ planned the project. FB developed and implemented the method, performed the cross-validation, interpreted the clustering results and annotated the hits. MBP assisted with the implementation of the method. FB and EK drafted the manuscript. The work was supervised by EK, AJ and DGJL. All authors read and approved the final manuscript.

REFERENCES

1. Davies J, Davies D: Origins and evolution of antibiotic resistance. Microbiol Mol Biol Rev. 2010, 74: 417-433. 10.1128/MMBR.00016-10..
2. Neu HC: The crisis in antibiotic resistance. Science (New York, N.Y.). 1992, 257: 837-842..
3. Martinez J, Baquero F: Mutation frequencies and antibiotic resistance. Antimicrobial agents. 2000, 44: 1771-1777. 10.1128/AAC.44.7.1771-1777.2000..
4. Stokes HW, Gillings MR: Gene flow, mobile genetic elements and the recruitment of antibiotic resistance genes into Gram-negative pathogens. FEMS Microbiol Rev. 2011, 35: 790-819. 10.1111/j.1574-6976.2011.00273.x..
5. Boucher Y, Labbate M, Koenig JE, Stokes HW: Integrons: mobilizable platforms that promote genetic diversity in bacteria. Trends Microbiol. 2007, 15: 301-309. 10.1016/j.tim.2007.05.004..
6. Gillings M, Boucher Y, Labbate M, Holmes A, Krishnan S, Holley M, Stokes HW: The evolution of class 1 integrons and the rise of antibiotic resistance. J Bacteriol. 2008, 190: 5095-5100. 10.1128/JB.00152-08..
7. Wright GD: The antibiotic resistome: the nexus of chemical and genetic diversity. Nat Rev Microbiol. 2007, 5: 175-186. 10.1038/nrmicro1614..
8. Cantón R: Antibiotic resistance genes from the environment: a perspective through newly identified antibiotic resistance mechanisms in the clinical setting. Clin Microbiol Infect. 2009, 15 (Suppl 1): 20-25..
9. D'Costa VM, Griffiths E, Wright GD: Expanding the soil antibiotic resistome: exploring environmental diversity. Curr Opin Microbiol. 2007, 10: 481-489. 10.1016/j.mib.2007.08.009..
10. D'Costa VM, McGrann KM, Hughes DW, Wright GD: Sampling the antibiotic resistome. Science (New York, N.Y.). 2006, 311: 374-377. 10.1126/science.1120800..
11. D'Costa VM, King CE, Kalan L, Morar M, Sung WWL, Schwarz C, Froese D, Zazula G, Calmels F, Debruyne R, Golding GB, Poinar HN, Wright GD: Antibiotic resistance is ancient. Nature. 2011, 477: 457-461. 10.1038/nature10388..
12. Martínez JL: Antibiotics and antibiotic resistance genes in natural environments. Science (New York, N.Y.). 2008, 321: 365-367. 10.1126/science.1159483..
13. Allen HK, Donato J, Wang HH, Cloud-Hansen KA, Davies J, Handelsman J: Call of the wild: antibiotic resistance genes in natural environments. Nat Rev Microbiol. 2010, 8: 251-259. 10.1038/nrmicro2312..
14. Von Groll A, Martin A, Jureen P, Hoffner S, Vandamme P, Portaels F, Palomino JC, da Silva PA: Fluoroquinolone resistance in Mycobacterium tuberculosis and mutations in gyrA and gyrB. Antimicrob Agents Chemother. 2009, 53: 4498-4500. 10.1128/AAC.00287-09..
15. Shah SQA, Nilsen H, Bottolfsen K, Colquhoun DJ, Sørum H: DNA Gyrase and Topoisomerase IV Mutations in Quinolone-Resistant Flavobacterium psychrophilum Isolated from Diseased Salmonids in Norway. Microb Drug Resist (Larchmont, N.Y.). 2012, 207-214.
16. Martínez-Martínez L, Pascual A, Jacoby GA: Quinolone resistance from a transferable plasmid. Lancet. 1998, 351: 797-799. 10.1016/S0140-6736(97)07322-4..
17. Robicsek A, Jacoby GA, Hooper DC: The worldwide emergence of plasmid-mediated quinolone resistance. Lancet Infect Dis. 2006, 6: 629-640. 10.1016/S1473-3099(06)70599-0..
18. Strahilevitz J, Jacoby GA, Hooper DC, Robicsek A: Plasmid-mediated quinolone resistance: a multifaceted threat. Clin Microbiol Rev. 2009, 22: 664-689. 10.1128/CMR.00016-09..
19. Vetting MW, Hegde SS, Fajardo JE, Fiser A, Roderick SL, Takiff HE, Blanchard JS: Pentapeptide repeat proteins. Biochemistry. 2006, 45: 1-10. 10.1021/bi052130w..
20. Bateman A, Murzin AG, Teichmann SA: Structure and distribution of pentapeptide repeats in bacteria. Protein Sci. 1998, 7: 1477-1480. 10.1002/pro.5560070625..
21. Xiong X, Bromley EHC, Oelschlaeger P, Woolfson DN, Spencer J: Structural insights into quinolone antibiotic resistance mediated by pentapeptide repeat proteins: conserved surface loops direct the activity of a Qnr protein from a gram-negative bacterium. Nucleic Acids Res. 2011, 39: 3917-3927. 10.1093/nar/gkq1296..
22. Vetting MW, Hegde SS, Wang M, Jacoby GA, Hooper DC, Blanchard JS: Structure of QnrB1, a plasmid-mediated fluoroquinolone resistance factor. J Biol Chem. 2011, 286: 25265-25273. 10.1074/jbc.M111.226936..
23. Handelsman J: Metagenomics: application of genomics to uncultured microorganisms. Microbiol Mol Biol Rev. 2004, 68: 669-10.1128/MMBR.68.4.669-685.2004..
24. Kristiansson E, Hugenholtz P, Dalevi D: ShotgunFunctionalizeR: an R-package for functional comparison of metagenomes. Bioinformatics (Oxford, England). 2009, 25: 2737-2738. 10.1093/bioinformatics/btp508..
25. Hugenholtz P, Goebel BM, Pace NR: Impact of culture-independent studies on the emerging phylogenetic view of bacterial diversity. J Bacteriol. 1998, 180: 4765-4774.
26. Streit WR, Schmitz RA: Metagenomics–the key to the uncultured microbes. Curr Opin Microbiol. 2004, 7:

492-498. 10.1016/j.mib.2004.08.002..

27. Wommack KE, Bhavsar J, Ravel J: Metagenomics: read length matters. Appl Environ Microbiol. 2008, 74: 1453-1463. 10.1128/AEM.02181-07..

28. Fonseca ÉL, Santos Freitas F, Vicente ACP: New qnr Gene Cassettes Associated with Superintegron Repeats in Vibrio cholerae O1. Emerg Infect Dis. 2008, 14: 1129-1131. 10.3201/eid1407.080132..

29. Sánchez MB, Hernández A, Rodríguez-Martínez JM, Martínez-Martínez L, Martínez JL: Predictive analysis of transmissible quinolone resistance indicates Stenotrophomonas maltophilia as a potential source of a novel family of Qnr determinants. BMC Microbiol. 2008, 8: 148-10.1186/1471-2180-8-148..

30. Rodríguez-Martínez JM, Velasco C, Briales A, García I, Conejo MC, Pascual A: Qnr-like pentapeptide repeat proteins in gram-positive bacteria. J Antimicrob Chemother. 2008, 61: 1240-1243. 10.1093/jac/dkn115..

31. qnr Numbering and Sequence.http://www.lahey.org/qnrStudies,

32. Benson DA, Boguski MS, Lipman DJ, Ostell J, Ouellette BF, Rapp BA, Wheeler DL: GenBank. Nucleic Acids Res. 1999, 27: 12-17. 10.1093/nar/27.1.12..

33. Seshadri R, Kravitz SA, Smarr L, Gilna P, Frazier M: CAMERA: a community resource for metagenomics. PLoS Biol. 2007, 5: e75-10.1371/journal.pbio.0050075..

34. Meyer F, Paarmann D, D'Souza M, Olson R, Glass EM, Kubal M, Paczian T, Rodriguez A, Stevens R, Wilke A, Wilkening J, Edwards RA: The metagenomics RAST server - a public resource for the automatic phylogenetic and functional analysis of metagenomes. BMC Bioinforma. 2008, 9: 386-10.1186/1471-2105-9-386..

35. Qin J, Li R, Raes J, Arumugam M, Burgdorf KS, Manichanh C, Nielsen T, Pons N, Levenez F, Yamada T, Mende DR, Li J, Xu J, Li SSS, Li D, Cao J, Wang B, Liang H, Zheng H, Xie Y, Tap J, Lepage P, Bertalan M, Batto J, Hansen T, Le D, Linneberg A, Nielsen HB, Pelletier E, Renault P, Sicheritz-Ponten T, Turner K, Zhu H, Yu C, Jian M, Zhou Y, Li Y, Zhang X, Guarner F, Qin N, Yang H, Wang JJ, Brunak S, Dore J, Le Paslier D, Doré J, Kristiansen K, Pedersen O, Parkhill J, Weissenbach J, Bork P, Ehrlich SD: A human gut microbial gene catalogue established by metagenomic sequencing. Nature. 2010, 464: 59-65. 10.1038/nature08821..

36. Leinonen R, Sugawara H, Shumway M: The sequence read archive. Nucleic Acids Res. 2011, 39: D19-D21. 10.1093/nar/gkq1019..

37. Kristiansson E, Fick J, Janzon A, Grabic R, Rutgersson C, Weijdegård B, Söderström H, Larsson DGJ: Pyrosequencing of antibiotic-contaminated river sediments reveals high levels of resistance and gene transfer elements. PLoS One. 2011, 6: e17038-10.1371/journal.pone.0017038..

38. Baquirin MHC, Barlow M: Evolution and recombination of the plasmidic qnr alleles. J Mol Evol. 2008, 67: 103-110. 10.1007/s00239-008-9131-3..

39. Jacoby GA, Griffin CM, Hooper DC: Citrobacter spp. as a source of qnrB Alleles. Antimicrob Agents Chemother. 2011, 55: 4979-4984. 10.1128/AAC.05187-11..

40. Wang MM, Guo Q, Xu X, Wang X, Ye X, Wu S, Hooper DC: New plasmid-mediated quinolone resistance gene, qnrC, found in a clinical isolate of Proteus mirabilis. Antimicrob Agents Chemother. 2009, 53: 1892-1897. 10.1128/AAC.01400-08..

41. Velasco C, Rodríguez-Martínez JM, Briales A, de Díaz Alba P, Calvo A, Pascual A: Smaqnr, a new chromosome-encoded quinolone resistance determinant in Serratia marcescens. J Antimicrob Chemother. 2010, 65: 239-242. 10.1093/jac/dkp424..

42. Overbeek R, Begley T, Butler RM, Choudhuri JV, Chuang H-Y, Cohoon M, de Crécy-Lagard V, Diaz N, Disz T, Edwards R, Fonstein M, Frank ED, Gerdes S, Glass EM, Goesmann A, Hanson A, Iwata-Reuyl D, Jensen R, Jamshidi N, Krause L, Kubal M, Larsen N, Linke B, McHardy AC, Meyer F, Neuweger H, Olsen G, Olson R, Osterman A, Portnoy V, et al: The subsystems approach to genome annotation and its use in the project to annotate 1000 genomes. Nucleic Acids Res. 2005, 33: 5691-5702. 10.1093/nar/gki866..

43. Morowitz MJ, Denef VJ, Costello EK, Thomas BC, Poroyko V: Strain-resolved community genomic analysis of gut microbial colonization in a premature infant. Proc Natl Acad Sci. 2010, 108: 1128-1133..

44. Yooseph S, Sutton G, Rusch DB, Halpern AL, Williamson SJ, Remington K, Eisen JA, Heidelberg KB, Manning G, Li W, Jaroszewski L, Cieplak P, Miller CS, Li H, Mashiyama ST, Joachimiak MP, van Belle C, Chandonia J-M, Soergel DA, Zhai Y, Natarajan K, Lee S, Raphael BJ, Bafna V, Friedman R, Brenner SE, Godzik A, Eisenberg D, Dixon JE, Taylor SS, Strausberg RL, Frazier M, Venter JC: The Sorcerer II Global Ocean Sampling expedition: expanding the universe of protein families. PLoS Biol. 2007, 5: e16-10.1371/journal.pbio.0050016..

45. Hooper SD, Dalevi D, Pati A, Mavromatis K, Ivanova NN, Kyrpides NC: Estimating DNA coverage and abundance in metagenomes using a gamma approximation. Bioinformatics (Oxford, England). 2010, 26: 295-301. 10.1093/bioinformatics/btp687..

46. Gilbert JA, Dupont CL: Microbial Metagenomics: Beyond the Genome. Ann Rev Mar Sci. 2011, 3: 347-371. 10.1146/annurev-marine-120709-142811..

47. Gilbert JA, Meyer F, Jansson J, Gordon J, Pace N, Ley R, Fierer N, Field D, Kyrpides N, Glöckner F: The Earth Microbiome Project: Meeting report of the " 1st EMP meeting on sample selection and acquisition " at Argonne National Laboratory October 6th 2010. 2010, 249-253.

48. Gilbert JA, Bailey M, Field D, Fierer N, Fuhrman JA, Hu B, Jansson J, Knight R, Kowalchuk GA, Kyrpides NC, Meyer F, Stevens R: The Earth Microbiome Project: The Meeting Report for the 1st International Earth Microbiome Project Conference, Shenzhen, China, June 13th-15th 2011. Stand Genomic Sci. 2011, 5: 243-247. 10.4056/sigs.2134923.

49. Eddy SR: Accelerated Profile HMM Searches. PLoS Comput Biol. 2011, 7: e1002195-10.1371/journal.

pcbi.1002195..

50. Metzker ML: Sequencing technologies - the next generation. Nat Rev Genet. 2010, 11: 31-46. 10.1038/nrg2626..

51. Katoh K, Misawa K, Kuma K, Miyata T: MAFFT: a novel method for rapid multiple sequence alignment based on fast Fourier transform. Nucleic Acids Res. 2002, 30: 3059-3066. 10.1093/nar/gkf436..

52. Rice P, Longden I, Bleasby A: The European Molecular Biology Open Software Suite EMBOSS: The European Molecular Biology Open Software Suite. Trends Genet. 2000, 16: 276-277. 10.1016/S0168-9525(00)02024-2..

53. Altschul SF, Madden TL, Schäffer AA, Zhang J, Zhang Z, Miller W, Lipman DJ: Gapped BLAST and PSI-BLAST: a new generation of protein database search programs. Nucleic Acids Res. 1997, 25: 3389-3402. 10.1093/nar/25.17.3389..

CHAPTER 16

INTEGRATIVE ANALYSIS OF FUNCTIONAL GENOMIC ANNOTATIONS AND SEQUENCING DATA TO IDENTIFY RARE CAUSAL VARIANTS VIA HIERARCHICAL MODELING

Marinela Capanu and Iuliana Ionita-Laza

Keywords: Causal variants, hierarchical modeling, sequencing studies, functional score, CADD score

Identifying the small number of rare causal variants contributing to disease has been a major focus of investigation in recent years, but represents a formidable statistical challenge due to the rare frequencies with which these variants are observed. In this commentary we draw attention to a formal statistical framework, namely hierarchical modeling, to combine functional genomic annotations with sequencing data with the objective of enhancing our ability to identify rare causal variants. Using simulations we show that in all configurations studied, the hierarchical modeling approach has superior discriminatory ability compared to a recently proposed aggregate measure of deleteriousness, the Combined Annotation-Dependent Depletion (CADD) score, supporting our premise that aggregate functional genomic measures can more accurately identify causal variants when used in conjunction with sequencing data through a hierarchical modeling approach.

Identifying a small number of variants most likely to be causal in a specific genetic region (such as a gene) is a challenging problem, but of fundamental importance to the understanding of precise biological mechanisms that influence disease (MacArthur et al., 2014). Rare causal variants, by definition, are only seen a small number of times in any given dataset and therefore are hard to distinguish from the abundant natural variation that occurs in any particular gene. This is a difficult setting, where the causal variants are sparse and tend to be weak as well. Experimental functional studies are the gold-standard, but they are expensive and difficult to implement for large number of variants. Statistical methods to help us distinguish between a true causal variant and a null variant are therefore of great interest.

For those causal variants that are rare but appear at sufficient frequency in a dataset, it is possible to prioritize them over other variants in a gene using genetic (i.e., frequency) data alone. However, for those causal variants that are observed only a few times (e.g., singletons, doubletons etc.), clearly these frequencies on their own are insufficient to provide meaningful risk predictions and no method will perform better than random guessing based on genetic data alone. It is for these variants that functional genomic annotations are essential. Large-scale studies such as the Encyclopedia of DNA Elements (ENCODE) project (ENCODE Project Consortium et al., 2012) provide rich functional genomics annotations that can complement genetic data and help identify likely causal variants. Aggregate measures (Frousios et al., 2013; Johansen et al., 2013; Kircher et al., 2014; Ritchie et al., 2014) that combine information across many annotations in a single measure of deleteriousness for a variant have been shown to outperform individual annotations. The usefulness of such functional measures depends on how well they correlate with pathogenicity. Clearly this correlation will depend on the disease or trait under study and possibly the gene or region of interest (e.g., the degree to which a gene is intolerant to functional variation Petrovski et al., 2013). It seems natural to expect that combining these two pieces of evidence: (1) the genetic score measuring the

Citation: Marinela Capanu and Iuliana Ionita-Laza, Integrative analysis of functional genomic annotations and sequencing data to identify rare causal variants via hierarchical modeling, http://dx.doi.org/10.3389/fgene.2015.00176.

statistical evidence for a variant being associated with a disease of interest, and (2) various functional scores for the variant, can enhance the ability to identify rare causal variants. In Supplementary Figure 1 we show three possible outcomes for correctly classifying a true causal variant as likely causal as a function of both genetic and functional scores. Evidently, causal variants with low functional scores and low support from genetic data (e.g., singletons or doubletons) will be impossible to classify correctly. At the other extreme, the causal variants with strong support from both genetic and functional scores will be easy to identify. For causal variants falling in-between these two extremes for which neither the genetic data nor the functional scores on their own provide sufficient evidence of their deleteriousness we believe that integrative methods that combine genetic data with functional scores would be most useful for correctly identifying these variants. Indeed, a recent report by a working group of researchers convened by the NHGRI discussed the challenges in reliably implicating sequence variants in human disease, and highlighted the importance of performing "a combined assessment of the genetic, experimental and informatic support for individual candidate variants" (MacArthur et al., 2014).

Hierarchical models (Gelman et al., 2003) provide a natural approach for such an integrative analysis. They offer a formal statistical framework that can be used in this setting to incorporate sequencing data and functional annotations with the goal of identifying rare causal variants. The strength of the hierarchical modeling approach comes from the fact that it draws upon the information contained in functional annotations to augment the weak information from the case/control frequencies for rare variants, thus improving the risk estimation for individual variants. In our setting, the hierarchical model has two levels: the first level contains the parameters of fundamental interest, namely the relative risks conferred by the individual genetic variants, and also individual-level confounding factors. In the second level, the individual log relative risks of the variants are modeled as linear functions of relevant functional scores. More details on the hierarchical modeling approach and its properties as well as applications to two large population-based case-control studies of melanoma and breast cancer can be found in Capanu et al. (2008), Capanu and Begg (2011), Capanu et al. (2011). A recent application of hierarchical modeling to *VPS13B*, a gene involved in Cohen syndrome and autism can be found in Ionita-Laza et al. (2014).

We conjecture that a hierarchical modeling approach incorporating the sequencing data with an aggregate functional measure more accurately classifies rare causal variants compared to a ranking based solely on the variants' functional score. We focus here on the recently proposed deleteriousness measure, the Combined Annotation-Dependent Depletion (CADD) score or C-score (Kircher et al., 2014), but our method can include any such genomic annotations. We investigate the discriminatory ability of this hierarchical modeling approach and that of the ranking based on the C-scores alone using simulations based on exome sequencing data for 861 individuals (part of the ARRA Autism Sequencing Collaborative project) for one gene, *VPS13B*, containing 166 observed single nucleotide variants (SNVs). We assumed 10% of SNVs to be truly causal variants, with relative risks of 1.1, 2, or 4 for the association of the C-score and the causal status of a variant. We then generated the case-control status following the same data generating mechanism as inLadouceur et al. (2012). Specifically, for carriers of causal variants we generated a continuous phenotype from a normal distribution with mean $\mu = 0.5$ and a standard deviation of 0.2 while for non-carriers we used a standard normal distribution. This corresponds to a moderate standardized effect size of 0.5 (Cohen, 1988). Note that smaller standardized effect sizes were also examined and the results were qualitatively the same (data not shown). Furthermore, individuals with phenotype values above the median were classified as cases, and the remaining individuals as controls.

The ROC curves for the two different methods are displayed in Figure 1 under different degrees of associations between the causal status and the C-scores and assuming $\mu = 0.5$. Solid curves correspond to ROC curves based on the z-values estimated from a hierarchical model in which the C-scores were the solely functional predictor, while dashed curves correspond to rankings based on the C-scores of variants that occurred in at least one of the cases. In all configurations, the hierarchical modeling approach has superior discriminatory ability to the C-score method, with biggest improvements observed when the functional score is weakly associated with the causal status ($RR = 1.1$, blue curves). As the association of the C-scores with the causal status gets stronger, the discriminatory ability of the two methods also improves. Similar trends are observed for larger values of μ such as 1, 1.5, and 2 (data not shown).

In conclusion, aggregate functional measures such as the C-score can identify causal variants more accurately when used in conjunction with sequencing data through a hierarchical modeling approach than when used on their own. Therefore, hierarchical models and other integrative methods are promising tools in this context, and further work in developing such methods is warranted to take full advantage of rich functional annotation data and large scale sequencing studies for many complex diseases in order to understand the nature of the causal variants involved in these diseases.

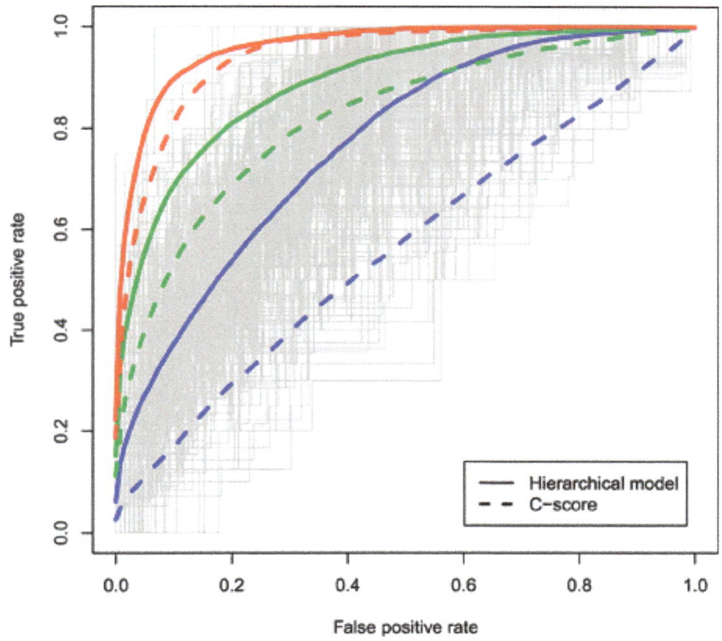

Figure 1. ROC curves of the z-values estimated from a hierarchical model with the C-scores included as a functional predictor (solid curves) and ROC curves based on the ranking of the C-scores of variants carried in at least one of the cases (dashed curves); 10% of variants are assumed truly causal variants; associations between the C-score and the causal status of a variant vary from relative risks of 1.1 (blue), to 2 (green), and 4 (red); μ, the effect size as a function of standard deviations, is assumed to be 0.5; estimates are averaged across 400 simulations.

Author Contributions

MC and II-L wrote and reviewed the manuscript.

Conflict of Interest Statement

The authors declare that the research was conducted in the absence of any commercial or financial relationships that could be construed as a potential conflict of interest.

REFERENCES

1. Capanu, M., Orlow, I., Berwick, M., Hummer, A. J., Thomas, D. C., and Begg, C. B. (2008). The use of hierarchical models for estimating relative risks of individual genetic variants: an application to a study of melanoma. *Stat. Med.* 27, 1973–1992. doi: 10.1002/sim.3196
2. Capanu, M., and Begg, C. B. (2011). Hierarchical modeling for estimating relative risks of rare genetic variants: properties of the pseudo-likelihood method. *Biometrics* 67, 371–380. doi: 10.1111/j.1541-0420.2010.01469.x
3. Capanu, M., Concannon, P., Haile, R. W., Bernstein, L., Malone, K. E., Lynch, C. F., et al. (2011). Assessment of rare *BRCA1* and*BRCA2* variants of unknown significance using hierachical modeling. *Genet. Epidemiol.* 35, 389–397. doi: 10.1002/gepi.20587
4. Cohen, J. (1988). *Statistical Power Analysis for the Behavioral Sciences, 2nd Edn*. Hillsdale, NJ: Lawrence Erlbaum Associates.
5. ENCODE Project Consortium, Dunham, I., Kundaje, A., Aldred, S. F., Collins, P. J., Davis, C. A., et al. (2012). An integrated encyclopedia of DNA elements in the human genome. *Nature* 489, 57–74. doi: 10.1038/nature11247
6. Frousios, K., Iliopoulos, C. S., Schlitt, T., and Simpson, M. A. (2013). Predicting the functional consequences of non-synonymous DNA sequence variants evaluation of bioinformatics tools and development of a consensus strategy. *Genomics* 102, 223–228. doi: 10.1016/j.ygeno.2013.06.005
7. Gelman, A., Carlin, J. B., Stern, H. S., and Rubin, D. B. (2003). *Bayesian Data Analysis, 2nd Edn*. Boca Raton, FL: Chapman and Hall/CRC.
8. Ionita-Laza, I., Capanu, M., De Rubeis, S., McCallum, K., and Buxbaum, J. D. (2014). Identification of rare causal variants in sequence-based studies: methods and applications to *VPS13B*, a gene involved in cohen syndrome and autism. *PLoS Genet.* 10:e1004729. doi: 10.1371/journal.pgen.1004729
9. Johansen, M. B., Izarzugaza, J. M., Brunak, S., Petersen, T. N., and Gupta, R. (2013). Prediction of disease causing non-synonymous SNPs by the artificial neural network predictor NetDiseaseSNP. *PLoS ONE* 8:e68370. doi: 10.1371/journal.pone.0068370
10. Kircher, M., Witten, D. M., Jain, P., O›Roak, B. J., Cooper, G. M., and Shendure, J. (2014). A general framework for estimating the relative pathogenicity of human genetic variants. *Nat. Genet.* 46, 310–315. doi: 10.1038/ng.2892
11. Ladouceur, M., Dastani, Z., Aulchenko, Y. S., Greenwood, C. M., and Richards, J. B. (2012). The empirical power of rare variant association methods: results from sanger sequencing in 1,998 individuals. *PLoS Genet.* 8:e1002496. doi: 10.1371/journal.pgen.1002496
12. MacArthur, D. G., Manolio, T. A., Dimmock, D. P., Rehm, H. L., Shendure, J., Abecasis, G. R., et al. (2014). Guidelines for investigating causality of sequence

variants in human disease. *Nature* 508, 469–476. doi: 10.1038/nature13127

13. Petrovski, S., Wang, Q., Heinzen, E. L., Allen, A. S., and Goldstein, D. B. (2013). Genic intolerance to functional variation and the interpretation of personal genomes. *PLoS Genet.* 9:e1003709. doi: 10.1371/journal.pgen.1003709

14. Ritchie, G. R. S., Dunham, I., Zeggini, E., and Flicek, P. (2014). Functional annotation of noncoding sequence variants. *Nat. Methods* 11, 294–296. doi: 10.1038/nmeth.2832

CHAPTER 17

GENOME SEQUENCING

Megan H. Brewer, Rabia Chaudhry, Jessica Qi, Aditi Kidambi, Alexander P. Drew , Manoj P. Menezes, Monique M. Ryan, Michelle A. Farrar, David Mowat, Gopinath M. Subramanian, Helen K. Young, Stephan Zuchner, Stephen W. Reddel, Garth A. Nicholson, Marina L. Kennerson

INTRODUCTION

Charcot-Marie-Tooth (CMT) disease is the collective name given to a group of clinically and genetically heterogeneous inherited peripheral neuropathies that affect both motor and sensory neurons. Over 80 genes have been associated with CMT and other related inherited peripheral neuropathies, which account for up to 80% of CMT cases [1–4]. In our Australian cohort, after extensive whole exome sequencing (WES) analysis of multiple family members, a proportion of these unsolved families also have no detectable protein-coding mutation in the exome. This suggests that point mutations and small insertions/deletions of non-coding DNA and DNA structural variations may account for some of the unsolved cases.

CMTX3, a subtype of X-linked CMT, is one such locus which has remained unsolved after extensive molecular analyses. The CMTX3 locus was initially mapped to the long arm of chromosome X in two American families [5]. The locus was confirmed and refined to a 5.7 Mb region on chromosome Xq26.3-q27.3 in a large United Kingdom/New Zealand family (CMT623) [6] and an Australian family (CMT193-ext) [7]. Affected males from these two families generally presented a slightly milder phenotype than the more common X-linked CMT subtype, CMTX1. However the degree of severity varied. Onset of disease generally started in the first decade, initially presenting in the lower limbs. Sensory symptoms included marked pain and paraethesia in hands and feet as well as sensory loss. Tremor in hands and spastic paraparesis was not observed. Nerve conduction velocities data suggested these patients have an intermediate CMT. Female carriers were considered asymptomatic with normal nerve conduction velocities, however the observation of subtle clinical signs including high-arched feet, weakness in foot dorsiflexion and loss of ankle reflexes suggested female carriers may present very mild symptoms [6].

The two families carry the same CMTX3 haplotype, suggesting they share an identical genetic mutation inherited from a common ancestor. Genotype analysis of one of the original American families (US-PED2) initially suggested this family also carried the distal portion of the CMTX3 haplotype [7]. However, re-examination of family US-PED2 by whole exome sequencing (WES) identified a known BSCL2 mutation (c.263A>G, p.Asn88Ser) as the genetic cause of disease in the family [8]. Mutation screening families CMT623 and CMT193-ext excluded all coding sequences mapping within the 5.7 Mb locus for pathogenic mutations [6, 9]. Therefore, we employed whole genome sequencing (WGS) to interrogate the disease locus for pathogenic non-coding single nucleotide variants and structural variations in these families.

RESULTS/DISCUSSION

Two affected males and an unaffected male control from each of the families CMT623 and CMT193-ext (i.e. four patients and two controls) underwent WGS. An average of 134 Gb of sequence was generated for each individual. On average, 96% of total reads mapped to the reference genome and all samples had a minimum depth of coverage (DOC) of 44X across the whole genome (Table 1). The CMTX3 locus had an average DOC of 24X, which reflected the males being hemizygous for chromosome X.

Citation: Brewer MH, Chaudhry R, Qi J, Kidambi A, Drew AP, Menezes MP, et al. (2016) Genome Sequencing. PLoS Genet 12(7): e1006177. doi:10.1371/journal.pgen.1006177

Table 1. Whole genome sequence quality data analysis.

	Individual	Total Reads	Mapped Reads	% Mapped Reads	Average Coverage Genome	Average Coverage ChrX	MapQ Score
CMT193	Affected 1	1,767,871,080	1,745,034,895	99	56.3	29.4	52.3
	Affected 2	1,398,881,966	1,377,234,225	98	44.4	22.8	51.6
	Control 1	1,415,254,852	1,389,518,446	98	44.8	23.4	51.5
CMT623	Affected 3	1,404,391,674	1,375,198,612	98	44.5	23.2	51.5
	Affected 4	1,423,140,198	1,372,077,383	96	44.3	23.1	49.4
	Control 2	1,419,371,166	1,392,511,028	98	45.1	23.3	51.7

Patient and control sequence alignments revealed the presence of split-reads at Xq27.1 (Table 2). The four affected males consistently showed split reads at the genomic location chrX:139,502,948. The corresponding paired ends for the split reads mapped both upstream and downstream of the suggestive breakpoint at chromosome Xq27.1. Split-reads at this location were not identified in the two unaffected males. The unaligned sequences of these split-reads mapped to two genomic regions (chr8:145,768,312 and chr8:145,848,158). These genomic positions are located 78 kb apart on chromosome 8q24.3 and represent the boundaries of the DNA region that has been inserted into chromosome Xq27.1 in the CMTX3 patients. Patient WGS data also showed split-reads on chromosome 8 that contained Xq27.1 sequence and paired with reads anchoring to these two locations on chromosome 8q24.3. Further analysis also identified discordant paired ends in which one read pair mapped to Xq27.1 and the other read pair mapped to 8q24.3. This was observed in all four patients and absent from the two control samples. Table 2 summarizes the number of split-reads and discordant paired ends identified for each patient. Based on these data we predicted that a 78 kb sequence from 8q24.3 had been inserted into chromosome Xq27.1 in CMTX3 patient DNA.

Table 2. Split-reads and discordant paired ends mapping to Xq27.1 and 8q24.3 in whole genome sequencing data from affected males.

	Individual	Read Type	Proximal Breakpoint	Distal Breakpoint
CMT193	Affected 1	Split-reads Paired end maps to chrX	7	9
		Split-reads Paired end maps to chr8	7	6
		Discordant paired ends	14	15
	Affected 2	Split-reads Paired end maps to chrX	8	7
		Split-reads Paired end maps to chr8	3	5
		Discordant paired ends	10	11
CMT623	Affected 3	Split-reads Paired end maps to chrX	7	13
		Split-reads Paired end maps to chr8	4	6
		Discordant paired ends	15	16
	Affected 4	Split-reads Paired end maps to chrX	6	6
		Split-reads Paired end maps to chr8	3	6
		Discordant paired ends	8	12

To determine whether the entire 78 kb region from chromosome 8q24.3 had been duplicated and inserted into Xq27.1 we assessed the DOC across the genomic interval chr8:145,700,000–145,900,000 (Table 3). Control males showed a uniform DOC across the entire 200 kb region with a mean DOC of 40X. The affected males, however, showed a 1.6-fold increase in DOC (mean DOC of 64X) within the boundaries of the insertion breakpoints (chr8:145,768,312–145,846,158). The DOC for the genomic regions immediately flanking the 8q24.3 insert sequence were similar to the controls (Fig 1A). These data suggested that patients with CMTX3 carry an extra copy of the 78 kb region from chromosome 8q24.3 through the interchromosomal insertion event at the CMTX3 locus.

Table 3. Average depth ± SD of sequence coverage across 8q24.3.

	CMT193-ext			CMT623		
Genomic Region	Affected 1	Affected 2	Control 1	Affected 3	Affected 4	Control 2
Upstream[a]	45 (±7)	36 (±6)	34 (±6)	36 (±6)	36 (±6)	37 (±5)
Insert[b]	76 (±14)	61 (±11)	39 (±8)	60 (±12)	60 (±11)	41 (±8)
Downstream[c]	50 (±8)	41 (±7)	39 (±7)	39 (±7)	40 (±7)	40 (±7)

[a]—chr8:145,700,000–145,768,311
[b]—chr8:145,768,312–145,846,158
[c]—chr8145,846,159–145,900,000

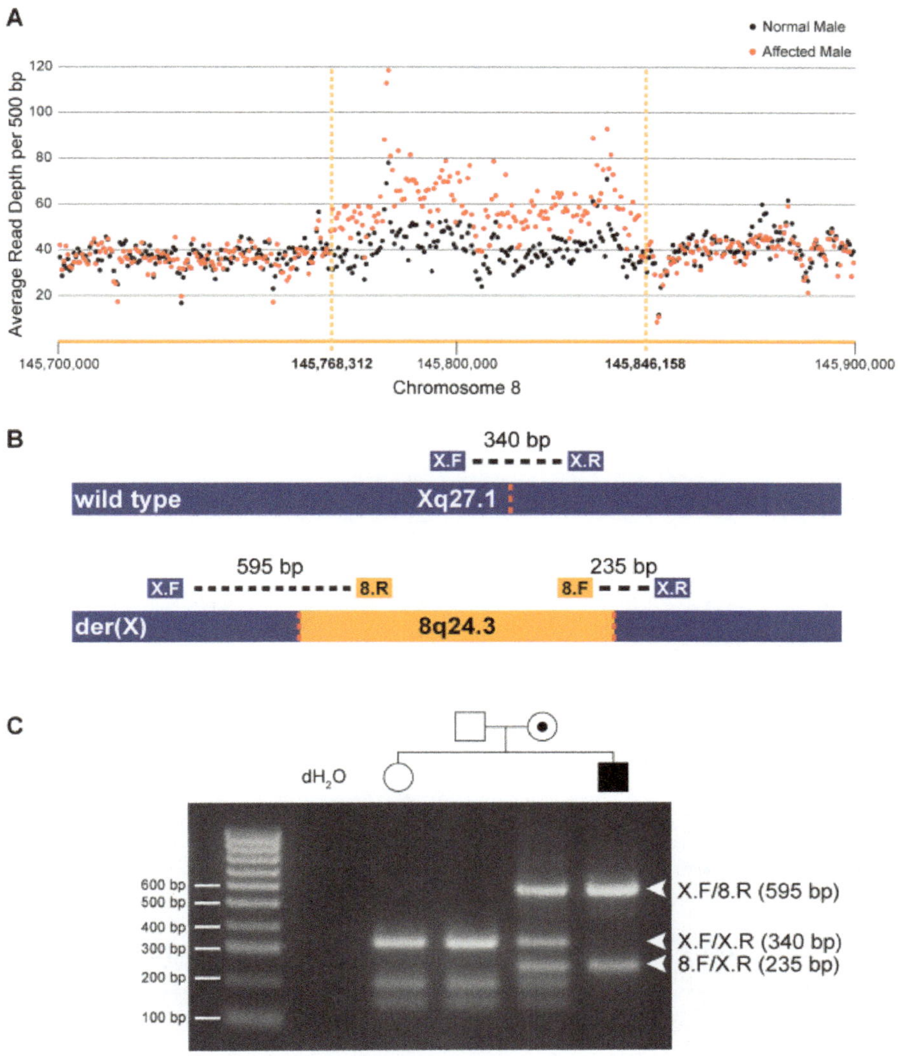

Figure 1. Identification and confirmation of a 78 kb chromosome 8q24.3 insertion in patients with CMTX3.

(A) Whole genome sequencing depth of coverage for affected (red) and normal (black) males across the 8q24.3 insertion and flanking sequence. (B) Depiction of wild type chromosome X (top) and mutant chromosome X (bottom). The location of primers and amplicon sizes for the multiplex PCR genotyping assay are shown. Dotted red lines represent insertion breakpoints. (C) Size fractionation of multiplex PCR genotyping assay for a subset of family members from CMT623. Individual genotypes are depicted above the gel lane. Expected band sizes for the various primer combinations are listed to the right. Unaffected hemizygous males and homozygous females generate a single 340 bp amplicon; affected hemizygous males generate 595 bp and 235 bp amplicons crossing the proximal and distal breakpoints, respectively; carrier females amplify all three amplicons.

We next assessed whether the interchromosomal insertion segregated with the disease in our two distantly related families using a multiplex PCR genotyping assay (Fig 1B). Genotyping results for a subset of family members from CMT623 are shown (Fig 1C). The different sized amplicons were confirmed via Sanger sequencing (S1 Fig). The 78 kb insertion segregated in 55 individuals (25 affected males and 30 carrier females) from families CMT623 and CMT193-ext. The 78 kb insertion was not seen in the 50 unaffected members (30 males, 20 females) from families CMT623 and CMT193-ext that were available for testing. All individuals were clinically diagnosed and genotyped for the CMTX3 haplotype prior to this study. The 8q24.3 interchromosomal insertion was absent in 627 control X chromosomes from neurologically normal females (n = 252) and males (n = 123).

Sanger sequencing the amplicons spanning the insertion breakpoints confirmed the WGS predictions (Fig 2A and 2B). The 8q24.3 sequence inserted directly between the genomic locations chrX:139,502,948–139,502,949. For the proximal breakpoint, the exact location of the end sequence from chromosome X and start position of the 8q24.3 insertion sequence could not be unambiguously defined due to a 2 bp overlap (AA) in the sequence (Fig 2A). For the purposes of defining breakpoints, we have designated the chromosome 8 insertion start position as chr8:145,768,312. The distal breakpoint is more complex (Fig 2B). The 8q24.3 insertion sequence ends at position chr8:145,848,158 followed by a small insertion from chromosome 12q13.12, which maps within an intron of the FAIM2 gene. A total of 19 bp from the small insertion sequence maps to 12q13.12 however the first 10 bp also overlap with chromosome 8 (green sequence, Fig 2B). Adjacent to the 12q13.12 insertion, the first 12 bps of chromosome X at the distal breakpoint are inverted. There is also a single nucleotide variant (T>G) at chrX:139,502,968 and a single nucleotide deletion at chrX:139,502,976 (Fig 2B). These variants appear to be unique to the two CMTX3 families and have not been reported in variant databases including the 1000 Genomes Project [10] or dbSNP [11].

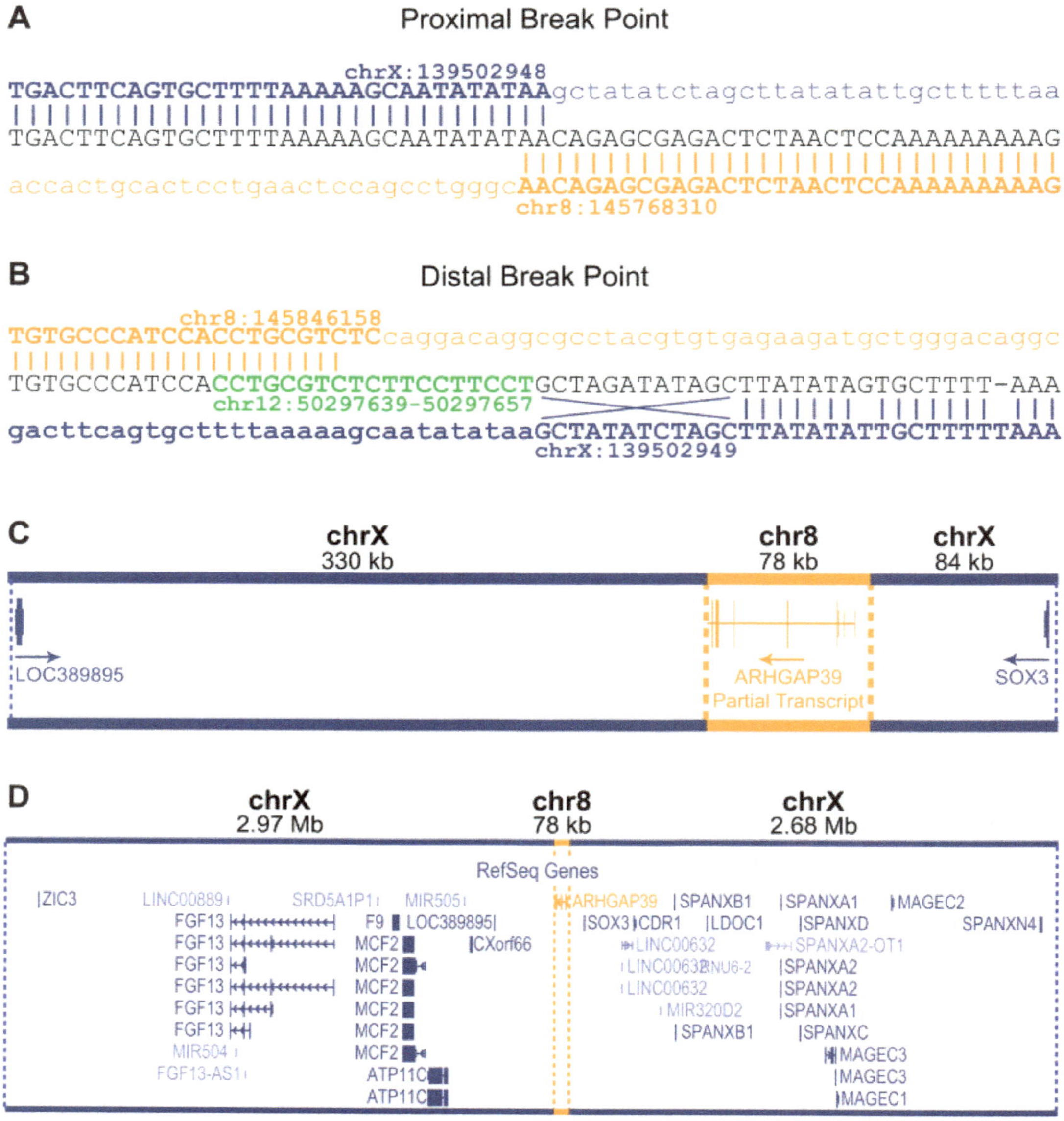

Figure 2. Characterization of the CMTX3 insertion. Sequence analysis of the proximal (A) and distal (B) breakpoints. Reference sequence for chromosome X and chromosome 8 are indicated in blue and orange, respectively. The distal breakpoint includes additional sequence from chromosome 12 (in green) and small rearrangements of the chromosome X sequence including an inversion of 12 bp, and a base pair substitution and a base pair deletion. (C) The 78 kb 8q24.3 sequence (in orange) contains the partial 5'ARHGAP39 transcript which has been inserted 330 kb downstream and 84 kb upstream of the genes LOC389895 and SOX3, respectively (in blue). The direction of transcripts are indicated by the arrow. (D) Location of the 78kb 8q24.3 insertion sequence (in orange) relative to the whole of the 5.7 Mb CMTX3 locus (in blue).

The 8q24.3 insertion region is 77,856 bp and contains a partial transcript of the ARHGAP39gene (exons 1–7) encoded on the negative strand (Fig 2C). The duplicated 8q24.3 sequence has inserted into an intergenic region of Xq27.1 with the nearest flanking genes beingLOC389895 (located 329 kb downstream proximal to the 78 kb insertion) and SOX3 (located 84 kb distal to of the insertion) (Fig 2C and 2D).

Based on the genomic architecture of the CMTX3 interchromosomal insertion, we hypothesized two possible mechanisms that could lead to peripheral neuropathy: 1) overexpression of the partial ARHGAP39 transcript due to 8q24.3 trisomy; or 2) transcriptional dysregulation of one or more genes mapping within the CMTX3 locus.

Aberrant splicing with the ARHGAP39 partial transcript may also be a possible mechanism. However this is unlikely, as the inserted ARHGAP39 partial transcript is predicted to be transcribed on the negative strand and the nearest downstream gene, LOC389895, is a single exon gene transcribed from the positive strand (Fig 2C).

Copy number variations (CNVs) that result in the duplication or deletion of a gene is a well-known cause of CMT neuropathy, indicating that peripheral nerves are sensitive to gene dosage. A 1.5 Mb duplication on chromosome 17p12 [12, 13], resulting in trisomy of thePMP22 gene [14–17], causes the most common form of CMT (CMT1A). This was the seminal example of a CNV causing disease. The reciprocal 1.5 Mb 17p12 deletion causes hereditary neuropathy with liability to pressure palsies (HNPP) [18]. Although relatively rare [19–21], a small number of individual cases describing whole and partial gene duplications or deletions for other CMT loci including MPZ [21–23], GJB1 [24–26], MFN2 [27], and NDRG1 [28] have also been reported. Currently there are no interchromosomal insertions reported as a cause of CMT.

To assess whether the CMTX3 insertion affects gene expression, quantitative RT-PCR analysis was used to assess the mRNA expression levels of candidate genes in patient and control lymphoblasts. No difference in ARHGAP39 expression was observed between the patient and controls (Fig 3A). This suggested that trisomy of the ARHGAP3 partial transcript is unlikely the underlying cause of neuropathy.

Large rearrangements disrupting non-coding DNA sequences are likely to cause disease by dysregulating the transcriptional expression of one or more nearby genes [29]. Duplication of a 186 kb sequence located 3 kb distal to the PMP22 gene [30, 31], harboring Schwann cell-specific transcription factor binding sites [32], was found to cause CMT1A by dysregulatingPMP22 expression [30, 31]. Non-coding DNA structural variations can disrupt the interaction between a gene and its functional non-coding DNA sequences (such as promoters, enhancers and silencers) or introduce new interactions, resulting in dysregulated temporal and spatial gene expression [29, 33, 34]. Recent studies have shown that regulatory elements and their target genes cluster within local chromatin interaction domains or "topologically associated domains" [35]. Genomic rearrangements that physically disrupt the boundaries of these domains introduce ectopic interactions between regulatory elements and genes that can cause disease [29]. However, based on Hi-C profile data from human embryonic stem cells [35] the 78 kb sequence from 8q24.3 appears to have inserted into a topologically associated domain without disrupting the boundaries (S2 Fig) suggesting that if the CMTX3 mutation dysregulates a nearby gene it is likely through some other mechanism.

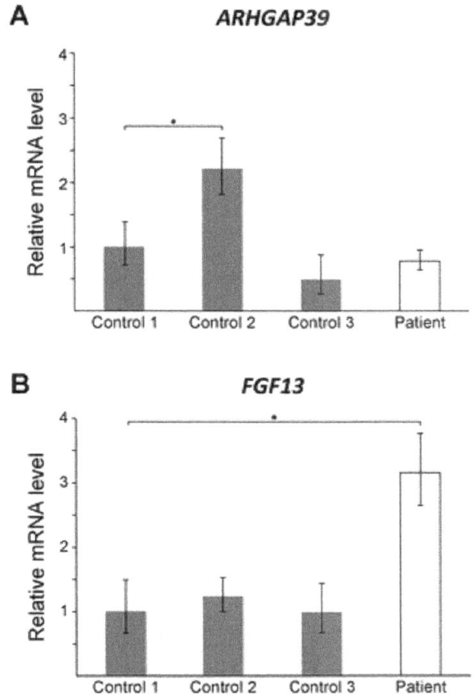

Figure 3. FGF13 mRNA expression is elevated in patient lymphoblasts. Quantitative RT-PCR showing mRNA levels for ARHGAP39 (A) and FGF13 (B) from patient lymphoblasts relative to three normal controls. Bars show the mean mRNA levels (± SD; error bars) relative to Control 1, which has been set to +1. A student t-test was performed comparing each value to Control 1 (*, $p < 0.05$).

To explore the possible mechanism of transcriptional dysregulation of one or more genes mapping within the CMTX3 locus, we assessed the expression of SOX3 and FGF13. Large DNA interchromosomal insertions at the Xq27.1 locus have been previously reported to cause a range of phenotypes [36–40] and these two genes are known to be dysregulated in patients with other Xq27.1 interchromosomal insertions [38, 40].

SOX3 encodes the sex determining region Y-box 3 transcription factor. In an XX sex reversal patient carrying a 774 kb interchromosomal insertion from chromosome 1q25.3, an increase inSOX3 expression was observed in the patient lymphoblasts [40]. SOX3 expression however was not detected in the control lymphoblasts. In both our patient and control lymphoblast cell lines, SOX3 mRNA expression could not be detected (S3 Fig). These results reflect previous reports of SOX3 expression in control lymphoblasts [40] and it is likely that SOX3 is silenced by methylation in lymphoblasts [41]. Unlike the 1q25.3 interchromosomal insertion, the presence of the 8q24.3 interchromosomal insertion does not appear to affect SOX3 expression in lymphoblasts.

FGF13 encodes the fibroblast growth factor 13 protein that is part of the fibroblast growth factor homologous family [42]. Hypertrichosis patients carrying a 389 kb interchromosomal insertion from chromosome 6p21.1 showed reduced FGF13 expression in patient hair follicles [38]. We observed a 3-fold increase in expression in lymphoblast cells from the CMTX3 patient (Fig 3B). Although the assay could not distinguish between the different FGF13 isoforms, our preliminary finding demonstrates that the 8q24.3 interchromosomal insertion dysregulatesFGF13 expression in CMTX3 patient lymphoblasts. We hypothesize that if similar dysregulation of FGF13 gene expression were to be observed in patient neurons this could be the underlying cause of disease in CMTX3 patients. It is also possible that the observed dysregulation of FGF13 is a benign, bystander effect of the 78 kb interchromosomal insertion. Further gene expression studies on FGF13 and the remaining genes mapping to the CMTX3 locus, will be required to fully determine the pathogenic consequence of the CMTX3 8q24.3 insertion.

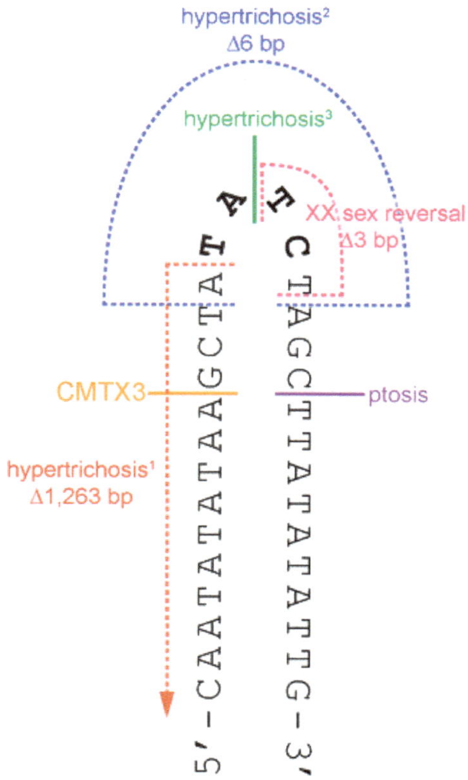

Figure 4. The breakpoints of disease-associated interchromosomal insertions at Xq27.1 localize near the center of 180 bp palindrome sequence.

There have been six large interchromosomal insertions previously reported; each originating from unique genomic regions and ranging from 124–774 kb [36–40]. These interchromosomal insertions have been shown to cause hypoparathyroidism [36], hypertrichosis [37, 38], ptosis [39], and XX male sex reversal [40]. CMTX3 is the fifth disease phenotype to be associated with an Xq27.1 interchromosomal insertion, clearly suggesting there is a recurrent mutation mechanism at the Xq27.1 locus. There are several mutation mechanisms that give rise to structural variations (recently reviewed in [43, 44]). We propose that this recurring mutation mechanism is possibly due to double stranded DNA breaks occurring in the 180 bp palindrome sequence at Xq27.1 [37] followed by incorrect repair of the DNA break through microhomology-mediated break-induced replication [45, 46]. For most of the interchromosomal insertions, including the CMTX3 insertion, at least one breakpoint is located near the center of the 180 bp palindrome sequence, close to where the hairpin loop is predicted to form (Fig 4) [37–40]. Hairpin loops are susceptible to double stranded DNA breaks due to endonuclease activity and are common hotspots for translocations [47]. Since the chromosome X breakpoints of these interchromosomal insertions localize within this hairpin structure, this suggests that hairpin formation of the palindrome sequence and endonuclease activity may be the initial process of the recurrent mutation mechanism.

Cartoon depicts a portion of the palindrome sequence (chrX:139,502,939–139,502,970) with the positive strand folded upon itself in a hairpin loop (black). The four non-palindromic bases in the middle of the 180 bp sequence (TATC, bolded black) are predicted to form the head of the hairpin loop. The locations of the breakpoints on chromosome Xq27.1 for CMTX3 (orange); hypertrichosis[1] (red, [37]); hypertrichosis[2](blue, [37]); hypertrichosis[3] (green,[38]); ptosis (pink; Bunyan [39]); and XX sex reversal (purple, Haines [40]) are marked out on the hairpin structure. Single breakpoints are depicted by a solid line. Multiple breakpoints are indicated by broken lines.

Microhomology-mediated break-induced replication (MMBIR) coupled with fork stalling and template switching (FoSTeS) has been proposed as an alternative model for the formation of genomic rearrangements that cannot be explained by non-allelic homologous recombination [45, 48, 49]. In this model, microhomology-induced template switching occurs where nearby single-stranded DNA is used as template to repair DNA breaks. Depending on the template, this results in the formation of deletions, duplications, triplications inversions or translocations that are flanked by minimal sequence homology of 2–6 bp at the breakpoints [45]. Further complexity at the genomic rearrangement breakpoints, involving small deletions and/or small insertions of unlinked or unknown sequences, are also commonly observed and is likely due to multiple template-switching events occurring during the repair process [49].

Sequencing the breakpoints of the CMTX3 rearrangement revealed an additional 19 bp from chromosome 12q13.12, an inversion of 12 bp from chromosome Xq27.1 and microhomology between chromosome X and chromosome 8 sequence as well as between the chromosome 8 and chromosome 12 sequence (Fig 2A and 2B). Microhomology, small deletions at the Xq27.1 sequence and additional small inserted sequences, from unlinked (i.e. from another chromosome) or unknown sources, also feature in the other disease-associated interchromosomal insertions at Xq27.1 [36–40] suggesting these insertions arose through MMBIR/FoSTeS.

Since each unique DNA insertion causes different disease phenotypes this suggests that the inserted genomic sequence is important. Based on the varying gene dysregulation observed for patients with hypertrichosis [38], XX sex reversal [40] and CMTX3, we predict the disease specificity from each interchromosomal insertion into Xq27.1 arises from the introduction of DNA regulatory elements that interact with the nearby genes in a tissue-specific manner. Unsolved Mendelian diseases mapping to the Xq27.1 region should therefore be assessed for large interchromosomal insertions using WGS analysis.

With 20% of our CMT families remaining genetically unsolved after WES [2], finding the causes of disease in these families is an important goal for inherited peripheral neuropathies. Our discovery suggests that structural variation involving non-coding DNA may explain a portion of the unsolved families. It also highlights the importance of looking beyond CNV when analyzing the genome for structural variation. Although the CMTX3 mutation represents trisomy of 8q24.3, given that this does not result in a dosage change for ARHGAP39, it is likely that the insertion itself underlies the peripheral neuropathy.

WGS provides a powerful tool to detect the full spectrum of DNA variation including all classes of structural variations [50, 51]. Given that structural variations are found throughout the general population [52, 53] distinguishing pathogenic and benign structural variations will be difficult without large families to confirm segregation. In time, improved annotation of benign genomic rearrangements in SV databases, that go beyond CNV and map the location and orientation of all SV subtypes, will assist in delineating pathogenic structural variations in patients. Pathogenic structural variations identified in families that are large enough for segregation analyses, as we have shown for the CMTX3 mutation, will provide genomic landmarks in which WGS data from smaller families can be mined for structural variation sequencing signatures (such as split reads and discordant paired ends). This strategy will, however, have limited use if structural variations causing inherited peripheral neuropathy prove to be rare private mutations. With decreasing WGS costs and improved sensitivity of WGS alignment algorithms, we predict that more structural variations are likely to be identified as the pathogenic cause of CMT. However, we acknowledge that the detection of these mutations in both the research and clinical diagnostic settings will be a challenge with no immediate solution.

In conclusion, we have provided compelling data supporting the likely genetic cause of CMTX3 neuropathy as a 78 kb interchromosomal insertion at Xq27.1 [der(X)dir ins(X;8)(q27.1;q24.3)]. Based on genealogy studies we believe this founder insertion originated prior to the early 1800s in a Scottish family. Our discovery is the first neuropathy caused by an Xq27.1 interchromosomal insertion. We propose that large structural variations involving non-coding DNA, similar to the CMTX3 mutation, may account for a proportion of the unsolved CMT cases.

MATERIALS AND METHODS

Research participation

Participating family members gave informed consent according to the protocols approved by the Sydney Local Health District Human Ethics Review Committee, Concord Repatriation General Hospital, Sydney, Australia (reference number: HREC/11/CRGH/105).

Genomic DNA extraction

Genomic DNA was extracted from peripheral blood using the PureGene Kit (Qiagen) following manufacturer's instructions. Extractions were performed by Molecular Medicine Laboratory, Concord Repatriation General Hospital (Sydney, Australia).

Whole genome sequencing

Genomic DNA samples (3 μg) were dispatched to NextCODE (Massachusetts, USA) who outsourced WGS of samples to Macrogen (South Korea). Paired-end (101 bp) sequencing was performed on a HiSeq 2000 sequencer (Illumina) following standard protocols.

WGS bioinformatics analyses

Raw WGS data was returned to NextCODE who performed the following bioinformatics analyses. Access to all pipeline output files and visual representation of WGS data was made available through the Sequence Miner (NextCODE) application.

Sequence alignment.

Sequence reads were aligned to the human reference sequence (hg19) using the Burrows-Wheeler Aligner (BWA) version 0.5.9 [54]. Alignments were merged into a single BAM file and marked for duplicates using Picard 1.55. Non-duplicate reads were selected for further downstream analyses.

Discordant paired end and split read detection.

WGS data was assessed for discordant paired end reads and split reads using in house pipelines developed by NextCODE. For discordant paired end detection, scripts were developed to identify high quality read pairs mapping to different chromosomes or with inserts greater than 700 bp (more than twice the library mean insert size). Using a 200 bp window, the local maximum rearrangement position was identified and regions with generally poor read alignment were excluded. For split read detection, algorithms were used to extract reads whereby one half of the read mapped to the genome and the second half did not map locally.

PCR amplification

Primers (X.F: 5'-CTCCAGCTTTGTTCTTTGGAC-3'; X.R: 5'-TCACCAACATTTCCAATCTCC-3'; 8.F: 5'-CAAACCCAATTCAGGTCCAG-3'; 8.R: 5'-GCCTAGGAGGTGTCCCTTTC-3') were designed to amplify wild type chromosome X and the distal and proximal breakpoints of the 8q24.3 interchromosomal insertion. Multiplex PCR was performed in a 15 μl reaction containing 25 ng genomic DNA, 1X MyTaq Red Mix (Bioline), 8 pmol primer X.F, 8 pmol primer X.R, 2 pmol primer 8.F and 4 pmol primer 8.R. All PCR thermocycling was performed on an Eppendorf MasterCycler using a touchdown cycling protocol. Specific cycling temperatures are available on request. Amplicons were size fractionated on 1.5% (w/v) agarose gel at 40 V/cm. Amplified DNA was purified using the Isolate PCR and Gel Kit (Bioline) after gel electrophoresis following manufacturer's instructions. Purified amplicons were submitted to Garvin Molecular Genetics (Sydney, Australia) for Sanger sequencing.

Tissue culture of patient lymphoblasts

Patient EBV-transformed lymphoblast cell lines were prepared using standard procedures at Genetic Repositories Australia (Sydney, Australia). Sex and aged matched controls were obtained from the Genetic Repositories Australia. Lymphoblasts were maintained in RPMI 1640 (Invitrogen) supplemented with 10% fetal bovine serum (Scientifix) and 2 mM L-glutamine (Gibco).

RNA isolation and cDNA synthesis

Total RNA was isolated from patient lymphoblast cells using Trizol (Life Technologies) according to the manufacturer's instructions. RNA was eluted in 50 µl RNAse-free water, DNase-treated with Turbo DNase (Life Technologies) and stored at -80°C until required. RNA (1 µg) was converted to cDNA using iScript cDNA Synthesis Kit (Biorad) following manufacturer's protocols.

Gene expression analysis

Isolated cDNA (100 ng) was subjected to quantitative RT-PCR analysis using TaqMan Gene Expression Assays (Invitrogen) following manufacturer's protocols. Quantitative RT-PCR was performed on a Step One Plus (Applied Biosystems) and relative fold difference was calculated using the comparative Ct method [55]. Target gene expression was determined relative to the housekeeping gene 18S. For each RNA extraction (n = 3 per sample), quantitative RT-PCR reactions were performed in triplicate.

SUPPORTING INFORMATION

S1 Figure Sanger sequencing confirms the CMTX3 interchromosomal insertion breakpoint sequences as predicted by whole genome sequencing (WGS).

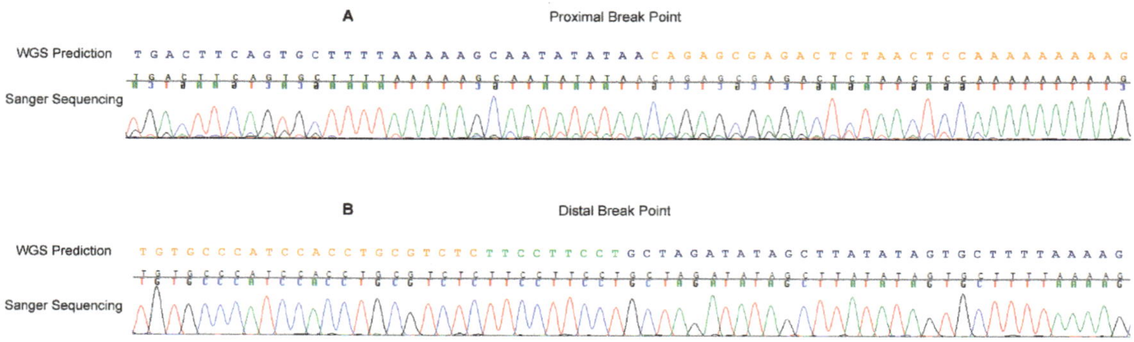

Predicted sequence based on WGS data are shown on top and corresponding Sanger sequencing trace profile is displayed underneath for the proximal (A) and distal (B) breakpoints. WGS prediction data are color-coded blue for chromosome X sequence, orange for chromosome 8 sequence, and green for chromosome 12 sequence.

S2 Figure The CMTX3 interchromosomal insertion maps within a topological associated domain (TAD) on Xq27.1.

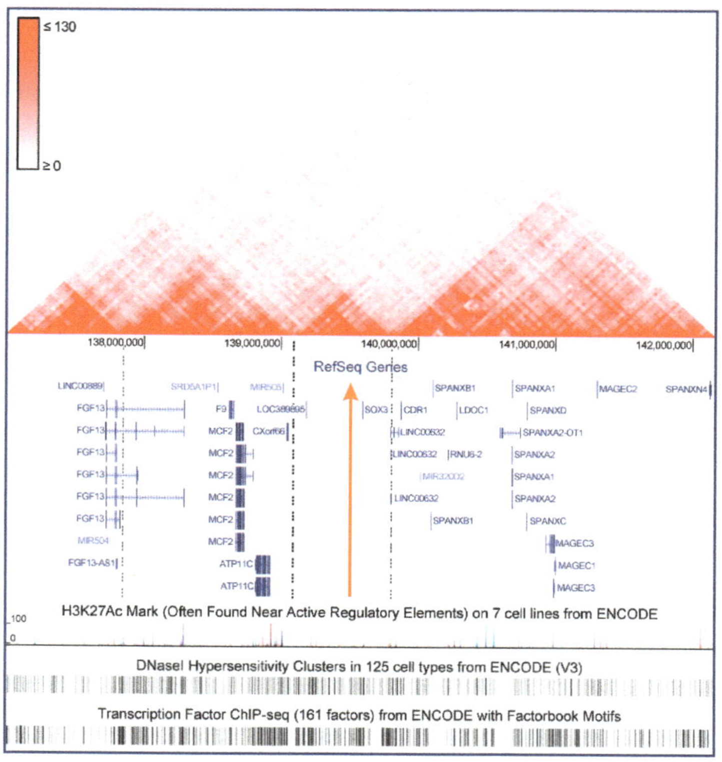

Hi-C data from human embryonic stem cells [35] across the CMTX3 locus from chrX:13137,000,000–142,000,000 (top panel). Middle panel depicts the location of genes mapping within the locus, adapted from the UCSC Genome Browser. Dotted lines indicate the TAD boundaries based on the Hi-C data. Position of the CMTX3 insertion is indicated by the orange arrow. H3K27Ac marks, DNaseI hypersensitivity clusters and transcription factor ChIP-seq data from ENCODE are depicted (as visualized in UCSC Genome Browser) in the bottom panel.

S3 Figure SOX3 mRNA expression is undetectable in patient and control lymphoblast cells.

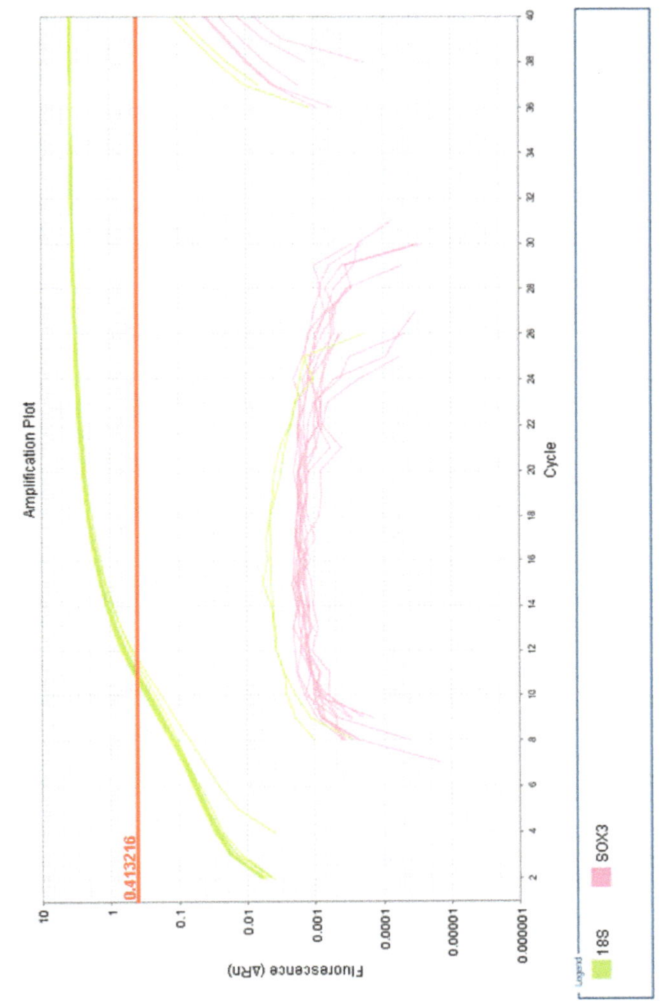

Real-time PCR amplification plot for SOX3 (pink) and 18S (green). The horizontal red line indicates the threshold value of fluorescence for calculating the Ct for 18S.

ACKNOWLEDGMENTS

The authors thank families CMT193-ext and CMT623 and the CMT Association of Australia for their ongoing participation, patience and support of this investigation, which has lasted over a decade. We thank Professor Robert Ouvrier for his invaluable clinical contribution to the families over the years. The authors also thank Mrs. Annette Berryman for tracing the genealogy of the families, and Dr. Jim Lund and Dr. Daniel Su from NextCODE for WGS and bioinformatics support.

Author Contributions

Conceived and designed the experiments: MHB GAN MLK. Performed the experiments: RC JQ AK APD. Analyzed the data: MHB MLK. Contributed reagents/materials/analysis tools: MPM MMR MAF DM GMS HKY SZ SWR GAN MLK. Wrote the paper: MHB GAN MLK.

REFERENCES

1. Saporta ASD, Sottile SL, Miller LJ, Feely SME, Siskind CE, Shy ME. Charcot-Marie-Tooth disease subtypes and genetic testing strategies. Ann Neurol. 2011;69: 22–33. doi: 10. 1002/ana. 22166. pmid:21280073
2. Drew AP, Zhu D, Kidambi A, Ly C, Tey S, Brewer MH, et al. Improved inherited peripheral neuropathy genetic diagnosis by whole-exome sequencing. Mol Genet Genomic Med. 2015;3: 143–154. doi: 10. 1002/mgg3. 126. pmid:25802885
3. Choi B-O, Koo SK, Park M-H, Rhee H, Yang S-J, Choi K-G, et al. Exome sequencing is an efficient tool for genetic screening of Charcot-Marie-Tooth disease. Hum Mutat. 2012;33: 1610–1615. doi: 10. 1002/humu. 22143. pmid:22730194
4. Schabhüttl M, Wieland T, Senderek J, Baets J, Timmerman V, De Jonghe P, et al. Whole-exome sequencing in patients with inherited neuropathies: outcome and challenges. J Neurol. 2014;261: 970–982. doi: 10. 1007/s00415-014-7289-8. pmid:24627108
5. Ionasescu VV, Trofatter J, Haines JL, Summers AM, Ionasescu R, Searby C. Heterogeneity in X-linked recessive Charcot-Marie-Tooth neuropathy. Am J Hum Genet. 1991;48: 1075–1083. pmid:1674639 doi: 10. 1002/mus. 880150317
6. Huttner IG, Kennerson ML, Reddel SW, Radovanovic D, Nicholson GA. Proof of genetic heterogeneity in X-linked Charcot-Marie-Tooth disease. Neurology. 2006;67: 2016–2021. pmid:17159110 doi: 10. 1212/01. wnl. 0000247271. 40782. b7
7. Brewer MH, Changi F, Antonellis A, Fischbeck K, Polly P, Nicholson G, et al. Evidence of a founder haplotype refines the X-linked Charcot-Marie-Tooth (CMTX3) locus to a 2. 5 Mb region. Neurogenetics. 2008;9: 191–195. doi: 10. 1007/s10048-008-0126-4. pmid:18458969
8. Chaudhry R, Kidambi A, Brewer MH, Antonellis A, Mathews K, Nicholson G, et al. Re-analysis of an original CMTX3 family using exome sequencing identifies a known BSCL2 mutation. Muscle Nerve. 2013;47: 922–924. doi: 10. 1002/mus. 23743. pmid:23553728
9. Brewer MH. Molecular genetics of X-linked Charcot-Marie-Tooth neuropathy (CMTX3). Ph. D. Thesis, University of Sydney. 2011. Available:http://opac. library. usyd. edu. au:80/record=b3855774~S4.
10. Abecasis GR, Altshuler D, Auton A, Brooks LD, Durbin RM, Gibbs RA, et al. A map of human genome variation from population-scale sequencing. Nature. 2010;467: 1061–1073. doi: 10. 1038/nature09534. pmid:20981092
11. Sherry ST, Ward MH, Kholodov M, Baker J, Phan L, Smigielski EM, et al. dbSNP: the NCBI database of genetic variation. Nucleic Acids Res. 2001;29: 308–

311. pmid:11125122 doi: 10. 1093/nar/29. 1. 308

12. Raeymaekers P, Timmerman V, Nelis E, De Jonghe P, Hoogendijk JE, Baas F, et al. Duplication in chromosome 17p11. 2 in Charcot-Marie-Tooth neuropathy type 1a (CMT 1a). The HMSN Collaborative Research Group. Neuromuscul Disord. 1991;1: 93–97. pmid:1822787 doi: 10. 1016/0960-8966(91)90055-w

13. Lupski JR, De Oca-Luna RM, Slaugenhaupt S, Pentao L, Guzzetta V, Trask BJ, et al. DNA duplication associated with Charcot-Marie-Tooth disease type 1A. Cell. 1991;66: 219–232. pmid:1677316 doi: 10. 1016/0092-8674(91)90613-4

14. Matsunami N, Smith B, Ballard L, Lensch MW, Robertson M, Albertsen H, et al. Peripheral myelin protein-22 gene maps in the duplication in chromosome 17p11. 2 associated with Charcot-Marie-Tooth 1A. Nat Genet. 1992;1: 176–179. pmid:1303231 doi: 10. 1038/ng0692-176

15. Patel PI, Roa BB, Welcher AA, Schoener-Scott R, Trask BJ, Pentao L, et al. The gene for the peripheral myelin protein PMP-22 is a candidate for Charcot-Marie-Tooth disease type 1A. Nat Genet. 1992;1: 159–165. pmid:1303228 doi: 10. 1038/ng0692-159

16. Timmerman V, Nelis E, Van Hul W, Nieuwenhuijsen BW, Chen KL, Wang S, et al. The peripheral myelin protein gene PMP-22 is contained within the Charcot-Marie-Tooth disease type 1A duplication. Nat Genet. 1992;1: 171–175. pmid:1303230 doi: 10. 1038/ng0692-171

17. Valentijn LJ, Bolhuis PA, Zorn I, Hoogendijk JE, Van Den Bosch N, Hensels GW, et al. The peripheral myelin gene PMP-22/GAS-3 is duplicated in Charcot-Marie-Tooth disease type 1A. Nat Genet. 1992;1: 166–170. pmid:1303229 doi: 10. 1038/ng0692-166

18. Chance PF, Alderson MK, Leppig KA, Lensch MW, Matsunami N, Smith B, et al. DNA deletion associated with hereditary neuropathy with liability to pressure palsies. Cell. 1993;72: 143–151. pmid:8422677 doi: 10. 1016/0092-8674(93)90058-x

19. Huang J, Wu X, Montenegro G, Price J, Wang G, Vance JM, et al. Copy number variations are a rare cause of non-CMT1A Charcot-Marie-Tooth disease. J Neurol. 2010;257: 735–741. doi: 10. 1007/s00415-009-5401-2. pmid:19949810

20. Høyer H, Braathen GJ, Eek AK, Nordang GBN, Skjelbred CF, Russell MB. Copy Number Variations in a Population-Based Study of Charcot-Marie-Tooth Disease. Biomed Res Int. 2015;2015: 1–7. doi: 10. 1155/2015/960404

21. Pehlivan D, Beck CR, Okamoto Y, Harel T, Akdemir ZHC, Jhangiani SN, et al. The role of combined SNV and CNV burden in patients with distal symmetric polyneuropathy. Genet Med. 2015: 725–726. doi: 10. 1038/gim. 2015. 124

22. Høyer H, Braathen GJ, Eek AK, Skjelbred CF, Russell MB. Charcot-Marie-Tooth caused by a copy number variation in myelin protein zero. Eur J Med Genet. 2011;54: e580–e583. doi: 10. 1016/j. ejmg. 2011. 06. 006. pmid:21787890

23. Maeda MH, Mitsui J, Soong B-W, Takahashi Y, Ishiura H, Hayashi S, et al. Increased gene dosage of myelin protein zero causes Charcot-Marie-Tooth disease. Ann Neurol. 2012;71: 84–92. doi: 10. 1002/ana. 22658. pmid:22275255

24. Ainsworth PJ, Bolton CF, Murphy BC, Stuart JA, Hahn AF. Genotype/phenotype correlation in affected individuals of a family with a deletion of the entire coding sequence of the connexin 32 gene. Hum Genet. 1998;103: 242–244. pmid:9760211 doi: 10. 1007/s004390050812

25. Lin C, Numakura C, Ikegami T, Shizuka M, Shoji M, Nicholson G, et al. Deletion and nonsense mutations of the connexin 32 gene associated with Charcot-Marie-Tooth disease. Tohoku J Exp Med. 1999;188: 239–244. pmid:10587015 doi: 10. 1620/tjem. 188. 239

26. Nakagawa M, Takashima H, Umehara F, Arimura K, Miyashita F, Takenouchi N, et al. Clinical phenotype in X-linked Charcot-Marie-Tooth disease with an entire deletion of the connexin 32 coding sequence. J Neurol Sci. 2001;185: 31–37. pmid:11266688 doi: 10. 1016/s0022-510x(01)00454-3

27. Østern R, Fagerheim T, Hjellnes H, Nygård B, Mellgren SI, Nilssen Ø. Diagnostic laboratory testing for Charcot Marie Tooth disease (CMT): the spectrum of gene defects in Norwegian patients with CMT and its implications for future genetic test strategies. BMC Med Genet. 2013;14: 94. doi: 10. 1186/1471-2350-14-94. pmid:24053775

28. Okamoto Y, Goksungur MT, Pehlivan D, Beck CR, Gonzaga-Jauregui C, Muzny DM, et al. Exonic duplication CNV of NDRG1 associated with autosomal-recessive HMSN-Lom/CMT4D. Genet Med. 2013;16. doi: 10. 1038/gim. 2013. 155

29. Lupiáñez DG, Kraft K, Heinrich V, Krawitz P, Brancati F, Klopocki E, et al. Disruptions of topological chromatin domains cause pathogenic rewiring of gene-enhancer interactions. Cell. 2015;161: 1012–1025. doi: 10. 1016/j. cell. 2015. 04. 004. pmid:25959774

30. Weterman MaJ, Van Ruissen F, De Wissel M, Bordewijk L, Samijn JPA, Van Der Pol WL, et al. Copy number variation upstream of PMP22 in Charcot-Marie-Tooth disease. Eur J Hum Genet. 2010;18: 421–428. doi: 10. 1038/ejhg. 2009. 186. pmid:19888301

31. Zhang F, Seeman P, Liu P, Weterman MaJ, Gonzaga-Jauregui C, Towne CF, et al. Mechanisms for nonrecurrent genomic rearrangements associated with CMT1A or HNPP: rare CNVs as a cause for missing heritability. Am J Hum Genet. 2010;86: 892–903. doi: 10. 1016/j. ajhg. 2010. 05. 001. pmid:20493460

32. Jones EA, Brewer MH, Srinivasan R, Krueger C, Sun G, Charney KN, et al. Distal enhancers upstream of the Charcot-Marie-Tooth type 1A disease gene PMP22. Hum Mol Genet. 2012;21: 1581–1591. doi: 10. 1093/hmg/ddr595. pmid:22180461

33. Kleinjan DA, Van Heyningen V. Long-range control of gene expression: emerging mechanisms and disruption in disease. Am J Hum Genet. 2005;76: 8–32. pmid:15549674 doi: 10. 1086/426833

34. Spielmann M, Mundlos S. Structural variations, the regulatory landscape of the genome and their alteration in human disease. Bioessays. 2013;35: 533–543. doi: 10. 1002/bies. 201200178. pmid:23625790

35. Dixon JR, Selvaraj S, Yue F, Kim A, Li Y, Shen Y, et al. Topological domains in mammalian genomes identified by analysis of chromatin interactions. Nature. 2012;485: 376–380. doi: 10. 1038/nature11082. pmid:22495300

36. Bowl MR, Nesbit MA, Harding B, Levy E, Jefferson A, Volpi E, et al. An interstitial deletion-insertion involving chromosomes 2p25. 3 and Xq27. 1, near SOX3, causes X-linked recessive hypoparathyroidism. J Clin Invest. 2005;115: 2822–2831. pmid:16167084 doi: 10. 1172/jci24156

37. Zhu H, Shang D, Sun M, Choi S, Liu Q, Hao J, et al. X-linked congenital hypertrichosis syndrome is associated with interchromosomal insertions mediated by a human-specific palindrome near SOX3. Am J Hum Genet. 2011;88: 819–826. doi: 10. 1016/j. ajhg. 2011. 05. 004. pmid:21636067

38. Destefano GM, Fantauzzo KA, Petukhova L, Kurban M, Tadin-Strapps M, Levy B, et al. Position effect on FGF13 associated with X-linked congenital generalized hypertrichosis. Proc Natl Acad Sci U S A. 2013;110: 7790–7795. doi: 10. 1073/pnas. 1216412110. pmid:23603273

39. Bunyan DJ, Robinson DO, Tyers AG, Huang S, Maloney VK, Grand FH, et al. X-Linked Dominant Congenital Ptosis Cosegregating with an Interstitial Insertion of a Chromosome 1p21. 3 Fragment into a Quasipalindromic Sequence in Xq27. 1. Open Journal of Genetics. 2014;04: 415–425. doi: 10. 4236/ojgen. 2014. 46039

40. Haines B, Hughes J, Corbett M, Shaw M, Innes J, Patel L, et al. Interchromosomal insertional translocation at Xq26. 3 alters SOX3 expression in an individual with XX male sex reversal. J Clin Endocrinol Metab. 2015;100: jc. 2014-4383. doi: 10. 1210/jc. 2014-4383

41. Cotton AM, Avila L, Penaherrera MS, Affleck JG, Robinson WP, Brown CJ. Inactive X chromosome-specific reduction in placental DNA methylation. Hum Mol Genet. 2009;18: 3544–3552. doi: 10. 1093/hmg/ddp299. pmid:19586922

42. Smallwood PM, Munoz-Sanjuan I, Tong P, Macke JP, Hendry SH, Gilbert DJ, et al. Fibroblast growth factor (FGF) homologous factors: new members of the FGF family implicated in nervous system development. Proc Natl Acad Sci U S A. 1996;93: 9850–9857. pmid:8790420 doi: 10. 1073/pnas. 93. 18. 9850

43. Weckselblatt B, Rudd MK. Human Structural Variation: Mechanisms of Chromosome Rearrangements. Trends Genet. 2015;31: 587–599. doi: 10. 1016/j. tig. 2015. 05. 010. pmid:26209074

44. Carvalho CMB, Lupski JR. Mechanisms underlying structural variant formation in genomic disorders. Nature reviews Genetics. 2016;17: 224–238. doi: 10. 1038/nrg. 2015. 25. pmid:26924765

45. Hastings PJ, Ira G, Lupski JR. A microhomology-mediated break-induced replication model for the origin of human copy number variation. PLoS Genet. 2009;5: e1000327. doi: 10. 1371/journal. pgen. 1000327. pmid:19180184

46. Onozawa M, Zhang Z, Kim YJ, Goldberg L, Varga T, Bergsagel PL, et al. Repair of DNA double-strand breaks by templated nucleotide sequence insertions derived from distant regions of the genome. Proc Natl Acad Sci U S A. 2014;111: 7729–7734. doi: 10. 1073/pnas. 1321889111. pmid:24821809

47. Kurahashi H, Inagaki H, Ohye T, Kogo H, Kato T, Emanuel BS. Palindrome-mediated chromosomal translocations in humans. DNA repair. 2006;5: 1136–1145. pmid:16829213 doi: 10. 1016/j. dnarep. 2006. 05. 035

48. Zhang F, Khajavi M, Connolly AM, Towne CF, Batish SD, Lupski JR. The DNA replication FoSTeS/MMBIR mechanism can generate genomic, genic and exonic complex rearrangements in humans. Nat Genet. 2009;41: 849–853. doi: 10. 1038/ng. 399. pmid:19543269

49. Sakofsky CJ, Ayyar S, Deem AK, Chung WH, Ira G, Malkova A. Translesion Polymerases Drive Microhomology-Mediated Break-Induced Replication Leading to Complex Chromosomal Rearrangements. Mol Cell. 2015;60: 860–872. doi: 10. 1016/j. molcel. 2015. 10. 041. pmid:26669261

50. Belkadi A, Bolze A, Itan Y, Cobat A, Vincent QB, Antipenko A, et al. Whole-genome sequencing is more powerful than whole-exome sequencing for detecting exome variants. Proc Natl Acad Sci U S A. 2015: 1418631112-. doi: 10. 1073/pnas. 1418631112

51. Zhang Y, Haraksingh R, Grubert F, Abyzov A, Gerstein M, Weissman S, et al. Child Development and Structural Variation in the Human Genome. Child Dev. 2013;84: 34–48. doi: 10. 1111/cdev. 12051. pmid:23311762

52. Redon R, Ishikawa S, Fitch KR, Feuk L, Perry GH, Andrews TD, et al. Global variation in copy number in the human genome. Nature. 2006;444: 444–454. pmid:17122850 doi: 10. 1038/nature05329

53. Feuk L, Carson AR, Scherer SW. Structural variation in the human genome. Nat Rev Genet. 2006;7: 85–97. pmid:16418744 doi: 10. 1038/nrg1767

54. Li H, Durbin R. Fast and accurate short read alignment with Burrows-Wheeler transform. Bioinformatics (Oxford, England). 2009;25: 1754–1760. doi: 10. 1093/bioinformatics/btp324

55. Livak KJ, Schmittgen TD. Analysis of relative gene expression data using real-time quantitative PCR and the 2(-Delta Delta C(T)) Method. Methods. 2001;25: 402–408. pmid:11846609 doi: 10.1006/meth.2001.1262

CHAPTER 18

IDENTIFICATION OF NOVEL CANDIDATE GENES FOR EARLY-ONSET COLORECTAL CANCER SUSCEPTIBILITY

Richarda M. de Voer, Marc-Manuel Hahn, Robbert D. A. Weren, Arjen R. Mensenkamp, Christian Gilissen, Wendy A. van Zelst-Stams, Liesbeth Spruijt, C. Marleen Kets, Junxiao Zhang, Hanka Venselaar , Lilian Vreede, Nil Schubert, Marloes Tychon, Ronny Derks , Hans K. Schackert , Ad Geurts van Kessel , Nicoline Hoogerbrugge, Marjolijn J. L. Ligtenberg, Roland P. Kuiper

INTRODUCTION

Colorectal cancer (CRC) is a heterogeneous disease with an estimated heritable component of 25–30%. About 5–10% of CRC cases are currently explained by germline mutations in genes that predispose to Mendelian cancer syndromes, such as Lynch syndrome, Familial Adomatous Polyposis, Peutz-Jeghers syndrome, Juvenile Polyposis syndrome, MUTYH-associated polyposis, NTHL1-associated polyposis, and Polymerase Proofreading-associated Polyposis syndrome.[1–5] Typically, these CRC syndromes are marked by a strong family history, a high-penetrance of the disease, and the development of multiple tumors at an early age.[1] An additional 10% of the heritability of CRC may be explained by a growing list of common, low penetrant risk factors.[5–7] In spite of this, a large part of the heritability of CRC still remains unexplained and may well result from the presence of rare variants with a moderate risk.[8]

Moderately penetrant risk factors do not necessarily result in dominant traits, since their phenotypic effects may rely on an interplay with other genetic and/or environmental factors.[2] However, these genetic factors may play a role in individuals with an early-onset of the disease, one of the hallmarks of hereditary cancer.[9] In addition, unexplained early-onset CRC cases differ from late-onset sporadic CRC cases based on their distinct clinical, molecular, and pathological etiology.[10]

Citation: de Voer RM, Hahn M-M, Weren RDA, Mensenkamp AR, Gilissen C, van Zelst-Stams WA, et al. (2016) Identification of Novel Candidate Genes for Early-Onset Colorectal Cancer Susceptibility. PLoS Genet 12(2): e1005880. doi:10.1371/journal.pgen.1005880

Here, we used whole-exome sequencing to identify novel moderately penetrant CRC risk factors. Since we expect such factors to follow non-Mendelian inheritance patterns, we focused specifically on individuals with an early onset of the disease, which frequently manifests in the absence of a clear family history. We selected recurrent rare variants in genes with a low burden of comparable variants in controls, and identified PTPN12 and LRP6 as novel candidate risk factors for early-onset CRC.

RESULTS

Whole-exome sequencing of early-onset CRC cases

To identify rare genetic variants involved in CRC susceptibility, we performed whole-exome sequencing on germline DNA from 55 CRC cases, diagnosed at age 45 years or younger. The average age at diagnosis was 35 years [range: 23–45] and 22 cases (40%) had a positive family history for cancer (Table 1 and S1 Table). The average coverage per target region was 76x [range: 46-127x] with on average 43,124 identified variants [range: 29,040–49,929] per exome (detailed metrics per exome are listed in S2 Table). In total 2,381,720 variants were identified. After quality assessment, common variants were excluded, which were defined as variants that are present in our in-house database with 2,037 exomes from mostly Western-European ancestry or the Exome variant server (EVS) with minor allele frequencies (MAF) >0.001.[11] Subsequently, we selected variants that result in protein truncation (i.e. frameshift or nonsense mutations and variants at canonical splice sites) and missense substitutions at highly conserved positions (non-synonymous variants with a PhyloP score $\geq$3; see Materials and Methods for a detailed description). We identified on average 34 [range: 10–89] rare variants per sample, including on average 5 [range: 1–10] protein truncating variants and 29 [range: 8–83] missense variants. In total, 279 protein truncating and 1,584 missense variants were identified. These potentially pathogenic variants were subjected to a subsequent filtering strategy to identify known and novel CRC predisposing gene variants (Fig 1).

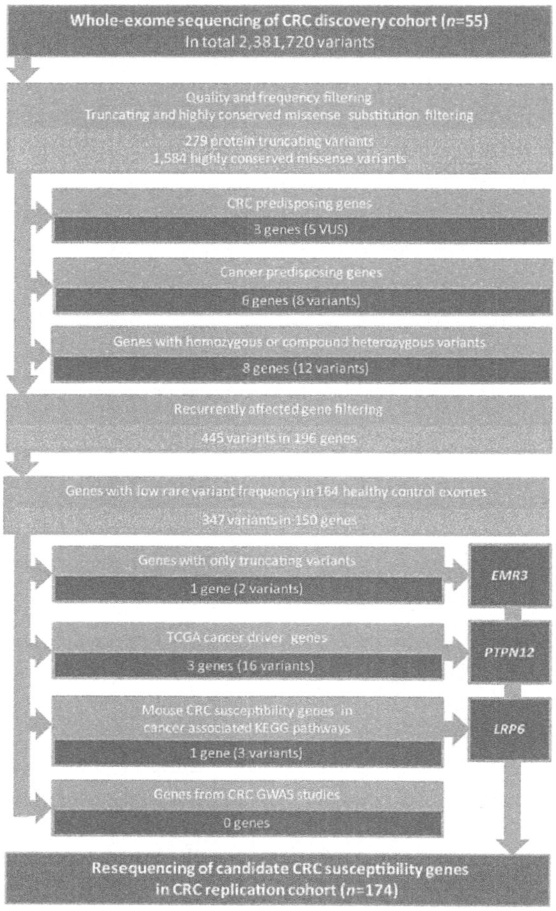

Figure 1. Study design, variant filtering and candidate gene prioritization.

Whole-exome sequencing was performed on germline DNA of 55 early-onset CRC cases. The exome data were first filtered for quality and frequency, followed by filtering for protein truncating and highly conserved missense variants. Next, we removed all known loss-of-function-tolerant genes from this list and searched for known and novel CRC predisposing gene variants.[12,13,57] An additional filtering was applied to identify genes that were affected by two or more potentially pathogenic variants and to remove genes that are frequently affected by protein-truncating or highly conserved missense variants in healthy controls. The remaining set of recurrent variants was filtered for (i) genes recurrently affected by protein truncating variants; (ii) cancer driver genes in CRC [23]; (iii) genes identified as CRC susceptibility genes in mice [29,30] and involved in cancer-related KEGG pathways [hsa04310 (WNT signaling), hsa04350 (TGF-beta signaling), hsa03430 (mismatch repair), hsa03410 (base excision repair), hsa03420 (nucleotide excision repair), map03450 (non-homologous end-joining), hsa03460 (Fanconi anemia), and hsa05200 (pathways in cancer)] (iv) genes identified in CRC GWAS studies [5–7,32]. Genes that remained after these filter steps were selected for re-sequencing in a replication cohort of 174 CRC cases. CRC: colorectal cancer; VUS: variant of unknown significance.

Table 1. Clinical characteristics of the discovery and replication cohorts with mismatch-repair proficient colorectal cancer.

Characteristic	Exome cohort (%) $N = 55$	Dutch replication cohort (%) $N = 82$	German replication cohort (%) $N = 92$
Average age of onset (SD)	35 (4)	40.4 (4.5)	37.7 (5.6)
Average age			
≤25 yr	2 (4)	1 (1)	1 (1)
25–30 yr	8 (15)	2 (2)	12 (13)
31–35 yr	17 (31)	10 (12)	16 (17)
36–40 yr	26 (47)	21 (26)	27 (29)
40–45 yr	2 (4)	46 (56)	35 (38)
45–50 yr	-	2 (2)	1 (1)
Family history for cancer			
None	27 (49)	23 (28)	4 (4)
≥one first degree relative	10 (18)	33 (40)	37 (3)
≥one second degree relative	10 (18)	13 (16)	20 (22)
≥one third degree relatives	2 (4)	1 (1)	1 (1)
Unknown	6 (11)	12 (15)	30 (33)
Tumor location			
Right colon	8 (15)	7 (9)	15 (16)
Transverse colon	4 (7)	8 (10)	9 (10)
Left colon	13 (24)	13 (16)	25 (27)
Rectum	25 (46)	32 (39)	33 (36)
Unknown	6 (11)	19 (23)	10 (11)

Variants in (colorectal) cancer predisposing genes

Within the list of potentially pathogenic variants, we analyzed whether these variants were present in any of the known CRC predisposing genes, i.e, mismatch repair (MMR) genes,APC, POLD1, POLE, SMAD4, BMPR1A, MUTYH, NTHL1. In three individuals, variants in the MMR genes MSH2, MSH6 (three variants) and PMS2 were identified, but based on microsatellite instability or immunohistochemistry analyses none of these variants resulted in MMR deficiency. Therefore, these variants were allocated to be of unknown significance.

Next, we focused on variants in genes known to predispose to other types of cancer or to cause cancer syndromes when present in a biallelic state.[12,13] We identified eight variants in six different genes. Two of these genes, BLM and ATM, were found to harbor rare variants in two patients. BLM encodes a RECQL-DNA helicase and is involved in the recessive Bloom syndrome, which predisposes to CRC. Although current literature on the risk of CRC development in carriers of pathogenic BLM alleles is contradictory [14–16], we recently found by targeted re-sequencing of a validation cohort that monoallelic pathogenic BLMvariants were enriched in these cases.[17] ATM is involved in double-strand break repair and mutations in its encoding gene are associated with ataxia telangiectasia, another autosomal recessive disorder. Somatic nonsense mutations in ATM occur frequently in CRC, but monoallelic germline mutations have thus far only been shown to increase the risk for gastric, breast and pancreatic cancers, and mostly when they result in truncated proteins.[18–20] Potentially pathogenic missense variants in ATM were also found twice in a cohort of 164 healthy individuals (Control dataset 1; see Materials and Methods and below) and we, therefore, conclude that ATM is not enriched in our cohort of CRC cases. The remaining four variants represent highly conserved missense or protein truncating variants that occurred in four different genes: BRIP1, EGFR, ERCC3 and WRN.

Identification of novel CRC susceptibility genes

To identify novel candidate CRC susceptibility genes, we first focused on genes with biallelic mutations (recessive inheritance pattern). Therefore, we analysed our list of potentially pathogenic variants for the presence of autosomal homozygous (≥95% variant reads) or compound heterozygous variants and, subsequently, performed Sanger validation. We identified biallelic variants in eight individuals, all affecting different genes (Fig 1). However, these genes were either found to be be linked to other phenotypes, to contain many rare variants in the general population, or to have a function that remains to be elucidated. Therefore, these variants were excluded from further analysis.

Subsequently, we filtered our list of potentially pathogenic variants for genes with at least two variants in unrelated individuals (see Materials and Methods for details). In total, we identified 445 rare potentially pathogenic variants in 196 recurrently affected genes. Some of these genes contain many rare variants that occur in the general population and are, thus, unlikely to provoke an increased risk for CRC. Therefore, we selected an exome sequencing data set from healthy individuals (Control dataset 1; n = 164) that were subjected to the same procedure as our CRC cohort and were found to be comparable based on genotyping accuracy and population. This 'Control dataset 1' was used to remove genes from our list that were not significantly enriched in the CRC cohort after a χ^2 goodness of fit test. The remaining variants, i.e., 347 variants in 150 genes, were subjected to a four-step prioritization as outlined below and depicted in Fig 1.

First, we investigated whether genes were recurrently affected by rare protein truncating variants. Only one gene, EMR3, was found to fulfill this criterion with two splice site mutations (Table 2), each predicted to result in skipping of an exon. EMR3 belongs to the EGF-TM7 protein family of G-protein coupled receptors and is specifically expressed in granulocytes and data from 'The Human Protein Atlas' suggest that EMR3 is not or only very lowly expressed in colonic tissue.[21,22] EMR3 has been suggested to function as a mediator of invasive phenotypic variation in glioblastoma.[23]

Second, we selected variants in genes that were identified as potential CRC driver genes.[24] We identified 16 variants in three genes: MSH6 (3 variants), TTN (10 variants) andPTPN12 (3 variants). The tumors of the carriers of the MSH6 variants do not reveal MMR deficiency and TTN is known to harbor an excess of rare private variants, is mainly expressed in cardiac and skeletal muscle, and is associated with cardiomyopathies (MIM: 188840).

Table 2. Variants in candidate CRC susceptibility genes identified by whole-exome sequencing and targeted re-sequencing.

Gene	Sample Names	Transcript	Variant			Pathogenicity				Variant Frequency (*n*; MAF)					
		Refseq. accession	Nucleotide (cDNA)	Amino acid (protein)	dbSNP	PhyloP	SIFT	Poly Phen-2	A-AVGD[a]	Discovery cohort (*n* = 55)	In-house DB (*n* = 2,037)	EVS (*n* = 6,503)	Control cohort 2 (*n* = 2,329)	ExAC (*n* = 60,706)	Replication cohort (*n* = 174)
EMR3	P025	NM_032571	c.882 +1G>A	p.?	N/A	2.427	N/A	N/A	N/A	1 (0.009091)	0	1 (0.0000769)	0	11 (0.0000914)	0
	P002		c.1249-2A>C	p.?	N/A	3.787	N/A	N/A	N/A	1 (0.009091)	0	0	1 (0.0002147)	0	0
PTPN12	P014	NM_002835	c.1565G>T	p.R522M	N/A	4.531	Del.	Prob. dam.	C25	1 (0.009091)	0	0	2 (0.0004294)	0	0
	P045 & P054		c.2051C>T	p.S684L	rs201001953	3.958	Del.	Prob. dam.	C0	2 (0.018182)	0	3 (0.0002307)	3 (0.0006441)	111 (0.000914)	0
	RC204		c.314C>T	p.A105V	N/A	4.24	Del.	Prob. dam.	C65	0	0	0	0	0	1
LRP6	P002	NM_002336	c.716C>A	p.W239L	N/A	5.103	Del.	Prob. dam.	C65	1 (0.009091)	0	0	0	0	0
	P001		c.2366T>C	p.N789S	N/A	6.244	Del.	Benign	C55	1 (0.009091)	0	0	0	0	0
	P008		c.2599A>G	p.T867A	rs141458215	5.13	Del	Benign	C55	1[b] (0.009091)	0	0	3 (0.0006441)	14 (0.000115)	0

[a] Align-GVGD scores vary from C0 (benign) to C65 (damaging).

[b] Did not pass the original quality settings.

N/A, not applicable; ND, not done; Del., deleterious; Prob.dam., probably damaging; Pos.dam., possibly damaging; EVS, exome variant server [11]; ExAC, Exome Aggregation Consortium [33].

Therefore, we investigated the three rare variants in PTPN12 in more detail (Table 2). PTPN12encodes the protein tyrosine phosphatase PTP-PEST that functions as a suppressor of epithelial cell motility in CRC cells and has been linked to breast cancer development.[25–27] The identified variants p.S684L (2 cases, subjects P045 and P054) and p.R522K (1 case, subject P014) were found to be located adjacent to the proline-rich regions of PTP-PEST (Fig 2), which have been shown to interfere with the kinase activity of PTP-PEST.[25–28] A data search in 'The Human Protein Atlas' revealed that PTPN12 is expressed at high levels in colonic tissue.[22] Somatic mutations that have been reported in PTPN12 were found to result in truncations of the protein or in amino acid substitutions (Fig 2A).[24]

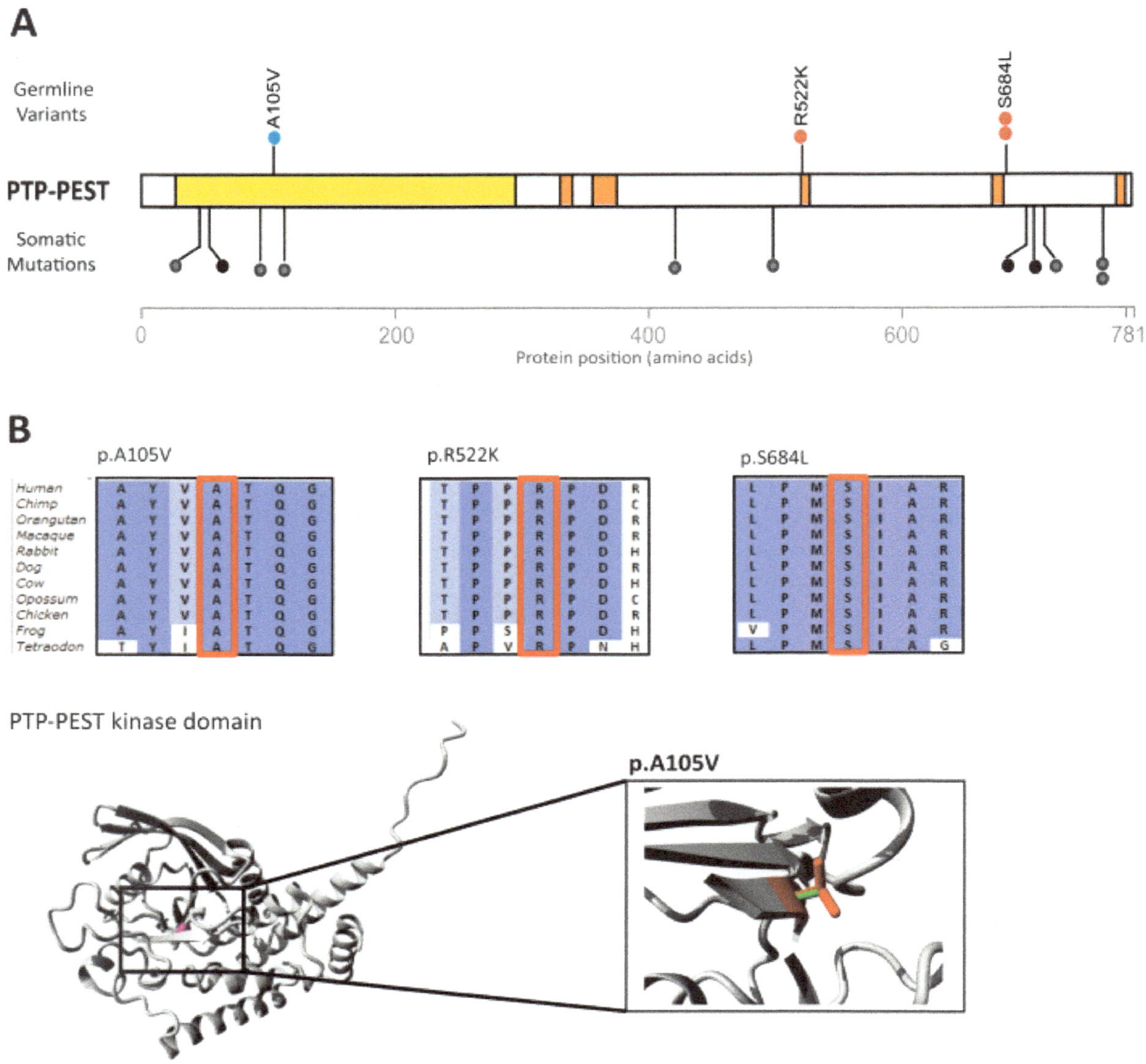

Figure 2. Rare variants in PTPN12 **encoding PTP-PEST in four cases.**

(A) Distribution of missense variants identified in the CRC discovery cohort (red dots) and CRC replication cohort (blue dots) in PTP-PEST. Somatic PTPN12 mutations identified in colorectal tumors [24] are indicated with black (missense) and green (protein truncating) dots. The kinase domain is shown in yellow and the proline-rich-regions are shown in orange. (B) Amino acid conservation of the three regions with missense variants (indicated with the red box) among 11 species, and the 3D protein structure of the kinase domain with the p.A105V variant. The close up shows the structural difference between the mutant (red) and wild-type (green) residue. The mutant residue at position 105 is bigger and may cause bumps during protein folding. The mutant residue at position 522 is smaller, which can result in loss of interactions. The mutant residue at position 684 is more hydrophobic than the wild-type residue, this may disturb correct protein folding.

Third, we filtered for variants in genes that were identified as mouse CRC susceptibility genes in transposon-based studies [29,30]. We identified 18 variants in eight such genes. Since most of these genes did not exhibit a clear link to cancer development, we filtered our list for genes for those that are described in KEGG pathways implicated in CRC development. This resulted in one remaining candidate, namely LRP6. In three CRC patients diagnosed before the age of 30 highly conserved LRP6 missense variants with a predicted pathogenicity, p.W239L (subject P002), p.N789S (subject P001) and p.T867A (subject P008), were identified (Table 2). LRP6 encodes a receptor of the WNT-FZD-LRP5-LRP6 complex that triggers β-catenin signaling. The LRP6 protein consists of four β-propeller domains, a transmembrane domain, and a cytoplasmic domain. All variants were located in β-propeller domains (Fig 3A and 3B), which are involved in the binding of WNT ligands and antagonists, such as WNT3a and Dickkopf-1, respectively.[31] Data from 'The Human Protein Atlas' revealed that LRP6 is expressed at high levels in colonic tissue.[22] Interestingly, LRP6 has also been found to be affected by somatic mutations in colorectal adenocarcinomas,[24] in which most of these mutations appear to occur within in the β-propeller domains (Fig 3A), thus supporting a role of missense variants in this gene in CRC development.

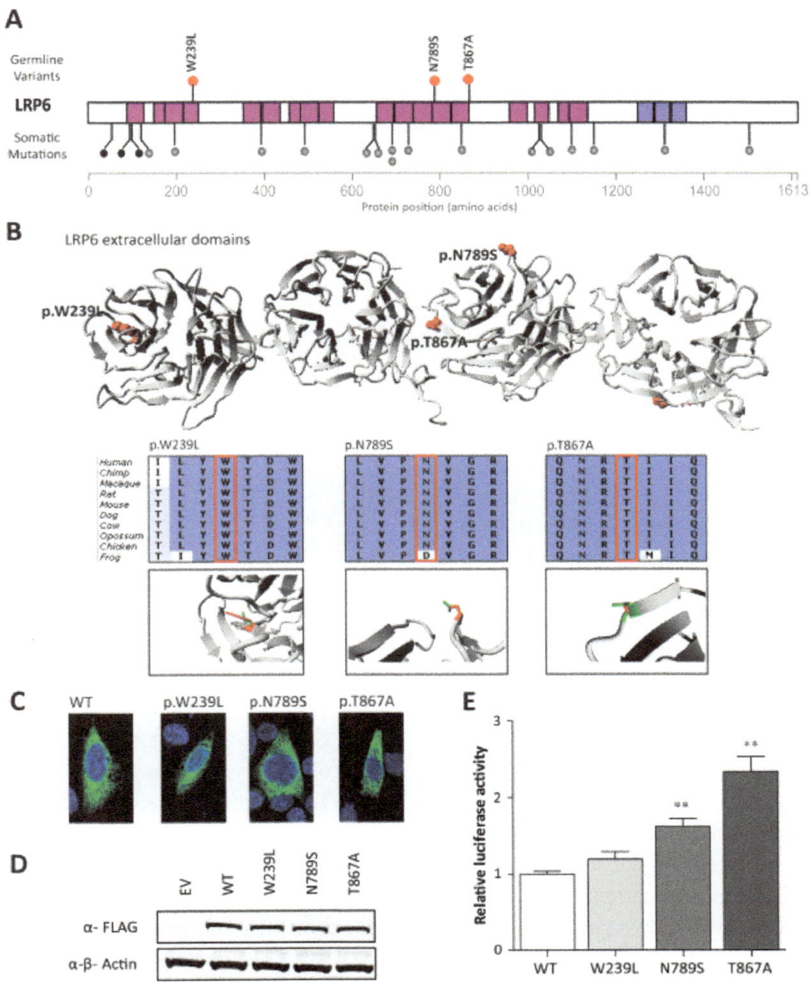

Figure 3. Rare variants in LRP6 **in three cases.**

(A) Distribution of missense LRP6 variants identified in the CRC discovery cohort (red dots). Somatic LRP6 mutations identified in colorectal tumors [24] are indicated with grey (missense) and black (protein truncating) dots. Structural domains include the β-propeller domains that are used to form the receptor complex (pink bars), and the transmembrane domain (purple). (B) 3D protein structure of the β-propeller domains of LRP6 with the positions of the identified missense variants in red. Insets show conservation of the region in which the missense variants (indicated with the red box) are located with, underneath, close ups of the local 3D protein structure with mutant (red) and wild-type (green) residues. The mutant residue at position 239 is predicted to disturb the protein structure (project HOPE; http://www.cmbi.ru.nl/hope/). The mutant residue at position 789 is much smaller than the wild-type residue and may disturb the binding of Dickkopf-1. Residue 867 is located on the surface of the protein and the mutant residues are not expected to disturb protein structure, but may influence protein binding. (C) Immunofluorescence analyses of LRP6 wild-type and mutant proteins showing similar subcellular localizations. (D) LRP6 protein expression levels normalized to β-actin are similar between wild-type and mutant LRP6. (E) TOPflash analyses of wild-type and mutant LRP6 to determine their effects on the WNT signaling pathway. Luciferase activity was normalized to control and wild-type constructs. Both p.N789S and p.T867A mutants reveal a significant increase in activation compared to the wild-type LRP6 protein. Experiments were performed three times in triplicate. $**P < 0.001$; error bars represent the standard error of the mean.

Fourth, we examined whether any of the genes that were previously identified in familial CRC genome-wide association studies (GWAS)[32] were present in our list of genes recurrently affected by rare variants, but none were identified.

Frequency of identified variants in control populations

We analyzed the frequency of the potentially pathogenic variants that we identified in theEMR3, PTPN12 and LRP6 genes in an additional cohort of locally sequenced control individuals without any suspicion for hereditary cancer, and in data from the Exome Aggregation Consortium.[33] The local control individuals were sequenced at a high coverage and exhibited sufficient read depth for our three candidate genes (Control dataset 2; n = 2,329;and Materials and Methods for a detailed description). All variants that we identified inEMR3, PTPN12 and LRP6 were either absent or present at an extremely low frequency in both these data sets (MAF of ≤0.001; Table 1). Next, we determined the number of variants in these three genes with a similar predicted effect in 'Control dataset 2'. This analysis revealed that protein-truncating variants in EMR3 and missense variants with a PhyloP $\geq$3.0 in PTPN12 andLRP6 are indeed enriched in our cohort of CRC patients, which remained significant after correcting for multiple testing for three genes. After correcting for exome-wide multiple testing, none of the genes were significantly enriched.

Resequencing of novel candidate CRC susceptibility genes

Next, we performed targeted resequencing of the novel candidate CRC susceptibility genesEMR3, PTPN12 and LRP6 using an Ion Ampliseq custom panel (Life technologies, seeMaterials and Methods for details) and a replication cohort of 174 CRC cases (Table 1). With an average read-depth of 530-fold per targeted region [range: 21–1,852] per sample, one additional rare potentially damaging variant in the kinase domain of the PTPN12 protein was identified (p.A105V, subject RC204, age 45 years) and confirmed by Sanger sequencing (Table 2 and Fig 2). This is not a significant increase compared to 'Control dataset 2'. No additional variants in EMR3 and LRP6 were identified.

Missense variants in LRP6 activate WNT signaling pathway

The three LRP6 variants identified were all encountered in individuals with a very early-onset of the disease: 23, 24 and 29 years of age. To assess whether these LRP6 variants may have an effect on the WNT signaling pathway, we performed TOPflash assays with LRP6 wild-type (WT) and mutant proteins. Immunofluoresence and Western blot analyses revealed similar localization patterns and equal expression levels of the WT and mutant LRP6 proteins (Fig 3C and 3D). Overexpression of the mutant LRP6 proteins (p.N789S and p.T867A) induced 1.6-fold ($P = 0.0003$) and 2.4-fold ($P < 0.0001$) increases in WNT signaling activity in the TOPflash assay compared to the LRP6 WT protein, respectively (Fig 3E).

Cosegregation analysis

Based on the availability of suitable material, a cosegregation analysis could only be performed for subject P002 (p.W239L; age 23 years). P002 did not have a clear family history of CRC, but her mother, two sisters and an aunt developed breast cancer. We found that the mother also carried the p.W239L variant. As we were unable to perform a complete cosegregation analysis in this family, or in any of the other PTPN12 or LRP6 families, it remains to be established to what extend carriers of variants in these genes tend to develop cancer at a young age.

Discussion

In this study we have performed whole-exome sequencing on germline DNA from 55 mismatch repair-proficient early-onset CRC cases and identified multiple potentially damaging variants in two colon-expressed genes: PTPN12 and LRP6. The germline variants identified in these genes appeared to affect highly conserved amino acids and were absent, or present at extremely low frequencies, in control populations. Targeted re-sequencing of a replication cohort of 174 individuals with early-onset CRC revealed one additional variant in PTPN12. We also found that two of the three missense variants in LRP6 can activate the WNT pathway in vitro. Based on these results, we propose that PTPN12 and LRP6 serve as novel moderately penetrant CRC susceptibility genes.

Within our discovery cohort, we focused on genes that were recurrently affected by rare potentially damaging variants. Rare variants represent the vast majority of normal variation in the human genome and they are unequally distributed between genes and between biological pathways,[34–37] illustrating that a comparison with exome sequence data from a geographically matched control cohort is crucial. We, therefore, selected only variants with a MAF $\leq$0.001 in locally sequenced control individuals, and applied the entire analysis pipeline to a dataset of 164 healthy controls that were sequenced using the same exome enrichment and sequencing procedures. This approach allowed us to reduce the risk of selecting locally common benign variants, to prevent the selection of false-positives by technical errors, and to focus only on genes that are protected from gathering pathogenic mutations in the normal population.[38] Furthermore, we analyzed an additional, more recent, high quality exome sequencing dataset from local individuals to confirm that our identified variants were indeed extremely rare.

One of the candidate genes, PTPN12, encodes the widely expressed cytoplasmic protein tyrosine phosphatase PTP-PEST, which regulates epithelial cell adhesion and migration.[25,39–41] In colon carcinoma cells, PTP-PEST has been shown to control cell motility and adherence junction assembly by regulating the intracellular localization of p120 catenin and, consequently, its interaction with E-cadherin.[27] Therefore, PTP-PEST may play a role in the tightly controlled migration of epithelial cells of the colonic crypts. The highly conserved variants identified in our study may result in diminished phosphatase activity, as has been demonstrated for comparable missense variants in the same domains,[26,28] resulting in aberrant crypt formation and possibly invasion.

LRP6 is a core-component of the WNT-FZD-LRP5-LRP6 receptor complex of the WNT signaling cascade, which is commonly activated in colon cancer.[42] Previously, this gene was also identified in a screen for mouse CRC susceptibility loci.[30] Remarkably, we found that the rare LRP6 variants were present in three of the youngest diagnosed individuals in our cohorts (age 23, 24 and 29). Furthermore, two of the identified missense variants in LRP6 were found to be located at positions of the protein that interact with the WNT antagonist Dickkopf-1 [43] and to result in significantly increased activations of the WNT pathway in in vitro TOPflash reporter assays. This finding is intriguing, as it was recently shown that missense variants inLRP6 can abrogate activation of the WNT pathway.[44]

Despite the fact that EMR3 is recurrently affected by rare protein truncating variants in our discovery cohort, we do not consider EMR3 a strong candidate gene for CRC susceptibility, since the protein is not or only very lowly expressed in tissue from colon and rectum, and we could not establish a functional link to CRC development.[21–23]

Several recent whole-exome sequencing studies have revealed novel candidate CRC susceptibility genes and variants,[45–51] but the concordance between these findings, including our own, is as yet limited, and statistical evidence for these correlations in case-control studies was not obtained. This limited concordance may be due to different patient inclusion criteria used, ranging from the selection of predominantly familial cases to individuals with isolated CRC at young age. In addition, it cannot be excluded that non-genetic (environmental) risk factors may have played a role in the development of CRC at a younger age in individual cases. Clearly, the genetic heterogeneity of CRC susceptibility may also, at least partly, explain the limited concordance between studies, and points out that statistical validation required very large case and control cohorts. Optimal phenotypic pre-selection, including genetic or histologic abnormalities in the tumor, or even the presence of additional congenital features as we recently identified in individuals with BUB1 and BUB3 abnormalities,[52] may limit this heterogeneity. Furthermore, variant selection varies between studies. So far, most studies have put a primary focus on high-penetrance germline mutations by showing cosegregation within families and second-hit mutations in the tumor,[45–50] but this approach may not be valid for predisposing variants with a moderate penetrance.

The inclusion of missense variants as potential candidates is challenging, because their effect is difficult to predict, and can vary widely between variants in a particular gene. Nevertheless, the putative relevance of missense variants in functionally important domains should not be underestimated, as was recently illustrated by the discovery of missense POLE and POLD1variants.[4] Functionally important domains are conserved both at the nucleic acid and the amino acid level. Currently, there is no consensus on the best strategy to discriminate pathogenic missense variants from benign missense variants, which poses a challenge to this type of cohort studies. We have used PhyloP scores as the first prioritization cut-off in the pathogenicity assessments, as it was previously shown that pathogenic variants have higher scores than benign variants,[53] This prioritization step was followed by other in silico steps to predict pathogenicity based on the biophysical amino acid characteristics and multiple protein sequence alignments. Finally, essential evidence for the role of damaging variants in novel genes may results from the presence of these variants in independent families, but their frequency is expected to be low. Therefore, large replication series are needed that encompass comparable cases to replicate the findings. Additionally, more and better candidates are likely to be identified when datasets from different studies are merged and re-analyzed. We did, however, identify several rare variants in single individuals in candidate CRC susceptibility genes previously reported by others. The same may, in reverse, turn out to be true for PTPN12 and LRP6.

In conclusion, we and others have shown by whole-exome sequencing that the genetic susceptibility to CRC is heterogeneous. Our findings are in line with a polygenic model of CRC susceptibility in which multiple risk factors in known and novel CRC pathways may contribute to additive risks.[54] Future studies, such as functional assessments of the candidate genes and replications in larger CRC and control cohorts, are needed to firmly establish the role ofPTPN12 and LRP6 in CRC susceptibility.

MATERIALS AND METHODS

Study samples

The discovery cohort used consists of 55 non-polyposis DNA mismatch repair (MMR)-proficient CRC cases, diagnosed at ≤45 years of age, which were referred to the Radboud university medical center, Nijmegen, the Netherlands (Table 1 and S1 Table).[12,52] The replication cohort used consists of 174 MMR-proficient CRC cases from both Nijmegen, The Netherlands, and Dresden, Germany, that fulfilled one of the following two criteria: (i) diagnosed with CRC ≤40 years of age (n = 90) regardless of family history, or (ii) diagnosed with CRC ≤50 years of age with at least two first-degree relatives with CRC (n = 84). All individuals provided written informed consent. The study was approved by the CMO (study number 2009/256), Arnhem and Nijmegen, the Netherlands.

Whole-exome sequencing

Whole-exome sequencing was performed on genomic DNA extracted from peripheral blood cells of cases included in the CRC discovery cohort with SOLiD4 (n = 10) and 5500xl (n = 45) sequencing platforms (Life technologies, Carlsbad, CA, USA) using the SOLiD-optimized SureSelect Human All Exon kit V1 (30Mb set, n = 1), V2 (50Mb set, n = 44) and V4 (50Mb set,n = 10; Agilent Technologies, Santa Clara, CA, USA) as described previously.[12,52,55] Sequencing reads were mapped to the hg19 reference genome using SOLiD LifeScope V2.1 software (Life technologies, Carlsbad, CA, USA).

Prioritization of variants

Variants were annotated using an in-house annotation pipeline, as described previously.[12,52,55] High-confidence calls (i.e. ≥10 reads, ≥5 variant reads, ≥5 unique starts (available only for substitutions) and ≥28% variant reads) were filtered for non-synonymous variants that were absent in our in-house variant database. This in-house variant database consists of variants identified by exome sequencing in 2,037 individuals from mostly Western European Ancestry (>95%) that were sequenced using SureSelect Human All Exon kit V2 and SOLiD4 sequencers (~64% of exomes), Exon kit V4 and 5500xl sequencers (~25% of exomes), or Exon kit V4 and Illumina HiSeq 2500 sequencers (~11% of exomes). All SOLiD4 and 5500xl exomes were mapped and called with LifeScope V2.1 software and the Illumina exomes were mapped with BWA and called using GATK. All exomes were sequenced at a median coverage of at least 50-fold. Next, we removed all variants present with a MAF of >0.001 in The National Heart, Lung, and Blood Institute Exome Sequencing Project database (6,503 exomes),[11] and genes that were described to be loss-of-function tolerant.[56]

Subsequently, variants that resulted in protein truncations (i.e. putative frameshifts, nonsense mutations and variants at canonical splice-sites), and non-synonymous variants with a PhyloP score ≥3.0 (missense mutations) were selected. The remaining list was analyzed for variants in known CRC predisposing genes and genes that predispose to other types of cancer and/or cause recessive cancer syndromes.[12,13,57]

In the next filter step, all recurrent variants and genes recurrently affected were selected. This list of variants was subsequently filtered based on the occurrence of rare potentially pathogenic variants in a whole-exome sequence data set of 164 anonymous healthy controls (Control dataset 1) that were extracted from a study reported by de Ligt et al.[55] These exomes were sequenced using a SureSelect Human All Exon kit V2 and SOLiD4 sequencers, mapped and called using SOLiD LifeScope V2.1 software, after which a filtering appoach identical to the one described for our CRC discovery cohort was applied. Analysis by a genotype-weighted metric described by Heinrich et al. [58] revealed that the exomes of the CRC patients and those from 'Control dataset 1' were comparable, both in terms of genetic origin and sequencing performance. Significance of differences between the frequencies of variants in our CRC discovery cohort and this dataset of 164 controls were calculated using the χ^2 goodness of fit test and a Benjamini-Hochberg (BH) correction for multiple testing was performed (corrected for 196 genes that harbored recurrent variants or were recurrently affected in our CRC discovery cohort). A P-value of ≤ 0.05 was considered significant before correction. After correction a χ^2 P-value less than the BH critical value was considered significant. None of the genes were significantly enriched in our CRC discovery cohort after correcting for multiple testing. Therefore, we continued with the genes that revealed a χ^2 goodness of fit P-value of ≤ 0.05 before multiple testing. This remaining list of variants was subjected to the following prioritization (Fig 1): (i) genes recurrently affected by protein-truncating variants solely; (ii) potential CRC driver genes [24]; (iii) genes identified in transposon-based CRC susceptibility studies in mice [29,30] and involved in CRC-related KEGG pathways [pathways hsa04310 (WNT signaling), hsa04350 (TGF-beta signaling), hsa03430 (mismatch repair), hsa03410 (base excision repair), hsa03420 (nucleotide excision repair), map03450 (non-homologous end-joining), hsa03460 (Fanconi anemia), and hsa05200 (pathways in cancer)]; and (iv) genes identified through GWAS studies [5–7,32]. Prioritized variants were further analyzed in silico using software packages Align-GVGD, SIFT and Polyphen-2 integrated in the Alamut 2.0 software package (Interactive Biosoftware), and 'HOPE' (http://www.cmbi.ru.nl/hope) was used to assess the structural effects of missense variants at the protein level.[59] All selected variants were validated using Sanger sequencing.

Comparisons to control populations

To investigate whether the variants we identified were truly rare, we analyzed their frequency in the dataset from the Exome Aggregation Consortium [33] and in an independent exome data set from a cohort of individuals of mostly Western-European/Dutch ancestry (Control dataset 2; n = 2,329) from which paired-end exome sequencing data were available with an average >90-fold coverage for our candidate genes (Agilent V4 kit; Illumina HiSeq 2500). This cohort did not contain any cases with a suspected hereditary form of cancer. In addition, we assessed the frequency of potentially pathogenic variants with a MAF ≤ 0.001 in our candidate genes in the latter dataset. Comparisons between the Discovery cohort and 'Control dataset 2' were performed using the Fisher's exact test followed by a Benjamini-Hochberg correction for the three candidate genes and for exome-wide multiple testing. A P-value of ≤ 0.05 was considered significant.

Targeted re-sequencing

A multiplex AmpliSeq panel (Ion AmpliSeq Designer, Life technologies) was designed, targeting all coding exons of EMR3, PTPN12 and LRP6. For library preparation, four DNA samples from the replication cohort were equimolarly pooled and used for amplification. Libaries were barcoded using Ion Xpress Barcode adapters, run on an OneTouch emulsion PCR system (Life Technologies), and sequenced using three Ion 318 chips (Life Technologies). Variant calling and annotation were performed using SeqNext (JSI Medical Systems, Kippenheim, Germany). Variants with a MAF of ≤ 0.001 in the EVS that resulted in protein truncations, splice-site defects, or missense mutations with a PhyloP ≥ 3.0 were selected and validated by Sanger sequencing in the four samples of the subsequent pool. The frequencies of variants in this CRC replication cohort and the 'Control dataset 2' were calculated using the Fisher's exact test, and a Benjamini-Hochberg correction for multiple testing was performed. A P-value of ≤ 0.05 was considered significant.

LRP6 localization and expression analyses

The human image clone IRCMp5012G1125D (Source BioScience, Nothingham, UK) was used to amplify the full-length cDNA of LRP6. This cDNA was subcloned into a cTAP vector in front of an in-frame C-terminal Flag-tag using the Gateway cloning system (Invitrogen, Carlsbad, CA, USA). Mutations were introduced using site-directed mutagenesis, and the open reading frames were confirmed by Sanger sequencing. For localization studies, CHO cells were grown on microscope glass slides and transfected with the wild-type or mutant LRP6 constructs using an X-tremeGENE tranfection reagent (Invitrogen). After 48 hrs, cells were fixed, incubated with a rabbit polyclonal anti-Flag antibody (Sigma Aldrich, St. Louis, USA), embedded in Vectashield with DAPI, and analyzed by fluorescence microscopy. Expression of wild-type or mutant LRP6 was compared by Western blot analyses using a rabbit polyclonal anti-Flag antibody and a goat polyclonal anti-actin antibody (Santa Cruz) and visualized using an Odyssey infrared system (Li-cor Biosciences, NE, USA).

TOPflash reporter assay

CHO cells were transfected in 96-well plates with wild-type or mutant LRP6 constructs together with TOP- or FOPflash reporter constructs (plasmid 12456 and 12457; Addgene, Cambridge, MA, USA) using an X-tremeGENE transfection reagent (Invitrogen).[60] The culture medium was refreshed 24 hrs post-transfection with normal or WNT3a-conditioned medium, and luciferase activity was measured after 16 hrs using a Dual-Glo Luciferase kit (Promega) and an InfiniteM200-Pro plate reader (Tecan). The expression of the reporter was normalized to co-transfected Renilla luciferase. Differences between wild-type or mutant LRP6 were assessed using a student's t-test. A P-value of ≤ 0.05 was considered significant.

SUPPORTING INFORMATION

S1 Table. Clinical characteristics of CRC discovery cohort.

Sample Name	Gender	Age of onset	Familial history for cancer[a]	Polyps	Location	Tumor type[b]	LN[c] Metastasis
P001	Male	23	No FHC	NO	Rectum	Adeno (NS)	NO
P002	Female	24	1B45; 1B/OV63-64; ?GC26; 2B60	NO	Sigmoid	Adeno (M)	YES
P003	Female	28	No FHC	YES	Rectum	Adeno (NS)	NO
P004	Female	28	No FHC	YES	Sigmoid	Adeno (M)	YES
P005	Male	28	No FHC	NO	Rectum	Signetring cell (NS)	YES
P006	Female	28	Unknown	NO	Unknown	Unknown	NO
P007	Female	29	2CRC?	NO	Caecum	Squamous cell (NS)	NO
P008	Female	29	No FHC	YES	Unknown	Unknown	NO
P009	Female	29	Unknown	NO	Rectum	Adeno (NS)	YES
P010	Female	30	2CRC80	NO	Caecum	Adeno (NS)	YES
P011	Male	31	No FHC	NO	Rectosigmoid	Adeno (M)	YES
P012	Male	31	No FHC	NO	Rectum	Adeno (NS)	NO
P013	Female	32	2CRC71/72; 2CRC?	NO	Rectum	Intramucosal (NS)	NO
P014	Male	32	No FHC	YES	Unknown	Unknown	NO
P015	Female	33	1OV39; 2CRC56; 2CRC80	NO	Rectosigmoid	Adeno (M)	NO
P016	Female	33	No FHC	YES	Rectum	Adeno (M/W)	YES
P017	Male	33	No FHC	NO	Rectum	Adeno (NS)	YES
P018	Male	33	No FHC	NO	Sigmoid	Adeno (M)	NO
P019	Male	33	Unknown	NO	Rectum	Adeno (NS)	NO
P020	Male	34	1CRC60; 2CRC70	NO	Rectum	Adeno (M)	NO
P021	Male	34	No FHC	NO	Appendix	Adeno (NS)	YES
P022	Male	34	No FHC	NO	Caecum/ Ascending	Adeno (M/W)	NO
P023	Female	34	No FHC	NO	Rectum	Adeno (P)	YES
P024	Female	34	No FHC	NO	Rectum	Adeno (M)	YES
P025	Female	34	Unknown	NO	Rectum	Adeno (NS)	NO
P026	Female	35	1CRC76	NO	Sigmoid	Adeno (M)	NO
P027	Female	35	No FHC	NO	Rectum	Adeno (M)	NO

P028	Female	36	?B35	NO	Ascending	Unknown	NO
Supplementary Table S1 continued							
P029	Female	36	1CRC71	NO	Descending	Adeno (NS)	NO
P030	Female	36	2CRC60	NO	Sigmoid	Adeno (M)	YES
P031	Female	36	2CRC74;2CRC70	NO	Rectum	Adeno (NS)	NO
P032	Female	36	3CRC45;3CRC50	NO	Rectum	Adeno (NS)	NO
P033	Male	36	No FHC	YES	Rectum	Adeno (W)	NO
P034	Male	37	1CRC63; 1CRC67	NO	Sigmoid	Adeno (M)	NO
P035	Male	37	2CRC81; 2CRC75	NO	Sigmoid	Adeno (NS)	YES
P036	Female	37	No FHC	NO	Descending	Adeno (NS)	NO
P037	Female	37	No FHC	NO	Descending/ Sigmoid	Adeno (NS)	NO
P038	Female	37	No FHC	NO	Rectum	Adeno (NS)	NO
P039	Female	37	No FHC	NO	Sigmoid	Adeno (W)	NO
P040	Male	37	No FHC	NO	Sigmoid	Adeno (NS)	NO
P041	Male	37	No FHC	NO	Sigmoid	Adeno (W)	NO
P042	Female	37	No FHC	NO	Unknown	Unknown	NO
P043	Female	38	1CRC70;2CRC80	NO	Rectosigmoid	Adeno (NS)	NO
P044	Male	38	2CRC80	YES	Sigmoid	Adeno (M)	YES
P045	Male	38	2EC79	NO	Rectum	Adeno (M)	YES
P046	Female	39	1SC30; 1SC>50	NO	Ascending	Adeno (W)	YES
P047	Male	39	2CRC?	NO	Rectum	Adeno (NS)	NO
P048	Female	39	2CRC59	NO	Unknown	Adeno (NS)	NO
P049	Female	39	3CRC42	NO	Rectosigmoid	Adeno (NS)	NO
P050	Male	39	?CRC53	NO	Sigmoid	Adeno (P)	YES
P051	Male	39	No FHC	NO	Transverse	Adeno (P)	YES
P052	Male	39	No FHC	NO	Unknown	Unknown	NO
P053	Female	40	1CRC79; 2CRC52; 2CRC/OV64	NO	Transverse	Adeno (M)	NO
P054	Male	43	No FHC	YES	Rectum	Adeno (M/W)	NO
P055	Male	45	1CRC60; 3CRC30	NO	Ascending	Adeno (M)	YES

S2 Table. Exome performance of CRC discovery cohort.

Sample	Enrichment	Total bases (Gb)	Total bases on/near target (Gb)	Average Coverage of targets	Median Coverage	% regions >= 10x	% regions >= 20x	Variants called
P001	V4-50Mb	6.33	4.74	75.14	55.00	92.02	82.85	49929
P002	V4-50Mb	4.36	3.50	56.97	45.00	91.22	80.68	48581
P003	V4-50Mb	4.39	3.62	58.41	45.00	91.08	79.96	49019
P004	V2-50Mb	7.28	5.72	97.59	75.00	87.08	81.83	43114
P005	V2-50Mb	7.94	5.92	99.60	75.50	86.80	81.13	43786
P006	V2-50Mb	5.84	4.89	85.07	68.00	86.11	80.49	43601
P007	V2-50Mb	6.79	4.00	67.51	52.00	83.37	75.44	39883
P008	V2-50Mb	8.72	5.36	87.13	68.00	84.89	78.93	37792
P009	V2-50Mb	6.47	3.85	65.37	51.00	82.57	74.55	38656
P010	V2-50Mb	5.18	4.37	75.85	60.50	85.00	78.58	45053
P011	V2-50Mb	6.66	5.37	92.20	70.50	88.54	83.44	40992
P012	V2-50Mb	6.26	5.21	89.21	71.00	86.55	80.94	44788
P013	V2-50Mb	6.12	3.35	56.43	42.50	80.71	71.48	29040
P014	V2-50Mb	6.54	5.18	83.75	65.00	85.79	79.68	44146
P015	V2-50Mb	5.87	4.55	77.65	60.00	83.39	76.65	41954
P016	V2-50Mb	5.01	3.93	63.22	48.00	83.43	75.25	40174
P017	V2-50Mb	6.90	4.06	69.18	54.00	84.58	76.85	39804
P018	V2-50Mb	5.91	3.29	54.93	43.00	81.94	72.68	38176
P019	V2-50Mb	6.62	5.54	95.66	77.00	86.51	81.13	44406
P020	V2-50Mb	5.32	3.30	57.15	44.00	83.96	74.91	38551
P021	V2-50Mb	7.06	4.24	70.27	53.00	84.91	77.66	40331
P022	V2-50Mb	6.59	5.12	87.23	67.00	85.18	79.00	42542
P023	V4-50Mb	5.79	4.52	76.15	60.00	92.89	85.59	47370
P024	V2-50Mb	4.37	3.52	56.12	44.00	83.06	74.98	43396
P025	V2-50Mb	9.49	6.00	101.65	77.00	87.63	82.61	39429
P026	V2-50Mb	N/A	4.46	74.74	57.50	85.02	78.49	38803
P027	V2-50Mb	6.25	4.85	81.59	61.00	83.77	76.98	42404
P028	V4-50Mb	4.60	3.76	60.80	48.00	92.05	82.15	49423
P029	V2-50Mb	4.34	3.40	57.79	45.00	82.50	74.34	39716
P030	V2-50Mb	6.85	5.78	101.89	82.00	87.99	83.28	44805
P031	V4-50Mb	5.25	4.25	69.45	54.00	92.47	84.04	49502
P032	V4-50Mb	6.24	5.06	81.03	63.00	93.99	87.15	49800
Supplementary Table S2 continued								

P033	V1-30Mb	N/A	2,78	46.68	48.50	73.47	65.36	36324
P034	V2-50Mb	6.20	4.57	76.86	59.50	83.28	76.65	41507
P035	V2-50Mb	6.98	5.74	98.44	78.00	87.47	82.36	45328
P036	V2-50Mb	6.66	5.48	93.47	74.00	87.16	82.02	45973
P037	V2-50Mb	8.86	6.76	114.35	87.00	86.94	81.87	43724
P038	V2-50Mb	8.53	7.16	127.29	102.0	89.46	85.59	45725
P039	V2-50Mb	6.90	5.37	91.72	72.00	86.39	80.92	42867
P040	V2-50Mb	6.29	5.14	84.90	67.00	87.11	81.51	46267
P041	V2-50Mb	7.18	6.03	105.27	84.00	87.58	82.60	45089
P042	V2-50Mb	5.37	4.15	70.45	54.50	83.28	76.03	40257
P043	V2-50Mb	6.15	4.94	78.50	62.00	85.73	79.92	44700
P044	V2-50Mb	6.39	5.07	85.36	64.00	85.44	79.14	41855
P045	V2-50Mb	6.13	4.73	81.03	62.00	83.48	76.65	41743
P046	V2-50Mb	5.48	4.23	74.32	57.00	84.70	77.65	41289
P047	V4-50Mb	4.66	3.70	57.02	41.00	89.08	75.98	47408
P048	V2-50Mb	5.72	4.45	70.99	56.00	84.85	78.39	45070
P049	V2-50Mb	6.71	5.40	86.62	68.00	86.89	81.73	45210
P050	V2-50Mb	4.01	3.25	53.35	42.00	83.37	74.55	43623
P051	V2-50Mb	4.38	3.26	53.54	42.00	80.43	71.11	40509
P052	V2-50Mb	5.78	4.14	67.90	53.00	82.14	75.06	41337
P053	V4-50Mb	3.83	3.03	47.44	35.00	87.42	72.12	46226
P054	V2-50Mb	5.92	4.19	66.33	51.00	83.39	76.05	41973
P055	V4-50Mb	4.29	3.46	56.71	44.00	90.56	79.20	48893

ACKNOWLEDGMENTS

The authors thank all individuals included in this study for their cooperation, Eveline Kamping, Nienke Wieskamp and Maartje van de Vorst for expert technical and bioinformatic assistance.

Author Contributions

Conceived and designed the experiments: RMdV MMH AGvK NH MJLL RPK. Performed the experiments: RMdV MMH RDAW ARM JZ CG HV LV NS MT RD. Analyzed the data: RMdV MMH RDAW CG MJLL RPK. Contributed reagents/materials/analysis tools: NH WAvZS LS CMK HKS. Wrote the paper: RMdV MMH RPK.

REFERENCES

1. Lynch HT, de la Chapelle A. (2003) Hereditary colorectal cancer. N Engl J Med 348:919–932. pmid:12621137 doi: 10. 1056/nejmra012242
2. De la Chapelle A. (2004) Genetic predisposition to colorectal cancer. Nat Rev Cancer 4:769–780. pmid:15510158 doi: 10. 1038/nrc1453
3. Weren RD, Ligtenberg MJ, Kets CM, de Voer RM, Verwiel ET, et al. (2015) A germline homozygous mutation in the base-excision repair gene NTHL1 causes adenomatous polyposis and colorectal cancer. Nat Genet. 47:668–671. doi: 10. 1038/ng. 3287. pmid:25938944
4. Palles C, Cazier JB, Howarth KM, Domingo E, Jones AM, et al. (2013) Germline mutations affecting the proofreading domains of POLE and POLD1 predispose to colorectal adenomas and carcinomas. Nat Genet 45:136–144. doi: 10. 1038/ng. 2503. pmid:23263490
5. Dunlop MG, Dobbins SE, Farrington SM, Jones AM, Palles C, et al. (2012) Common variation near CDKN1A, POLD3 and SHROOM2 influences colorectal cancer risk. Nat Genet 44:770–776. doi: 10. 1038/ng. 2293. pmid:22634755
6. Zhang B, Jia WH, Matsuda K, Kweon SS, Matsuo K, et al. (2014) Large-scale genetic study in East Asians identifies six new loci associated with colorectal cancer risk. Nat Genet 6:533–542. doi: 10. 1038/ng. 2985
7. Theodoratou E, Montazeri Z, Hawken S, Allum GC, Gong J, et al. (2012) Systematic meta-analyses and

field synopsis of genetic association studies in colorectal cancer. J Natl Cancer Inst 104:1433–1457. doi: 10. 1093/jnci/djs369. pmid:23019048

8. Manolio TA, Collins FS, Cox NJ, Goldstein DB, Hindorff LA, et al. (2009) Finding the missing heritability of complex diseases. Nature 461:747–753. doi: 10. 1038/ nature08494. pmid:19812666

9. Gryfe R, Kim H, Hsieh ET, Aronson MD, Holowaty EJ, et al. (2000) Tumor microsatellite instability and clinical outcome in young patients with colorectal cancer. N Engl J Med 342:69–77. pmid:10631274 doi: 10. 1056/ nejm200001133420201

10. Chang DT, Pai RK, Rybicki LA, Dimaio MA, Limaye M, et al. (2012) Clinicopathologic and molecular features of sporadic early-onset colorectal adenocarcinoma: an adenocarcinoma with frequent signet ring cell differentiation, rectal and sigmoid involvement, and adverse morphologic features. Mod Pathol 25:1128–1139. doi: 10. 1038/modpathol. 2012. 61. pmid:22481281

11. Exome Variant Server. NHLBI GO Exome Sequencing Project (ESP), Seattle, WA. 2014. Available at: http:// evs. gs. washington. edu/EVS.

12. Neveling K, Feenstra I, Gilissen C, Hoefsloot LH, Kamsteeg EJ, Mensenkamp AR, et al. (2013) A post-hoc comparison of the utility of sanger sequencing and exome sequencing for the diagnosis of heterogeneous diseases. Hum Mutat 34:1721–1726. doi: 10. 1002/ humu. 22450. pmid:24123792

13. Rahman N. (2014) Realizing the promise of cancer predisposition genes. Nature 505:302–308. doi: 10. 1038/nature12981. pmid:24429628

14. Gruber SB, Ellis NA, Scott KK, Almog R, Kolachana P, et al. (2002) BLM heterozygosity and the risk of colorectal cancer. Science 297:2013. pmid:12242432 doi: 10. 1126/science. 1074399

15. Cleary SP, Zhang W, Di Nicola N, Aronson M, Aube J, et al. (2003) Heterozygosity for the BLMAsh mutation and cancer risk. Cancer Res 63:1769–1771. pmid:12702560

16. Baris HN, Kedar I, Halpern GJ, Shohat T, Magal N, et al. (2007) Prevalence of breast and colorectal cancer in Ashkenazi Jewish carriers of Fanconi anemia and Bloom syndrome. Isr Med Assoc J 9:847–850. pmid:18210922

17. de Voer RM, Hahn MM, Mensenkamp AR, Hoischen A, Gilissen C, et al (2015) Deleterious Germline BLM Mutations and the Risk for Early-onset Colorectal Cancer. Sci Rep. 5:14060. doi: 10. 1038/srep14060. pmid:26358404

18. Helgason H, Rafnar T, Olafsdottir HS, Jonasson JG, Sigurdsson A, et al. (2015) Loss-of-function variants in ATM confer risk of gastric cancer. Nat Genet. 47:906–910. doi: 10. 1038/ng. 3342. pmid:26098866

19. Paglia LL, Lauge A, Weber J, Champ J, Cavaciuti E, et al. ATM germline mutations in women with familial breast cancer and a relative with haematological malignancy. Breast Cancer Res Treat 2010;119:443–452. doi: 10. 1007/s10549-009-0396-z. pmid:19404735

20. Roberts NJ, Jiao Y, Yu J, et al. (2012) ATM mutations in patients with hereditary pancreatic cancer. Cancer Discov 2:41–46. doi: 10. 1158/2159-8290. CD-11-0194. pmid:22585167

21. Matmati M, Pouwels W, van Bruggen R, Jansen M, Hoek RM et al. (2007) The human EGF-TM7 receptor EMR3 is a marker for mature granulocytes. J Leukoc Biol. 81:440–448. pmid:17108056 doi: 10. 1189/jlb. 0406276

22. The Human Protein Atlas. Available at: http://www. proteinatlas. org

23. Kane AJ, Sughrue ME, Rutkowski MJ, Phillips JJ, Parsa AT. (2010) EMR-3: a potential mediator of invasive phenotypic variation in glioblastoma and novel therapeutic target. Neuroreport 21:1018–1022. doi: 10. 1097/WNR. 0b013e32833f19f2. pmid:20827226

24. The Cancer Genome Atlas Network. (2012) Comprehensive molecular characterization of human colon and rectal cancer. Nature 487:330–337. doi: 10. 1038/nature11252. pmid:22810696

25. Sun T, Aceto N, Meerbrey KL, Kessler JD, Zhou C, et al. (2011) Activation of multiple proto-oncogenic tyrosine kinases in breast cancer via loss of the PTPN12 phosphatase. Cell 144:703–718. doi: 10. 1016/j. cell. 2011. 02. 003. pmid:21376233

26. Espejo R, Jeng Y, Paulucci-Holthauzen A, Rengifo-Cam W, Honkus K, et al. (2014) PTP-PEST targets a novel tyrosine site in p120 catenin to control epithelial cell motility and Rho GTPase activity. J Cell Sci 127:497–508. doi: 10. 1242/jcs. 120154. pmid:24284071

27. Espejo R, Rengifo-Cam W, Schaller MD, Evers BM, Sastry SK. (2010) PTP-PEST controls motility, adherens junction assembly, and Rho GTPase activity in colon cancer cells. Am J Physiol Cell Physiol 299:C454–C463. doi: 10. 1152/ajpcell. 00148. 2010. pmid:20519451

28. Streit S, Ruhe JE, Knyazev P, Knyazeva T, Iacobelli S, et al. (2006) PTP-PEST phosphatase variations in human cancer. Cancer Genet Cytogenet 170:48–53. pmid:16965954 doi: 10. 1016/j. cancergencyto. 2006. 05. 013

29. Starr TK, Allaei R, Silverstein KA, Staggs RA, Sarver AL, et al. (2009) A transposon-based genetic screen in mice identifies genes altered in colorectal cancer. Science 323:1747–1750. doi: 10. 1126/science. 1163040. pmid:19251594

30. March HN, Rust AG, Wright NA, ten Hoeve J, de Ridder J, et al. (2011) Insertional mutagenesis identifies multiple networks of cooperating genes driving intestinal tumorigenesis. Nat Genet 43:1202–1209. doi: 10. 1038/ ng. 990. pmid:22057237

31. Cheng Z, Biechele T, Wei Z, Morrone S, Moon RT, et al. (2011) Crystal structures of the extracellular domain of LRP6 and its complex with DKK1. Nat Struct Mol Biol 18:1204–1210. doi: 10. 1038/nsmb. 2139. pmid:21984209

32. Welter D, MacArthur J, Morales J, Burdett T, Hall P, et al. (2014) The NHGRI GWAS Catalog, a curated resource of SNP-trait associations. Nucleic Acids Res. 42: D1001–1006. doi: 10. 1093/nar/gkt1229. pmid:24316577

33. Exome Aggregation Consortium (ExAC), Cambridge, MA. 2014. Available at:http://exac. broadinstitute. org.

34. Marth GT, Yu F, Indap AR, Garimella K, Gravel S, et al. (2011) The functional spectrum of low-frequency coding variation. Genome Biol 12:R84. doi: 10. 1186/gb-2011-12-9-r84. pmid:21917140

35. Keinan A, Clark AG. (2012) Recent explosive human population growth has resulted in an excess of rare genetic variants. Science 336:740–743. doi: 10. 1126/science. 1217283. pmid:22582263

36. Tennessen JA, Bigham AW, O'Connor TD, Fu W, Kenny EE, et al. (2012) Evolution and functional impact of rare coding variation from deep sequencing of human exomes. Science 337:64–69. doi: 10. 1126/science. 1219240. pmid:22604720

37. The 1000 Genomes Project Consortium. (2012) An integrated map of genetic variation from 1,092 human genomes. Nature 491:56–65. doi: 10. 1038/nature11632. pmid:23128226

38. MacArthur DG, Manolio TA, Dimmock DP, Rehm HL, Shendure J, et al. (2014) Guidelines for investigating causality of sequence variants in human disease. Nature. 508:469–76. doi: 10. 1038/nature13127. pmid:24759409

39. Mathew S, George SP, Wang Y, Siddiqui MR, Srinivasan K, et al. (2008) Potential molecular mechanism for c-Src kinase-mediated regulation of intestinal cell migration. J Biol Chem 283:22709–22722. doi: 10. 1074/jbc. M801319200. pmid:18482983

40. Taieb D, Roignot J, Andre F, Garcia S, Masson B, et al. (2008) ArgBP2-dependent signaling regulates pancreatic cell migration, adhesion, and tumorigenicity. Cancer Res 68:4588–4596. doi: 10. 1158/0008-5472. CAN-08-0958. pmid:18559503

41. Zheng Y, Xia Y, Hawke D, Halle M, Tremblay ML, et al. (2009) FAK phosphorylation by ERK primes ras-induced tyrosine dephosphorylation of FAK mediated by PIN1 and PTP-PEST. Mol Cell 35:11–25. doi: 10. 1016/j. molcel. 2009. 06. 013. pmid:19595712

42. Clevers H, Nusse R. (2012) Wnt/β-catenin signaling and disease. Cell 149: 1192–11205. doi: 10. 1016/j. cell. 2012. 05. 012. pmid:22682243

43. Mao B, Wu W, Li Y, Hoppe D, Stannek P, et al. (2001) LDL-receptor-related protein 6 is a receptor for Dickkopf proteins. Nature 411:321–325. pmid:11357136 doi: 10. 1038/35077108

44. Massink MP, Créton MA, Spanevello F, Fennis WM, Cune MS et al. (2015) Loss-of-Function Mutations in the WNT Co-receptor LRP6 Cause Autosomal-Dominant Oligodontia. Am J Hum Genet. 97:621–6. doi: 10. 1016/j. ajhg. 2015. 08. 014. pmid:26387593

45. DeRycke MS, Gunawardena SR, Middha S, Asmann YW, Schaid DJ, et al. (2013) Identification of novel variants in colorectal cancer families by high-throughput exome sequencing. Cancer Epidemiol Biomarkers Prev 22:1239–1251. doi: 10. 1158/1055-9965. EPI-12-1226. pmid:23637064

46. Gylfe AE, Katainen R, Kondelin J, Tanskanen T, Cajuso T, et al, (2013) Eleven candidate susceptibility genes for common familial colorectal cancer. PLoS Genet 9: e1003876. doi: 10. 1371/journal. pgen. 1003876. pmid:24146633

47. Smith CG, Naven M, Harris R, Colley J, West H, et al. (2013) Exome resequencing identifies potential tumor-suppressor genes that predispose to colorectal cancer. Hum Mutat 34:1026–1034. doi: 10. 1002/humu. 22333. pmid:23585368

48. Esteban-Jurado C, Vila-Casadesús M, Garre P, Lozano JJ, Pristoupilova A, et al. (2015) Whole-exome sequencing identifies rare pathogenic variants in new predisposition genes for familial colorectal cancer. Genet Med. 17:131–42. doi: 10. 1038/gim. 2014. 89. pmid:25058500

49. Schulz E, Klampfl P, Holzapfel S, Janecke AR, Ulz P, et al. (2014) Germline variants in the SEMA4A gene predispose to familial colorectal cancer type X. Nat Commun. 5:5191. doi: 10. 1038/ncomms6191. pmid:25307848

50. Tanskanen T, Gylfe AE, Katainen R, Taipale M, Renkonen-Sinisalo L, et al. (2015) Systematic search for rare variants in Finnish early-onset colorectal cancer patients. Cancer Genet. 208:35–40. doi: 10. 1016/j. cancergen. 2014. 12. 004. pmid:25749350

51. Zhang JX, Fu L, de Voer RM, Hahn MM, Jin P, et al. (2015) Candidate colorectal cancer predisposing gene variants in Chinese early-onset and familial cases. World J Gastroenterol. 21:4136–4149. doi: 10. 3748/wjg. v21. i14. 4136. pmid:25892863

52. De Voer RM, Geurts van Kessel A, Weren RD, Ligtenberg MJ, Smeets D, et al. (2013) Germline mutations in the spindle assembly checkpoint genes BUB1 and BUB3 are risk factors for colorectal cancer. Gastroenterology 145: 544–547. doi: 10. 1053/j. gastro. 2013. 06. 001. pmid:23747338

53. Vissers LE1, de Ligt J, Gilissen C, Janssen I, Steehouwer M, et al. (2010) A de novo paradigm for mental retardation. Nat Genet. 42:1109–1112. doi: 10. 1038/ng. 712. pmid:21076407

54. Fletcher O, Houlston RS. (2010) Architecture of inherited susceptibility to common cancer. Nat Rev Cancer 10:353–361. doi: 10. 1038/nrc2840. pmid:20414203

55. De Ligt J, Willemsen MH, van Bon BW, Kleefstra T, Yntema HG, et al. (2012) Diagnostic exome sequencing in persons with severe intellectual disability. N Engl J Med 20:1921–1929. doi: 10. 1056/nejmoa1206524

56. MacArthur DG, Balasubramanian S, Frankish A, Huang N, Morris J, et al. (2012) A systematic survey of loss-of-function variants in human protein-coding genes. Science 335:823–828. doi: 10. 1126/science. 1215040. pmid:22344438

57. Vogelstein B, Papadopoulos N, Velculescu VE, Zhou S, Diaz LA, et al. (2013) Cancer genome landscapes. Science 339:1546–1558. doi: 10. 1126/science. 1235122. pmid:23539594

58. Heinrich V, Kamphans T, Stange J, Parkhomchuk D, Hecht J, et al. (2013) Estimating exome genotyping accuracy by comparing to data from large scale sequencing projects. Genome Med. 5:69. doi: 10. 1186/

gm473. pmid:23902830

59. Venselaar H1, Te Beek TA, Kuipers RK, Hekkelman ML, Vriend G. (2010) Protein structure analysis of mutations causing inheritable diseases. An e-Science approach with life scientist friendly interfaces. BMC Bioinformatics. 11:548. doi: 10. 1186/1471-2105-11-548. pmid:21059217

60. Veeman MT, Slusarski DC, Kaykas A, Louie SH, Moon RT. (2003) Zebrafish prickle, a modulator of noncanonical Wnt/Fz signaling, regulates gastrulation movements. Curr Biol. 13:680–685. pmid:12699626 doi: 10.1016/s0960-9822(03)00240-9

CHAPTER 19

MUTATIONS IN MAB21L2 RESULT IN OCULAR COLOBOMA, MICROCORNEA AND CATARACTS

Brett Deml, Ariana Kariminejad, Razieh H. R. Borujerdi, Sanaa Muheisen, Linda M. Reis, Elena V. Semina

INTRODUCTION

Coloboma is a congenital segmental ocular defect which can affect one or more structures of the eye; typical coloboma results in an inferior deficiency of iris, chorioretinal, and/or optic nerve tissue [1–3]. Ocular coloboma is believed to result from failure of normal closure of the optic fissure during embryonic eye development, Oermed optic fissure closure defect (OFCD) [1,2]. Coloboma can occur as an isolated anomaly (simple coloboma) but in most cases it is associated with additional ocular defects, including microphthalmia, cataract, retinal detachment, and ocular motility disorders [1–4]. Microcornea, a reduction in the diameter of the cornea, is common in colobomatous eyes and can be associated with normal or even increased (macrophthalmic) axial length [2,3,5]. Additional systemic anomalies are present in a large proportion of patients with OFCDs including brain, skeletal, cardiac, or urogenital anomalies [3,4].

A number of genes have been associated with coloboma including transcriptional regulatorsSOX2, OTX2, PAX2, PAX6, CHD7 and SALL2; secreted signaling factor-encoding gene SHH; members of the transforming growth factor-beta (TGF-beta) superfamily GDF6 and GDF3;members of the retinoic acid synthesis pathway STRA6 and ALDH1A3; as well as membrane porphyrin transporter ABCB6, and a member of the HIPPO growth control pathway, YAP1[6–19].

Citation: Deml B, Kariminejad A, Borujerdi RHR, Muheisen S, Reis LM, Semina EV (2015) Mutations in MAB21L2 Result in Ocular Coloboma, Microcornea and Cataracts. PLoS Genet 11(2): e1005002. doi:10.1371/journal.pgen.1005002

Due to the number of genes involved and the large proportion of unexplained cases, whole exome sequencing has been used with increasing frequency to screen families with coloboma and other ocular conditions [16–21]. Since whole exome sequencing generates a large number of variants and often involves genes with unexplored/unknown function, studies in animal models can be invaluable in providing further insight into the functional roles of candidate genes/variants and their possible involvement in the studied phenotype [17,22]. Recent advances in genomic editing technologies using engineered nucleases empowered researchers with tools for the functional exploration of these genes/variants of interest [23].

In this manuscript we present evidence for the role of MAB21L2 in human coloboma and further investigate its role in vertebrate ocular development by generation and analysis of zebrafish mab21l2 mutants.

RESULTS

Identification of a MAB21L2 mutation in a human pedigree affected with ocular disease

The proband (Patient 1) was diagnosed with bilateral microcornea, iris and chorioretinal coloboma, corectopia, nystagmus and cataract (Fig. 1); the cataractous lens of his right eye was removed at age 24. Based on ultrasound measurements at age 32, the axial length was 29.02 mm (right eye) and 24.67 mm (left eye), thus showing no signs of microphthalmia (normal axial length for adult males is approximately 23 mm) [24]. Evaluation of other systems identified mild contracture in the knees and elbows and rhizomelia of the upper and lower limbs: the lengths of the femur (40.3 cm, left and 40.6 cm, right), tibia (34.5cm, left and 34.3 cm, right), humerus (26 cm, left and 26.3 cm, right), ulna (23.5 cm, left and 23.4 cm, right) and radius (22.2 cm, left and 22.6 cm, right) were determined by scanography and the observed femur/tibia (1.18) and humerus/radius (1.17) ratios were found to deviate from the normal reference numbers of 1.23 and 1.31, respectively. No signs of cardiac, brain or other abnormalities were identified. Analysis of family history identified a similarly affected sister, brother, and two nephews, while his father, mother, and two additional sisters were unaffected (Fig. 2A).

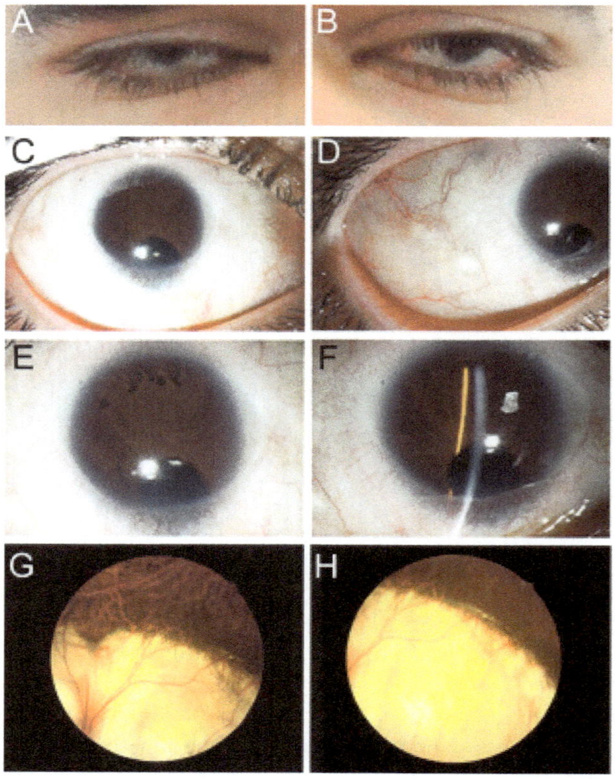

Figure 1. Ocular Images of Patient 1. Photographs of the right (A, C, E, G) and the left (B, D, F, H) eyes showing bilateral iris coloboma with microcornea and corectopia (C-F) as well as chorioretinal coloboma (G, H) in the proband (Patient 1).

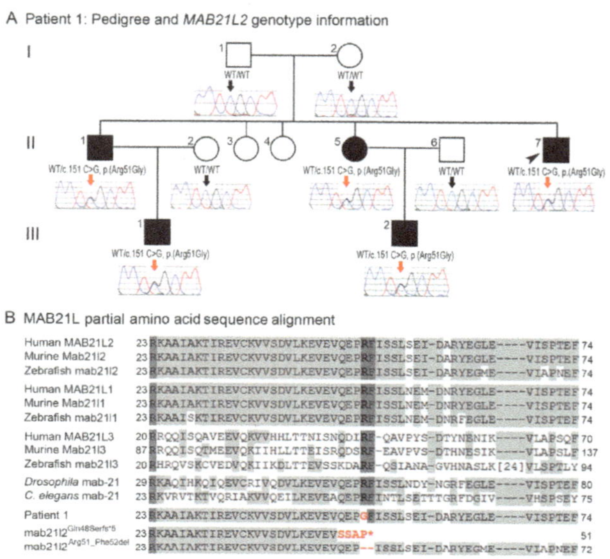

Figure 2. MAB21L2 **mutations and protein sequence conservation.**

A. Three-generation pedigree of Patient 1 with MAB21L2 genotype information. DNA chromatograms for all tested family members are shown with c.151C position indicated with black (WT allele) or red (heterozygous mutant allele) arrows. The proband (Patient 1) is indicated with a black arrowhead. Please note the presence of the mutant allele in all affected individuals, its absence in unaffected family members, and the presence of a low 'G' peak in addition to the normal 'C' nucleotide at the mutant position in the proband's unaffected mother. **B.** Amino acid alignment of the MAB21L1-3 and mab-21 regions surrounding the arginine at position 51; amino acids identical between different homologs are highlighted with a light grey color, three invariant residues are shown in dark grey; the glycine (G) predicted to replace arginine 51 in Patient 1 is shown in red font; the positions and predicted effects of the zebrafish mab21l2 mutations involving the same region are also shown in red font. Accession numbers for sequences utilized in the alignment are provided in Methods.

Independent whole exome sequencing of DNA samples from the proband's two affected nephews (III-1 and III-2, Fig. 2A) yielded a mean coverage of 63.9X ± 4.0 for the two samples with 96.25% ± 0.49 of bases having >10X coverage. Initial analysis of the whole exome data excluded mutations in 72 known factors involved in anophthalmia, microphthalmia, and/or coloboma [25]. Comparison of whole exome data of the two nephews identified 16 shared heterozygous variants that were novel or rare (<1%): one splicing, one frameshift indel, one inframe indel, and 13 missense alleles (three novel and ten rare) that were found to be damaging by at least 4 functional effect prediction programs (S1 Table). The five novel alleles and one rare frameshift variant were tested for cosegregation in the pedigree; only the heterozygous MAB21L2 missense mutation c.151 C>G, p.(Arg51Gly), was present in all five affected individuals (II-1, -5, -7 and III-1, -2) and absent in the unaffected parents (a low 'G' peak at position c.151 was seen in the mother's sample (I-2) in addition to the wild-type 'C' on sequencing of two independent PCR reactions, suggesting that she is likely to have low-level mosaicism for this mutation) (Fig. 2A). The MAB21L2 variant was further identified as a strong candidate based on its absence in all control populations (EVS, dbSNP, and 1000 genomes) and having the highest Genomic Evolutionary Rate Profiling (GERP++) score, as well as enrichment of both human MAB21L2 and mouse Mab21l2 transcripts in ocular structures based in BioGPS (http://biogps.org). The mutation was predicted to be damaging by SIFT, Polyphen2, Mutation Taster and MutationAssessor, and demonstrated high conservation scores for the affected nucleotide with a GERP++ score of 6.16 and a PhyloP score of 2.94 (of note, the highest possible GERP++ score is 6.17 (most conserved) [26]).

The MAB21L2 gene, located at 4q31.3, encodes a 359-a.a. protein similar to C. elegans mab-21 cell fate-determining factor [27], with the mab-21 domain predicted to span amino acids 62–346 (based on Pfam (Protein FAMilies database) [28]. Alignment of MAB21L amino acid sequences from different species revealed that the arginine residue at position 51 is conserved in all MAB21L human, mouse and zebrafish proteins as well as fruit fly and C. elegans mab-21 (Fig. 2B). The function and domain structure of MAB21L proteins are largely unknown; the most similar protein with a known structure is human MB21D1 (Mab-21 domain containing 1, also known as cyclic GMP-AMP synthase (cGAS)), a protein involved in innate immunity and binding to cytosolic double stranded DNA to activate interferon production [29]. The domain structure of MB21D1 includes a mab-21 domain and two DNA-binding domains, one located N-terminally to the mab-21 domain (with a three-residue overlap) and the other situated within the C-terminal portion of the mab-21 domain [29,30]. If MAB21L2 structure is similar to MB21D1, then the arginine at position 51 of MAB21L2 would be located in proximity to the predicted mab-21 domain and within the N-terminal DNA-binding domain; this is consistent with the fact that arginine represents the most basic amino acid and is often observed at protein-nucleic acid interaction sites.

Analysis of additional human patients affected with ocular disease

To further explore the role of MAB21L2 in human coloboma phenotypes, we examined 276 patients with developmental ocular conditions from our collection as well as whole exome data from 125 cases derived from the UK10K_Rare_Coloboma (EGA Study ID: EGAS00001000127) project of the UK10K Consortium study [18,31]. We identified no additional mutations in our population that included 39 patients affected with A/M and coloboma, 16 patients with coloboma and normal eye size, 104 patients with A/M without coloboma, 50 with aniridia, 37 with various anterior segment dysgenesis conditions, 12 with cataract, and 18 with other developmental ocular conditions. Analysis of the UK10K_Rare_Coloboma cohort identified a heterozygous mutation affecting the same arginine residue described above (Fig. 2B), c.152 G>A, p.(Arg51His), in two samples: UK10K_COL5001067 (the c.152 G>A change was present in 10 out of 23 high quality reads) and UK10K_COL5001068 (the c.152 G>A change was seen in 21 out of 32 high quality reads). While the publicly available UK10K data does not specify family relationships, the presence of identical mutations in consecutively numbered samples suggests that these individuals may be family members. Similar to the c.151 C>G, p.(Arg51Gly) allele, this mutation was not reported in the Exome Variant Server (0/13,006 alleles), the 1000 Genomes Browser (0/2,194 alleles), or dbSNP, and is predicted to be damaging by SIFT, Polyphen2, Mutation Taster and Mutation Assessor. These data indicate a small contribution of MAB21L2 mutations to human coloboma phenotypes (<2%) and suggest no role for MAB21L2 mutations in the other ocular disorders that were examined in this study.

Zebrafish mab21l2 expression studies

To investigate the role of MAB21L2/mab21l2 in ocular development, we performed careful evaluation of mab21l2 expression in zebrafish using in situ hybridization. At 18-hpf, expression was seen in the presumptive eye field and midbrain (Fig. 3A, B). At 24-hpf, mab21l2expression was seen in the retina (ventral and dorsal periphery), lens, spinal cord, midbrain and pharyngeal arch region (Fig. 3C, D, I). In 48–72-hpf, the transcripts could be detected in the ciliary marginal zone (CMZ) (or germinal zone) of the retina that contains multipotent retinal progenitors, in the inner nuclear and ganglion cell layers of the retina, and around the optic fissure in the eye, as well as the midbrain, hindbrain, developing fins, and branchial arches (Fig. 3E-H, J, K).

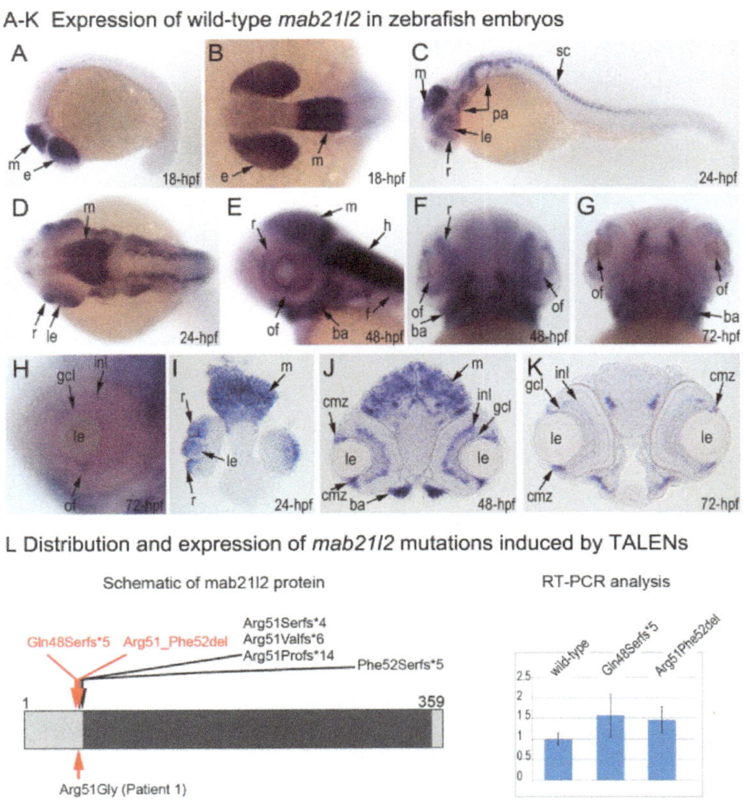

Figure 3. Expression and mutations of zebrafish mab21l2. **A-K.** Expression pattern of mab21l2 in zebrafish 18–72-hpf embryos. Whole mount images (A-H) and sections (I-K) are shown. **A, B.** At 18-hpf, expression in the presumptive eye field (e) and midbrain

(m) is observed. **C, D, I.** At 24-hpf, mab21l2expression is seen in the periphery of the retina (r), lens (le), spinal cord (sc), midbrain (m) and pharyngeal arch region (pa). **E-H, J, K.** At 48–72-hpf, expression in the ciliary marginal zone (cmz), inner nuclear layer (inl) and ganglion cell layer (gcl) of the retina, and the region of the optic fissure (of) in the eye as well as the midbrain (m), hindbrain (h), developing fins (f), and branchial arches (ba) is shown with arrows. **L.** Distribution and expression of mab21l2 mutations induced by TALENs. On the left, a schematic of the zebrafish mab21l2 protein is shown as a light grey box with the mab-21 domain (amino acids 62–346) indicated in dark grey color; the positions of the zebrafish mutations identified in the progeny of TALEN-injected fish are shown at the top of the box and the position of the human mutation identified in Patient 1 is indicated at the bottom; the positions of the p.(Gln48Serfs*5) and p.(Arg51_Phe52del) mutations are shown with red arrows. On the right, a graph summarizing results of semi-quantitative RT-PCR analysis of wild-type and mutant mab21l2 transcript levels in 48-hpf homozygous embryos is shown.

Generation and gross morphological analysis of mab21l2 zebrafish mutants

To determine the effect of mab21l2 deficiency on ocular development, the mab21l2 gene was disrupted using TALEN genome editing technology. DNA sequencing of mab21l2 mutant fish identified the following alleles: c.141_153delCCAAGAGCCCCGT, p.(Gln48Serfs*5); c.150_156delCCGTTTC, p.(Arg51Serfs*4); c.151delC, p.(Arg51Valfs*6); c.151dupC, p.(Arg51Profs*14); and c.155delT, p.(Phe52Serfs*5) frameshift mutations (all predicted to result in truncation of the mab21l2 protein at ~14% of its total length) and an in-frame deletion of two amino acids including the arginine at position 51, c.151_156delCGTTTC, p.(Arg51_Phe52del) (Fig. 3L, S1 Fig.).

Zebrafish carrying heterozygous frameshift alleles were crossed to generate homozygous or compound heterozygous mab21l2 mutants and heterozygous fish with the c.151_156delCGTTTC, p.(Arg51_Phe52del) in-frame deletion were bred to obtain homozygous embryos; the resulting embryos were examined to determine the associated phenotypes (seeFig. 4 for embryonic phenotypes associated with wild-type (A-F), frameshift (G-L) and in-frame deletion (M-R) alleles). Crosses involving frameshift mutations resulted in a distinct phenotype in 26 out of 101 (26%) embryos, consistent with a recessive mode of inheritance. The phenotype of homozygous frameshift mutants included microphthalmia with small or absent lens in 100% of affected embryos, as well as coloboma and shortened body/curved tail in 76% and 56% of affected fish, respectively (Fig. 4G-I, S2 Fig.). The phenotype was first evident in 24–48-hpf embryos and became progressively worse over time. All 26 abnormal fish from these crosses were found to either be compound heterozygous for the c.150_156delCCGTTTC, p.(Arg51Serfs*4) and c.151dupC, p.(Arg51Profs*14) alleles (9 embryos), homozygous for the c.155delT, p.(Phe52Serfs*5) allele (3), homozygous for the c.150_156delCCGTTTC, p.(Arg51Serfs*4) allele (2), homozygous for c.141_153delCCAAGAGCCCCGT p.(Gln48Serfs*5) mutation (9) or homozygous for the c.151delC, p.(Arg51Valfs*6) allele (3) by restriction digest and/or Sanger sequencing. Crosses involving heterozygous carriers of the c.151_156delCGTTTC, p.(Arg51_Phe52del) allele produced 12 out of 57 (21%) abnormal embryos, also consistent with a recessive mode of inheritance. The abnormal phenotype was first evident at 72-hpf and involved severe ocular coloboma in all affected embryos and corneal defects in 42% (5/12), while lenses and eye size appeared to be only mildly affected (Fig. 4M-O).

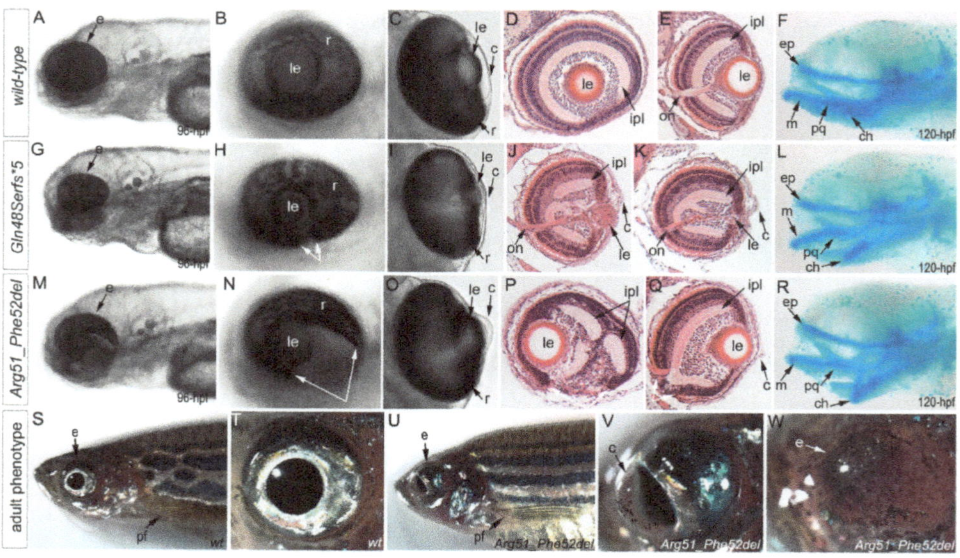

Figure 4. Phenotypic analysis of homozygous embryos carrying mutant mab21l2alleles encoding p.(Gln48Serfs*5) truncation (mab21l2Q48Sfs*5) and p.(Arg51_Phe52del) in-frame deletion (mab21l2R51_F52del) proteins. A-R. Embryonic phenotypes. Images of wild-type larvae at 96-hpf (A-E) and 120-hpf (F), as well as embryos carrying the p.(Gln48Serfs*5) frameshift (G-L) or p.(Arg51_Phe52del) in-frame deletion (M-R) alleles are shown. Whole mount images (A-C, G-I, and M-O), as well as frontal (E, J, K, Q) and sagittal (D, P) ocular sections are presented. Please notice reduced eye size (G-K), coloboma (white arrows in H), degenerative (H-J) or absent (K) lens, disorganized retina and irregular cornea (J, K) in embryos with frameshift mutations, as well as severe coloboma (white arrows in N) with disorganized retina, discontinuous RPE (white arrows in P, Q), and corneal defects (O) but overall comparable to wild-type eye size and lenses (M-Q) in embryos

that are homozygous for the in-frame deletion. Alcian blue stain of wild-type (F) and mutant embryos (L, R) identified defects in craniofacial development with primary defects in the development of the ceratohyal cartilage of the hyoid arch (or the second pharyngeal arch). S-W. Adult phenotype. Images of adult wild-type (S, T) and Arg51_Phe52del mutant (U-W) fish: please notice microphthalmic highly disorganized eye with pigmented cornea (V) and anophthalmic contralateral eye with residual abnormal pigmented tissue (W). Please also note normal appearance of pectoral fins in the mutant fish (U). ch, ceratohyal; ep, ethmoid plate; m, Meckel›s cartilage; pq, palatoquadrate; e, eye; c, cornea; le, lens; ipl, inner plexiform layer; on, optic nerve; pf, pectoral fins; r, retina.

Mutant lines were established for the c.141_153delCCAAGAGCCCCGT, p.(Gln48Serfs*5) frameshift mutation (mab21l2^{Q48Sfs*5}) and the c.151_156delCGTTTC, p.(Arg51_Phe52del) in-frame deletion (mab21l2^{R51_F52del}) alleles (Fig. 3L and S1 Fig.) and were further characterized. Expression of mutant mab21l2 transcripts was examined by RT-PCR using RNA extracted from 48-hpf embryos. Both mutant transcripts were found to be expressed at slightly higher levels than wild-type transcript, but this increase was not statistically significant (Fig. 3L, S1 Fig.).

Histological analysis of the 96–120-hpf homozygous embryos with mab21l2^{Q48Sfs*5} and other frameshift mutations demonstrated a small degenerative (Fig. 4J) or absent (Fig. 4K) lens, disorganized retina (particularly the inner plexiform layer), and irregular cornea (Fig. 4J, K). Histological analysis of the mab21l2^{R51_F52del} homozygous embryos confirmed severe coloboma, abnormally formed retina (inner plexiform layer) and cornea, discontinuous RPE (retinal pigmented epithelium), as well as generally normal eye size and lens appearance (Fig. 4P, Q). Alcian blue staining identified craniofacial defects in some mab21l2^{Q48Sfs*5} (3/7; 43%) and mab21l2^{R51_F52del} (3/6; 50%) 120-hpf homozygous fish: the cartilage elements of the pharyngeal arches, particularly the ceratohyal cartilage of the hyoid arch (or the second pharyngeal arch), were malformed and displaced (Fig. 4L, R) while the ethmoid plate cartilage of the upper jaw appeared to be largely unaffected. Analysis of the pectoral fin did not identify any obvious malformations in mab21l2^{Q48Sfs*5} or mab21l2^{R51_F52del} 120-hpf embryos ormab21l2^{R51_F52del} adult fish (Fig. 4U).

Homozygous mab21l2^{Q48Sfs*5}embryos demonstrated 100% lethality with no embryos surviving into adulthood while two out of fifteen (13%) mab21l2^{R51_F52del} homozygous larvae developed into adults. Gross morphological examination of adult fish revealed a severe ocular phenotype with anophthalmia of one eye and microphthalmia of the contralateral eye (see Fig. 4S, T for wild-type and 4U-W for mutant fish phenotypes). In addition to small size, the ocular structures appeared to be highly disorganized with an expanded anterior segment and pigmented cornea (Fig. 4V).

Comparative analysis of apoptosis, proliferation and ocular markers in wild-type and mab21l2 embryos

Analysis of apoptosis with TUNEL assay (that detects terminal deoxynucleotidyl transferase dUTP nick end labeling) identified an excessive number of TUNEL-positive cells in 24–72-hpf homozygous mab21l2^{Q48Sfs*5} embryos in comparison to wild-type (Fig. 5A-D; S3 Fig.): at 24- hpf, the increased number of TUNEL-positive cells was observed in the developing lens and ventral retina (Fig. 5C, D); at 48–72-hpf clusters of TUNEL-positive cells continued to be found in lens, margins of the open optic fissure and other regions of the retina (possibly the outer nuclear layer) (S3 Fig.). In mab21l2^{R51_F52del} mutants carrying the in-frame deletion allele, a moderate increase in TUNEL-positive cells was observed: at 24-hpf an increase in TUNEL-positive cells was detected in the ventral region of the retina with some staining in other retinal regions and in the lens (Fig. 5E, F); at 48–72-hpf, TUNEL staining continued to be seen primarily the retina and not in the lens (S3 Fig.). A moderate increase in TUNEL staining was also observed in the brain and other embryonic tissues in both mutants (Fig. 5D, S3 Fig.).

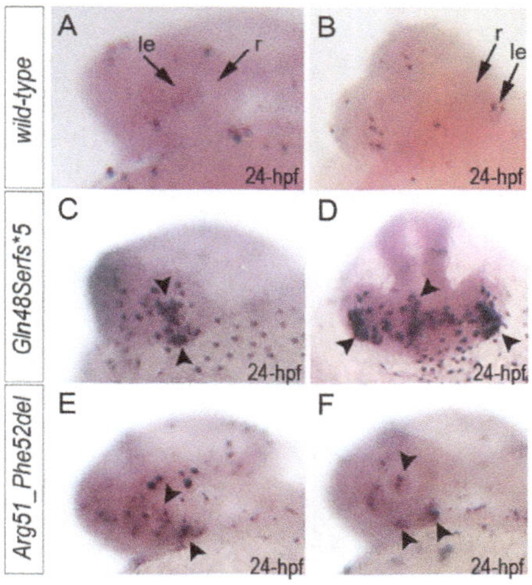

Figure 5. Summary of TUNEL assays in zebrafish wild-type and mab21l2 **mutant embryos.** TUNEL results in 24-hpf wild-type (A-B), mab21l2^{Q48Sfs*5} embryos (C-D) andmab21l2^{R51_F52del} mutants (E-F) are shown. An increase in TUNEL staining was observed in both mab21l2 mutants with remarkably high levels in the mab21l2^{Q48Sfs*5}embryos, particularly in the lens and ventral retina (C-D), and moderately increased levels in the mab21l2^{R51_F52del} embryos (E-F); arrowheads indicate sites of increased TUNEL staining in the eye and brain; le, lens; r, retina.

Immunohistochemistry with PCNA (Proliferating Cell Nuclear Antigen) was performed to compare proliferation patterns in 24–72-hpf wild-type and both mab21l2^{Q48Sfs*5} andmab21l2^{R51_F52del} mutant embryos; the monoclonal antibody ZL-1 was used to examine zebrafish fiber cell differentiation and the sections were counterstained with wheat germ agglutinin (WGA) and/or DAPI and to visualize cell membranes and nuclei, correspondingly (Fig. 6 and S4 and S5 Fig.). Strong nuclear PCNA immunoreactivity indicating robust proliferation was observed in the retinal marginal zone in 24-, 48- and 72-hpf wild-type embryos (Fig. 6A-F) as well as the developing lens, particularly in the anterior lens epithelium at 48- and 72-hpf (Fig. 6D, F). In mab21l2^{Q48Sfs*5} mutant embryos, the intensity of PCNA staining appears to be diminished at early stages (Fig. 6G, H) with a disorganized pattern being observed in the retina at 48–72-hpf (Fig. 6I-L); no proliferation activity was detected in the anterior lens epithelium of either 48- or 72-hpf embryos (Fig. 6J and L) in these mutants. In themab21l2^{R51_F52del} deletion mutant, strong PCNA staining in the peripheral parts of the developing retina was observed at 24-hpf (Fig. 6M, N); disordered patterns were evident in 48- and 60-hpf embryos (Fig. 6O-R) with patches of PCNA-positive cells seen in the central regions of the retina (arrowheads in Fig. 6Q); in contrast to the frameshift mutant, PCNA staining was observed in the cells of anterior lens epithelium in both 48- and 60-hpfmab21l2^{R51_F52del} embryos (Fig. 6P, R). ZL-1 positive cells were observed in wild-type embryos starting from 24-hpf (S5 Fig.); this staining was not noted in the abnormal eyes ofmab21l2^{Q48Sfs*5} mutants at 24-hpf but was detected in 48- and 72-hpf mab21l2^{Q48Sfs*5}embryos and 72-hpf mab21l2^{R51_F52del} mutants (S5 Fig.).

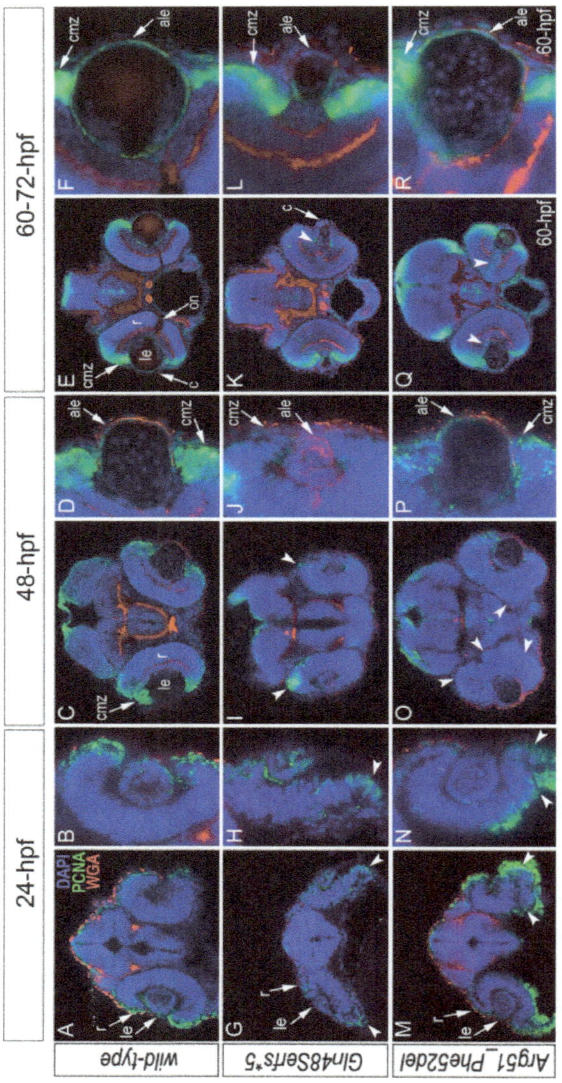

Figure 6. Analysis of proliferation patterns and differentiation markers in wild-type and mutant embryos. Immunostaining with PCNA (Proliferating Cell Nuclear Antigen) (green), DAPI (blue), wheat germ agglutinin (WGA) (red) was performed using 24–72-hpf wild-type embryos (A-F) as well as mab21l2^{Q48Sfs*5} (G-L) and mab21l2^{R51_F52del} (M-R) mutant tissues. Embryonic stages are indicated above; overlay fluorescence images are shown and single immunoreactivity data is available in S4 Fig. White arrowheads point to defects in retinal invagination and regions of abnormal retinal folding (H,M,N) observed in bothmab21l2^{Q48Sfs*5} and mab21l2^{R51_F52del} embryos (please see text), as well as areas of aberrant PCNA labeling (I,K,O,Q). Please also note the absence of PCNA staining in the anterior lens epithelium of 48- and 72-hpf mab21l2^{Q48Sfs*5} mutants (J,L). ale, anterior lens epithelium; c, cornea; cmz, ciliary marginal zone; le, lens; on, optic nerve; r, retina.

Both mutants demonstrated abnormal retinal shape at 24-hpf (Fig. 6G, H, M, N) suggesting a possible invagination defect; a shallow optic cup, particularly at its ventral region, was detected in the mab21l2^{Q48Sfs*5} frameshift mutants (Fig. 6G, H) and a smaller, more constricted, optic vesicle was present in the mab21l2^{R51_F52del} deletion mutants (Fig. 6M, N); abnormal retinal folding was evident in both mutants at 24- and 48-hpf (arrowheads in Fig. 6G, H, M-O).

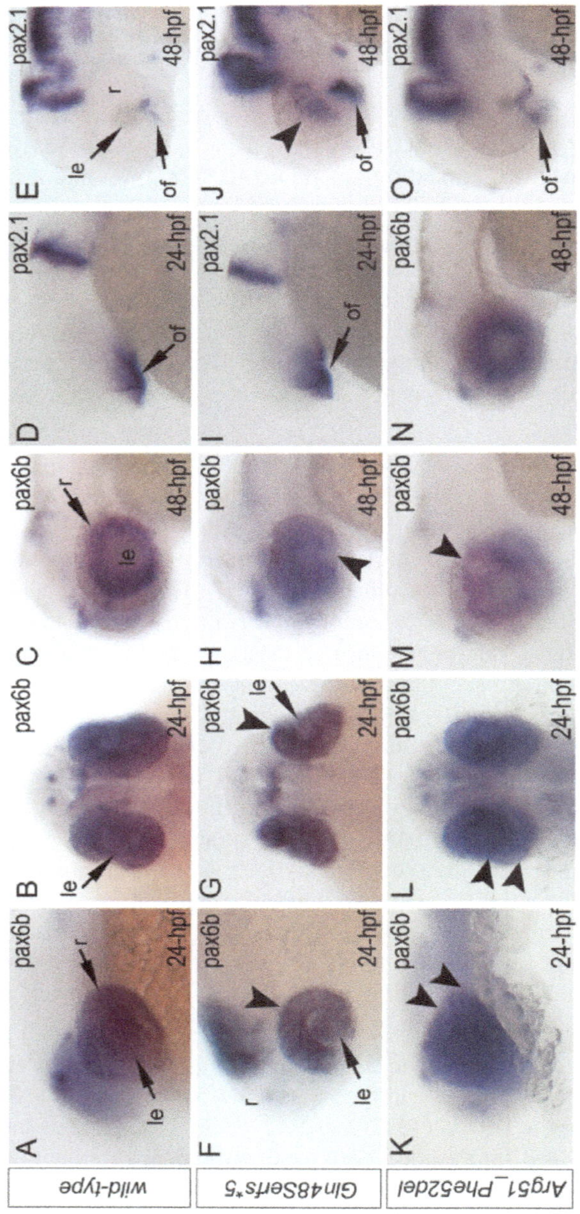

Figure 7. Analysis of pax6b, pax2.1 and foxe3 **expression in wild-type,**mab21l2^{Q48Sfs*5} **and** mab21l2^{R51_F52del} **embryos.**

Expression of the pax6b, pax2.1 and foxe3 genes was examined in wild-type and mutant fish (Fig. 7, S5 Fig.). Expression of pax6b in wild-type embryos was detected throughout the developing eye at 24-hpf (Fig. 7A, B) with a more restricted pattern in the retinal ganglion cells and inner nuclear layer neurons at 48-hpf (Fig. 7C). In mab21l2^{Q48Sfs*5} mutants, pax6bexpression was detected in both the developing lens and retina but appeared to be downregulated in the ventral/temporal versus dorsal/nasal domain (arrowhead in Fig. 7F, G); at 48-hpf pax6b expression was not present in the region of the coloboma (arrowhead in Fig. 7H). In the mab21l2^{R51_F52del} mutants, pax6b expression was detected throughout the abnormally folded retina at 24-hpf (Fig. 7K, L); at 48-hpf, 50% (2/4) of the embryos showed patchy pattern of pax6b expression (Fig. 7M) while others (2/4) demonstrated a grossly normal pax6bdistribution (Fig. 7N). We also examined zebrafish pax2.1 expression, which normally shows robust staining at the opposite edges of the open fissure at early embryonic stages (24-hpf) (Fig. 7D) and becomes diminished and more restricted to the optic nerve and the site of choroid fissure as the fissure begins to close (by 48-hpf) (Fig. 7E, S5 Fig.). In mab21l2^{Q48Sfs*5}homozygous mutants, pax2.1 expression appears to be unaffected at 24-hpf (Fig. 7I) but an altered pattern is observed at later stages with broad and intense expression continuing in the region of optic fissure (Fig. 7J, S5 Fig.) and abnormal areas of pax2.1-positive cells being noticeable in the central retina (arrowheads in Fig. 7J and S5 Fig.). In the mab21l2^{R51_F52del}mutants, pax2.1 expression is expanded in 48-hpf embryos and continues to be observed at the edges of the retina at the site of coloboma at 72-hpf (Fig. 7O, S5 Fig.); no pax2.1 positive patches were detected in other retinal regions. Expression of foxe3 (which marks the lens epithelial layer) in the developing 48-hpf lens seemed to be somewhat downregulated in both mutants with mutant lenses also appearing smaller than wild-type lenses (S5 Fig.).

Wild-type (A-E) and mutant (F-O) zebrafish embryos at 24–48-hpf were analyzed as indicated in the right bottom corner of each image. Please note a change in pax6btranscript distribution at 24-hpf and 48-hpf in mab21l2^{Q48Sfs*5} (arrowheads in F-H), retinal folding defect in mab21l2^{R51_F52del} embryos at 24-hpf (arrowheads in K, L) and visibly abnormal pax6b pattern at 48-hpf in some (arrowheads in M) but not all (N) mab21l2^{R51_F52del} embryos. pax2.1 expression seems to be unaffected in 24-hpf frameshift mutant embryos (I) but shows an abnormal pattern in both mutants at 48-hpf (J,O). At 48-hpf, in addition to more broad and intense pax2.1 expression in the region of optic fissure, abnormal pax2.1 staining was detected in central retina inmab21l2^{Q48Sfs*5} embryos (arrowheads in J). le, lens; of, optic fissure; retina.

Analysis of wild-type and mutant MAB21L2/ mab21l2 proteins

To examine the effect of the p.(Arg51Gly) mutation on the MAB21L2 protein, we tested the expression, localization and protein stability of the wild-type and mutant proteins via transfections of the corresponding FLAG-tagged constructs into human lens epithelial B3 (HLE-B3) cells [32]; MAB21L2 was also found to be endogenously expressed in these cells (S1 Fig.).

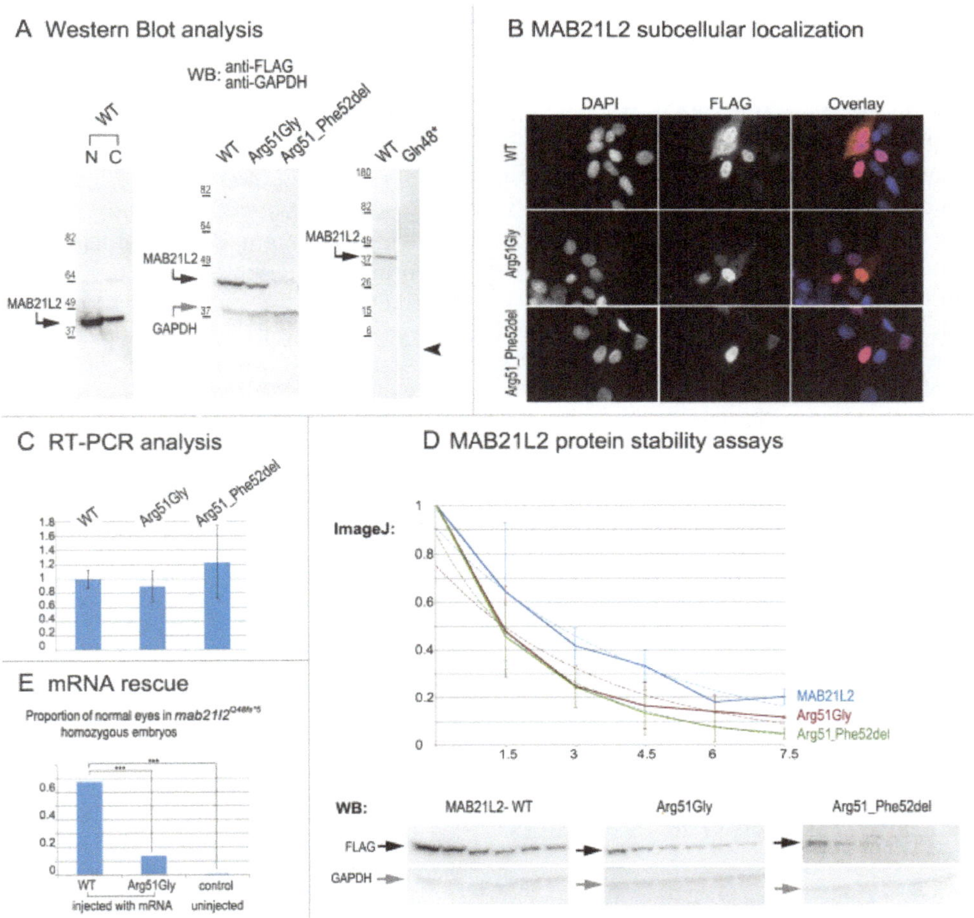

Figure 8. MAB21L2 wild-type and mutant protein studies. **A.** Western Blot analyses of MAB21L2 wild-type and mutant proteins (with N-terminal FLAG tag) in HLE-B3 cells. Please note the presence of wild-type MAB21L2 in both nuclear (N) and cytoplasmic (C) fractions (left), decreased expression of Arg51Gly and Arg51_Phe52del mutants (center) and the absence of Gln48* mutant protein (right; arrowhead indicates region corresponding to 5.5kDa, the predicted molecular weight for this peptide); predicted molecular weight for MAB21L2 is ~41kDa and for GAPDH is ~36 kDa; positions and corresponding molecular weights of protein ladder are shown for every blot.

B. Cellular immunofluorescence analysis demonstrated no significant alteration in the localization pattern between wild-type and mutant (Arg51Gly and Arg51_52del) proteins with predominant nuclear localization and some cytoplasmic staining for all forms. **C.** RT-PCR analysis of MAB21L2 wild-type and mutant transcripts in human lens epithelial cells transfected with corresponding expression constructs. **D.**Protein stability assays with cycloheximide showed a more rapid decrease in the amount of Arg51Gly and Arg51_Phe-52del mutant proteins in comparison to wild-type protein. Western blots signals were measured using ImageJ software, and obtained values were graphed to produce degradation curves represented by solid blue (wild-type), red (Arg51Gly) and green (Arg51_Phe52del) lines (standard deviations for every time point are indicated as thin vertical lines and exponential decay curves fitted into each graph are shown as dotted lines of corresponding colors); representative Western blot (WB) images are shown on the bottom (stability assays were performed in triplicate; 0, 1.5, 3, 4.5, 6, and 7.5 correspond to hours of exposure to cycloheximide). **E.**Summary of mRNA rescue experiments. Proportions of embryos with normal eyes in homozygous mab21l2Q48fs*5 embryos injected with wild-type human MAB21L2 mRNA, mRNA encoding the p.(Arg51Gly) mutant protein, and uninjected control larvae are shown; statistically significant ($p<0.0005$) differences are indicated with asterisks (***).

Mab21l proteins were previously shown to localize primarily to the nucleus [33]. Western Blot analysis of nuclear and cytoplasmic fractions confirmed the presence of ~41kDa wild-type MAB21L2 protein in both cellular compartments with greater nuclear localization (Fig. 8A). Western blot analysis of whole-cell extracts detected a decreased amount of the p.(Arg51Gly) mutant in comparison to wild-type protein (Fig. 8A); the mutant protein was found to be present at 31.97% ± 9.36% of wild-type based on three independent experiments. Cellular immunofluorescence analysis demonstrated no significant alteration in the localization pattern between wild-type and mutant protein with predominant nuclear localization and some cytoplasmic staining for both forms (Fig. 8B). Since the levels of recombinant MAB21L2transcript encoding for wild-type and p.(Arg51Gly) mutant proteins detected by RT-PCR did not show a significant difference (Fig. 8C, S1 Fig.), we proceeded to perform protein stability assays using a series of cycloheximide treatments of HLE-B3 cells transfected with MAB21L2 constructs (Fig. 8D). Protein stability assays showed a more rapid decrease in the amount of p.(Arg51Gly) mutant in comparison to wild-type protein at all examined time points, with 11% of the mutant protein being present after 7.5 hours of cycloheximide treatment in comparison to 20% of the wild-type MAB21L2 (Fig. 8D). Calculation of the proteins' half-life identified a statistically significant difference ($p<0.05$) in stability of wild-type (2.64±0.25 hours) versus the p.(Arg51Gly) mutant (1.91±0.36). These data suggest that the substitution of the arginine at position 51 to glycine affects MAB21L2 stability.

Functional analysis of the p.(Gln48*) (to represent the zebrafish p.(Gln48Serfs*5) mutant) and p.(Arg51_Phe52del) proteins was also undertaken in HLE-B3 cells. The p.(Gln48*) mutant was found to be highly unstable as no detectable level of this protein (estimated to have a molecular weight of ~5.5 kDa) was identified via Western blot analysis (Fig. 8A). The p.(Arg51_Phe52del) mutant also demonstrated a reduction in the amount of detected protein to 2.57% ± 2.20% of wild-type MAB21L2 protein based on three independent experiments (Fig. 8A); cellular immunofluorescence analysis demonstrated predominantly nuclear staining similar to wild-type distribution (Fig. 8B). Protein stability assays confirmed increased instability of the p.(Arg51_Phe52del) protein with less than 5% of mutant protein being detected after 7.5 hours of cycloheximide exposure versus 20% for the wild-type (Fig. 8D). The half-life of the p.(Arg51_Phe52del) mutant was estimated to be 1.91±0.27 hours versus 2.64±.25 for wild-type, which represented a statistically significant difference ($p<0.05$). The half-life values of the p.(Arg51_Phe52del) and p.(Arg51Gly) proteins were not significantly different from each other despite the observed reduced level of p.(Arg51_Phe52del) in comparison to p.(Arg51Gly) in replicate Western blots of untreated cells (see above, Fig. 8A); this suggests that there may be additional factors affecting the stability of the p.(Arg51_Phe52del) mutant which may require alternative assays to uncover [34].

To further test the pathogenicity of the human p.(Arg51Gly) allele, we injected embryos generated by heterozygous mab21l2^{Q48Sfs*5} crosses with either wild type MAB21L2 mRNA or mRNA encoding for the p.(Arg51Gly) mutant; a small number of embryos were left uninjected as a control. The embryos were carefully examined for ocular anomalies at 72-hpf, divided into affected and normal groups, and then genotyped. In total, out of 104 surviving embryos injected with wild type MAB21L2, 68% (21/31) of homozygous fish developed normal eyes and lenses while out of 108 surviving embryos injected with the mutant mRNA encoding for p.(Arg51Gly), only 14% (3/22) of homozygous fish developed normal eyes and lenses; in the control group, none of the 9 uninjected homozygous embryos (out of 36 surviving) had normal eyes and lenses. The difference in the proportion of normal phenotypes seen in the homozygous mab21l2^{Q48Sfs*5} fish injected with wild-type mRNA versus embryos injected with either mutant mRNA or left uninjected was statistically significant ($p<.0005$), while the difference between the mutant RNA- injected and the uninjected embryos was not statistically significant ($p>.20$) by chi-squared analysis (Fig. 8E). The efficient rescue by wild typeMAB21L2 mRNA confirms that the ocular phenotype in the mutant line is caused by themab21l2 deficiency and demonstrates functional conservation between zebrafish and human mab21l2/MAB21L2 proteins. The absence of robust rescue by mRNA encoding for the p.(Arg51Gly) mutant supports the pathogenic role of this MAB21L2 allele in human disease.

To investigate the possibility of dominant-negative effects for the mutant allele, MAB21L2 wild type mRNA or mRNA encoding for the p.(Arg51Gly) mutant were injected (at the same concentrations as in rescue experiments) into wild-type embryos and observed for phenotypes up to 120-hpf. Among the 39 surviving embryos that were injected with wild-type MAB21L2, no embryos displayed an eye phenotype (9 fish showed moderate-severe overall malformations). Similarly, among the 61 surviving embryos that were injected with the mutant mRNA encoding for the p.(Arg51Gly) protein, no embryos showed an eye phenotype (10 fish showed moderate-severe overall malformations). Thus, these experiments identified no dominant-negative effect for the p.(Arg51Gly) mutant allele in zebrafish at concentrations that are sufficient for phenotypic rescue of the mab21l2-deficient phenotype.

DISCUSSION

In this manuscript we present evidence for the conserved function of MAB21L2/mab21l2 in vertebrate ocular development through demonstration of abnormal phenotypes associated with mutations in this gene in humans and zebrafish. Human MAB21L2, located at 4q31.3, is a member of the MAB21L gene family that consists of three members, MAB21L1-3. MAB21L proteins are related to the mab-21 (male abnormal 21) nuclear factor [33] associated with thinning of ray 6 and frequent fusions of rays 4 and 6 of a set of nine bilateral peripheral rays in male C. elegans [27]. The molecular function of MAB21L2 is largely unknown. Previous reports involving double mutants of mab-21 and sma members (SMAD family) in C. elegans indicated that mab-21 is positioned downstream of sma and is negatively regulated by dbl-1, a homolog of human BMP5, thus placing mab-21 in the TGF-β signaling cascade [35,36]. The TGF-β signaling cascade plays an important role in ocular development and mutations in many associated factors, such as BMP4, BMP7, GDF3, and GDF6, lead to an overlapping spectrum of phenotypes in humans [13,14, 37–39]. Additionally, mab-18 (PAX6 ortholog) mutants demonstrate a phenotype that is highly similar to mab-21 C. elegans mutants [27] and Mab21l2expression was found to be upregulated in embryonic mouse lenses heterozygous for a Pax6loss-of-function allele [40] suggesting a possible conserved genetic interaction.

In mouse, Mab21l2 ocular expression was reported in the dorsal optic vesicle and head surface ectoderm in E8.5–9.5 embryos and the neural retina, optic nerve and RPE at E12 [41,42]; homozygous Mab21l2 knockout mice demonstrated a rudimentary retina and aphakia due to improper invagination of the optic vesicle as well as ventral body wall defects, improper formation of the heart and liver, and embryonic lethality [41,42]. Previously published reports of lens expression in animal models are somewhat inconsistent: four studies reported lack of lens expression for Mab21l2/mab21l2 (with many showing the presence of lens expression for its close homolog, Mab21l1/ mab21l1) [41,43–45] while three other manuscripts notedMab21l2/mab21l2 transcripts in the developing lens [33,46,47], which is consistent with the results of our study. In zebrafish, morpholino-mediated knockdown of mab21l2 resulted in microphthalmia and incomplete retinal development including discontinuous inner and outer plexiform layers [47]. In the zebrafish genetic mutants that we developed, severe defects in the development of both the lens and retina were observed consistent with strong expression of mab21l2 in both tissues. While the phenotypes of mab21l2 morphants and mutants show overlap, some ocular features, including severe lens degeneration, coloboma, and early retinal invagination defects, appear to be more pronounced or observed primarily in genetic mutants; this may be due to incomplete disruption of mab21l2 function via morpholino, the transient nature of morpholino-induced effects, and/or genetic background differences.

Both of the mab21l2 mutants generated in this study demonstrated variable retinal invagination defects. In zebrafish, retinal invagination, which occurs upon contact of the optic vesicle (formed as an extension of the forebrain neuroepithelium) with the surface ectoderm, is completed with formation of the cup-shaped optic vesicle by ~22-hpf. In mab21l2^{Q48Sfs*5}embryos, a shallow misshapen optic cup, especially at its ventral part, was detected in 24-hpf embryos; the lens mass (similar to the mammalian lens vesicle) was also visibly smaller than normal at this stage. In the mab21l2^{R51_F52del} in-frame deletion mutant, a more constricted optic cup with some ventral and dorsal retinal folding was observed, while the developing lens appeared to have normal size and shape in most embryos. The observed defects in early optic cup formation indicate a possible conserved role for mab21l2 in this process in vertebrates.

Studies of proliferation and cell death in zebrafish wild-type and mab21l2^{Q48Sfs*5} ormab21l2^{R51_F52del} homozygous mutant embryos identified multiple deviations from normal patterns. The most remarkable finding was a significant increase in TUNEL staining in the developing retina and lens of mab21l2^{Q48Sfs*5} mutants at early embryonic stages. An increase in TUNEL staining was also observed at later stages of development and was, to a lesser degree, present in the mab21l2^{R51_F52del} embryos carrying homozygous in-frame deletion alleles. Both increased cell death (through apoptosis and/or necroptosis) and defects in cellular proliferation have been linked to optic fissure closure defects in other genetic models of coloboma [48–59]; since the TUNEL assay may not discriminate between apoptotic and other cell death mechanisms [60], further studies are needed to evaluate the possible involvement of necroptosis in mab21l2 deficient phenotypes. Additionally, the expression of several ocular markers including pax6b, pax2.1, foxe3 and ZL-1 was altered in mab21l2 mutants. These observed differences seem more likely to be caused by the severe disorganization of mutant ocular tissues rather than direct regulation of expression of those markers by mab21l2.

The distinct phenotypes associated with the mab21l2^{Q48Sfs*5} frameshift truncation andmab21l2^{R51_F52del} in-frame deletion mutations suggest different molecular mechanisms. Themab21l2^{R51_F52del} in-frame deletion demonstrated milder features in comparison to themab21l2^{Q48Sfs*5} mutant, such as less affected lens development, less pronounced cell death and incomplete embryonic lethality. These observations support the possibility that this mutation results in a hypomorphic allele retaining some of its normal function, particularly in relation to lens development. The severe coloboma observed in mab21l2^{R51_F52del} embryos may point to the particular importance of domains located in the N-terminal region of mab21l2 for its proper functioning in the developing retina. Since the zebrafish p.(Arg51_Phe52del) in-frame deletion and the human p.(Arg51Gly) missense alleles affect homologous regions of the MAB21L2/mab21l2 proteins, the mechanism(s) of these mutations may be similar to each other. Understanding of these mechanisms requires additional studies into the domain structure and function of MAB21L2/mab21l2 protein.

Analysis of wild-type and mutant proteins in human lens epithelial cells identified a range of protein stability defects among mutant forms with the human p.(Arg51Gly) mutant stability mildly reduced, the zebrafish p.(Arg51_Phe52del) mutant stability highly affected, and the p.(Gln48*) truncation protein (similar to the p.(Gln48Serfs*5) mutant) being entirely unstable. This analysis suggested that the zebrafish p.(Gln48Serfs*5) mutation results in a complete loss-of-function allele, since the similar mutant protein p.(Gln48*) was completely unstable and any protein produced would be missing the entire mab-21 domain. These experiments also indicated the likely importance of arginine 51 and the immediately adjacent amino acids for normal conformation and stability of the MAB21L2/mab21l2 protein because disruptions of this region resulted in decreased stability for both the human p.(Arg51Gly) and the zebrafish p.(Arg51_Phe52del) proteins. Further studies demonstrated that, in contrast to wild-type humanMAB21L2 mRNA, mutant mRNA encoding for the p.(Arg51Gly) protein failed to efficiently rescue the ocular phenotype of homozygous mab21l2^{Q48Sfs*5} embryos, suggesting functional deficiency for the identified human mutation. In addition, overexpression of mutant MAB21L2mRNA in zebrafish embryos resulted in no obvious ocular phenotype, implying absence of a dominant-negative effect. However, it is possible that the full impact of the p.(Arg51Gly) mutation was not discernable due to insufficient dosage, its acting later in development, or other factors; this needs to be further investigated by additional approaches, including development of zebrafish mutants carrying this specific allele.

No abnormal phenotype was seen in heterozygous zebrafish for either the frameshift truncation or in-frame deletion mutations, while a dominant phenotype was observed in human patients with the p.(Arg51Gly) alteration. This may be explained by variability in gene dosage requirements between species [61] or a different mechanism for the human mutation. The presence of mild rhizomelia/ contractures in human patients with MAB21L2 mutations suggests its involvement in skeletal development. Additional phenotypes such as shortened body/curved tail, craniofacial malformations and lethality were present in the zebrafish mab21l2mutants while heart, liver, embryonic lethality and other anomalies were previously reported in mouse Mab21l2 mutants [41,42]. Considering these observations and the fact that multiple pleiotropic effects of mab-21 mutations have been previously noted [27], additional MAB21L2-associated phenotypes are likely to be identified and may present with broad interfamilial variability.

While this paper was in revision, four families with mutations in MAB21L2 were described by Rainger et al [62]. This manuscript reports three heterozygous mutations (p.(Arg51Cys), p.(Arg51His), and p.(Glu49Lys) affecting the same region as the mutation reported here and resulting in similar phenotypes (anophthalmia or colobomatous microphthalmia with rhizomelic skeletal dysplasia in two families); one of the reported families includes the UK10K_COL5001067 and UK10K_COL5001068 cases with the p.(Arg51His) mutation that we presented in results from the publically available data. In addition, one family with a recessiveMAB21L2 mutation affecting the C-terminal region of the protein was identified. Functional assays of the mutant alleles using an inducible HEK293 cell system expressing wild-type or mutant MAB21L2 as GFP fusion proteins suggested a possible gain-of-function effect for the dominant mutations based on observed increased protein stability; an increase in phospho-ERK1 was detected with induction of either wild-type or p.(Arg51His) mutant MAB21L2 protein [62]. This differs from the proposed mechanism of the mutation identified in our study which revealed a decrease in protein stability for the p.(Arg51Gly) mutant tagged with FLAG epitope and absence of a dominant phenotype in zebrafish embryos injected with mRNA encoding for this protein. This may be due to diverse effects of the studied amino acid substitutions (Arg51Gly versus Arg51His, Arg51Cys, and Glu49Lys) on MAB21L2 protein structure, different effects of tags on protein stability (GFP versus FLAG), or other factors, and needs to be investigated further. Rainger and co-authors (2014) also suggested an involvement of MAB21L2 in ssRNA binding [62]. In our manuscript, we developed an allelic series of zebrafishmab21l2 mutants, uncovered an early onset optic cup apoptosis phenotype in affected embryos, and demonstrated a decrease in protein stability, as well as functional deficiency and no dominant-negative effect for the p.(Arg51Gly) mutation in zebrafish embryos.

Taken as a whole, the complete co-segregation of the identified MAB21L2 allele with the ocular phenotype in the family, the de novo appearance of the mutation in the affected progeny of unaffected parents with low-level mosaicism present in the mother, the in silico and experimental indications of the functional importance of the arginine at position 51, the development of ocular defects in mab21l2 mutant zebrafish embryos, as well as rescue of the ocular phenotype of homozygous mab21l2^{Q48Sfs*5} embryos with injection of wild-type but not the p.(Arg51Gly)-encoding mutant mRNA, provide strong support for the pathogenicity of the identified MAB21L2 allele and the involvement of MAB21L2 in human ocular development and disease. The developed zebrafish mab21l2 mutants will help to further explore the developmental roles and molecular function of this conserved ocular factor.

MATERIALS AND METHODS

Ethics statement

The human study was approved by the Children's Hospital of Wisconsin Institutional Review Board (protocol number CHW 03/56) with written informed consent obtained from each participant and/or their legal representative, as appropriate. This study also utilized data generated by the UK10K Consortium, derived from samples from UK10K_Rare_Coloboma (EGA Study ID: EGAS00001000127); a full list of the investigators who contributed to the generation of the data is available from http://www.UK10K.org. Access to data generated by the UK10K_Rare_Coloboma (EGA Study ID: EGAS00001000127) project of the UK10K Consortium study (http://www.UK10K.org) was obtained through a Data Access Agreement. The animal protocol was approved by the Institutional Animal Care and Use Committee at the Medical College of Wisconsin (protocol number AUA00000351_AR_5).

Human sequencing studies

Whole exome sequencing of DNA samples of the proband's two affected nephews was undertaken. Library capture was completed using the Agilent Sure Select v4 capture kit (Santa Clara, CA) and 100 base pair paired end sequencing was performed using the Illumina HiSeq 2000 at Axeq Technologies (Rockville, MD). The obtained data were aligned using the Burrows-Wheeler Aligner (BWA) and variants were called using the SAMTOOLS analysis pipeline available through Axeq. Exome data were analyzed using the SNP & Variation

Suite (Golden Helix, Bozeman, MT) to identify variants that are shared between the affected individuals and then prioritized based on their absence/rarity in the general population (as reported in publicly available databases dbSNP (http://www.ncbi.nlm.nih.gov/snp), NHLBI Exome Sequencing Project Exome Variant Server (EVS; http://evs.gs.washington.edu/EVS/), and 1000 Genomes (http://www.1000genomes.org/data), as well as our own data) and possible effect on protein function; for missense variants, functional profiling was performed using SIFT, Polyphen2, Mutation Taster, MutationAssessor, and FATHMM as well as nucleotide conservation scores GERP++ and PhyloP as accessed through dbNSFP [63].

To confirm the identified MAB21L2 changes and perform cosegregation analysis, DNA from all available family members was amplified using the primers and conditions provided in S2 Table. PCR products were sequenced bidirectionally using Big Dye Terminator chemistry and the ABI 3730XL sequencer (Applied Biosystems/Life Technologies, Carlsbad, CA, USA). Sequences were reviewed manually and using Mutation Surveyor (SoftGenetics, State College, PA) and compared to the NM_006439.4 transcript.

Variant Call Format (VCF) files from the UK10K_Rare_Coloboma (EGA Study ID: EGAS00001000127) project of the UK10K Consortium study (http://www.UK10K.org) were analyzed using the SNP & Variation Suite (Golden Helix, Bozeman, MT) with filtering for theMAB21L2 gene only. DNA samples from this cohort were not available for independent confirmation of the identified variants.

Additional human samples were screened using Sanger sequencing of the 1362-bp PCR product encompassing the full MAB21L2 coding region using PCR primers and two extra internal primers (S2 Table). Sequences were analyzed by manual inspection and Mutation Surveyor software as described above.

MAB21L2 protein studies

Protein sequences were aligned using the Kalign multiple sequence alignment tool (http://www.ebi.ac.uk/Tools/msa/kalign). The accession numbers for the MAB21L sequences used in the protein alignment are as follows: human MAB21L2 (AF155219.1), murine Mab21l2 (AF223425.1), zebrafish mab21l2 (AY038031.1), human MAB21L1 (NM_005584), murine Mab21l1 (AF228913.1), zebrafish mab21l1 (NM_152974.2), human MAB21L3 (NM_152367.2), murine Mab21l3 (NM_172295.4), zebrafish mab21l3 (NM_001110025.1), Drosophila melanogaster mab-21 (NP_651971.2), Caenorhabditis elegans mab-21 (NP_497940.2).

The expression construct for MAB21L2 wild-type protein with N-terminal FLAG (Cat. #EX-V1703-M11) was purchased from GeneCopoiea (Rockville, MD). The mutations were introduced using the Agilent QuikChange Lightning (Cat. #210519) site directed mutagenesis kit (Santa Clara, CA). Mutagenesis primers were designed using the online QuikChange Primer Design tool. HPLC purified mutagenesis primers were ordered from Thermo Fisher Scientific (Waltham, MA) and sequences were as follows: MAB21L2-p.R51G-Sense—5'-gaggtgcaggagcctggcttcatcagct-3', MAB21L2-p.R51G-Antisense—5'-agctgatgaagccaggctcctgcacctc-3', MAB21L2-p.51_52del-Sense—5'-gctcaaggagctgataggctcctgcacctc-3', MAB21L2-p.51_52del-Antisense—5'-gaggtgcaggagcctatcagctccttgagc-3', MAB21L2-Q48X-Sense—5'- gaagcgaggctcctacacctccacttcct-3', MAB21L2-Q48X-Antisense—5'- aggaagtggaggtgtaggagcctcgcttc-3'.

Human lens epithelial B3 (HLE-B3) cells (ATCC, CRL-11421) were maintained in MEM (Life Technologies) supplemented with 20% FBS (Life Technologies), 2 mM glutamine (Life Technologies), and 1 mM sodium pyruvate (Life Technologies). All transfections were performed by transfecting HLE-B3 cells with 15 μg of DNA and 30 μl of Lipofectamine 2000 (Life Technologies) in Opti-MEM in 100 mm petri dishes.

For Western blot analysis, nuclear and cytoplasmic fractions were generated using the CelLytic NuCLEAR Extraction kit (Cat#NXTRACT Sigma-Aldrich,). 48 hours after transfection, cells were washed with PBS, collected, and resuspended in 0.5 ml of hypotonic lysis buffer and incubated on ice for 15 minutes, 30 μl of 10% IGEPAL was added to the cell suspension. Cells were then vortexed and spun at 10,000 xg for 30 seconds at 4°C. The supernatant (cytoplasmic fraction) was decanted and saved. The nuclear fraction was generated by adding 70 μl of nuclear extraction buffer to the pellet, incubating on ice for 25 minutes, spun at 20,000 xg for 5 minutes at 4°C and the supernatant was saved (nuclear fraction). Molecular weights for wild-type and mutant proteins were estimated using Protein Molecular Weight calculator (http://bioinformatics.org/sms/prot_mw.html). The BenchMark Pre-stained Protein Ladder (Cat. #10748-010) (Life Technologies) was utilized as the protein molecular weight standard.

The stability of the MAB21L2 wild type and mutant proteins were characterized using a modified protocol previously described by Alur et al. 2010 [64]. In these experiments, cycloheximide, which is known to block translational elongation and thus to inhibit protein biosynthesis in eukaryotic organisms, was used to treat cells transfected with MAB21L2 expression constructs in a time-course analysis to allow for protein degradation rates to be revealed in the absence of new protein production. Briefly, cells were split 24 hours after transfection into 35 mm petri dishes. After an additional 24 hours, cells were treated with 100 μg/ml cycloheximide (Cat. #C4859; Sigma-Aldrich) and collected at the indicated time points (0-, 1.5-, 3-, 4.5-, 6, and 7.5-hours after exposure). Whole cell lysates were generated by washing with PBS, cells were scraped in PBS and collected in 1.5 ml tubes, cells were spun at 1,000 xg for 1.5 minutes and PBS was removed. Cells were then resuspended in 40 μl of 1x RIPA buffer (50 mM Tris-HCL pH 8.0, 150 mM NaCL, 0.1% SDS, 0.5% sodium deoxycholate, 1% Triton X-100) and incubated on ice for 15 minutes, vortexing every 5 minutes. Cells were spun down for 10 minutes at 20,000 xg at 4°C and the supernatant was used for Western Blot analysis (see below). Western blots signals for MAB21L2 were quantified using ImageJ software and normalized to GAPDH levels (also measured by ImageJ) and the obtained values were graphed to produce degradation curves. Stability assays were performed in triplicate. Exponential decay curves were fitted to each replicate stability assay and the half-lives were determined. A two-tailed student›s t-test was used to determine if the groups were different.

Lysates were denatured by adding equal volume of 2x sample buffer (65.8 mM Tris-HCl, pH 6.8, 26.3% (w/v) glycerol, 2.1% SDS, and 0.01% bromophenol blue) (Cat. #161-0737) (Bio-Rad, Hercules, CA) followed by boiling for 4 minutes at 95°C and run on a 10% Criterion Tris-HCl Gel (Cat. #345-1018) (Bio-Rad). Gels were immunobloted with anti-FLAG (Cat. #F1804) (Sigma-Aldrich) antibody at a 1:1000 dilution or anti-GAPDH (Cat#ab8245) (Abcam, Cambridge, MA) antibody at 1:5000 dilution. The secondary antibody was goat anti-mouse IgG HRP conjugate (Cat. #12-349) (Upstate Cell Signaling Solutions) at a 1:2500 dilution. The blots were developed using the Chemiluminescent Nucleic Acid Detection Module Kit (Thermo Fisher Scientific).

For cellular immunofluorescence experiments cells were split 24 hours after transfection and seeded onto coverslips. After 24 hours the cells were fixed with 4% paraformaldehyde for 15 minutes at room temperature, washed twice with PBS, permeabilized with 0.25% Triton X-100 in PBS, washed twice with PBS, blocked with 10% normal donkey serum in PBS for 30 minutes at 37°C, incubated with 1:1000 anti-FLAG antibody in 10% normal donkey serum in PBS for 2 hours at 37°C, washed three times with PBS, incubated in 1:1000 Alexa Flour 568 donkey anti-mouse IgG (Cat. #A10037) (Life Technologies), washed twice with PBS, incubated for 5 minutes at room temp with 1:1000 DAPI in PBS, washed twice with PBS and mounted on glass slides.

Expression studies, histology, apoptosis assays and immunohistochemistry in zebrafish

Zebrafish (Danio rerio) maintenance and developmental staging were performed as previously described [65]. The protocol was approved by the Institutional Animal Care and Use Committee at the Medical College of Wisconsin. The expression of mab21l2, pax6b, pax2 andfoxe3 was studied in 18–72-hpf zebrafish embryos using transcript-specific antisense riboprobes and previously described protocols [65]. For the mab21l2 probe, a 698-bp fragment covering the sequence between nucleotides 788 and 1485 (GenBank# AY038031.1; primers provided in S2 Table) was utilized; clones for pax6b (AL915181) and pax2.1 (AL906738) were purchased from Open Biosystems (Huntsville, Alabama) and linearized with EcoRv and BamHI, respectively; for the foxe3 probe, a full length 1369-bp fragment covering the sequence between nucleotides 16 and 1384 (GenBank #BC163348.1) was utilized.

Gross morphological and histological analysis of zebrafish embryos was performed as previously described [65]. For apoptosis analysis, whole mount TUNEL assay as described by Eimon was followed [66]. For immunohistochemistry, immunohistochemical staining of zebrafish frozen sections was performed with DAPI (Cat. #62247) (Thermo Scientific), PCNA at 1:100 (Cat. #P8825) (Sigma-Aldrich), ZL-1 at 1:100 (ZIRC), and wheat germ agglutinin at 5 μg/ml (Cat. #W32464) (Life Technologies) following the previously published protocols [67–70].

Generation of mab21l2 mutant lines

TALENs were constructed following the Sanjana et al (2012) protocol [23]. Briefly, mab21l2TALENs were designed to target the region surrounding the nucleotide corresponding to the mutation site in human patients (left TALEN—5'-GAAGGAGGTGGAGGTCCAA-3' and right TALEN—5'-CTATCTCGCTCAGGGAGCT-3'). Interruption of the mab21l2 target sequence was predicted to affect the BanII restriction site (GRGCYC) located between the left and right TALENs; thus BanII digestion of the PCR-amplified genomic fragment involving this region was utilized to determine TALEN cutting efficiencies as well as to identify mutant embryos/adult fish and was followed by DNA sequencing for confirmation. Zebrafish embryos at the 1–4 cell stage were injected with TALEN RNA; initial analysis of injected larvae confirmed genome editing events and ~200 injected embryos were raised to adulthood to generate mosaic founders; these fish were then bred to produce embryos carrying germlinemab21l2 mutations that were raised to adulthood, genotyped using the primers provided in S2 Table, and bred to generate homozygous/compound heterozygous embryos.

RNA isolation, RT-PCR and mRNA injections

To detect transcript levels in HLE-B3 cells, RNA from cells was isolated following transfection with expression plasmids containing sequences encoding for either wild type, or p.(Arg51Gly) or p.(Arg51_Phe52del) MAB21L2 alleles using TRIzol Reagent (Cat. #15596-026) (Life Technologies) 48-hours after transfection. Each sample was treated with DNase I (Cat. #18068) and reverse transcribed in triplicate using the SuperScript III Reverse Transcriptase system (Cat. #18080) (Life Technologies). Following reverse transcription the samples were treated with RNase H (Cat. #18021). Samples were amplified for MAB21L2 using the following primers: MAB21L2-FLAG-F 5'-CAAAGACGATGACGACAAGG-3' and MAB21L2-rt-R 5'-GGTAGAGCACCACCTCAAATTC-3' (PCR product equal 305 bp). The following GAPDHprimers were used as a loading control: GAPDH-F 5'- CCAAGGTCATCCATGACAACT-3' and GAPDH-R 5'- GAGGCAGGGATGATGTTCTG-3' (PCR product equal 148 bp). Endogeneous expression of MAB21L2 transcript in the human lens epithelial cell line was detected with the following primers MAB21L2-endogenous-F, 5'-CCAGGTGGAAAACGAGAGTG-3' and MAB21L2-rt-R, 5'-GGTAGAGCACCACCTCAAATTC-3' (PCR product equal 384 bp).

To detect mab21l2 transcript levels in zebrafish RNA, three independent samples, each containing two embryos of either homozygous mab21l2^{Q48Sfs*5} and mab21l2^{R51_F52del}mutants or wildtype, were isolated using the RNAqueous-Micro Total RNA Isolation Kit (Cat. #AM1931) (Life Technologies). Each sample was reverse transcribed as described previously. Samples were amplified for mab21l2 using the following primers: mab21l2-zf-T-F 5'-TCTTTTCCTGGGAGTTGTGC-3' and mab21l2-zf-T-R 5'- CCCCATCTGGTTCAGGTAAA-3' (PCR product equal 350 bp). Because MAB21L2/mab21l2 represents a single exon gene, a minus-reverse transcriptase control was included in each RT-PCR experiment to assure absence of contaminating DNA in each RNA sample. Amplification of the zebrafish gene for translation elongation factor 1 alpha (loading control) was performed with the following primers:ef1ax1-2F 5'-TCTCTCAATCTTGAAACTTATCAATCA-3' and ef1ax3R 5'- AACACCCAGGCGTACTTGAA-3' (PCR product equal 205 bp). The 1 Kb Plus DNA Ladder was utilized as nucleic acid standard (Cat. #10787-018) (Life Technologies). The PCR products were analyzed by electrophoresis and bands were quantitated using Image J software.

For rescue and overexpression experiments, mRNA was generated using the T7 mMESSAGE mMACHINE Transcription kit (Cat. #AM1344) (Life Technologies). 300 pg of mRNA was injected into 1–4 cell stage embryos produced by wild-type or c.141_153delCCAAGAGCCCCGT heterozygous mutant crosses. The injected embryos were observed for up to 5 days of fertilization, separated into groups based on observed presence/absence of ocular phenotype and then genotyped.

Supporting Information

S1 Table. Summary of novel or rare heterozygous variants predicted to be functionally significant.

Gene 1	Transcript 1	Variant	EVS frequency	SNP#	HGVS Nucleotide	Amino acid	Damaging Predictions*	GERP++	PhyloP	BioGPS	Co-segregation
Nonsense, splicing or frameshift											
DISP2	NM_033510	15:40657155	0/13006	-	c.719+1G>A	NA	NA	4.7	2.44	++	No
FAM200B	NM_001145191	4:15688985	1/6582	-	c.386_387del	p.Lys129Ilefs*8	NA	NA	NA	NA	No
Inframe indels											
TCEB3B	NM_016427	18:44560827	0/13006	-	c.792_809del	p.Arg264_ Ala269del	NA	NA	NA	+	No
Novel Missense											
DHFR	NM_000791	5:79949838	0/12154	-	c.125C>T	p.Ser42Phe	5/5	5.67	2.68	++	No
MAB21L2	**NM_006439**	**4:151504332**	**0/13006**	**-**	**c.151C>G**	**p.Arg51Gly**	**4/5**	**6.16**	**2.94**	**++++**	**Yes**
PGAP2	NM_001145438	11:3832586	0/12998	-	c.268G>A	p.Ala90Thr	4/5	4.92	1.48	++	No
Rare Missense											
ABCC2	NM_000392	10:101594176	7/13006	rs142715085	c.3298C>T	p.Arg1100Cys	5/5	4.38	1.23	+	ND
ASPM	NM_018136	1:197073196	122/13002	rs41299623	c.5185C>T	p.Arg1729Trp	4/5	5.98	2.84	++	ND
KCNG4	NM_172347	16:84256128	66/13000	rs140124801	c.1255G>A	p.Val419Met	5/5	5.61	2.63	+	ND
KIF25	NM_030615	6:168443258	1/13006	-	c.847G>A	p.Gly283Arg	4/5	4.27	2.09	+	ND
NNT	NM_012343	5:43700321	56/13006	rs78818665	c.2977A>G	p.Ile993Val	5/5	5.76	2.2	+	ND
PIWIL3	NM_001008496	22:25124155	45/13006	rs148034582	c.1921G>A	p.Val641Met	4/5	1.68	0.5	+	ND
PKN2	NM_006256	1:89299123	3/12320	-	c.2947T>C	p.Trp983Arg	4/5	5.84	2.23	++	ND
SI	NM_001041	3:164764786	13/13006	rs121912615	c.1730T>G	p.Val577Gly	5/5	5.36	2.04	-	ND
SPATA17	NM_138796	1:217955553	8/13004	rs145637899	c.761G>A	p.Arg254His	4/5	4.73	2.35	+	ND
SLC5A4	NM_014227	22:32616985	17/13006	rs139861447	c.1690C>T	p.Arg564Trp	4/5	3.34	1.05	+	ND

S2 Table. PCR conditions and oligonucleotides utilized for amplification of gene regions in this study.

Gene	Sequence (5'→3')	Annealing Temp.	Product size
Human primers to amplify the region around c.151 C>G p.(Arg51Gly) allele			
MAB21L2	AGACGCCGGTGTATAGCC (forward)	60°C	415 bp
MAB21L2	TTACGCGCTGAGAGATAGCC (reverse)	60°C	
Human primers to amplify full coding region of MAB21L2			
MAB21L2	ccaggtggaaaacgagagtg (forward)	60°C	1362 bp
MAB21L2	gaaggtcttctgccggattc (reverse)	60°C	
MAB21L2	CGGTGGACAAGTGCAGCTAT (internal 1)	N/A	
MAB21L2	AGGGATGTGGGGCATAGG (internal 2)	N/A	
Zebrafish primers for genotyping of TALEN alleles			
mab21l2	TCTTTTCCTGGGAGTTGTGC (forward)	60°C	350 bp
mab21l2	CCCCATCTGGTTCAGGTAAA (reverse)	60°C	
Zebrafish primers surrounding the region utilized for in situ probe			
mab21l2	GGGACGTGGTTAAGATGGTG (forward)	60°C	698 bp
mab21l2	GCAAACGTCCGTAAATAGGC (reverse)	60°C	
WES Confirmation Primers for other genes			
DISP2	CTTCCCTGCTCTGAGGAGTC (forward)	60°C	389 bp
DISP2	TATGCCAGGCACCATTAGG (reverse)	60°C	
FAM200B	AAGTAAGTGCAAGACGTTATAATGAAG (forward)	60°C	338 bp
FAM200B	TTTTTCAGCAGCTGTGTTAGC (reverse)	60°C	
TCEB3B	GGCCTCTGCTGTGTCCAG (forward)	60°C	382 bp
TCEB3B	CCGTGTGTCCCATTTCCTG (reverse)	60°C	
DHFR	AGGCCCAGTTGCTGATTTC (forward)	60°C	400 bp
DHFR	TTTTAATAATGGTAAATGAACCTTGG (reverse)	60°C	
PGAP2	GACTGAGCACAAGGGCTGAC (forward)	60°C	376 bp
PGAP2	CAGCCCCGTATGTTTGATG (reverse)	60°C	

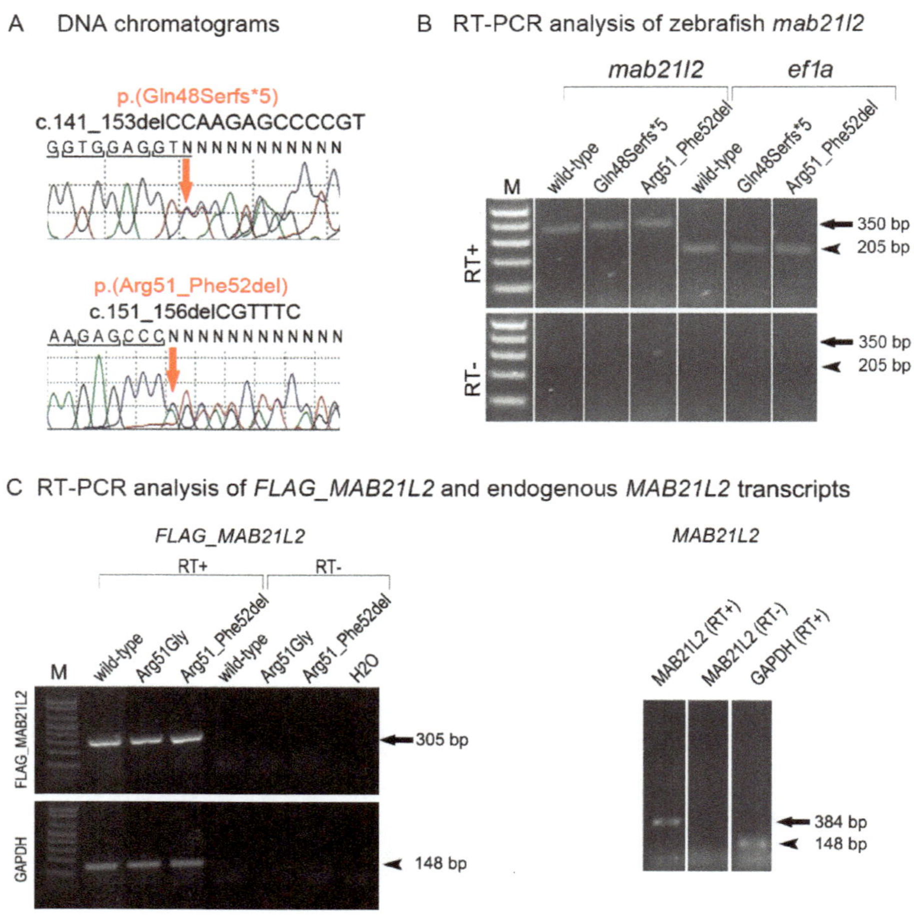

S1 Figure (A) DNA chromatograms that illustrate sequences of c.141_153delCCAAGAGCCCCGT, p. (Gln48Serfs*5) and c.151_156delCGTTTC, p.(Arg51_Phe52del) alleles (in heterozygous fish). (B) Agarose gel analysis of zebrafish mab21l2 transcript- specific amplification from 48-hpf homozygous zebrafish wild-type and mutant embryos; **(C)** Agarose gels representing RT-PCR expression analysis of recombinant FLAG-MAB21L2 wild-type and mutant transcripts (left) as well as endogenous MAB21L2 transcript in human lens epithelial cells (HLE-B3). RT minus (RT-) control refers to a mock reverse transcription containing all the

RT-PCR reagents, except the reverse transcriptase, to demonstrate the absence of contaminating DNA in the corresponding RNA samples; ef1a and GAPDH amplification was performed for loading control in zebrafish and human samples correspondingly; the reactions were run on the same gel but irrelevant lanes were removed when needed; M- molecular marker, black arrow indicates-mab21l2-, FLAG-MAB21L2 or MAB21L2-specific bands of 350, 305 and 384 bp, correspondingly; black arrowhead points to ef1a- and GAPDH- specific products of 205 and 148 bp, respectively.

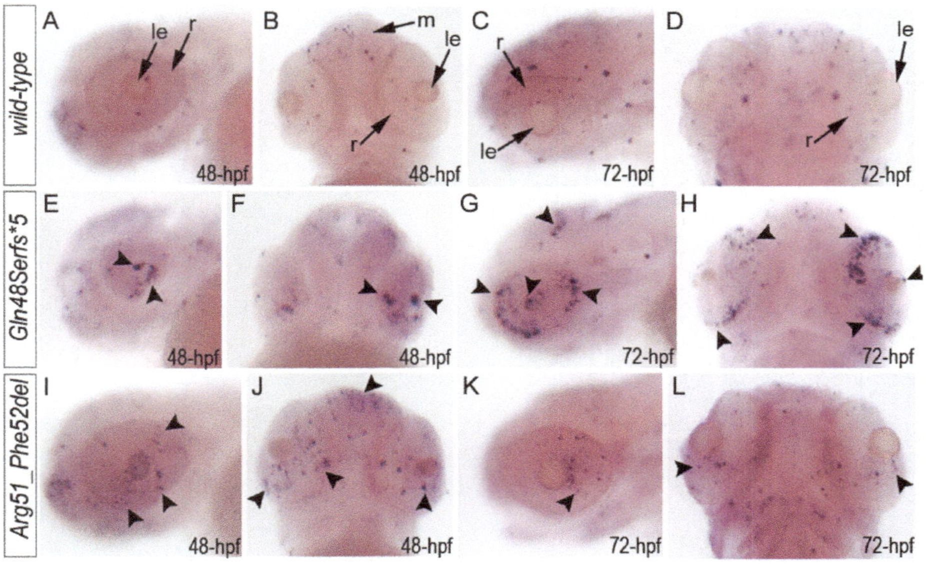

S2 Figure mab21l2 compound heterozygous embryos generated by the cross of c.150_156delCCGTTTC, p.(Arg51Serfs*4) and c.151dupC, p.(Arg51Profs*14) heterozygous carriers.

A wild-type fish from the same progeny is shown at the top and followed by 7 compound heterozygous embryos. Please note small eye (black arrowheads) in all mutant embryos and shortened tail (black arrows) in 4 out of 7 fish.

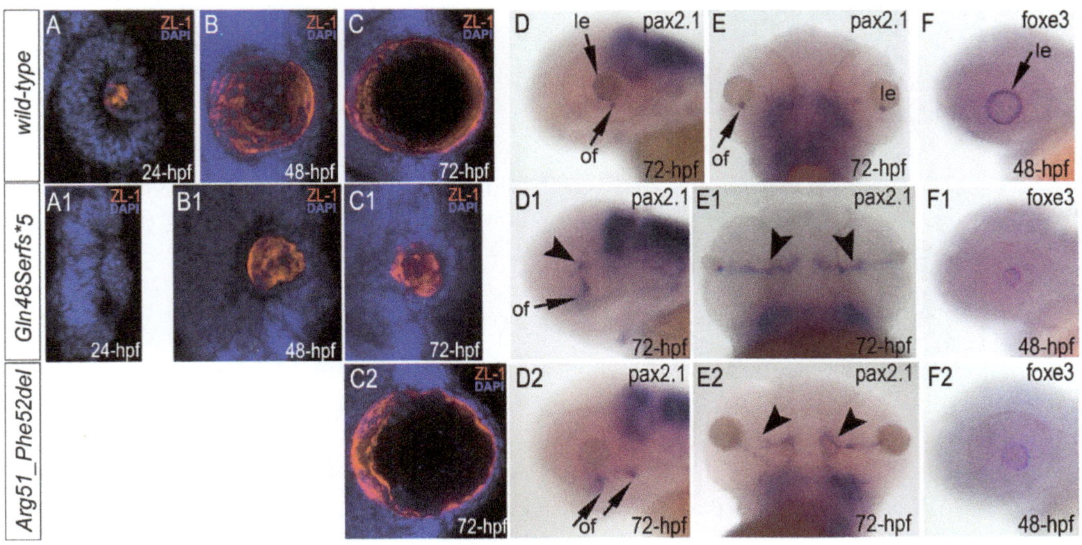

S3 Figure TUNEL results in 48–72-hpf wild-type (A-D), mab21l2^{Q48Sfs*5} embryos (E-H) andmab21l2^{R51_F52del} mutants (I-L) are shown.

An increase in TUNEL staining was observed in both mab21l2 mutants with remarkably high levels in the mab21l2^{Q48Sfs*5} embryos (E-H) and moderately increased levels in themab21l2^{R51_F52del} embryos (I-L); arrowheads indicate sites of increased TUNEL staining in the eye and brain; le, lens; r, retina; m, midbrain.

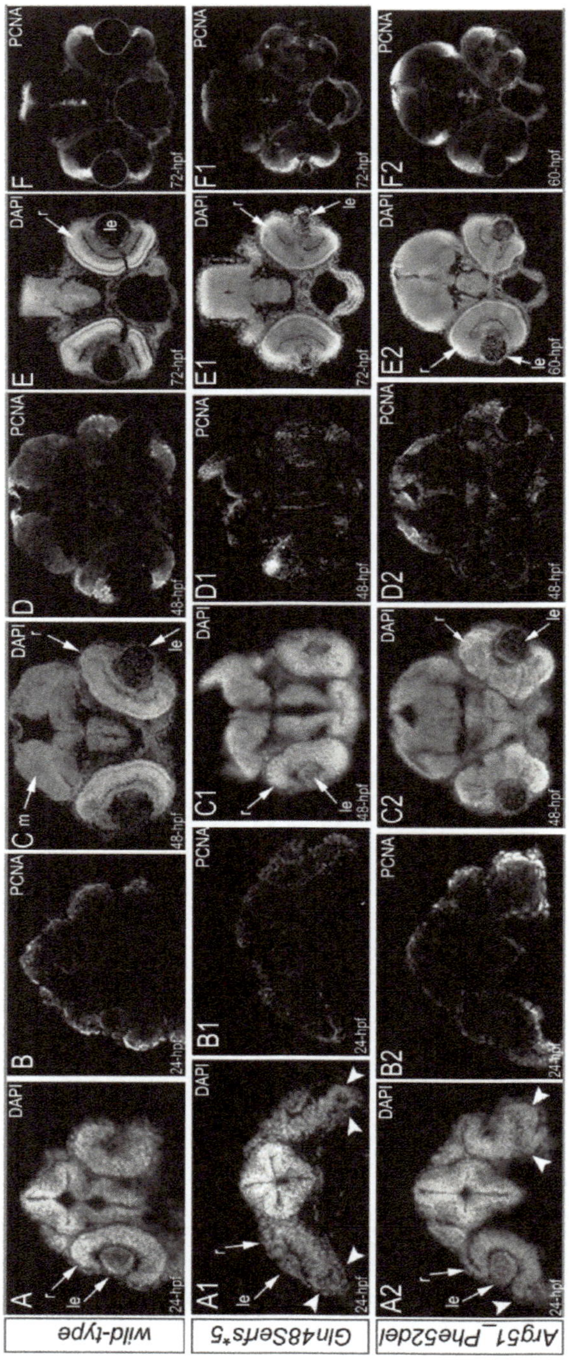

S4 Figure Immunostaining with PCNA (Proliferating Cell Nuclear Antigen) and DAPI in 24–72-hpf wild-type (A-F), mab21l2^{Q48Sfs*5} (A1-F1), and mab21l2^{R51_F52del} (A2-F2) embryos.

Overlay images of the PCNA and DAPI immunostaining are shown in Fig. 6. The arrowheads in A1 and A2 indicate abnormal retinal folding;le, lens; m, midbrain; r, retina.

The ZL-1 staining is absent in 24-hpf (A1) but present in 48–72-hpf mutant embryos (B1, C1, C2), pax2.1 pattern is abnormal in 72-hpf mutant embryos (D1, E1, D2, E2), arrowhead in D1 shows abnormal areas of pax2.1-positive cells in the central retina and arrowheads in E1 show broad and intense expression in the region of optic fissure; foxe3 expression is decreased in 48-hpf mutants (F1, F2); le, lens; of, optic fissure.

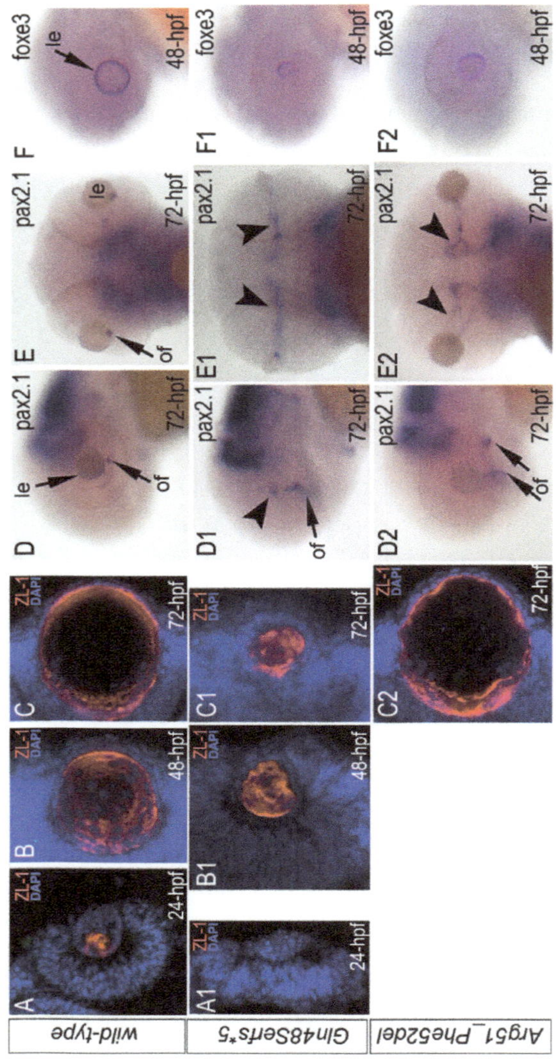

S5 Figure Immunostaining with ZL-1 (red) and in situ hybridization with pax6b, pax2.1 andfoxe3 antisense riboprobes in wild-type (A-F), mab21l2^{Q48Sfs*5} (A1-F1) andmab21l2^{R51_F52del} (C2-F2) embryos.

ACKNOWLEDGMENTS

The authors gratefully acknowledge the patients and their families for their participation in research studies.

Author Contributions

Conceived and designed the experiments: BD EVS. Performed the experiments: BD SM. Analyzed the data: BD SM EVS. Contributed reagents/materials/analysis tools: AK RHRB LMR. Wrote the paper: BD LMR EVS. Oversaw human subject recruitment and ethical approvals: LMR. Performed clinical evaluation of patients and participated in enrollment: AK RHRB.

REFERENCES

1. Morrison D. , FitzPatrick D. , Hanson I. , Williamson K. , van Heyningen V. , et al. (2002). National study of microphthalmia, anophthalmia, and coloboma (MAC) in Scotland: Investigation of genetic aetiology. J. Med.

Genet. 39, 16–22. pmid:11826019 doi: 10. 1136/jmg. 39. 1. 16

2. Hornby S. J. , Adolph S. , Gilbert C. E. , Dandona L. , Foster A. (2000). Visual acuity in children with coloboma: Clinical features and a new phenotypic classification system. Ophthalmology 107, 511–520. pmid:10711890 doi: 10. 1016/s0161-6420(99)00140-2

3. Skalicky S. E. , White A. J. , Grigg J. R. , Martin F. , Smith J. , et al. (2013) Microphthalmia, anophthalmia, and coloboma and associated ocular and systemic features: understanding the spectrum. JAMA Ophthalmol. , 131, 12, 1517–1524. doi: 10. 1001/jamaophthalmol. 2013. 5305. pmid:24177921

4. Nakamura K. M. , Diehl N. N. , Mohney B. G. (2011) Incidence, ocular findings, and systemic associations of ocular coloboma: a population-based study. Arch Ophthalmol. 129(1), 69–74. doi: 10. 1001/archophthalmol. 2010. 320. pmid:21220631

5. Toker E. , Elcioglu N. , Ozcan E. , Yenice O. , Ogut M. (2003). Colobomatous macrophthalmia with microcornea syndrome: report of a new pedigree. Am J Med Genet A. 121A, 25–30. pmid:12900897 doi: 10. 1002/ajmg. a. 20083

6. Schneider A. , Bardakjian T. , Reis L. M. , Tyler R. C. , Semina E. V. (2009). Novel SOX2 mutations and genotype-phenotype correlation in anophthalmia and microphthalmia. Am. J. Med. Genet. A 149A, 2706–2715. doi: 10. 1002/ajmg. a. 33098. pmid:19921648

7. Schilter K. F. , Schneider A. , Bardakjian T. , Soucy J. F. , Tyler R. C. , et al. (2011). OTX2 microphthalmia syndrome: four novel mutations and delineation of a phenotype. Clin. Genet. 79,158–168. doi: 10. 1111/j. 1399-0004. 2010. 01450. x. pmid:20486942

8. Sanyanusin P. , Schimmenti L. A. , McNoe L. A. , Ward T. A. , Pierpont M. E. , et al. (1995). Mutation of the PAX2 gene in a family with optic nerve colobomas, renal anomalies and vesicoureteral reflux. Nat. Genet. 9, 358–64. pmid:7795640 doi: 10. 1038/ng0495-358

9. Azuma N. , Yamaguchi Y. , Handa H. , Tadokoro K. , Asaka A. , et al. (2003). Mutations of the PAX6 gene detected in patients with a variety of optic-nerve malformations. Am. J. Hum. Genet. 72, 1565–1570. pmid:12721955 doi: 10. 1086/375555

10. Vissers L. E. , van Ravenswaaij C. M. , Admiraal R. , Hurst J. A. , de Vries B. B. , et al. (2004). Mutations in a new member of the chromodomain gene family cause CHARGE syndrome. Nature Genet. , 36, 955–957. pmid:15300250 doi: 10. 1038/ng1407

11. Wang L. , He F. , Bu J. , Zhen Y. , Liu X. , et al. (2012) ABCB6 mutations cause ocular coloboma. Am. J. Hum. Genet. , 90, 1, 40–48. doi: 10. 1016/j. ajhg. 2011. 11. 026. pmid:22226084

12. Schimmenti L. A. , de la Cruz J. , Lewis R. A. , Karkera J. D. , Manligas G. S. , et al. (2003). Novel mutation in sonic hedgehog in non-syndromic colobomatous microphthalmia. Am. J. Med. Genet. A 116A, 215–221. pmid:12503095 doi: 10. 1002/ajmg. a. 10884

13. Asai-Coakwell M. , French C. R. , Berry K. M. , Ye M. , Koss R. , et al. (2007). GDF6, a novel locus for a spectrum of ocular developmental anomalies. Am. J. Hum. Genet. 80, 306–15. pmid:17236135 doi: 10. 1086/511280

14. Ye M. , Berry-Wynne K. M. , Asai-Coakwell M. , Sundaresan P. , Footz T. , et al. (2010). Mutation of the bone morphogenetic protein GDF3 causes ocular and skeletal anomalies. Hum. Mol. Genet. 19,287–98. doi: 10. 1093/hmg/ddp496. pmid:19864492

15. Casey J. , Kawaguchi R. , Morrissey M. , Sun H. , McGettigan P. , et al. (2011) First implication of STRA6 mutations in isolated anophthalmia, microphthalmia, and coloboma: a new dimension to the STRA6 phenotype. Hum. Mutat. 32, 1417–1426. doi: 10. 1002/humu. 21590. pmid:21901792

16. Fares-Taie L. , Gerber S. , Chassaing N. , Clayton-Smith J. , Hanein S. , et al. (2013). ALDH1A3 mutations cause recessive anophthalmia and microphthalmia. Am. J. Hum. Genet. 92, 265–270. doi: 10. 1016/j. ajhg. 2012. 12. 003. pmid:23312594

17. Kelberman D. , Islam L. , Lakowski J. , Bacchelli C. , Chanudet E. , et al. (2014) Mutation of SALL2 causes recessive ocular coloboma in humans and mice. Hum. Mol. Genet. , 23, 10, 2511–2526, doi: 10. 1093/hmg/ddt643. pmid:24412933

18. Williamson K. A. , Rainger J. , Floyd J. A. , Ansari M. , Meynert A. , et al (2014). Heterozygous loss-of-function mutations in YAP1 cause both isolated and syndromic optic fissure closure defects. Am. J. Hum. Genet. 94, 295–302. doi: 10. 1016/j. ajhg. 2014. 01. 001. pmid:24462371

19. Williamson K. A. , FitzPatrick D. R. (2014). The genetic architecture of microphthalmia, anophthalmia and coloboma. Eur. J. Med. Genet. 57, 369–80. doi: 10. 1016/j. ejmg. 2014. 05. 002. pmid:24859618

20. Kondo Y. , Koshimizu E. , Megarbane A. , Hamanoue H. , Okada I. , et al. (2013). Whole-exome sequencing identified a homozygous FNBP4 mutation in a family with a condition similar to microphthalmia with limb anomalies. Am. J. Med. Genet. A161A, 1543–1546. doi: 10. 1002/ajmg. a. 35983. pmid:23703728

21. Zahrani F. , Aldahmesh M. A. , Alshammari M. J. , Al-Hazzaa S. A. , Alkuraya F. S. (2013). Mutations in c12orf57 cause a syndromic form of colobomatous microphthalmia. Am. J. Hum. Genet. 92, 387–391. doi: 10. 1016/j. ajhg. 2013. 01. 008. pmid:23453665

22. Manzini M. C. , Tambunan D. E. , Hill R. S. , Yu T. W. , Maynard T. M. , et al (2012) Exome sequencing and functional validation in zebrafish identify GTDC2 mutations as a cause of Walker-Warburg syndrome. Am J Hum Genet. 91(3), 541–7. doi: 10. 1016/j. ajhg. 2012. 07. 009. pmid:22958903

23. Sanjana N. E. , Cong L. , Zhou Y. , Cunniff M. M. , Feng G. , et al. (2012). A transcription activator-like effector toolbox for genome engineering. Nat. Protoc. 7, 171–192. doi: 10. 1038/nprot. 2011. 431. pmid:22222791

24. Hashemi H. , Khabazkhoob M. , Miraftab M. , Emamian M. H. , Shariati M. , et al. (2012) The distribution of axial length, anterior chamber depth, lens thickness, and vitreous chamber depth in an adult population of

Shahroud, Iran. BMC Ophthalmol. 12, 50–57 doi: 10. 1186/1471-2415-12-50. pmid:22988958

25. Deml, B. , Reis, L. M. , Maheshwari, M. , Griffis, C. , Bick, D. , et al. (2014). Whole exome analysis identifies dominant COL4A1 mutations in patients with complex ocular phenotypes involving microphthalmia. Clin. Genet. [Epub ahead of print]

26. Davydov E. V. , Goode D. L. , Sirota M. , Cooper G. M. , Sidow A. , et al. (2010). Identifying a high fraction of the human genome to be under selective constraint using GERP++. PLoS Comput. Biol. 6, e1001025. doi: 10. 1371/journal. pcbi. 1001025. pmid:21152010

27. Baird S. E. , Fitch D. H. , Kassem I. A. , Emmons S. W. (1991). Pattern formation in the nematode epidermis: determination of the arrangement of peripheral sense organs in the C. elegans male tail. Development 113, 515–526. pmid:1782863

28. Finn R. D. , Bateman A. , Clements J. , Coggill P. , Eberhardt R. Y. , et al. (2014) Pfam: the protein families database. Nucleic Acids Res. 42, D222–D230. doi: 10. 1093/nar/gkt1223. pmid:24288371

29. Kranzusch P. J. , Lee A. S. , Berger J. M. , Doudna J. A. (2013). Structure of human cGAS reveals a conserved family of second-messenger enzymes in innate immunity. Cell Rep. 3, 1362–1368. doi: 10. 1016/j. celrep. 2013. 05. 008. pmid:23707061

30. Sun L. , Wu J. , Du F. , Chen X. , Chen Z. J. (2013). Cyclic GMP-AMP synthase is a cytosolic DNA sensor that activates the type I interferon pathway. Science. 339, 786–791. doi: 10. 1126/science. 1232458. pmid:23258413

31. Muddyman D. , Smee C. , Griffin H. , Kaye J. , the UK10K Project. (2013). Implementing a successful data-management framework: the UK10K managed access model. Genome Med. 5, 100. doi: 10. 1186/gm504. pmid:24229443

32. Andley U. P. , Rhim J. S. , Chylack L. T. Jr. , Fleming T. P. (1994). Propagation and immortalization of human lens epithelial cells in culture. Invest. Ophthalmol. Vis. Sci. 35, 3094–3102. pmid:8206728

33. Mariani M. , Baldessari D. , Francisconi S. , Viggiano L. , Rocchi M. , et al. (1999). Two murine and human homologs of mab-21, a cell fate determination gene involved in Caenorhabditis elegans neural development. Hum. Mol. Genet. 8, 2397–2406. pmid:10556287 doi: 10. 1093/hmg/8. 13. 2397

34. Alvarez-Castelao B. , Ruiz-Rivas C. , Castaño J. G. (2012) A critical appraisal of quantitative studies of protein degradation in the framework of cellular proteostasis. Biochem Res Int. 2012, 823597, 1–11. doi: 10. 1155/2012/823597. pmid:23119163

35. Morita K. , Chow K. L. , Ueno N. (1999). Regulation of body length and male tail ray pattern formation of Caenorhabditis elegans by a member of TGF-beta family. Development 126, 1337–1347. pmid:10021351

36. Baldessari D. , Badaloni A. , Longhi R. , Zappavigna V. , Consalez G. G. (2004). MAB21L2, a vertebrate member of the Male-abnormal 21 family, modulates BMP signaling and interacts with SMAD1. BMC Cell Biol. 5, 48. pmid:15613244 doi: 10. 1186/1471-2121-5-48

37. Reis L. M. , Tyler R. C. , Schilter K. F. , Abdul-Rahman O. , Innis J. W. , et al. (2011). BMP4 loss-of-function mutations in developmental eye disorders including SHORT syndrome. Hum. Genet. 130, 495–504. doi: 10. 1007/s00439-011-0968-y. pmid:21340693

38. Wyatt A. W. , Osborne R. J. , Stewart H. , Ragge N. K. (2010). Bone morphogenetic protein 7 (BMP7) mutations are associated with variable ocular, brain, ear, palate, and skeletal anomalies. Hum. Mutat. 31, 781–787. doi: 10. 1002/humu. 21280. pmid:20506283

39. French C. R. , Stach T. R. , March L. D. , Lehmann O. J. , Waskiewicz A. J. (2013). Apoptotic and proliferative defects characterize ocular development in a microphthalmic BMP model. Invest. Ophthalmol. Vis. Sci. 54, 4636–4647. doi: 10. 1167/iovs. 13-11674. pmid:23737474

40. Wolf L. V. , Yang Y. , Wang J. , Xie Q. , Braunger B. , et al. (2009). Identification of pax6-dependent gene regulatory networks in the mouse lens. PLoS One 4, e4159. doi: 10. 1371/journal. pone. 0004159. pmid:19132093

41. Yamada R. , Mizutani-Koseki Y. , Koseki H. , Takahashi N. (2004). Requirement for Mab21l2 during murine retina and ventral body wall. Dev. Biol. 274, 295–307. pmid:15385160 doi: 10. 1016/j. ydbio. 2004. 07. 016

42. Saito Y. , Kojima T. , Takahashi N. (2012). Mab21l2 is essential for embryonic heart and liver development. PLoS One. 7,e32991. doi: 10. 1371/journal. pone. 0032991. pmid:22412967

43. Wong R. L. , Chow K. L. (2002). Depletion of Mab21l1 and Mab21l2 messages in mouse embryo arrests axial turning, and impairs notochord and neural tube differentiation. Teratology. 65, 70–77. pmid:11857508 doi: 10. 1002/tera. 10018

44. Yamada R. , Mizutani-Koseki Y. , Hasegawa T. , Osumi N. , Koseki H. , et al. (2003). Cell-autonomous involvement of Mab21l1 is essential for lens placode development. Development. 130, 1759–1770. pmid:12642482 doi: 10. 1242/dev. 00399

45. Wong Y. M. , Chow K. L. (2002). Expression of zebrafish mab21 genes marks the differentiating eye, midbrain and neural tube. Mech Dev. 113, 149–152. pmid:11960703 doi: 10. 1016/s0925-4773(02)00012-6

46. Cederlund M. L. , Vendrell V. , Morrissey M. E. , Yin J. , Gaora P. Ó. , et al. (2011). mab21l2 transgenics reveal novel expression patterns of mab21l1 and mab21l2, and conserved promoter regulation without sequence conservation. Dev Dyn. 240, 745–754. doi: 10. 1002/dvdy. 22573. pmid:21360786

47. Kennedy B. N. , Stearns G. W. , Smyth V. A. , Ramamurthy V. , van Eeden F. , et al. (2004). Zebrafish rx3 and mab21l2 are required during eye morphogenesis. Dev Bio. 270, 336–349. doi: 10. 1016/j. ydbio. 2004. 02. 026

48. Viringipurampeer I. A. , Ferreira T. , DeMaria S. , Yoon J. J. , Shan X. , et al. (2012). Pax2 regulates a fadd-dependent molecular switch that drives tissue fusion during eye development. Hum. Mol. Genet. 21, 2357–

69. doi: 10. 1093/hmg/dds056. pmid:22357656

49. Masai I. , Lele Z. , Yamaguchi M. , Komori A. , Nishiwaki Y. , et al. (2003). N-cadherin mediates retinal lamination, maintenance of forebrain compartments and patterning of retinal neuritis. Development. 130, 2479–2494. pmid:12702661 doi: 10. 1242/dev. 00465

50. Yamaguchi M. , Imai F. , Tonou-Fujimori N. , Masai I. (2010). Mutations in N-cadherin and a Stardust homolog, Nagie oko, affect cell-cycle exit in zebrafish retina. Mech Dev. 127, 247–64. doi: 10. 1016/j. mod. 2010. 03. 004. pmid:20362667

51. Barbieri A. M. , Lupo G. , Bulfone A. , Andreazzoli M. , Mariani M. , et al. (1999) A homeobox gene, vax2, controls the patterning of the eye dorsoventral axis. Proc Natl Acad Sci USA, 96(19), 10729–34. pmid:10485894 doi: 10. 1073/pnas. 96. 19. 10729

52. Hallonet M. , Hollemann T. , Pieler T. , Gruss P. (1999) Vax1, a novel homeobox-containing gene, directs development of the basal forebrain and visual system. Genes Dev. 13, 3106–3114. pmid:10601036 doi: 10. 1101/gad. 13. 23. 3106

53. Take-uchi M. , Clarke J. D. , Wilson S. W. (2003) Hedgehog signalling maintains the optic stalk-retinal interface through the regulation of Vax gene activity. Development. 130, 955–68. pmid:12538521 doi: 10. 1242/dev. 00305

54. Mui S. H. , Kim J. W. , Lemke G. , Bertuzzi S. (2005). Vax genes ventralize the embryonic eye. Genes Dev. 19, 1249–1259. pmid:15905411 doi: 10. 1101/gad. 1276605

55. Ou J. , Bharti K. , Nodari A. , Bertuzzi S. , Arnheiter H. (2013). Vax1/2 genes counteract Mitf-induced respecification of the retinal pigment epithelium. PLoS One. 8, e59247. doi: 10. 1371/journal. pone. 0059247. pmid:23555005

56. Gestri G. , Osborne R. J. , Wyatt A. W. , Gerrelli D. , Gribble S. , et al. (2009). Reduced TFAP2A function causes variable optic fissure closure and retinal defects and sensitizes eye development to mutations in other morphogenetic regulators. Hum. Genet. 126, 791–803. doi: 10. 1007/s00439-009-0730-x. pmid:19685247

57. French C. R. , Stach T. R. , March L. D. , Lehmann O. J. , Waskiewicz A. J. (2013). Apoptotic and proliferative defects characterize ocular development in a microphthalmic BMP model. Invest Ophthalmol Vis Sci. 54, 4636–47. doi: 10. 1167/iovs. 13-11674. pmid:23737474

58. Asai-Coakwell M. , French C. R. , Ye M. , Garcha K. , Bigot K. , et al. (2009). Incomplete penetrance and phenotypic variability characterize Gdf6-attributable oculo-skeletal phenotypes. Hum Mol Genet. 18,1110–21. doi: 10. 1093/hmg/ddp008. pmid:19129173

59. Rosenbaum D. M. , Degterev A. , David J. , Rosenbaum P. S. , Roth S. , et al. (2010). Necroptosis, a novel form of caspase-independent cell death, contributes to neuronal damage in a retinal ischemia-reperfusion injury model. J. Neurosci. Res. 88, 1569–76. doi: 10. 1002/jnr. 22314. pmid:20025059

60. Grasl-Kraupp B. , Ruttkay-Nedecky B. , Koudelka H. , Bukowska K. , Bursch W. , et al. (1995). In situ detection of fragmented DNA (TUNEL assay) fails to discriminate among apoptosis, necrosis, and autolytic cell death: a cautionary note. Hepatology 21, 1465–8. pmid:7737654 doi: 10. 1002/hep. 1840210534

61. Zhang Z. 1. , Baldini A. (2008) In vivo response to high-resolution variation of Tbx1 mRNA dosage. Hum Mol Genet. 17(1), 150–7. pmid:17916582 doi: 10. 1093/hmg/ddm291

62. Rainger J. , Pehlivan D. , Johansson S. , Bengani H. , Sanchez-Pulido L. , et al. (2014). Monoallelic and biallelic mutations in MAB21L2 cause a spectrum of major eye malformations. Am. J. Hum. Genet. 94, 915–923. doi: 10. 1016/j. ajhg. 2014. 05. 005. pmid:24906020

63. Liu X. , Jian X. , Boerwinkle E. (2013). dbNSFP v2. 0: a database of human non-synonymous SNVs and their functional predictions and annotations. Hum. Mutat. 34, E2393–E2402. doi: 10. 1002/humu. 22376. pmid:23843252

64. Alur R. P. , Vijayasarathy C. , Brown J. D. , Mehtani M. , Onojafe I. F. , et al. (2010). Papillorenal syndrome-causing missense mutations in PAX2/Pax2 result in hypomorphic alleles in mouse and human. PLoS Genet. 6, e1000870. doi: 10. 1371/journal. pgen. 1000870. pmid:20221250

65. Liu Y. , Semina E. V. (2012). pitx2 Deficiency results in abnormal ocular and craniofacial development in zebrafish. PLoS One. 7, e30896. doi: 10. 1371/journal. pone. 0030896. pmid:22303467

66. Eimon P. M. (2014). Studying apoptosis in the Zebrafish. Methods Enzymol. 544, 395–431. doi: 10. 1016/B978-0-12-417158-9. 00016-9. pmid:24974299

67. Imai F. , Yoshizawa A. , Fujimori-Tonou N. , Kawakami K. , Masai I. (2010). The ubiquitin proteasome system is required for cell proliferation of the lens epithelium and for differentiation of lens fiber cells in zebrafish. Development. 137, 3257–3268. doi: 10. 1242/dev. 053124. pmid:20724448

68. French C. R. , Erickson T. , French D. V. , Pilgrim D. B. , Waskiewicz A. J. (2009). Gdf6a is required for the initiation of dorsal-ventral retinal patterning and lens development. Dev. Biol. 333, 37–47. doi: 10. 1016/j. ydbio. 2009. 06. 018. pmid:19545559

69. Collery R. F. , Link B. A. (2011). Dynamic smad-mediated BMP signaling revealed through transgenic zebrafish. Dev. Dyn. 240, 712–722. doi: 10. 1002/dvdy. 22567. pmid:21337469

70. Greiling T. M. , Aose M. , Clark J. I. (2010). Cell fate and differentiation of the developing ocular lens. IOVS. 51, 1540–1546. doi: 10. 1167/iovs.09-4388

INDEX

N

O

P

Q

R

S

T

V

W